# Learning
# Radiology

# Learning Radiology

## 5th Edition

**William Herring, MD, FACR**

Vice Chairman and Residency Program Director (Retired)
Einstein Healthcare Network
Philadelphia, Pennsylvania

ELSEVIER

**Elsevier**
1600 John F. Kennedy Blvd.
Ste. 1600
Philadelphia, PA 19103-2899

LEARNING RADIOLOGY, FIFTH EDITION ISBN: 978-0-323-87817-3

Previous editions copyrighted 2020, 2016, 2012, 2007.

*Senior Content Strategist:* Marybeth Thiel
*Publishing Services Manager:* Catherine Jackson
*Senior Project Manager:* John Casey
*Design Direction:* Bridget Hoette

Printed in India

9 8 7 6 5 4 3 2

In Remembrance of a Remarkable Radiologist, Great Teacher, and Friend

*Morrie Kricun, MD*
1938-2020

# CONTRIBUTORS

**William Herring, MD, FACR**
Vice Chairman and Residency Program
  Director (Retired)
Einstein Healthcare Network
Philadelphia, Pennsylvania

**Debra Copit, MD, FACR**
Former Director of Women's Imaging
Einstein Healthcare Network
Philadelphia, Pennsylvania

**Daniel J. Kowal, MD**
Chief and Medical Director of Ultrasound
  Baystate Health
Associate Professor
UMass Chan Medical School—Baystate
Springfield, Massachusetts

**Natasha Larocque, MD, FRCPC**
Assistant Professor
McMaster University
Hamilton, Ontario, Canada

**Susan L. Summerton, MD, FACR**
Associate Professor of Clinical Radiology
Penn Medicine
Philadelphia, Pennsylvania

**Peter S. Wang, MD**
Associate Chair of Informatics
Section Chief of Abdominal Imaging
Einstein Healthcare Network
Philadelphia, Pennsylvania

**Jeffrey L. Weinstein, MD, FSIR**
Program Director, Vascular and
  Interventional Radiology Residency
  Programs
Beth Israel Deaconess Medical Center
Assistant Professor
Harvard Medical School
Boston, Massachusetts

## REVIEWERS

**Richard Hicks, MD, FACR**
Chair, Department of Radiology
UMass Chan Medical School—Baystate
Springfield, Massachusetts

**David Saul, MD**
Department of Radiology
Nemours Children's Hospital
Wilmington, Delaware

# PREFACE

The fifth edition of *Learning Radiology: Recognizing the Basics* features numerous additions and improvements while adhering to its fundamental design of presenting essential material in a succinct, straightforward format.

**Two completely new online appendices** have been added to this edition.

One looks forward in time and addresses the fundamental principles of **artificial intelligence** and its importance in imaging (e-Appendix G).

The other is a look back at some of the early and, what might now seem, odd **history of radiology,** radiation, and how imaging changed the practice of medicine (e-Appendix E).

Radiology is a specialty with images at its core, so there are **more than 1,600 photos and illustrations** in the print and online components of this book. More than a third of the photos in the text are new to this edition and almost all the remaining images have been fine-tuned to highlight the findings.

There is a new, online section that provides images and descriptions of more than **200 imaging signs** from every organ system that can make it easier for you to reach a diagnosis for a myriad of diseases.

Each text chapter starts with a **pertinent quiz** question, answered at the end of the chapter, that highlights one of the core principles in that chapter. These questions invite you to discover the solution as you review the chapter, increasing your interactive understanding of the material.

Also available is an abundance of additional material online, some of it interactive, starting of course with full-access to the entire text and all of its photos. There are also full online chapters on **Nuclear Medicine, Radiation Safety,** and an in-depth algorithm for diagnosing **adult heart disease** using conventional radiography that could be very helpful.

There is an online **appendix of key terminology** and a new, interactive module that presents several common **clinical scenarios** that takes you through the best imaging test to order based on recommendations from expert panels of the American College of Radiology. This information should prove indispensable on clinical rounds.

With this new edition and its online supplements, you should hopefully be able to recognize abnormalities and interpret images better and, by so doing, perhaps participate in the care of patients with more assurance, confidence, and skill.

When you complete the text, you might begin diagnosing abnormalities with such astonishing skill that you unsuspectingly impress your mentors and peers while you simultaneously amaze your friends and relatives.

The path to being even more astounding begins on page 1.

*William Herring, MD*

# ACKNOWLEDGMENTS

I am again grateful to the many thousands of you whom I have never met but who have helped make this textbook so well-received that it is now in its 5th edition.

For his help and suggestions, I would like to thank Otto Schoeck, MD, who made invaluable suggestions about how this edition could be improved and assisted in expanding it. Peter Wang, MD, contributed two superb chapters on ultrasound, augmenting the material from the last edition. Daniel Kowal, MD, again did a wonderful job in simplifying the complexities of MRI for the chapter he wrote. Susan Summerton, MD, FACR skillfully assisted with the chapter on gastrointestinal, hepatic and urinary tract abnormalities. Debra Copit, MD, FACR, again contributed a terrific chapter on mammography. Jeffrey Weinstein, MD, FSIR, an attending physician at Beth Israel Deaconess Medical Center who, along with Natasha Larocque, MD, FRCPC, added important material on image-guided interventions in medicine.

I want to thank David Saul, MD, from Nemours Children's Hospital in Delaware for his contributions to the pediatrics chapter, and Richard Hicks, MD, FACR, University of Massachusetts Chan Medical School — Baystate, for his review of the neuroradiology chapter.

Morrie Kricun, MD, to whom this edition is posthumously dedicated, was professor emeritus of radiology at the University of Pennsylvania's Perelman School of Medicine and an attending radiologist when I was a radiology resident at Einstein. Many years later, he joined me on the faculty at Einstein as an associate. He had a kind and gentle manner, a wonderful sense of humor, and offered me unwavering support. He was probably more responsible than anyone else for teaching me how to teach.

I certainly want to recognize and thank Marybeth Thiel from Elsevier for her abundance of patience and valuable assistance in this project, as well as John Casey from Elsevier for his aid and expertise in managing the project.

I also wanted to acknowledge the hundreds of radiology residents and medical students who, over the years, provided me with an audience of motivated learners without whom a teacher would have no one to teach.

Finally, I want to thank my wonderful wife, Pat, who has encouraged me throughout the project, and my family.

*William Herring, MD*

# CONTENTS

# VIDEO CONTENTS

# Recognizing Anything: Past, Present, and Future

*William Herring, MD, FACR*

This chapter will briefly introduce you to the major imaging modalities: conventional radiography, computed tomography, ultrasound, magnetic resonance imaging, and the use of fluoroscopy. Nuclear medicine has its own online chapter (see **e-Appendix A**).

- In every chapter of this text, there will be a "Case Quiz" based on material in that chapter. The answer to each quiz question can be found in a special box at the end of that chapter. Don't be concerned if you don't know the correct answers to the quizzes—you are about to embark on learning the answers and much more.

**CASE QUIZ 1 QUESTION**

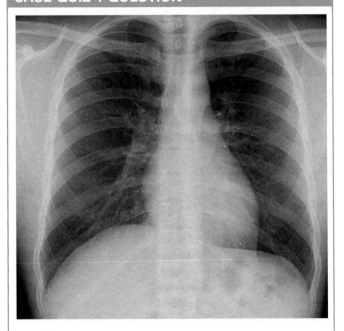

This is a 23-year-old male with a normal chest x-ray. We know there is blood inside the heart's muscular chambers. Why can't we see the blood itself inside the heart? The explanation is in this chapter and the answer appears at the end of the chapter.

## PAST: THE DISCOVERY

- In 1895, Wilhelm Röntgen (or Roentgen), working in a darkened laboratory in Würzburg, Germany, noticed that a screen painted with a fluorescent material and located in the same room a few feet away from a cathode ray tube he had energized and made light-proof started to glow (*fluoresce*). He also noticed that if he held his hand in front of the fluorescent screen, an image of the bones of his hand was visible. He initially thought he was hallucinating (Fig. 1.1).
- After repeating the experiment, he recognized that the screen was responding to the nearby production of a form of energy transmitted invisibly through the room. He named the new rays *x-rays* using the mathematical symbol "x" for something unknown. It didn't take long before almost everyone was taking x-rays of almost everything imaginable (see **e-Appendix E. Early History and Public Exuberance of the Discovery of X-rays**).

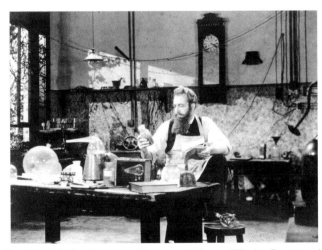

**Fig. 1.1 Wilhelm Roentgen Discovers X-Rays.** Wilhelm Roentgen in his laboratory in Germany is shown in this photograph from 1895, the year in which (on November 8) he discovered a new, invisible source of electromagnetic radiation he called "x-rays." For his discovery, he was awarded the very first Nobel Prize for Physics in 1901. (*Reused with permission from New York Public Library/Science Source.*)

# PRESENT: TODAY'S IMAGING MODALITIES

## Conventional Radiography (CR, Plain Films)

- Images produced through the use of ionizing radiation, i.e., the production of x-rays, but without added *contrast material* like **barium** or **iodine,** are called *conventional radiographs* or, more often, *plain films* or *x-rays,* as in *chest x-rays.*
- Such images require a **source** to produce the x-rays (the "x-ray machine"), a method to **record** the image (a film, cassette, or photosensitive plate) and a way to **process** the recorded image (either using chemicals or a digital reader).
- Conventional radiographic images were produced then, as they are today, by a combination of *ionizing radiation* and **light** striking a *photosensitive surface,* which, in turn, produces a *latent image* that is subsequently **processed** to become **visible.** For about a hundred years after the discovery of x-rays, conventional radiographic images survived their birth as a burst of ionizing radiation by relaxing comfortably on a piece of **film.**
- At first, the processing of film was carried out in a darkroom containing trays with various chemicals and the films were then, literally, hung up to dry. The term *wet reading,* now replaced by the expression "**stat interpretation,**" arose because the early films were interpreted while still dripping wet from their processing chemicals and water.
- The processed films were then viewed on **lighted view boxes** (if the image was being used as part of a movie or television show, it was almost always positioned backward or upside-down). In a few places, film is the medium still used, but it is much less common because it had some **major drawbacks.**
  - Archiving each patient's films required a great deal of **physical storage space** for their ever-growing number. Even though each film is very thin, many films in thousands of patients' folders take up a great deal of space (eFig. 1.1).
  - The other drawback was that radiographic studies could physically be in only **one place at a time,** which was not necessarily where they might be needed to help in the care of the patient.
- Eventually **digital radiography** came into being, in which the photographic film was replaced by a *photosensitive cassette* or *plate* that could be processed by an *electronic reader,* and that image could then be stored in a **digital format.** This electronic processing no longer required a darkroom to develop the films or a large room to store them. Countless images could be stored in the space of one, spinning, hard disk on a computer server. Even more importantly, the images could be viewed by **anyone** with the right to do so, **anywhere** in the world, at **any time.**
- Today, imaging studies are primarily maintained on computer servers on which the images can be **archived** for posterity, from which they can be **communicated** to others and in which they can be **stored.** This system is called a *PACS system,* for *Picture Archiving, Communications and Storage* system.
- With PACS systems (most often shortened to just "PACS"), images from all modalities can be stored and retrieved including conventional radiographs (**CR**), computed tomographic scans (**CT**), ultrasound images (**US**), magnetic resonance imaging studies (**MRI**), fluoroscopy studies, and nuclear medicine (**NM**) studies.

## Advantages, Disadvantages, and Uses of Conventional Radiography

- The major advantage of conventional radiographs is that the images are relatively **quick** to acquire and **inexpensive** to produce and can be obtained almost **anywhere** using portable or mobile machines. They are still the **most widely obtained** imaging studies.
- The major **disadvantages** of conventional radiography are the **limited range of densities** it can demonstrate and its reliance on **ionizing radiation.**
- Although conventional radiographs are produced by ionizing radiation in relatively low doses, radiation has the **potential** to produce cell mutations that could lead to many forms of cancer or anomalies. Public health data on lower levels of radiation vary as to their assessment of risk, but it is generally held that only **medically necessary diagnostic examinations** should be performed and studies using x-rays should be avoided during potentially teratogenic times, such as pregnancy (see **e-Appendix C. Radiation Dose and Safety**).
- **Common uses** for conventional radiography include the ubiquitous chest x-ray, plain films of the abdomen, and virtually every initial image of the skeletal system to evaluate for fractures or arthritis.

## The Five Basic Densities

- Conventional radiography is limited to demonstrating five basic densities, arranged in Fig. 1.2 from least to most dense.

## Computed Tomography (CT, CAT Scans)

- CT or CAT scanners, first introduced in the 1970s, brought a quantum leap to medical imaging.
- By means of a *gantry* containing a rotating x-ray beam and multiple detectors in various arrays (which themselves are rotating continuously around the patient), along with sophisticated computer algorithms to process the data, a complete three-dimensional set of images can be obtained (Fig. 1.3; Video 1.1).

| | Density | Appearance |
|---|---|---|
| | Air | Absorbs the least x-rays and appears "blackest" on conventional radiographs |
| | Fat | Gray, somewhat darker (blacker) than soft tissue |
| | Fluid or soft tissue | Both fluid (e.g., blood) and soft tissue (e.g., muscle) have the same density on conventional radiographs |
| | Calcium | The most dense, naturally occurring material (e.g., bones); absorbs most x-rays |
| | Metal | Usually absorbs all x-rays and appears the "whitest" (e.g., bullets, barium) |

Fig. 1.2 Five Basic Densities Seen on Conventional Radiography.

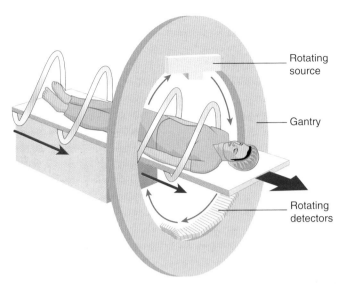

Fig. 1.3 Spiral (Helical) CT Scanner. Most CT scans today are acquired in a helical/spiral fashion. This involves a combination of movement of the scanning table *(red arrows)* upon which the patient lies at the same time the x-ray source and detectors in the gantry rotate *(blue arrows)* around the moving patient. From any point on the patient, the x-ray beam traces a helical path *(yellow band)*. This type of acquisition results in a three-dimensional data set from which virtually any image can be computer-reconstructed.

- The **CT scanner** is connected to a **computer** that processes the data through various **algorithms** to produce **images** of diagnostic quality.
- A **CT** image is composed of a matrix of thousands of tiny squares called *pixels,* each of which is computer-assigned a *CT number* from −1000 to +1000 measured in something called *Hounsfield units (HU),* after Sir Godfrey Hounsfield, the man credited with developing the first CT scanner (for which he won the Nobel Prize in Medicine in 1979 along with Allan Cormack).
  - The CT number will **vary according to the density of the tissue** scanned and is a **measure of how much of the x-ray beam is absorbed** by the tissues at each point in the scan. By convention, **water** is assigned a Hounsfield number of **zero** and other tissues are assigned a range of Hounsfield numbers/units depending on their density (Fig. 1.4).

| | Tissue | Hounsfield numbers |
|---|---|---|
| | Air | −1000 |
| | Fat | ~ −40 to −120 |
| | Water | 0 |
| | Soft tissue | ~ +20 to +100 |
| | Bone | ~ +400 to +600 |
| | Metal | ~ +1000 or higher |

Fig. 1.4 Hounsfield Unit Scale.

- CT images are displayed or viewed using a **range of Hounsfield numbers** pre-selected to best demonstrate the tissues being studied (e.g., the range of only those densities between −100 to +300). Anything within that range of CT numbers is displayed over the available gray scale. This range of displayed densities is called the *window.*

### ▶▶ IMPORTANT POINTS

- **Denser substances** that absorb more x-rays have **high CT numbers.** They are said to demonstrate *increased attenuation* and are displayed as **whiter** on CT scan images.
- On conventional radiographs, these substances (like **metal** and **calcium**) would also appear whiter and be said to have *increased density* or be *more opaque.*
- **Less dense substances** that absorb fewer x-rays have **low CT numbers.** They are said to demonstrate *decreased attenuation* and are displayed as **blacker** on CT scan images (see Fig. 1.4).
- On conventional radiographs, these substances (like **air** and **fat**) would also appear blacker and be said to have *decreased density* (or *increased lucency*).

- CT scans can also be windowed in a way that optimizes the visibility of different types of pathology **after** they are obtained, a benefit called *post-processing* that digital imaging, in general, markedly advanced. Post-processing allows for additional manipulation of the raw data to best demonstrate the abnormality **without repeating a study** and without re-exposing the patient (Fig. 1.5).

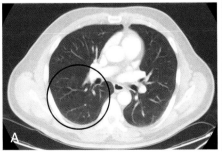
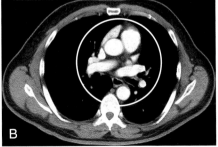
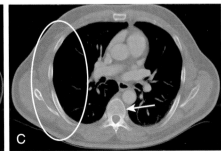

Fig. 1.5 Windowing the Thorax. Chest CT scans are usually "windowed" and displayed in several formats in order to optimize anatomic details. (A) **Lung windows** are chosen to maximize our ability to image abnormalities of the lung parenchyma and to identify normal and abnormal bronchial anatomy *(black circle).* (B) **Mediastinal windows** are chosen to display the mediastinal, hilar, and pleural structures to their best advantage *(white circle).* (C) **Bone windows** are utilized as a third way of displaying the data, visualizing the bony structures to their best advantage *(white arrow and oval).* It is important to recognize that the displays of these different windows are manipulations of the data obtained during the original scan and do not require re-scanning the patient.

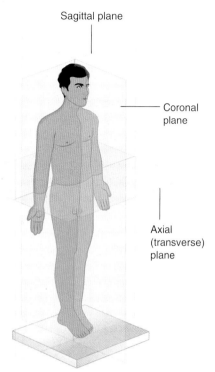

Sagittal plane

Coronal plane

Axial (transverse) plane

**Fig. 1.6 Standard Imaging Planes.** There are three standard imaging planes used in cross-sectional imaging. ***Axial*** (or ***transverse***) planes are very common and divide the body into upper and lower sections. The ***coronal*** plane divides the body into anterior and posterior sections. The ***sagittal*** plane divides the body into right and left sections. If the sagittal plane is located in the midline of the body, it is called the ***midsagittal*** (or ***median***) plane. Sections located to either the left or right side of the midline are called ***parasagittal.***

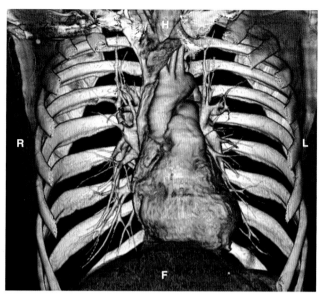

**Fig. 1.7 CT 3D Rendering of Thorax.** This is a color version of a 3D surface rendering of the thorax made possible by the volumetric acquisition of multiple CT sections through the body that can then be digitally reconstructed and computer-rendered to demonstrate surface anatomy. The same dataset could have been manipulated to show the entire rib cage or lungs (which are digitally removed here) rather than the heart. Such renderings are helpful in demonstrating the exact anatomic relationships of structures, especially for surgical planning for certain body parts. *F,* Foot; *H,* head; *L,* left; *R,* right.

- Traditionally, CT images were viewed mostly in the ***axial (transverse)*** plane. Now, because of ***volumetric acquisition*** of data, CT images can be shown in any plane: the most common being ***axial, sagittal, or coronal*** (frontal) (Fig. 1.6). Volumetric data consists of a data set so rich that it can be **reassembled** by computer for a 3-D reconstruction. ***Surface*** and ***volume rendering*** in 3D can produce CT images of amazing realistic quality (Fig. 1.7).
- Because of increasingly sophisticated arrays of detectors and acquisition of a large set of data points simultaneously, **multislice CT scanners permit very fast imaging** (head to toe in less than 10 seconds) that has allowed for development of new applications for CT like ***virtual colonoscopy*** and ***virtual bronchoscopy, cardiac calcium scoring,*** and ***CT coronary angiography*** (Video 1.2).
- These examinations can contain a thousand or more images so that the older method of filming each image for display on a view box became impractical and such examinations are now viewed on computer workstations where it is possible to study many images by scrolling.

## Advantages, Disadvantages, and Uses of Computed Tomography
- CT scanning markedly **expands the gray scale,** which enables us to differentiate many more than the five basic densities available on conventional radiographs. CT scans markedly reduce any overlapping of structures that may obscure underlying pathology. Patients with implanted devices that may prohibit the performance of an MRI, such as a cardiac pacemaker, can safely be scanned by CT. Although CT scanners are **widely available,** they are not truly portable.
- Like conventional radiography, CT scanners also must **utilize ionizing radiation** (x-rays) to produce their images. To produce CT images requires an expensive scanner, a space dedicated to its installation, and sophisticated computer processing power.
- **CT scans are the cornerstone of cross-sectional imaging,** now capable of displaying any body part in any plane, including three-dimensional rendering in color.

## Ultrasound (US)
- Ultrasound ***probes*** use **acoustical energy** above the audible frequency of humans to produce images, instead of using ionizing radiation as both conventional radiography and CT scans do (see Chapter 18).
- An ultrasound ***probe*** or ***transducer*** both produces the ultrasonic signal and records it. The signal is processed for its characteristics by an on-board computer. Ultrasound images are recorded digitally and are easily stored in a PACS system. Images are displayed as either static images or in the form of a video (cine) (Video 1.3).

## Advantages, Disadvantages, and Uses of US

- Ultrasound scanners are relatively **inexpensive** compared to CT and MRI scanners. They are **widely available** and can be made **portable** to the point they can be handheld. Because ultrasound utilizes no ionizing radiation, it is particularly useful in imaging women of **child-bearing age** and **during pregnancy** and in **children.**
- Ultrasound **cannot penetrate bones** and the presence of large, **gas-filled** structures disrupts the ultrasound signal. It can be difficult to visualize deep structures in **obese** patients. Finally, it is **operator-dependent,** meaning the person performing the scan must have sufficient training and knowledge to direct the probe correctly to visualize an abnormality.
- **Ultrasound is widely used in medical imaging.** It is usually **the study of first choice** in imaging the female pelvis and in pediatric patients, in differentiating cystic versus solid lesions in patients of all ages, in non-invasive vascular imaging, in imaging of the fetus and placenta during pregnancy, and in real-time, image-guided fluid aspiration and biopsies (Fig. 1.8).
- Other common uses are evaluation of breast masses, thyroid nodules, and tendons, and in assessing the brain, hips, and spine in newborns. Ultrasound can be used everywhere from intra-operative scanning in the hospital surgical suite to the medical tent in a battlefield and in locations as remote as Antarctica.
- Ultrasound is generally considered to be **a very safe imaging modality** without any known major side effects when used at medically diagnostic levels.

## Magnetic Resonance Imaging (MRI)

- Magnetic resonance imaging utilizes the **potential energy** stored in the body's **hydrogen atoms**, mostly those in water. Hydrogen atoms, whose nucleus contains a single proton that can be made to act like a small magnet, are manipulated by the scanner's extremely strong **magnetic fields** and **radio-frequency pulses** to produce enough localizing and tissue-specific energy to allow highly sophisticated computer programs to generate 2- or 3-dimensional images from that energy (see Chapter 20).
- Some patients undergoing MRI scans may receive an intra-venous dose of a chelated-form of a rare-earth metal called **gadolinium.** Gadolinium is used primarily for better detection of lesions such as tumors, abscesses, or metastases and for imaging of blood vessels as in MR angiography.

## Advantages, Disadvantages, and Uses of Magnetic Resonance Imaging

- MRI uses **no ionizing radiation.** It provides superior contrast between soft tissues to CT and can differentiate better between fat, water, muscle, and other soft tissues. It can characterize and discriminate among tissues using their physical and biochemical properties (e.g., water, iron, fat, and extravascular blood and its breakdown products). Blood flow, cerebrospinal fluid flow, and contraction and relaxation of organs, both physiologic and pathologic, can be evaluated.
- Because calcium emits no signal on most MRI images, tissues surrounded by bone, such as the contents of the posterior fossa and the spine, can be imaged. MRI can produce images of equal resolution in any projection without moving the patient, which adds to its diagnostic utility and offers special advantages for radiation and/or surgical treatment planning. MRI protocols can be programmed to acquire data on physiologic phenomena such as the velocity of moving blood or the diffusion of water (useful in detecting stroke).
- MR scanners are **not as widely available** as CT scanners. They are **expensive** to acquire and require careful site construction to operate properly. In general, they also have a relatively **high, ongoing operating cost.**
- There are **safety issues** associated with the extremely strong magnetic fields of an MRI scanner, both for objects within the body (e.g., cardiac pacemakers) and for ferromagnetic projectiles in the MRI scanner environment (e.g., metal oxygen tanks in the room which, due to the strength of the magnet, can become airborne "missiles"). There are also known side effects from the radio-frequency waves such scanners produce, and possible adverse effects from some MRI contrast agents.
- MRI is widely used in **neurologic imaging** and is particularly sensitive in imaging **soft tissues** like muscles, tendons, and ligaments (Fig. 1.9).

## Fluoroscopy (Fluoro)

- **Fluoroscopy** is a modality that utilizes **ionizing radiation** (x-rays) in performing **real-time visualization** of the body in a way that allows for evaluation of the motion of body parts and positioning changes of bones and joints. Images can be viewed in real-time on video screens and captured for archiving either as a series of static images or as motion (video) images (Video 1.4).
- Fluoroscopy requires an x-ray unit specially fitted to allow for controlled motion of not only the x-ray **source**, but also the imaging **sensor** and the **patient** in order to find the best projection to demonstrate the body part being

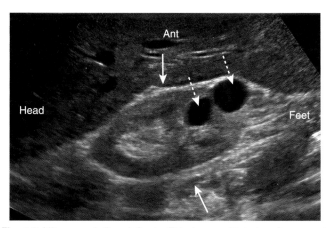

**Fig. 1.8 Ultrasound, Renal Cysts.** This is a sagittal view from an ultrasound examination of the right kidney *(solid arrows)*. There are two cysts located in the lower pole of this kidney *(dashed arrows)*. The cysts are fluid-filled, which accounts for them being devoid of any markings **(echoes)** (see Chapter 18). *Ant, Anterior.*

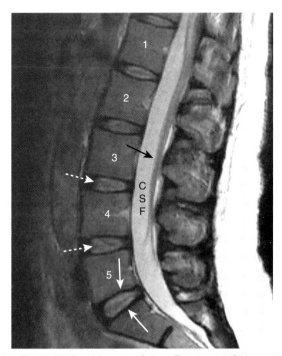

**Fig. 1.9 Sagittal MRI of Lumbar Spine.** This is an MRI image in the sagittal plane of the five lumbar vertebrae (1-5), their bodies being visible because of the marrow they contain. Cortical bone *(solid white arrows)* surrounding each vertebral body is black as it emits no competing signal, making MRI an excellent modality for visualizing soft tissue structures like the intervertebral discs *(dashed white arrows)*, fluids like the cerebrospinal fluid (CSF) in the lower spinal canal, and the nerves of the cauda equina *(black arrow).*

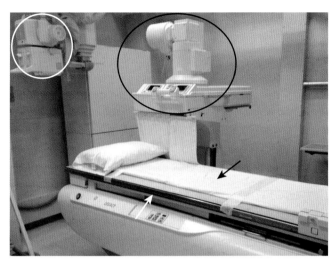

**Fig. 1.10 A Standard Radiology Room Equipped to Perform Both Conventional Radiographs and Fluoroscopy.** The patient lies on the tabletop *(black arrow)*, which has the capacity to tilt up or down. Images can be obtained using the sensor on the fluoroscopic carriage *(black oval)* that can be manipulated more-or-less freely by the operator in order to follow the barium column. Static images can be obtained using the overhead x-ray tube *(white circle)* that can be moved into place over an x-ray cassette that would be located under the patient *(white arrow).*

studied. To do this, fluoroscopic tables are made to tilt and the fluoroscopic tube is able to move freely back and forth to image the patient (Fig. 1.10).

- Instantaneous "snapshots" during a procedure are called ***spot films*** (usually obtained by the radiologist) and they are combined with other images obtained by an overhead x-ray machine in multiple projections (usually obtained by a radiologic technologist) during the performance of barium studies for whatever part of the GI tract is being studied, depending on the nature of the abnormality and the mobility of the patient (Fig. 1.11).
- In **interventional radiology**, iodinated contrast is selectively injected into blood vessels, tubes, or other ducts that can be fluoroscopically imaged to demonstrate normal anatomy, pathology, or the positioning of catheters or other devices (Video 1.5).

## Advantages, Disadvantages, and Uses of Fluoroscopy

- Fluoroscopy units can be made **mobile**, although they are still relatively large and heavy. They can provide real-time visualization for device placement (e.g., pacemakers) or foreign body localization for extraction.
- Fluoroscopy carries the same warnings of exposure to radiation as any modality using **ionizing radiation.** Radiation doses from fluoroscopy can be **substantially higher** than

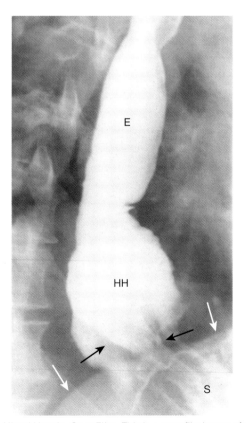

**Fig. 1.11 Hiatal Hernia, Spot Film.** This is a *spot film* image of a barium-filled distal esophagus (E) at the level of the diaphragm *(white arrows)*. The patient was swallowing barium (displayed here as white) while this image was obtained. There is a hiatal hernia (HH) present that contains rugal folds of the stomach *(black arrows)* extending into the herniated stomach above the diaphragm. *S,* Stomach below diaphragm.

for conventional radiography because the equivalent of many static images is acquired for every minute of fluoroscopy time. Therefore, the dose is reduced by using the **shortest possible fluoroscopy time** to obtain diagnostic images.

- Fluoroscopy is used extensively to follow the location and path of externally administered barium or iodine contrast agents in real-time through the gastrointestinal and genitourinary tracts and blood vessels. Because of its real-time acquisition of images, it can be used for localization of tissues for biopsy and for guidance and confirmation of medical device placement.

## Nuclear Medicine

- A **radioactive isotope** *(radioisotope)* is an unstable form of an element that emits radiation from its nucleus as it decays. Eventually, the end product is a stable, nonradioactive isotope of another element. Radioisotopes used in clinical nuclear medicine are also referred to as *radionuclides, radiotracers,* or sometimes simply *tracers.*
- Radioisotopes can be produced **artificially** (most frequently by neutron enrichment in a nuclear reactor or in a cyclotron) or may occur **naturally.** Naturally occurring radioisotopes include **uranium** and **thorium.** The **vast majority of radioisotopes** used in medicine are produced **artificially.**
- *Radiopharmaceuticals* are combinations of **radioisotopes** attached to a *pharmaceutical carrier* that is chosen for its binding properties, which allow the radiopharmaceutical to concentrate in *(i.e., target)* certain body tissues, e.g., the lungs, thyroid, or bones.
- Various body organs have a specific affinity for, or absorption of, different biologically active carriers. For example, the **thyroid** takes up **iodine,** the **brain** utilizes **glucose, bones** utilize **phosphates,** and **particles** of a **certain size** can be trapped in the **lung** capillaries (Fig. 1.12).
- After the radiopharmaceutical is carried to a tissue or organ in the body, usually via the bloodstream, its radioactive emissions can be measured and imaged using a detection device called a *gamma camera* (Fig. 1.13).
- **Single photon emission computed tomography** *(SPECT)* imaging is a nuclear medicine study performed by using a gamma camera to acquire many two-dimensional (2D) images from **multiple angles,** which are then reconstructed by computer into a **three-dimensional (3D) dataset** that can be manipulated to demonstrate thin slices in any projection. To acquire SPECT scans, the **gamma camera rotates around the patient.**
- **Positron emission tomography** *(PET)* scans operate on a molecular level to produce 3D images that depict the body's biochemical and metabolic processes. They are performed using a *positron* **(positive electron)**-producing radioisotope attached to a **targeting pharmaceutical.** The most commonly used target molecule in PET scanning is an analog of glucose called *fluorodeoxyglucose (FDG).* Oncologic PET scans used in the **diagnosis and treatment follow-up of cancer** make up about 90% of the clinical use of PET (Fig. 1.14, Video 1.6).

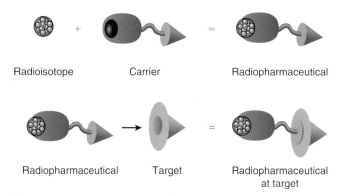

Radioisotope     Carrier     Radiopharmaceutical

Radiopharmaceutical     Target     Radiopharmaceutical at target

**Fig. 1.12 Nuclear Medicine Flow Chart.** The most common *radioisotope* used in nuclear medicine is artificially produced from the element *technetium* and is called Technitium-99m (shortened to Tc-99). Tc-99 is linked to chemical compounds *(carriers)* (e.g., pertechnetate, an anion similar in some properties to the iodide ion) to form a *radiopharmaceutical* (Tc-99m pertechnetate), which, when injected, permits specific anatomic or physiologic processes to be studied by being incorporated or trapped in its *target* at the organ of interest (e.g., thyroid gland).

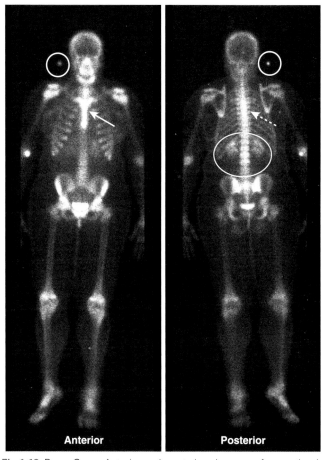

**Anterior**     **Posterior**

**Fig.1.13 Bone Scan.** Anterior and posterior views are frequently obtained for bone scans, because each view brings different structures closer to the gamma camera for optimum imaging, e.g., the sternum on the anterior view *(solid arrow)* and the spine on the posterior view *(dashed arrow).* Notice that the kidneys are normally visible on the posterior view *(oval).* Unlike the convention used in viewing other studies in radiology, the patient's right side is not always on your left in nuclear medicine scans. On posterior views, the patient's right side is on your right. This can be confusing, so make sure you look for the labels on the scan. In many cases a white marker dot will be placed on the patient's right side *(circles).*

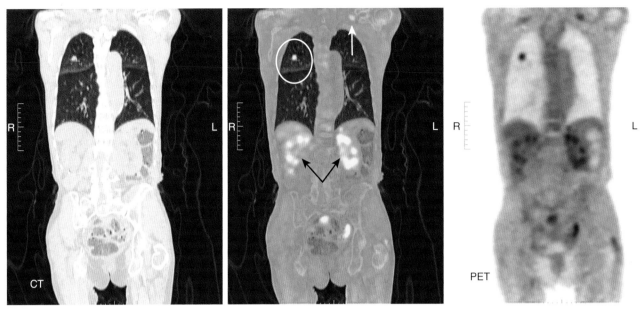

**Fig. 1.14 Positive PET Scan, Bronchogenic Carcinoma.** The CT scan (left) is superimposed on the PET image (right) to form the PET/CT fusion image (center). Uptake of FDG is depicted by varying intensities of red. An **FDG avid** lesion is seen in the right upper lobe *(circle)* on the fused PET/CT scan confirming what was suspected to be the malignant nature of this lesion. This was an adenocarcinoma of the lung. A metastatic lymph node is seen in the left supraclavicular region *(white arrow)*. Normal uptake of FDG is seen in the kidneys *(black arrows)*.

### Advantages, Disadvantages, and Uses of Nuclear Medicine Studies

- PET scans are frequently used **to locate hidden metastases** or to **detect recurrence** from a known tumor. Nuclear studies are used for cardiopulmonary imaging to assess function and anatomy of the heart and lungs. Nuclear imaging is also used to evaluate bones, especially for metastatic disease, fractures, and infections. Nuclear medicine has a long history in **treating** certain thyroid abnormalities.
- Compared to CT and fluoroscopy examinations, nuclear medicine studies, in general, produce **less patient exposure to radiation.** The types of scans that deliver the highest dose relative to other nuclear scans are cardiac studies and PET scans (see **e-Appendix A. Nuclear Medicine: Understanding the Principles and Recognizing the Basics**).
- Unlike other modalities that use **external** ionizing radiation, the patient can briefly be the **source** of radiation exposure to others (e.g., technologists) utilizing nuclear medicine studies. To limit exposure to others, the principles of **decreasing the time** in proximity to the patient, **increasing the distance** from the source (the patient), and **appropriate shielding** are used (see **e-Appendix C. Radiation Dose and Safety**).

## FUTURE: ARTIFICIAL INTELLIGENCE

- *Artificial intelligence (AI)* is defined as intelligence demonstrated by a machine.
- In radiology, AI has traditionally involved *supervised learning,* whereby a programmer or radiologist **teaches**

**the computer,** which is accomplished by providing the computer with examples of a diagnosis and then allowing the software to extrapolate its own rules for what constitutes that diagnosis (Fig. 1.15).
- The future of AI in radiology, though, lies beyond machine learning, with the development of *deep learning.* Deep learning allows the **software to teach itself** using a complex system that mirrors the workings of human neural networks.
- While there has been some form of **computer-aided technology** in use since the 1990s, AI has increasingly become a hot topic. As AI has improved, more and more questions arise about its application in radiology. How are radiologists using AI in day-to-day practice? How will AI change the practice of radiology in years to come? Perhaps the most daunting question of all is what will be the role of human radiologists?
- If we begin to understand how to use AI in the best way, our imaging interpretation skills will increase manyfold.
- For more information on the current and future uses of AI in radiology, see **e-Appendix G. Artificial Intelligence and Radiology.**

## CONVENTIONS USED IN THIS BOOK

- And now, a word from our sponsor. **Bold type** is used liberally throughout this text to **highlight important points,** and because this is a book filled with numerous amazingly important points, **there is much bold type.** New terms first appear in *bold italic.*

■ GGO (ground glass opacity)

■ Consolidation

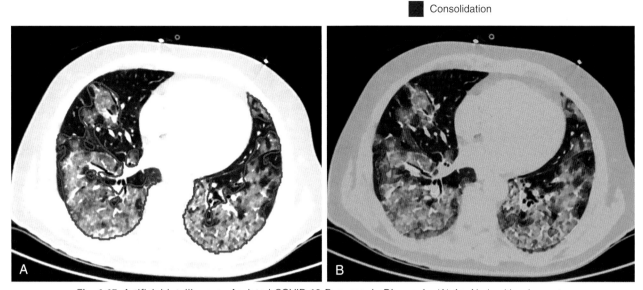

**Fig. 1.15** Artificial Intelligence–Assisted COVID-19 Pneumonia Diagnosis. (A) An AI algorithm has automatically outlined abnormal opacities at both lung bases in red on this axial CT image of the chest. (B) The algorithm has further characterized the opacities as **ground glass** *(red)* versus **consolidative** *(blue)*. Ground glass opacities are a feature of COVID-19 pneumonia.

- **Diagnostic pitfalls,** potential false-positive or false-negative traps on your intrepid journey to the correct interpretation of an image, are signaled by this icon: ⧉
- **Important points** that are so important not even **boldface** type does them justice are signaled by this icon: ⧉
- This symbol means there is additional or complementary instructional material available online (see inside front cover for instructions): ⧉ Online-only extras include chapters on Nuclear Medicine, Artificial Intelligence, Radiation Safety, an Early History of Radiology, videos, and a compendium of 200 radiology signs.
- **"Take home"** points at the end of chapters are signaled by this icon: ⧉
  - Notwithstanding its name, you may take these points anywhere, not only to your home.

**CASE QUIZ 1 ANSWER**

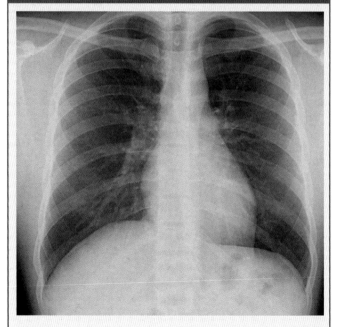

We can't see the blood inside the heart because conventional radiography displays only a limited number of densities. Fluid (blood) and soft tissue (muscle) are about the same density on conventional radiography so it is not possible to differentiate between the blood and muscle of the heart.

## TAKE HOME POINTS

- Today, almost all images are stored electronically on a picture archiving and communications system called **PACS.**
- **Conventional radiographs** (plain films) are produced using ionizing radiation generated by x-ray machines and viewed most commonly on a monitor.
- Such x-ray machines are relatively **inexpensive and widely available** and can be made **portable.** The images **are limited as to the range** of densities they can reveal and therefore to the scope of findings they are capable of displaying.
- There are **five basic radiographic densities**, arranged in order here from that which is displayed the whitest to that which is displayed as the blackest: metal, calcium (bone), fluid (soft tissue), fat, and air.
- **Computed tomography** utilizes rapidly spinning arrays of x-ray sources and detectors and sophisticated computer processing to increase the range of densities visible and displays them in any geometric plane.
- CT scanners **have become the foundation of cross-sectional imaging.** They are **moderately expensive** and also use **ionizing radiation** to produce their images.
- **Ultrasound** produces its images using the acoustical properties of tissue and **does not employ ionizing radiation.** It is thus safe for use in pregnancy, children, and women of child-bearing age. It is particularly useful in analyzing soft tissues and blood flow.

- Ultrasound units are **less expensive,** are in **widespread use,** and have been produced as small as **handheld devices.**
- **Magnetic resonance imaging** produces its images based on the energy derived from hydrogen atoms placed in a very strong magnetic field and subjected to radio-frequency pulsing. The data is analyzed by powerful computer algorithms to produce its images in any imaging plane.
- MRI units are **relatively expensive,** require site construction for their placement, and are usually **higher in cost to operate.** They have become the **cornerstone of neuroimaging** and are of particular use in studying muscles, ligaments, and tendons.
- **Fluoroscopy** uses **ionizing radiation** to produce real-time visualization of the body that allows for evaluation of motion and positioning and the visualization of barium or iodinated contrast agents moving through the gastrointestinal and genitourinary tracts and blood vessels.
- **Nuclear medicine** uses radioisotopes that have been given the property to "target" different organs of the body in order to evaluate the physiology and anatomy of those organs. Unlike other modalities using ionizing radiation, the **patient** can briefly be the source of radiation exposure in nuclear medicine studies.
- **Artificial intelligence (AI)** is already aiding radiologists in optimizing workflows, quantitating some disease processes, and assisting in certain diagnoses. Its role will expand and be continuously assessed in years to come.

 Additional content is available online including chapters on Nuclear Medicine, Artificial Intelligence, Radiation Dose and Safety, an Early History of Radiology, and a compendium of 200 Diagnostic Radiology Signs.

# 2

# Recognizing Normal Pulmonary Anatomy

*William Herring, MD, FACR*

In this chapter, you'll learn how to evaluate the normal anatomy (Fig. 2.1) and the technical adequacy (Fig. 2.2) of the lungs on conventional radiography as well as on computed tomography. To become more proficient interpreting images of the chest, you should first be able to recognize fundamental, normal anatomy in order to differentiate it from what is abnormal.

## CASE QUIZ 2 QUESTION

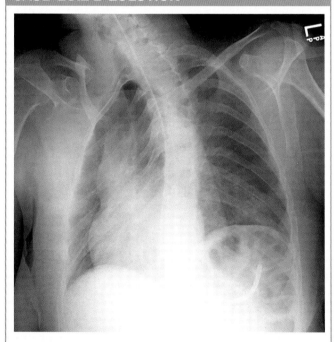

This is a 52-year-old male with a debilitating disease. Is this patient's heart really on the wrong side of the body or is there another explanation for the appearance of this image? The "L" marker (*at top right*) is in the correct location. The explanation appears in this chapter and the answer box is at the end of this chapter.

## THE NORMAL FRONTAL CHEST RADIOGRAPH

- Fig. 2.1 displays some of the normal anatomic features visible on the frontal chest radiograph.
- **Vessels and bronchi—normal lung markings**
  - **Virtually all of the branching white lines** you see in the lungs on a chest radiograph **are blood vessels.** Blood vessels characteristically branch and taper gradually from the

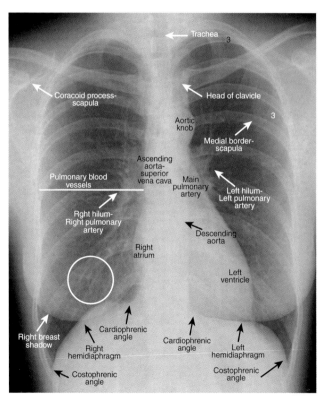

**Fig. 2.1 Normal Landmarks on Frontal View of Chest.** The spine is faintly visible through the heart shadow. Both the right and left lateral costophrenic angles (sulci) are sharply and acutely angled. The white line demarcates the approximate level of the minor or horizontal fissure that is usually visible on the frontal view. There is no minor fissure on the left side. The white circle contains lung markings that are blood vessels. Note that the left hilum is normally slightly higher than the right. The black numeral 3 lies on the posterior 3rd rib, and the white numeral 3 lies on the anterior 3rd rib.

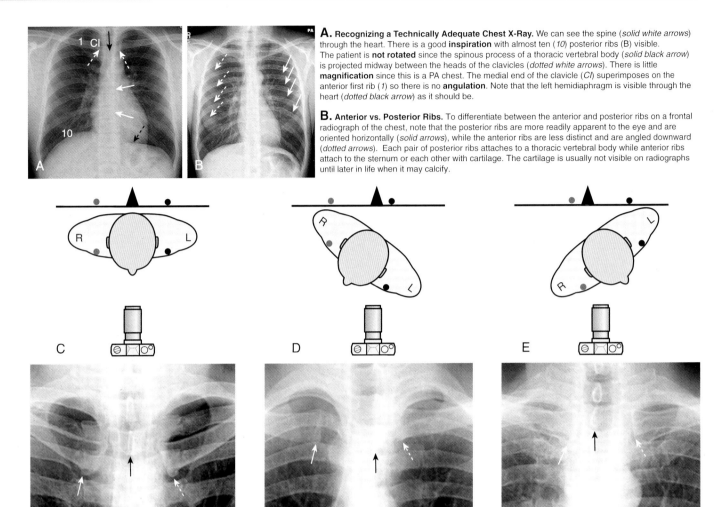

**A.** Recognizing a Technically Adequate Chest X-Ray. We can see the spine (*solid white arrows*) through the heart. There is a good **inspiration** with almost ten (*10*) posterior ribs (B) visible. The patient is **not rotated** since the spinous process of a thoracic vertebral body (*solid black arrow*) is projected midway between the heads of the clavicles (*dotted white arrows*). There is little **magnification** since this is a PA chest. The medial end of the clavicle (*Cl*) superimposes on the anterior first rib (*1*) so there is no **angulation**. Note that the left hemidiaphragm is visible through the heart (*dotted black arrow*) as it should be.

**B.** Anterior vs. Posterior Ribs. To differentiate between the anterior and posterior ribs on a frontal radiograph of the chest, note that the posterior ribs are more readily apparent to the eye and are oriented horizontally (*solid arrows*), while the anterior ribs are less distinct and are angled downward (*dotted arrows*). Each pair of posterior ribs attaches to a thoracic vertebral body while anterior ribs attach to the sternum or each other with cartilage. The cartilage is usually not visible on radiographs until later in life when it may calcify.

**C.-H.** How to Determine if the Patient is Rotated. (C) No rotation: The medial ends of the right (*orange dot*) and left (*black dot*) clavicles are projected on the radiograph (*depicted as a black line*) equidistant from the location of the spinous process (*black triangle*). (D) Rotated right. The medial end of the left clavicle (*black dot*) is projected closer to the spinous process than is the medial end of the right clavicle (*orange dot*). (E) Rotated left. The medial end of the right clavicle (*orange dot*) is projected closer to the spinous process than is the medial end of the left clavicle (*black dot*). The x-ray source (*depicted by the camera icon*) indicates this is an AP projection, but the same relationships would be true for a PA projection as well. The lower row of images are close-ups of chest radiographs. (F) No rotation: The heads of the clavicles (*white arrows*) are each about equidistant from the spinous process of the vertebral body between them (*black arrow*). (G) Rotated right. The spinous process (*black arrow*) projects much closer to the left clavicular head (*dotted white arrow*) than to the right clavicular head (*solid white arrow*). (H) Rotated left. The spinous process (*black arrow*) is much closer to the right clavicular head (*solid white arrow*) than it is to the left (*dotted white arrow*).

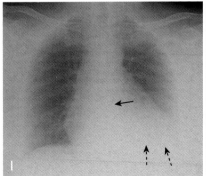 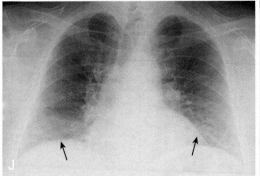 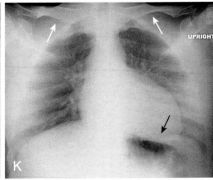

**I.** Underpenetrated Frontal Chest Radiograph. The spine (*solid black arrow*) is not visible through the cardiac shadow. The left hemidiaphragm is also not visible (*dotted black arrows*) but the degree of underpenetration makes it impossible to differentiate between actual disease at the left lung base versus non-visualization of the left hemidiaphragm from underpenetration. A lateral radiograph of the chest would help to differentiate between artifact of technique and true disease.

**J.** Sub-optimal Inspiration. Only eight posterior ribs are visible on this frontal chest radiograph. A poor inspiration may *crowd* and therefore accentuate the lung markings at the bases (*black arrows*) and may make the heart seem larger than it actually is. The crowded lung markings may mimic the appearance of aspiration or pneumonia. A lateral chest radiograph would help in eliminating or confirming the presence of basilar airspace disease suspected from the frontal radiograph.

**K.** Apical Lordotic Chest Radiograph. An apical lordotic view of the chest is most frequently obtained inadvertently using the portable technique in patients who are **semi-recumbent** because they are **bedridden** and cannot stand. Notice how the clavicles are projected above the first ribs and their usual "S" shape is now straightened (*white arrows*). The lordotic view also distorts the shape of the heart and produces spurious obscuration of the left hemidiaphragm (*black arrow*). Unless the artifacts of technique are understood, these findings could be mistaken for disease that doesn't exist.

**Fig. 2.2** Technical adequacy of a chest x-ray.

hila to the periphery of the lung. You cannot accurately differentiate between pulmonary arteries and pulmonary veins on a conventional radiograph (Fig. 2.3).

- **Bronchi are mostly invisible** on a normal chest radiograph because they are normally very **thin-walled**, they **contain air** and are **surrounded by air.**

## Pleura: Normal Anatomy

- The pleura is composed of two layers, the outer parietal and inner visceral layer with the pleural space between them. The visceral pleura is adherent to the lung and enfolds to form the *major (oblique)* and *minor (horizontal) fissures.*
- Normally there are **several milliliters of fluid, but no air, in the pleural space.**
- **Neither the parietal pleura nor the visceral pleura is routinely visible** on a conventional chest radiograph, except where the two layers of visceral pleura enfold to form the fissures. Even then, they are **usually no thicker than a line you could draw with the point of a sharpened pencil** (Fig. 2.4).

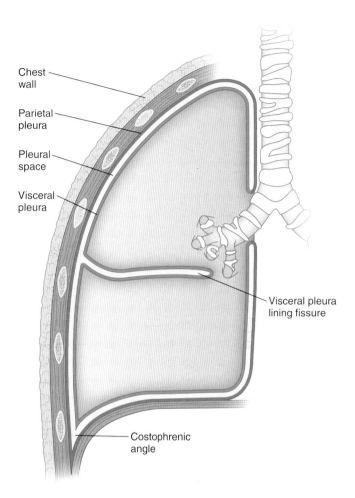

**Fig. 2.4 Diagram of Pleural Space.** The *visceral pleura* is attached to the lung and folds upon itself to form the *fissures.* A very small amount of fluid is present in the *pleural space* between the visceral and parietal pleurae. The *parietal pleura* lines the inner chest wall but is not normally attached to it. The *lateral costophrenic angle* is a sharp, deep sulcus present on both the right and left side.

## Normal Pulmonary Vasculature

> ### ▶ IMPORTANT POINTS
>
> - In the **upright position,** the blood flow to the **bases** is normally **greater** than the flow to the apices because of the effect of gravity. Therefore, the vessels at the **base are normally larger in size** than the **vessels at the apex** of the lung.

- Changes in pressure or flow can alter the normal dynamics of the pulmonary vasculature, some of which are described in Chapter 11.
- **Online extra:** For more on **recognizing normal pulmonary vasculature and an imaging approach to diagnosing heart disease in adults from the chest x-ray,** see e-Appendix B. The ABCs of Heart Disease.

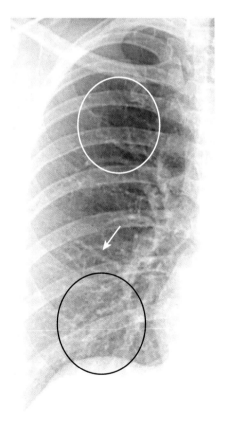

**Fig. 2.3 Normal Pulmonary Vasculature.** The right lung is shown. In the upright position, the lower lobe vessels *(black circle)* should be larger in **size** (not number) than the upper lobe vessels *(white circle)* and all vessels taper gradually from central to peripheral *(arrow).* Alterations in pulmonary flow or pressure may change these relationships.

# THE NORMAL LATERAL CHEST RADIOGRAPH (FIG. 2.5)

- As part of the standard two-view chest examination, patients usually have an **upright, frontal** chest radiograph and an **upright, left lateral** view of the chest. A **left lateral chest x-ray** (the patient's left side is against the detector) is of **great diagnostic value** but is **sometimes ignored by beginners** because of their lack of familiarity with the findings visible in that projection (Box 2.1, Fig. 2.5).

### BOX 2.1  Why Look at the Lateral Chest?

- It can help you **define** the **location** of disease you already identified as being present on the frontal image.
- It can **confirm** the **presence** of disease you may be unsure of on the basis of the frontal image alone, such as a mass or pneumonia.
- It can **demonstrate** the **existence** of disease **not visible** on the frontal image (Fig. 2.6).

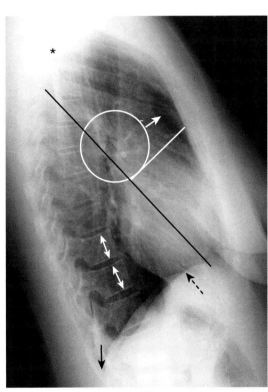

**Fig. 2.5 Normal Left Lateral Chest Radiograph.** There is a clear space behind the sternum *(solid white arrow)*. The hila produce no discrete shadow *(white circle)*. The vertebral bodies are approximately of equal height and their end plates are parallel to each other *(double white arrows)*. The **posterior costophrenic angles** *(solid black arrow)* are sharp. Notice how the thoracic spine *appears* to become blacker (darker) from the shoulder girdle *(asterisk)* to the diaphragm because there is less dense tissue for the x-ray beam to traverse at the level of the diaphragm. The superior surface of the right hemidiaphragm is frequently seen continuously from back to front *(dashed black arrow)* because it is not obscured by the heart, whereas the heart normally touches the anterior aspect of the left hemidiaphragm and obscures *(silhouettes)* it. Notice the normal space posterior to the heart and anterior to the spine; this will be important in assessing cardiomegaly (see Chapter 11). The black line represents the approximate location of the major fissure; the white line is the approximate location of the minor fissure. Both are frequently visible on the lateral view.

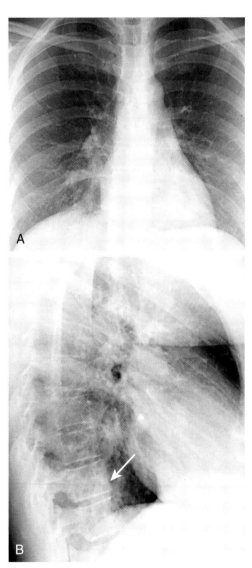

**Fig. 2.6 The Spine Sign.** Frontal (A) and lateral (B) views of the chest demonstrate airspace disease on the lateral image (B) in the left lower lobe that may not be immediately apparent on the frontal image (look closely at (A) and you may see the pneumonia in the left lower lobe behind the heart). Normally, the thoracic spine appears to get **"blacker"** as you view it from the neck to the diaphragm (see Fig. 2.5). In this case a **left lower lobe pneumonia** superimposed on the lower spine in the lateral view *(arrow)* makes the spine appear **"whiter"** (more dense) just above the diaphragm. This is called the **spine sign.**

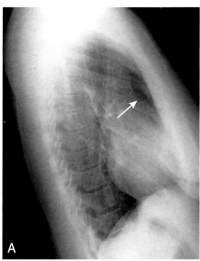

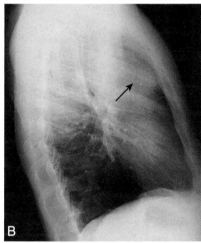

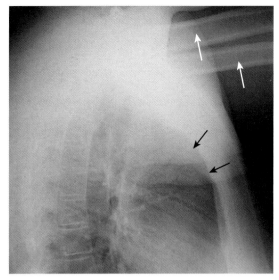

**Fig. 2.8 Arms Obscure Retrosternal Clear Space.** In this example, the patient was not able to hold her arms over her head for the lateral chest examination, as patients are instructed to do in order to eliminate the shadows of the arms from overlapping the lateral chest. The humeri are clearly visible *(white arrows)* so even though the soft tissue of the patient's arms appears to *fill-in* the retrosternal clear space *(black arrows)*, this should not be mistaken for an abnormality such as anterior mediastinal adenopathy (see Fig. 2.7).

**Fig. 2.7 Anterior Mediastinal Adenopathy.** (A) A normal lateral view shows a clear space behind the sternum—the ***retrosternal clear space*** *(arrow).* (B) Left lateral view of the chest demonstrates a soft tissue density that is filling-in this space behind the sternum *(arrow).* This represents anterior mediastinal lymphadenopathy in a patient with lymphoma. Adenopathy is probably the most frequent reason the retrosternal clear space is obscured. Thymoma, teratoma, and substernal thyroid enlargement also can produce anterior mediastinal masses but do not usually produce exactly this appearance.

## Five Key Areas on the Lateral Chest X-Ray (See Fig. 2.5)

### The Retrosternal Clear Space

- **Look for the normal lucency behind the upper sternum to "fill-in" with soft tissue density when there is an anterior mediastinal mass** present (Fig. 2.7).

---

**! DIAGNOSTIC PITFALLS**

- Be careful not to mistake the soft tissue of the patient's superimposed **arms** for "filling-in" of the retrosternal clear space. Although patients are asked to hold their arms over their head for a lateral chest exposure, many are too weak to raise their arms.
- To avoid this pitfall, you should be able to identify the location of the patient's arm by identifying the humerus (Fig. 2.8).

---

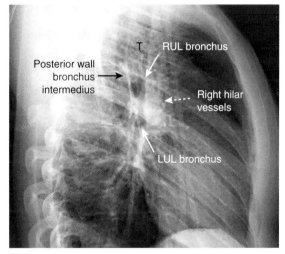

**Fig. 2.9 Normal Hilar Structures.** Left lateral chest x-ray shows the major normal hilar structures. The right pulmonary artery produces an opacity **anterior** to the distal trachea (T). Normally, only aerated lung is seen posterior to the bronchus intermedius. *LUL,* Left upper lobe; *RUL,* right upper lobe.

### The Hilar Region

- The hila may be difficult to assess on the frontal view, especially if **both** hila are slightly enlarged since comparison with the opposite normal side is impossible. The lateral view may help. Most of the normal hilar densities are made up of the pulmonary arteries. No discrete mass should be visible in the hilar region on the lateral view (Fig. 2.9).

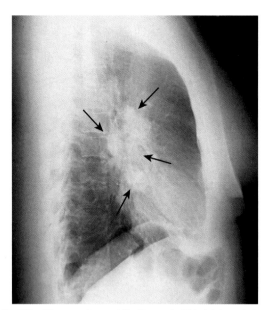

**Fig. 2.10** Hilar Mass on Lateral Radiograph. This left lateral view of the chest shows multiple, lobulated soft tissue masses in the region of the hila *(arrows)*. Compare this to the normal hilum in Fig. 2.9. This patient had bilateral hilar adenopathy from sarcoidosis, but any cause of hilar adenopathy or a primary tumor in the hilum might have a similar appearance.

- When there is a hilar mass, such as might occur with enlargement of hilar lymph nodes, the hilum (or hila) will cast a distinct, lobulated, soft tissue shadow on the lateral radiograph (Fig. 2.10).

### The Fissures
- On the **lateral** projection, both the **major and minor fissures may be visible** as smooth, fine, white lines. The fissures demarcate the upper and lower lobes on the left and the upper, middle, and lower lobes on the right.
- Because of the oblique plane of the major fissure, only the right-sided **minor fissure** is usually visible on the **frontal view.**
- The **major fissures** course obliquely, roughly **from the level of the fifth thoracic vertebra** to a point on the diaphragmatic surface of the pleura **a few centimeters behind the sternum.**
- The **minor fissure lies in a plane roughly at the level of the 4th anterior rib** (on the right side only) and is **horizontally oriented** (see Fig. 2.5).
- When a fissure contains fluid or develops fibrosis from a chronic process, it will become *thickened* (Fig. 2.11). Thickening of the fissure **by fluid** is almost always associated with other signs of fluid in the chest such as *Kerley B lines* and pleural effusions (see Chapter 11). Thickening of the fissure **by fibrosis** is the more likely cause if there are **no other signs of fluid in the chest.**

### The Thoracic Spine
- Normally, the **thoracic vertebral bodies are** roughly **rectangular in shape** and **each** vertebral body's **endplate parallels the endplate of the vertebral body above and below it.** Each intervertebral disk space remains **the same** or **slightly greater** in height as the one above it throughout the thoracic spine.

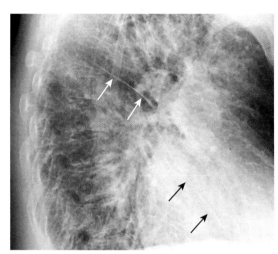

**Fig. 2.11** Fluid in the Major Fissures. Left lateral view of the chest shows thickening of both the right and left major fissures *(arrows)*. This patient was in congestive heart failure and this thickening represents **fluid** in the fissures. Normally, the fissures are either invisible or, if visible, they are fine, white lines of uniform thickness no thicker than a line made with the point of a sharpened pencil. The major fissure usually courses from the level of the 5th thoracic vertebral body to a point on the anterior diaphragm about 2 cm behind the sternum. Notice the increased interstitial markings that are visible throughout the lungs and are due to abnormal fluid in the interstitium of the lung.

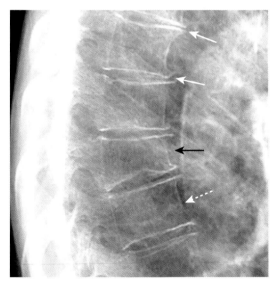

**Fig. 2.12** Osteoporotic Compression Fracture and Degenerative Disk Disease. Normally, the thoracic vertebral bodies are roughly rectangular in shape *(dashed white arrow)*. In this study, there is loss of stature of the 8th thoracic vertebral body due to osteoporosis *(black arrow)*. Compression fractures frequently involve the superior endplate of the vertebral body first. There are small **osteophytes** present at multiple levels from degenerative disk disease *(solid white arrows)*.

- **Degeneration** of the disk can lead to narrowing of the disk space and the development of small, bony spurs *(osteophytes)* at the margins of the vertebral bodies.
- When there is a *compression fracture,* most often from osteoporosis, the vertebral body loses height. Compression fractures very commonly first involve depression of the **superior endplate** of the vertebral body (Fig. 2.12).

- Don't forget to look at the thoracic spine when studying the lateral chest radiograph for valuable clues about systemic disorders (see Chapter 22).

## The Diaphragm

- Because the **diaphragm** is composed of soft tissue (muscle) and the abdomen below it contains soft tissue structures like the liver and spleen, only the **upper border** of the diaphragm, abutting the air-filled lung, is usually visible on conventional radiographs.
- Even though we have one diaphragm that separates the thorax from the abdomen, we do not normally see the entire diaphragm from the left-to-right side on conventional radiographs because of the position of the heart in the center of the chest. Therefore, **radiographically** we refer to the **right-half** of the diaphragm as the *right hemidiaphragm* and the **left-half** of the diaphragm as the *left hemidiaphragm.*

---

**⟫ IMPORTANT POINTS**

- **How to tell the right from the left hemidiaphragm on the lateral radiograph:**
  - The **right hemidiaphragm** is usually visible for its **entire length from front to back**. Normally, the **right hemidiaphragm** is slightly **higher than the left**, a relationship that tends to hold true on the lateral radiograph as well as the frontal.
  - The **left hemidiaphragm** is seen sharply posteriorly but **is *silhouetted* by the muscle of the heart anteriorly** (i.e., its edge disappears anteriorly because the heart and the diaphragm are both soft tissue density) (see Fig. 2.5).
  - **Air in the stomach or splenic flexure of the colon appears immediately below the left hemidiaphragm.** The liver lies below the right hemidiaphragm and bowel gas is usually not seen between the liver and the right hemidiaphragm.

---

## The Posterior Costophrenic Angles (Posterior Costophrenic Sulci)

- Each hemidiaphragm produces a rounded dome that indents the central portion of the base of each lung, like the bottom of a wine bottle. This produces a depression or *sulcus* that surrounds the base of each lung and represents the lowest point of the pleural space when the patient is upright.
- On a frontal chest radiograph, this sulcus is most easily viewed at the outer edge of the lung as the *lateral costophrenic sulcus* (also called the *lateral costophrenic angle*) and on the lateral radiograph as the *posterior costophrenic sulcus* (also known as the *posterior costophrenic angle*) (see Figs. 2.1 and 2.5).
- **Normally,** the **costophrenic sulci** are **sharply outlined** and **acutely angled.**
- **Pleural effusions** accumulate in the deep recesses of the costophrenic sulci with the patient upright, filling-in their acute angles. This is called ***blunting of the costophrenic angles*** (see Chapter 7).
- It requires only about **75 mL** of fluid (or less) to **blunt the posterior costophrenic angle** on the lateral projection, while it takes about **250 to 300 mL** to visibly **blunt the lateral costophrenic angles** on the frontal projection.

## NORMAL CT ANATOMY OF THE CHEST

- By convention, **CT scans of the chest**, like most other radiologic studies, **are viewed** with the **patient's right on your left and the patient's left on your right.** If the patient is scanned in the supine position, as most usually are, the **top** of each image is **anterior** and the **bottom** of each image is **posterior** unless marked otherwise (Fig. 2.13).

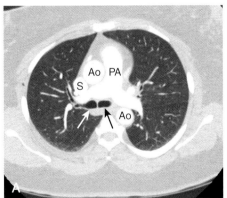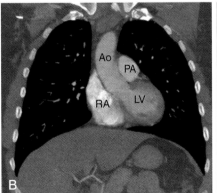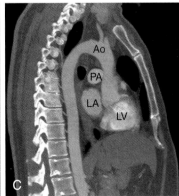

**Fig. 2.13** CT Axial (A), Coronal (B), and Sagittal Views (C) of the Thorax. The three standard planes for imaging the thorax are shown (see Fig. 1.6). Remember that this data was all acquired at the time of the same scanning session but volume acquisition allows digital **reformatting** in any plane. The left main bronchus *(black arrow)* and the right main bronchus *(white arrow)* are seen in (A). *Ao,* Aorta; *LA,* left atrium; *LV,* left ventricle; *PA,* pulmonary artery; *R,* right; *RA,* right atrium; *S,* superior vena cava.

- Chest CT scans are usually **windowed** and **displayed** in at least **two formats** designed to be viewed as parts of the same study, in order to optimize anatomic definition.
- **Lung windows** are chosen to maximize our ability to image abnormalities of **the lung parenchyma** and to identify **normal and abnormal bronchial anatomy.** The mediastinal structures frequently appear as a homogenous white density on lung windows.
- **Mediastinal windows** are chosen to display the **mediastinal, hilar, and pleural structures** to best advantage. The lungs usually appear completely black when viewed with mediastinal windows.
- **Bone windows** are also often used as a third way of displaying the data, demonstrating the **bony structures** to their best advantage.
- It is important to know that the displays of these different windows are manipulations of the data obtained **during the original scan** and **do not require re-scanning the patient** (see Fig. 1.5).

## NORMAL CT ANATOMY OF THE LUNGS

- CT scans of the lungs reveal additional and more detailed anatomy than conventional radiographs. With computer reconstruction of thin-section CT images, the lungs can be visualized in any plane, although the three most common planes are the *axial, sagittal,* and *coronal* (see Fig. 2.13; Fig. 1.6).
- Blood vessels are visible for almost their entire course from hilum to pleural surface. Pulmonary arteries can be differentiated from pulmonary veins (Fig. 2.14, Video 2.1).
- Bronchi and bronchioles are also visible and, as a rule, **bronchi are normally smaller** in diameter than their **accompanying pulmonary artery** (Fig. 2.15).
- The **trachea** is usually oval in shape and about 2 cm in diameter.
- In most people, there is a space present just underneath the arch of the aorta but above the pulmonary artery called the

*aortopulmonary window* (Fig. 2.16). The aortopulmonary window is an important landmark because it is a favorite location for **enlarged lymph nodes to appear.** At or slightly

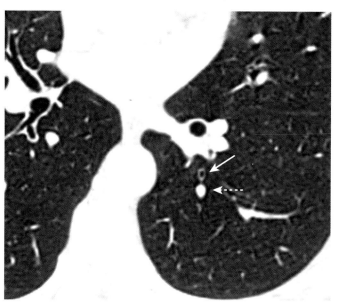

**Fig. 2.15 Bronchus-Artery Relationship.** The normal relationship between the **pulmonary artery** *(dashed arrow)* and its accompanying **bronchus** *(solid arrow)* is that the artery is usually larger than the bronchus. In **bronchiectasis,** that relationship is reversed with the bronchus becoming larger than the artery (see Chapter 10).

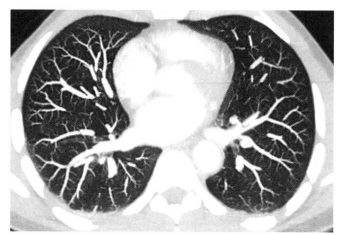

**Fig. 2.14 MIP of Pulmonary Vasculature.** *MIP* (or MIPs if pleural) stands for *maximum intensity projection* and is a way to display certain structures of a given density preferentially making them stand-out more easily. It is a computer post-processing manipulation of the same data acquired at the time of the original scan. It produces an image that looks like an angiogram and is used particularly for CT-angiography (as here) and is also utilized for finding pulmonary nodules (see Video 2.1).

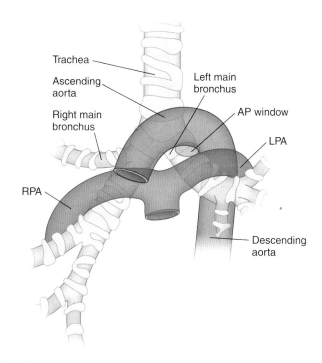

**Fig. 2.16 Aortopulmonary Window (Space).** The *aortopulmonary (aortic-pulmonary) window* (AP window) is a mediastinal space important in imaging because it is a common site of lymphadenopathy. It is bound superiorly by the aortic arch, inferiorly by the left pulmonary artery (LPA), medially by the trachea, and laterally by the left lung. Don't confuse the name for this space with the very rare congenital heart disesase, also called an aortopulmonary window. *RPA,* Right pulmonary artery.

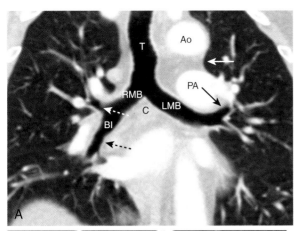

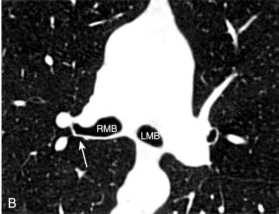

**Fig. 2.17 Coronal and Axial CT at Carina.** (A) The trachea (T) bifurcates at the carina (C) into the right main bronchus (RMB) and left main bronchus (LMB). After the origin of the right upper lobe bronchus *(dashed white arrow)*, the bronchus intermedius (BI) gives rise to the right lower lobe bronchus *(dashed black arrow)* and middle lobe bronchus (not shown). The left upper lobe bronchus is shown by the *solid black arrow*. The *solid white arrow* points to the aortopulmonary window (see Fig. 2.16). (B) Just distal to the carina, the right main bronchus (RMB) gives rise to the upper lobe bronchus *(white arrow)*. The left main bronchus (LMB) is also seen at this level.

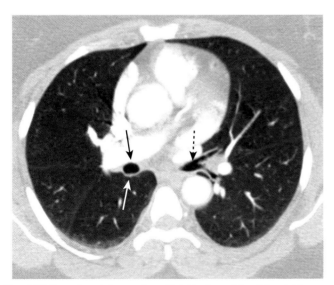

**Fig. 2.18 Bronchus Intermedius.** Distal to the origin of the right upper lobe bronchus is the short bronchial section called the ***bronchus intermedius*** *(solid black arrow)*. The bronchus intermedius divides into the middle and lower lobe bronchi more caudal to this image. There is normally only lung tissue posterior to the bronchus intermedius *(white arrow):* soft tissue in this location would be suspicious for a tumor or adenopathy. The **left main bronchus** is shown by the *dashed black arrow*.

below this level, the trachea bifurcates at the **carina** into the **right and left main bronchi** (Fig. 2.17).

- Slightly more inferior are the **right and left main bronchi** and the **bronchus intermedius.** The **right main bronchus** will appear as a circular, air-containing structure that will then become tubular as the **right upper lobe** bronchus comes into view. Only aerated lung should be seen posterior to the **bronchus intermedius.** The **left main bronchus** will appear as an air-containing circular structure on the left (Fig. 2.18).

## The Fissures

- Depending on slice thickness, the **fissures** will be visible either as **thin white lines or** by an **avascular band** up to 2 cm thick as they travel obliquely through the lungs (Fig. 2.19).

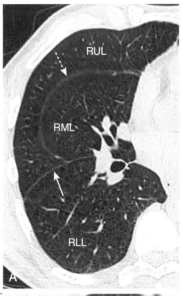

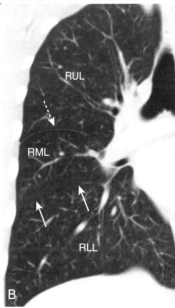

**Fig. 2.19 Fissures Seen on Axial and Coronal Reformatted Views.** (A) The major fissure is seen as a thin white line on the axial view of the right lung *(solid arrow)* and the minor fissure can be seen anterior to the major fissure *(dashed white arrow)*. (B) The minor fissure is a faint white line *(dashed white arrow)* while the major fissure travels obliquely at this level and is represented by an **avascular zone** that surrounds the fissure *(solid arrows)*. *RLL,* Right lower lobe; *RML,* right middle lobe; *RUL,* right upper lobe.

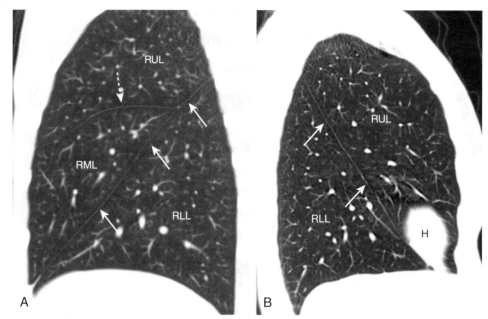

**Fig. 2.20** Lobes and Fissures—Sagittal of Right (A) and Left (B) Lungs. (A) The major fissure *(solid arrows)* demarcates the right lower lobe (RLL) from the upper (RUL) and middle lobes (RML). On the right, the minor fissure *(dashed white arrow)* demarcates the middle lobe, which separates the upper and lower lobes anteriorly. (B) The major fissure is seen on the left *(solid arrows)*. The analog of the middle lobe on the left is the lingula, part of the left upper lobe. A portion of the heart (H) is seen on the left.

- The **major fissure** demarcates the lower lobe from the upper lobe on the left. On the right, it separates the lower lobe from the upper and middle lobes. On the right, the **minor fissure** demarcates the upper from the middle lobe. The middle lobe's analog on the left is the lingular segment of the left upper lobe (Fig. 2.20).

- The **minor fissure** travels in the same horizontal plane as the plane of an axial CT image so the minor fissure is normally not visible on an axial image but is visible in the sagittal or coronal planes.
- In the coronal view, the **location of the major fissure can be inferred by an avascular zone** between the right upper and middle lobes (see Fig. 2.19B).

## Which System Works Best

- What is the best system to analyze any imaging study, like a chest x-ray?
- Some folks systematically look at imaging studies, such as chest x-rays, from the outside of the image to the inside of the image; others look at them from the inside out or from top to bottom. Some systems for reminding you to examine every part of an image have catchy acronyms and mnemonics.
- The fact is: **it doesn't matter what system you use as long as you look at everything** on the image. So, **use whatever system works** for you but be sure to look at everything. "Looking at everything," by the way, includes looking at **all of the views available in a given study**, not just everything on one view (don't forget the lateral chest radiograph on a two-view study of the chest).
- **Experienced radiologists usually have no system at all.** "Burned-in" images are bad for computer monitors but they're great for radiologists. "Burned" into the neurons of a radiologist's brain are mental images of what a normal frontal chest radiograph looks like, what thoracic sarcoidosis looks like, and so on. They frequently use a *gestalt* impression of a study that they see in their mind's eye within seconds of looking at an image. If the image does or does not correspond to the mental image that resides in their brains, **then** they systematically study the images. This is not magic; this ability

comes only with experience so, at least for now, you are probably not quite ready to use the gestalt approach.

- The most important component of the "system" you use in interpreting images is a **system in which you routinely increase your knowledge.** If the system tells you **where** to look but leaves out **what** you are looking for, you can stare at an image for days at a time and the end result will be the same: you won't see the findings. There is an axiom in radiology: **you only see what you look for and you only look for what you know.** So, if you don't know **what** to look for, you will never recognize the finding no matter what system you use or how long you stare at the image.
- But just in case you absolutely, positively MUST have a check-list for a chest x-ray, here's one that's hard to forget:
  1. Technical adequacy (see Fig. 2.2)
  2. Soft tissues
  3. Bones
  4. Heart
  5. Lungs
  6. Diaphragm
- By reading this book, you will gain the knowledge that will allow you to recognize **what it is you're looking for**—the best system of all.

## CASE QUIZ 2 ANSWER

No, this patient's heart is not really on the wrong side. This appearance is caused by marked rotation toward the patient's right projecting his heart over the right hemothorax. The ends of the clavicles *(arrows)* both project over the right hemithorax. Recognizing a technically adequate chest x-ray can help avoid possible pitfalls in diagnosis.

## 🏠 TAKE HOME POINTS

- **Penetration, inspiration, rotation, magnification, and angulation** are the parameters by which a technically adequate chest examination is measured. Their recognition is important to accurately differentiate true abnormalities from technically produced artifacts.
- If the chest is adequately penetrated, you should be able to see spine through the heart; **underpenetrated** (too light) studies may obscure the left lung base and tend to spuriously accentuate the lung markings; **overpenetrated** studies (too dark) may mimic emphysema or pneumothorax.
- If the patient has taken an **adequate inspiration**, you should see at least eight to nine posterior ribs above the level of the diaphragm; poor inspiratory efforts may mimic basilar lung disease and may make the heart appear larger.
- The spinous process should fall equidistant between the medial ends of the clavicles to indicate the patient is **not rotated.** Rotation can introduce numerous artifactual anomalies affecting the contour of the heart and the appearance of the hila and diaphragm.
- **Anteroposterior (AP)** films (mostly portable chest x-rays) will **magnify** the heart slightly compared with the standard **posteroanterior (PA)** chest radiograph (usually done in the radiology department).
- Frontal views of the chest obtained with the patient semi-upright in bed (i.e., tilted backward) may produce **apical lordotic** images that distort normal anatomy.
- Virtually all of the lung markings on chest radiographs are composed of **pulmonary blood vessels;** most **bronchi** are too thin-walled to be visible on conventional radiography.
- Normal pulmonary vasculature **tapers gradually** from central to peripheral and the vessels are normally larger at the base than apex on an **upright** chest radiograph.
- The **lateral chest radiograph** can provide invaluable information and should always be studied when available.

- **Five key areas** to inspect on the **lateral** projection include the retrosternal clear space, hilar region, fissures, thoracic spine, and diaphragm/costophrenic sulci.
- There is normally a **retrosternal "clear space"** on a lateral radiograph that can fill-in with a mediastinal mass or adenopathy, such as in lymphoma.
- Although the pulmonary arteries themselves can normally be seen in the hila on the lateral projection, a discrete mass in the hilum is abnormal and should alert to the possibility of tumor or adenopathy.
- The **minor fissure,** not the major fissure, will usually be visible on a frontal chest x-ray. On the lateral view, both the major and minor fissures can be seen normally. When visible, they are very thin lines of uniform size about 1 to 2 mm in thickness.
- On the lateral view, the **left hemidiaphragm** will be obscured (silhouetted) anteriorly by the heart. The **right hemidiaphragm** is usually higher than the left and can be seen in its entirety from front to back.
- The **costophrenic angles** are normally acute and sharply outlined. Pleural effusions and scarring may cause blunting of the costophrenic angles.
- CT scans of the chest display much more detail than conventional radiographs and, due to rapid acquisition of very thin slices, can be displayed in any plane using the original dataset. The planes most commonly used are the **axial, sagittal, and coronal.**
- The normal anatomy of the trachea and main bronchi is outlined.
- Both the major and minor fissures are visible on CT either as **thin, white lines** or **avascular bands** depending on the orientation of the fissure relative to the plane in which the scan is displayed.
- The best **system** to use for recognizing any abnormality is one based on solid knowledge of the appearance of **normal anatomy** and the most common deviations from normal.

📶 Additional content is available online including chapters on Nuclear Medicine, Artificial Intelligence, Radiation Dose and Safety, an Early History of Radiology, and a compendium of 200 Diagnostic Radiology Signs.

# 3

# Recognizing Normal Cardiac Anatomy

*William Herring, MD, FACR*

Starting with conventional radiography, we'll begin with an assessment of heart size, then describe the normal and abnormal contours of the heart on the frontal radiograph and, finally, discuss the normal anatomy of the heart as seen on computed tomography (CT) and magnetic resonance imaging (MRI).

## CASE QUIZ 3 QUESTION

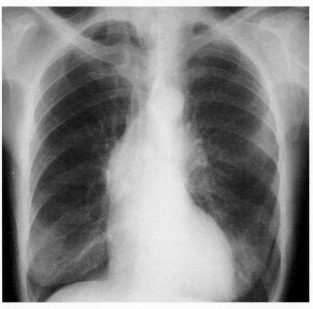

The image is a frontal chest x-ray of a 52-year-old female with a history of episodes of fainting, angina, and congestive heart failure. Besides the history, there is an abnormality of the cardiac contour that suggests the diagnosis. The explanation appears in this chapter and the answer box is at the end of this chapter.

## EVALUATING THE HEART ON CHEST RADIOGRAPHS

### Recognizing a Normal-Sized Heart

> #### IMPORTANT POINTS
>
> - You can estimate the size of the cardiac silhouette on the frontal chest radiograph using the ***cardiothoracic ratio,*** which is a measurement of the widest transverse diameter of the heart compared to the widest internal diameter of the rib cage (from inside of rib to inside of rib at the level of the diaphragm) (Fig. 3.1).

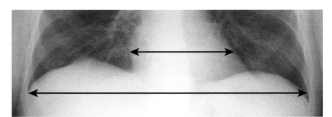

**Fig. 3.1 The Cardiothoracic Ratio.** The cardiothoracic ratio compares the widest diameter of the heart *(top double arrow)* to the widest **internal** diameter of the thoracic cage from the inside of rib to the inside of rib *(bottom double arrow)* at the level of the diaphragm. It should normally be less than 50%.

- In most normal adults at **full inspiration**, the cardiothoracic ratio is **less than 50%**. That is, the size of the heart is usually less than half of the internal diameter of the thoracic rib cage.

### The Normal Cardiac Contours

- The **normal cardiac contours** comprise a series of bumps and indentations visible on the frontal chest radiograph. They are demonstrated in Fig. 3.2.

## GENERAL PRINCIPLES

- As you interpret cardiac abnormalities, no matter what imaging modality is being used, the following principles hold true:
- The **ventricles respond to obstruction** to their outflow **by first undergoing hypertrophy** rather than dilatation. Therefore, the heart may **not** appear enlarged at first with lesions like **aortic stenosis, coarctation of the aorta, pulmonic stenosis, or systemic hypertension.** When the ventricular wall becomes thicker, the lumen actually becomes smaller and it is only when the muscle begins to fail and the heart decompensates that the heart visibly enlarges on chest radiographs.
- **Cardiomegaly,** as recognized on chest radiographs, refers to enlargement of the cardiac silhouette produced by **ventricular enlargement,** not by isolated enlargement of the atria. For example, the cardiac silhouette usually appears normal in size when there is isolated atrial enlargement, such as left atrial enlargement in early mitral stenosis.
- In general, **the most marked chamber enlargement will occur from volume overload** rather than **elevated pressure,** so that the largest chambers are usually produced by

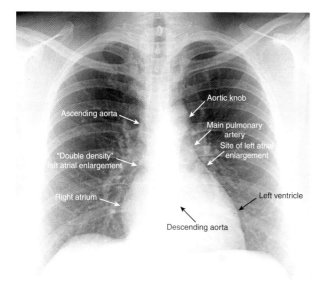

**Fig. 3.2 Normal Cardiac Contours Seen on the Frontal Projection.** On the right side of the heart, the first contour is the **ascending aorta**. Where the contour of the ascending aorta meets the contour of the right atrium, there is usually a **slight indentation,** which is where the left atrium may appear when it enlarges *(double-density)*. The right heart border is formed by the **right atrium**. On the left, the first contour is the **aortic knob**, a radiographic structure formed by the foreshortened aortic arch super-imposed on a portion of the proximal descending aorta. The next contour below the aortic knob is the **main pulmonary artery**, before it divides into a right and left pulmonary artery. Just below the main pulmonary artery segment there is normally a **slight indentation** where an enlarged left atrium/left atrial appendage may appear on the left side of the heart. The last contour of the heart on the left is formed by the **left ventricle**. The descending aorta almost disappears with the shadow of the spine.

---

**▶▶ IMPORTANT POINTS**

**Key points about the cardiac contours**

- The **ascending aorta** should normally not project farther to the right than the right heart border (i.e., the right atrium).
- The **aortic knob** is normally less than 35 mm (measured from the edge of the air-filled trachea) and will normally push the trachea slightly to the right.
- The **main pulmonary artery** segment is usually concave or flat. In **younger females** it may **normally be convex** outward.
- The **normal-sized left atrium** does not contribute to the border of the heart on a non-rotated frontal chest radiograph.
- An **enlarged left atrium** and left atrial appendage "fills-in" and **straightens** the normal concavity just inferior to the main pulmonary artery segment and may sometimes be visible on the right side of the heart as well.
- The lower portion of the left heart border is made up of the **left ventricle**. Remember that the left ventricle is really a **posterior** ventricle and the **right ventricle** is an **anterior** ventricle.
- Normally, the **descending aorta** parallels the spine and is barely visible on the frontal radiograph of the chest. When it becomes **tortuous** or **uncoiled**, it swings farther away from the thoracic spine toward the patient's left (Fig. 3.3).

**regurgitant valves** rather than **stenotic valves**. Therefore, the heart will usually be larger as a result of aortic regurgitation than aortic stenosis and the left atrium will usually be larger in mitral regurgitation than mitral stenosis (Fig. 3.4).

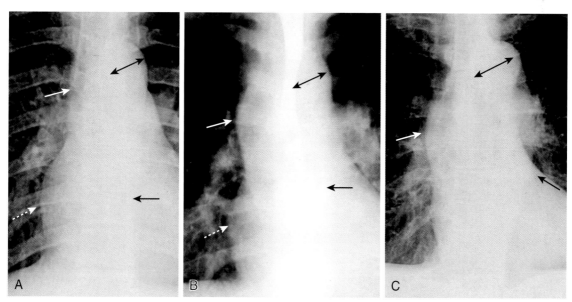

**Fig. 3.3 Appearances of the Aorta.** (A) **Normal.** The ascending aorta is a low-density, almost straight edge *(solid white arrow)* and does not project more lateral than the right heart border *(dashed white arrow)*. The aortic knob is not enlarged *(double arrow)* and the descending aorta *(solid black arrow)* almost disappears with the shadow of the thoracic spine. (B) **Aortic stenosis.** The ascending aorta is abnormal as it projects convex outward *(solid white arrow)* almost as far as the right heart border *(dashed white arrow)*. This is due to *post-stenotic dilatation*. The aortic knob *(double arrow)* and descending aorta *(solid black arrow)* remain normal. (C) **Systemic hypertension.** Both the ascending *(solid white arrow)* and descending aorta *(solid black arrow)* project too far to the right and left, respectively. The aortic knob is enlarged *(double black arrow)*.

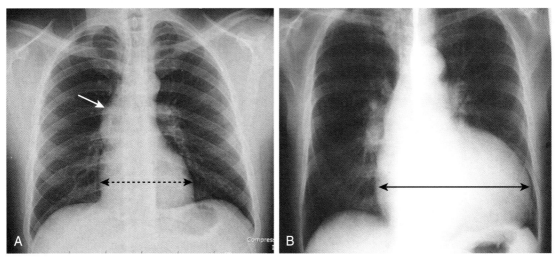

**Fig. 3.4 Heart Size with Stenotic Versus Regurgitant Valve.** (A) There is **post-stenotic dilatation** of the ascending aorta *(white arrow)* from turbulent flow in this patient with **aortic stenosis**. Notice that the cardiac silhouette is not enlarged *(dashed double black arrow)* even though this lesion produces left ventricular hypertrophy. (B) This patient has **aortic regurgitation**. Note the enlarged cardiac silhouette *(double black arrow)* due to an extremely large left ventricle. Volume overload will cause a greater increase in chamber size than will increased pressure alone.

## EVALUATING THE HEART ON CARDIAC CT

- **CT scanning of the heart** is done using a fast, multi-slice CT scanner, usually with intravenous iodinated contrast and electrocardiographic (ECG)-gated acquisition to reduce motion artifacts.
- Both cardiac CT and cardiac MRI use *ECG-gating,* which allows for a series of images to be obtained either prospectively or retrospectively only during a specified portion of the cardiac cycle when cardiac motion is at its least, usually during diastole. The images are then parsed together by powerful computer algorithms to produce images that are less degraded by the pulsations of the heart.
- Cardiac CT can be used to evaluate the **coronary arteries and valves** and search for cardiac **masses**. By reconstructing multiple phases of the cardiac cycle, it is also possible to analyze **wall motion** and evaluate **ejection fraction** and **myocardial perfusion**.
- The three standard planes for viewing CT images of the heart are the **axial, sagittal, and coronal**. Figs. 3.5 to 3.10 demonstrate the major normal CT anatomy of the heart and great vessels.

## Normal Cardiac CT Anatomy

- We will cover only a few of the major anatomic landmarks demonstrable on chest CT and all of the scans utilized will

be *contrast-enhanced* (i.e., in the scans shown the patient will have had an injection of intravenous contrast to opacify the heart chambers and blood vessels). It is best to read the text in conjunction with its associated photograph. Any references to "right" or "left" mean the patient's right or left side, not yours.
- We will start at the top of the chest and progress inferiorly, highlighting the major structures visible at **six key levels**. This is a good way to systematically study every CT examination of the chest.

### Five-Vessel Level (Fig. 3.5)

- At this level, you should be able to identify the **lungs, the trachea, and the esophagus**. The **trachea** is black because it contains air, is usually oval in shape, and is about 2 cm in diameter. The **esophagus** lies posterior and either to the left or right of the trachea. The esophagus is usually collapsed but may contain swallowed air.
- Depending on the exact level of the image, several of the great vessels will be visible. The larger **venous structures** tend to be more **anterior than the arterial**. The **brachiocephalic (innominate) veins** lie just posterior to the sternum.

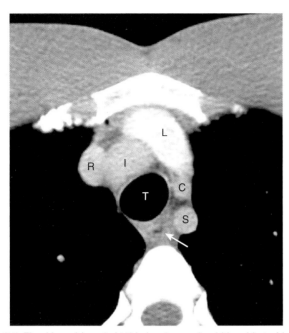

**Fig. 3.5** Five-Vessel Level. At this level, you should be able to identify the lungs, the **trachea (T)** and the **esophagus** *(arrow)*. Depending on the exact level of the image, several of the great vessels will be visible. The **right brachiocephalic vein (R)** is the vessel to the right of the **trachea (T)**. The **left brachiocephalic vein (L)** lies just posterior to the sternum. From the patient's right to the patient's left, the arteries visible may include the **innominate artery (I)**, **left common carotid (C)**, and **left subclavian arteries (S)**.

## Aortic Arch Level (Fig. 3.6)

- At this level, you should be able to identify the **aortic arch, superior vena cava, and azygos vein**.
- The *aortic arch* forms an upside-down "U"-shaped tube. If the scan skims the very top of the arch, it will appear as a comma-shaped tubular structure with roughly the same diameter anteriorly as posteriorly. To the right of the trachea will be the *superior vena cava* into which the *azygos vein* drains.

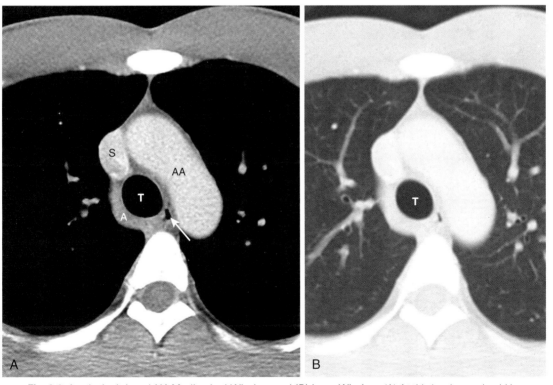

**Fig. 3.6** Aortic Arch Level (A) Mediastinal Window and (B) Lung Window. (A) At this level, you should be able to identify the **aortic arch (AA), superior vena cava (S)**, and **azygos vein (A)**. The arrow points to air in the esophagus. (B) The same image as (A) but windowed to better visualize lung anatomy. Lung windows are chosen to maximize our ability to image abnormalities of the lung parenchyma and to identify normal and abnormal bronchial anatomy. *T,* Trachea.

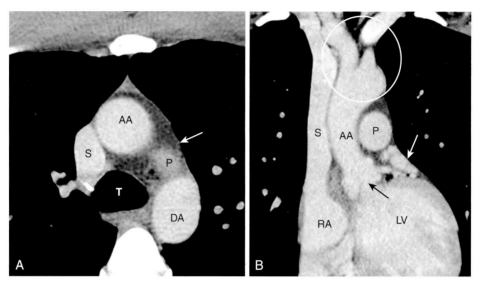

**Fig. 3.7** Aortopulmonary Window Level, Axial (A) and Coronal Views (B). (A) At this level you should be able to identify the **trachea (T), ascending (AA) and descending aorta (DA), superior vena cava (S),** and possibly the uppermost aspect of the **left pulmonary artery (P)**. In most people, there is a space visible just under the arch of the aorta and above the pulmonary artery called the ***aortopulmonary window*** *(arrow)* (see Fig. 2.16). (B) Coronal reformatted CT enables us to also see the **right atrium (RA), superior vena cava (S), pulmonary artery (P), left ventricle (LV), aortic valve** *(black arrow),* **left atrial appendage** *(white arrow),* and origin of the great vessels *(circle).*

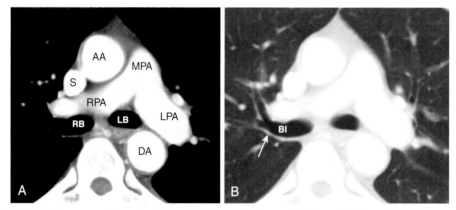

**Fig. 3.8** Main Pulmonary Artery Level (A) Mediastinal Window and (B) Lung Window. (A) At this level, you should be able to identify the **main (MPA), right (RPA), and left pulmonary arteries (LPA), the right (RB) and left main bronchi (LB),** and the **superior vena cava (S).** The left pulmonary artery passes anterior to the **descending aorta** (DA). The right pulmonary artery passes posterior to the **ascending aorta (AA)** and crosses to the right side. (B) Distal to the takeoff of the right upper lobe bronchus is the **bronchus intermedius (BI).** The posterior wall of the right upper lobe bronchus is 2 to 3 mm in thickness with only aerated lung normally posterior to it *(arrow).*

## Aortopulmonary Window Level (Fig. 3.7)

- At this level you should be able to identify the **ascending and descending aorta, superior vena cava,** and **uppermost aspect of the left pulmonary artery** (maybe).

> ## ⟫ IMPORTANT POINTS
>
> - As we scan lower and scan through the opening of the upside-down U-shaped aortic arch, the **ascending aorta** will appear as a rounded density **anteriorly** while the descending aorta will appear as a separate rounded density **posterior** and to the **left** of the spine. The **ascending aorta** usually measures **2.5 to 3.5 cm** in diameter and the **descending aorta** is slightly smaller at **2 to 3 cm**.

- In most people, there is a space visible just underneath the arch of the aorta but above the pulmonary artery called the *aortopulmonary window.* The aortopulmonary window is an important landmark because it is a favorite location for **enlarged lymph nodes** to appear (see Fig. 2.16).
- At or slightly below this level, the trachea bifurcates at the **carina** into the **right and left main bronchi.**

## Main Pulmonary Artery Level (Fig. 3.8)

- At these levels (it may require more than one image to see all of these structures), you should be able to identify the **main, right, and left pulmonary arteries,** the **right and left main bronchi,** and the **bronchus intermedius.**

- The **left pulmonary artery** is higher than the right and appears as a direct continuation of the main pulmonary artery. The **right pulmonary artery** originates at a 90° angle to the main pulmonary artery and crosses to the right side.
- On the **right**, the **main bronchus** will appear as a circular, air-containing structure that will then become tubular as the **right upper lobe** bronchus comes into view. The **bronchus intermedius** then gives rise to the right middle and lower lobe bronchi. Only lung tissue should be seen posterior to the bronchus intermedius (Fig. 3.8B). On the **left**, the **main bronchus** will appear as an air-containing circular structure.

## High Cardiac Level (Fig. 3.9)
- At this level, you should be able to identify the **left atrium, right atrium, aortic root, and right ventricular outflow tract**.

>> **IMPORTANT POINTS**

- The anatomic locations of the right ventricular outflow tract (and pulmonic valve) and the aortic root are important, especially in the diagnosis of congenital cardiac lesions. The **right ventricular outflow tract** normally lies **anterior, lateral, and superior** to the root of the aorta. A good way to remember that relationship is by using the acronym: **PALS**- **P**ulmonic valve lies **A**nterior, **L**ateral and **S**uperior to the aortic valve.

## Low Cardiac Level (Fig. 3.10)
- At this level, you should be able to identify the **right atrium, right ventricle, left ventricle, and interventricular septum**.
- The **right atrium** forms the right heart border. The **right ventricle** is anteriorly located, just behind the sternum, and demonstrates **more muscular trabeculation** than the **smoother-walled left ventricle**. The left ventricle produces the left heart border and normally has a thicker wall than the right ventricle.

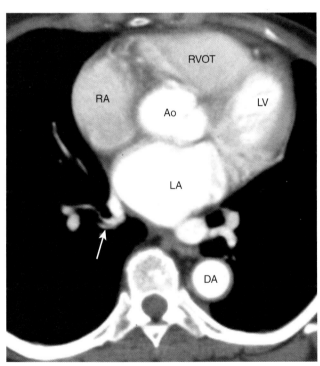

**Fig. 3.9** High Cardiac Level. At this level, you should be able to identify the **left atrium (LA), right atrium (RA), aortic root (Ao)**, and **right ventricular outflow tract (RVOT)**. The **left atrium** occupies the posterior and central portion of the heart. One or more **pulmonary veins** may be seen entering the left atrium *(arrow)*. The right atrium produces the right heart border and lies anteriorly and to the right of the left atrium. *DA*, Descending thoracic aorta; *LV*, left ventricle.

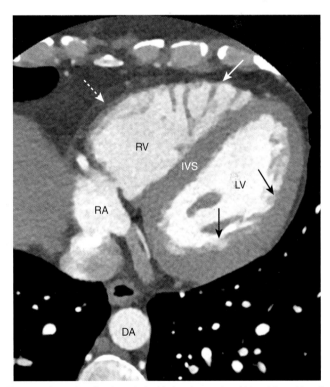

**Fig. 3.10** Low Cardiac Level. At this level, you should be able to identify the **right atrium (RA), right ventricle (RV), left ventricle (LV)**, and **interventricular septum (IVS)**. The right ventricle is more **heavily trabeculated** *(solid white arrow)* and has a **thinner wall** *(dashed white arrow)* than the wall of the left ventricle *(solid black arrows)*. *DA*, Descending thoracic aorta.

- With intravenous contrast filling the chambers, you should be able to see the **interventricular septum** between the right and left ventricles.
- When seen, the **normal pericardium** is about **2 mm thick** and is usually outlined by **mediastinal fat** outside the pericardium and **epicardial fat** on its inner surface.

## USES OF CARDIAC CT

- Cardiac CT scanning is used for evaluation of the coronary arteries, the presence of **cardiac masses**, abnormalities of the aorta (including **aortic dissection**), and **pericardial diseases**.
- Cardiac CT allows for the imaging and three-dimensional reconstruction of the **coronary arteries** and quantitative measurement of the amount of **coronary artery calcium**. The administration of intravenous contrast allows for evaluation of vessel patency with identification of thrombus in the lumen or plaque in the vessel wall.

### Calcium Scoring

- **Calcium scoring** is based on the premise that the amount of calcium detectable in the coronary arteries is related to the degree of coronary atherosclerosis and that quantifying the amount of calcium may help **predict** future cardiac events related to coronary artery disease, such as **heart attack**. The scoring is usually done by calculations that combine the amount and **density** of calcium in the coronary arteries visualized on unenhanced CT of the heart. The **absence** of coronary artery calcification has a **high negative predictive value** for significant luminal narrowing. The higher the calcium score, the greater the risk for a future cardiac event (Fig. 3.11).

- Although calcium scoring is primarily used for risk analysis of asymptomatic patients, **coronary CT angiography (CCTA)** is primarily used in patients with **acute or chronic chest pain**. Like calcium scoring, a **negative CCTA** has a **high negative predictive value**, i.e., a negative study effectively excludes obstructive coronary artery disease.

- One potential drawback to cardiac CT is the **radiation dose** delivered to the patient, which historically had been relatively high. Numerous methods are now being utilized to reduce that dose so that the procedure can now be performed at a dose well below the average annual background radiation dose.

### Coronary CT Angiography: Normal Anatomy

- Coronary CT angiography (CCTA) compares favorably in accuracy with invasive (catheter) coronary angiography, long held as the reference standard in studying the coronary arteries (Video 3.1).
- There are many variations of normal coronary artery anatomy. Only the most common branching is described here (Fig. 3.12).
- The two main coronary arteries are the **left** (also known as the left main) and the **right coronary artery**.

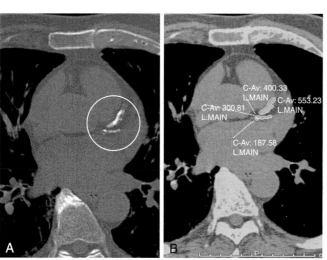

**Fig. 3.11 Coronary Artery Calcification and Scoring.** (A) There is dense calcification mostly in the left anterior descending coronary artery *(circle)*. (B) The **calcium scores** are shown superimposed on the areas of calcification. A score of zero means no calcium is detectable and correlates with a low likelihood of a cardiac event in the near future. The higher the calcium score, the higher the risk of adverse cardiac events in the long term. Scores of 100 to 300 correlate with a mild to moderate risk of a heart attack or other cardiac events over the next 3 to 5 years. As seen in this image, a score greater than 300 indicates a greater likelihood of severe disease and a heart attack risk.

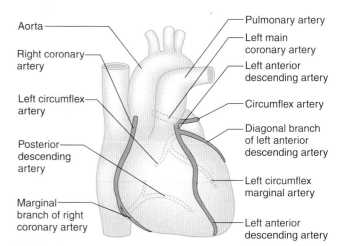

**Fig. 3.12 Coronary Arteries.** The two main coronary arteries are the **left** (also known as the **left main**) and the **right coronary artery**. The left coronary artery divides almost at once into the **circumflex artery** and **left anterior descending artery (LAD)**. The LAD, in turn, gives rise to **diagonal branches** and **septal branches** (not shown). The circumflex artery has **marginal branches**. The **right coronary artery** courses between the right atrium and right ventricle to the inferior part of the septum. It gives rise to a large acute **marginal branch** and, in most people, the **posterior descending artery (PDA)**. The PDA supplies the inferior wall of the left ventricle and inferior part of the septum. (From Bruce NH, Ray R. Cardiovascular disease. In: Kumar P, Clark M, eds. *Kumar and Clark's Clinical Medicine*, 8th ed. London: Elsevier; 2012, pg. 673.)

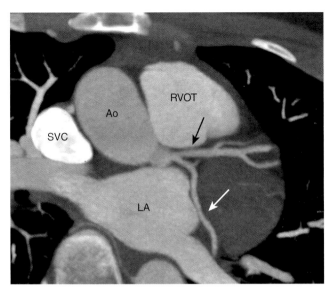

**Fig. 3.13** CT Coronary Angiogram, Left Coronary Artery. The **left coronary artery (LCA)** originates from the left coronary cusp at the aortic valve and divides almost immediately into the **circumflex artery** *(white arrow)* and **left anterior descending artery (LAD)** *(black arrow)*. *Ao,* Aorta; *LA,* left atrium; *RVOT,* right ventriclar outflow tract; *SVC,* superior vena cava.

- The **left coronary artery (LCA)** arises from the left coronary cusp at the aortic valve. It divides almost at once into the **circumflex artery** and **left anterior descending artery (LAD)** (Fig. 3.13). The LAD, in turn, gives rise to **diagonal branches** and **septal branches.** The **circumflex artery** has **marginal branches.**
- The LAD travels in the **anterior interventricular groove** and continues to the apex of the heart (Fig. 3.14). It supplies most of the left ventricle and also the atrioventricular (AV)-bundle, serving the anterior part of the septum with **septal branches** and the anterior wall of the left ventricle with **diagonal branches.**
- The **circumflex artery** (see Fig. 3.13) lies between the left atrium and left ventricle and supplies **obtuse marginal** vessels to the lateral wall of the left ventricle.
- The right aortic sinus gives rise to the **right coronary artery (RCA)**, which courses between the right atrium and right ventricle to the inferior part of the septum (Fig. 3.15).
- In most people, the first branch of the RCA is the **conus branch** that supplies the right ventricular outflow tract. In most people, a **sinus node artery** arises as a second branch of the RCA. The next branches are **diagonals** that supply the anterior wall of the right ventricle.
- The large **acute marginal branch** (AM) supplies the lateral wall of the right ventricle and runs along the *margin* of the right ventricle above the diaphragm. The RCA continues in the AV groove posteriorly and gives off a branch to the AV node (see Fig. 3.12).
- In most people, the **posterior descending artery (PDA)** is a **branch of the RCA.** The PDA supplies the inferior wall of the left ventricle and inferior part of the septum (see Fig. 3.15).

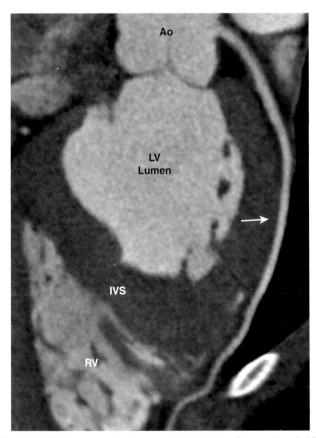

**Fig. 3.14** CT Coronary Angiogram, Left Anterior Descending (LAD) Coronary Artery. The LAD *(arrow)* sits in the **anterior interventricular groove** continuing to the apex of the heart and supplying most of the left ventricle and the AV-bundle. *Ao,* Aorta; *IVS,* interventricular septum; *LV,* left ventricular; *RV,* right ventricle.

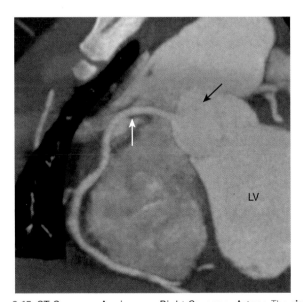

**Fig. 3.15** CT Coronary Angiogram, Right Coronary Artery. The **right aortic sinus** *(black arrow)* gives rise to the **right coronary artery (RCA)** *(white arrow),* which courses between the right atrium and right ventricle to the inferior part of the septum. In most people, as here, the RCA continues to the **posterior descending artery.** *LV,* Left ventricle.

### Coronary Artery Dominance

- The artery that supplies the **posterior descending artery** determines **coronary artery dominance**.
- If the **posterior descending artery** is supplied by the **right coronary artery**, then the coronary circulation is said to be **right dominant**.
- If the **posterior descending artery** is supplied by the **circumflex artery**, a branch of the left coronary artery, then the coronary circulation is called **left dominant**.
- If the **posterior descending artery** is supplied by **both** the **right coronary artery** and the **circumflex artery**, then the coronary circulation is called **co-dominant**.

> ### ▶ IMPORTANT POINTS
>
> - The **overwhelming majority** of the population is **right dominant**, about 10% are left dominant, and the remainder are co-dominant. A **left dominant** coronary artery system is associated with an **increased risk of non-fatal myocardial infarction** and increased overall mortality.

- It is possible to perform an emergent CT scan that will allow for the simultaneous evaluation of **coronary artery disease**, **aortic dissection**, and **pulmonary thromboembolic disease**, the so-called *triple scan (triple rule-out)* for patients who present with **acute chest pain**. Such scans have been shown to improve clinical decision-making and allow for earlier discharge from the hospital.

## CARDIAC MRI

- MRI can be used to obtain **anatomic** and **functional** images of the heart using a combination of ECG-gating and rapid acquisition of images. Respiratory motion, which would also contribute to blurring the image, can be reduced by having the patient hold their breath for short periods of time while the images are acquired (Video 3.2).
- **Cardiac MRI** can depict scarring from a myocardial infarction, perfusion of the heart, anatomic defects or masses, and can assess the function of the valves and cardiac chambers.
- Cardiac MRI can be performed without intravenous contrast or with intravenous contrast (**Gadolinium: see Chapter 20**). Cardiac MRI is particularly useful in children as a way of evaluating congenital heart disease after other studies (such as echocardiography) produce inconclusive or conflicting information.

### Normal Cardiac MRI Anatomy

- One of the benefits of MRI is that its images can be depicted in **any** plane. The anatomy of the heart in the **axial, sagittal**, and **coronal** planes is the same as that seen on CT scans displayed in those planes (Fig. 3.16).
- Besides the axial, sagittal, and coronal planes, there are several additional views that are typically used in cardiac MRI that allow for additional visualization of the heart. They are called the **horizontal long-axis (otherwise known as the four-chamber view), vertical long-axis, short-axis**, and **three-chamber views** (Fig. 3.17).
- The **horizontal long-axis (four-chamber) view** resembles an axial view and is best used for evaluating the left ventricle's septal and lateral walls and apex, the right ventricular

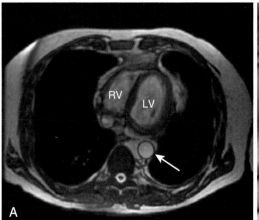 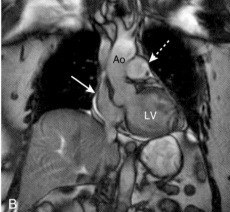 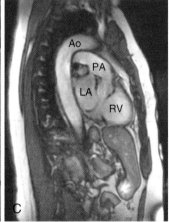

**Fig. 3.16 Cardiac MRI, Axial, Coronal, and Sagittal Planes.** These three planes produce images with a similar appearance as those on CT (see Fig. 2.13). (A) The axial view at this level shows the **right (RV) and left ventricles (LV)** and the **descending aorta** *(arrow)*. (B) This coronal image demonstrates the **right atrium** *(solid arrow)*, **left ventricle (LV)**, **aorta (Ao)**, and **main pulmonary artery** *(dashed arrow)*. (C) The sagittal image at this level shows the **right ventricle (RV), pulmonary artery (PA), left atrium (LA)**, and **aorta (Ao)**. In all of these images, the blood is depicted as "bright" (i.e., white).

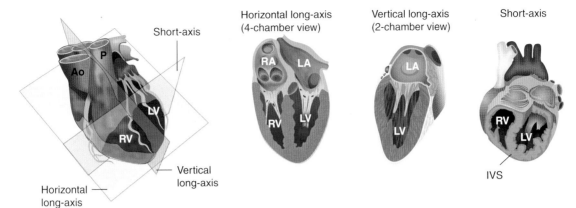

**Fig. 3.17 Common MRI Views of the Heart.** These standard imaging planes are similar to ones used for echocardiography and CT and are designed to demonstrate certain cardiac structures to their best advantage. An additional view, the three-chamber view, is similar to the coronal view (see Fig. 3.21). *Ao,* Aorta; *IVS,* interventricular septum; *LA,* left atrium; *LV,* left ventricle; *P,* pulmonary artery; *RA,* right atrium; *RV,* right ventricle.

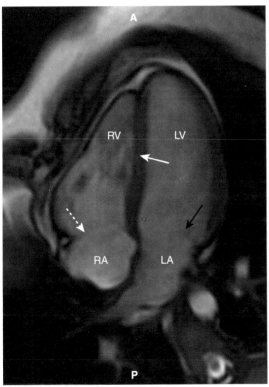

**Fig. 3.18** Cardiac MRI, Horizontal Long-Axis View. This is another standard view of the heart using MRI called the **horizontal long-axis** or **four-chamber view.** The **right (RV)** and **left ventricles (LV)** are separated by the **interventricular septum** *(solid white arrow).* Posterior to each of them are the **right atrium (RA)** and **left atrium (LA),** separated by the regions of the **tricuspid** *(dashed white arrow)* and **mitral valves** *(solid black arrow),* respectively. *A,* Anterior; *P,* posterior.

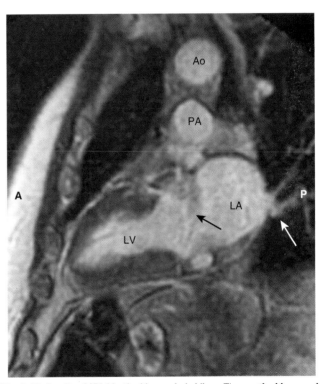

**Fig. 3.19** Cardiac MRI, Vertical Long-Axis View. The **vertical long-axis** or **two-chamber view** demonstrates the **left ventricle (LV)** separated from the more posterior **left atrium (LA)** by the **mitral valve area** *(black arrow).* **Pulmonary veins** drain into the left atrium *(white arrow).* The **aorta (Ao)** sits atop the **pulmonary artery (PA).** *A,* Anterior; *P,* posterior.

free wall, and for the size of the cardiac chambers. The mitral and tricuspid valves are especially well visualized in this view (Fig. 3.18).

- The **vertical long-axis view** resembles a sagittal view and is best used in the evaluation of the anterior and inferior walls and apex of the left ventricle (Fig. 3.19).

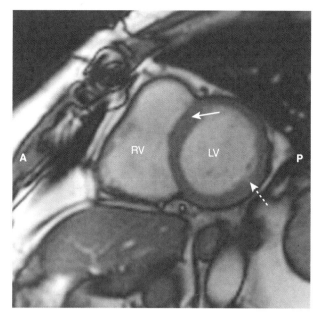

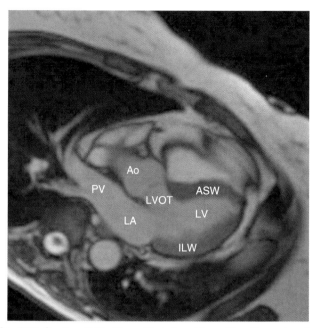

**Fig. 3.20** Cardiac MRI, Short-Axis View. This is a standard view of the heart using MRI called the **short-axis view**. The **right ventricle (RV)** lies anterior to the **left ventricle (LV)**, separated by the **interventricular septum** *(solid arrow)*. Note the normally thicker wall of the left ventricle *(dashed arrow)* than the right ventricle. *A,* Anterior; *P,* posterior.

**Fig. 3.21** Cardiac MRI, Three-Chamber View. The **three-chamber view** is similar in appearance to a coronal view and shows the **aorta (Ao)**, **left ventricular outflow tract (LVOT)**, **left ventricle (LV)**, **left atrium (LA)**, **pulmonary veins (PV)**, and the **anteroseptal (ASW)** and **inferolateral (ILW)** walls of the left ventricle (which are abnormally thickened in this person).

- The **short-axis view** depicts the left and right ventricles in a way that is useful for making **volumetric measurements** (Fig. 3.20).
  - Because MR images of the heart are already obtained with three-dimensional volumes in both end-systole and end-diastole, computer-based measurements of **ventricular mass, end-diastolic volume**, and **end-systolic volume** can be determined and, from them, **stroke volume** and **ejection fraction** can be calculated without other intervention.

- The **three-chamber view**, which is similar to a coronal view, is particularly helpful in assessing the mitral and aortic valves, left atrial size, and the walls of the left ventricle (Fig. 3.21).
- Depending on the MRI pulse sequence used to obtain the images, **blood** can be depicted as either **black** (usually using something called a *spin echo* pulse sequence), the mode **most often used for anatomic evaluation**, or bright, i.e., **white** (usually using something called a *gradient echo* pulse sequence), the mode most often used for **functional evaluation** (Fig. 3.22).

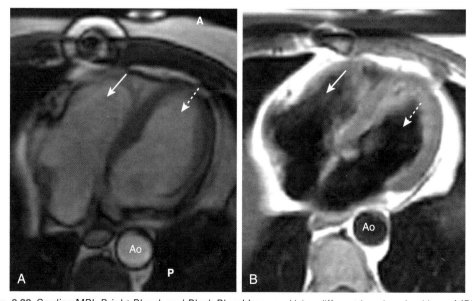

**Fig. 3.22** Cardiac MRI, Bright Blood, and Black Blood Images. Using different imaging algorithms, MRI is capable of displaying the same tissues with differing appearances. (A) and (B) are both axial sections through the heart, showing the **right ventricle** *(solid arrows)*, the **left ventricle** *(dashed arrows)*, and the **aorta (Ao)**. (A) The **bright blood** technique is utilized to assess **cardiac function,** while (B) the **black blood** technique usually is better at depicting **cardiac morphology**. *A,* Anterior; *P,* posterior.

## CASE QUIZ 3 ANSWER

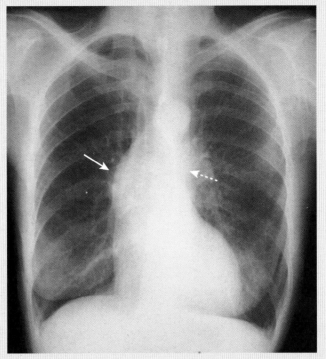

The ascending aorta *(solid arrow)* is enlarged. It normally should not extend farther than the right heart border below it. The remaining contour of the aorta *(dashed arrow)* is normal. Along with the patient's history, this finding is suggestive of post-stenotic dilatation seen in ***aortic valvular stenosis,*** which was proven by echocardiography.

## 🏠 TAKE HOME POINTS

- In adults, the frontal chest x-ray can serve for a quick assessment of heart size by using the **cardiothoracic ratio**, which is the ratio of the widest transverse diameter of the heart compared to the widest internal diameter of the rib cage. In normal adults, the cardiothoracic ratio is usually <50%.
- The normal contours of the heart on the frontal chest x-ray are reviewed.
- The ventricles respond to obstruction to their outflow by first undergoing hypertrophy rather than dilatation. On plain films, **cardiomegaly** is primarily produced by **ventricular enlargement.** The most marked chamber enlargement will occur from **volume overload** rather than pressure overload.
- Normal anatomy of the major structures is described at six levels in the chest (from top to bottom): five-vessel view, aortic arch, aortopulmonary window, main pulmonary artery, upper cardiac, and lower cardiac levels.
- **Cardiac CT** scanning uses a fast, multi-slice CT scanner, usually with intravenous iodinated contrast and electrocardiographic (ECG)-gated acquisition to reduce motion artifact.
- **Cardiac CT** scanning is used for evaluation of the coronary arteries, the presence of cardiac masses, abnormalities of the aorta (including aortic dissection), and pericardial diseases.

- Normal coronary artery anatomy is described. The artery that supplies the posterior descending artery (PDA) determines **coronary artery dominance.** The overwhelming majority of the population is **right dominant.**
- For patients who present with **acute chest pain,** it is possible to perform an emergent CT scan for the simultaneous evaluation of **coronary artery disease, aortic dissection,** and **pulmonary thromboembolic** disease (***triple rule-out scan***).
- MRI can be used to obtain anatomic and functional images of the heart. Cardiac MRI can show scarring from a myocardial infarction, depict perfusion of the heart and anatomic defects or masses, and can assess the function of the valves and cardiac chambers.
- Several specific views that are typically used in cardiac MRI that allow for the best visualization of the heart are described. They are called: the **horizontal long-axis** (otherwise known as the **four-chamber view), vertical long-axis, short-axis, and three-chamber** views.
- **Cardiac function** is usually evaluated using MRI sequences producing **"bright blood"** images, so-called because the blood is depicted with increased signal intensity.
- **Cardiac morphology** is usually evaluated using MRI sequences producing **"black blood"** images. These images allow for anatomic assessment of the cardiac structures without interference from the bright blood signal.

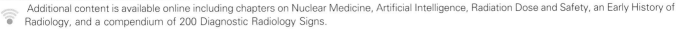

Additional content is available online including chapters on Nuclear Medicine, Artificial Intelligence, Radiation Dose and Safety, an Early History of Radiology, and a compendium of 200 Diagnostic Radiology Signs.

# 4

# Recognizing Airspace Versus Interstitial Lung Disease

*William Herring, MD, FACR*

Recognizing the difference between **normal anatomy** and what is **abnormal** is critical to your ability to make a correct diagnosis. This chapter begins your exploration into the realm of the abnormal, starting with recognizing patterns of parenchymal lung disease.

## CASE QUIZ 4 QUESTION

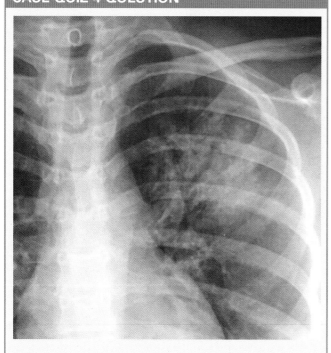

A close-up view of the left upper lobe is shown. Is this most likely airspace disease or interstitial lung disease? Given a history of cough, what is a likely diagnosis? See the answer at the end of the chapter.

## CLASSIFYING PARENCHYMAL LUNG DISEASE

- **Diseases** that affect the lung parenchyma **can be arbitrarily divided into two main categories** based in part on their **pathology** and in part on the **pattern** they typically produce on a chest imaging study.
  - **Airspace (alveolar) disease**

  - **Interstitial (infiltrative) disease**
- Why learn the difference?
  - While many diseases produce abnormalities that display both patterns, recognition of these two patterns frequently helps narrow the disease possibilities so that you can form a reasonable **differential diagnosis** (Box 4.1).

### BOX 4.1 Classification of Parenchymal Lung Diseases

**Airspace Diseases**

*Acute*
- Pneumonia
- Pulmonary alveolar edema
- Hemorrhage
- Aspiration
- Near-drowning

*Chronic*
- Adenocarcinoma (subtype formerly called bronchoalveolar carcinoma)
- Alveolar cell proteinosis
- Sarcoidosis
- Lymphoma

**Interstitial Diseases**

*Reticular*
- Pulmonary interstitial edema
- Interstitial pneumonia
- Scleroderma
- Sarcoid

*Nodular*
- Bronchogenic carcinoma
- Metastases
- Silicosis
- Miliary tuberculosis
- Sarcoid

## CHARACTERISTICS OF AIRSPACE DISEASE

- Airspace disease characteristically produces opacities in the lung that have a **fluffy, cloudlike,** or **hazy** appearance.

- The **margins of airspace disease are indistinct**, meaning it is frequently difficult to identify a clear demarcation point between the disease and the adjacent normal lung.
- These fluffy opacities also tend to be **confluent**, meaning they blend into one another with **imperceptible margins.**
- Airspace disease may be **distributed throughout the lungs**, as in pulmonary edema (Fig. 4.1), or it may **appear more localized,** as in a segmental or lobar pneumonia (Fig. 4.2).
- The **visibility of air in the bronchus because of surrounding airspace disease** is called an **air bronchogram.** Airspace disease may contain *air bronchograms.*
  - An air bronchogram is almost always a **sign of airspace disease.**
    - Bronchi are **normally not visible** because their walls are **very thin,** they **contain air,** and they are **surrounded by air.** When something like fluid or soft tissue replaces the air normally surrounding the bronchus, then the air inside of the bronchus becomes visible as **a series of black, branching tubular structures**—this is called an *air bronchogram* (Fig. 4.3).
  - What can fill the airspaces besides air?
    - **Fluid,** such as occurs in pulmonary edema
    - **Blood** (e.g., pulmonary hemorrhage)
    - **Gastric juices** (e.g., aspiration)
    - **Inflammatory exudate** (e.g., pneumonia)
    - **Water** (e.g., near-drowning)

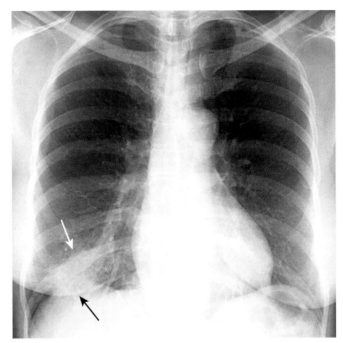

**Fig. 4.2 Right Lower Lobe Pneumonia.** There is an area of increased opacification in the right lower lobe *(white arrow)* characteristic of airspace disease. The disease silhouettes the mid portion of the right hemidiaphragm *(black arrow)* localizing it to the lower lobe.

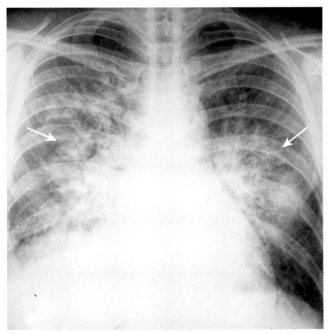

**Fig. 4.1 Diffuse Airspace Disease of Pulmonary Alveolar Edema.** Fluffy, confluent, bilateral, perihilar airspace disease with indistinct margins, sometimes described as having a ***bat-wing*** or ***angel-wing*** configuration, is present *(arrows)*. The heart is enlarged. This is a typical example of pulmonary alveolar edema.

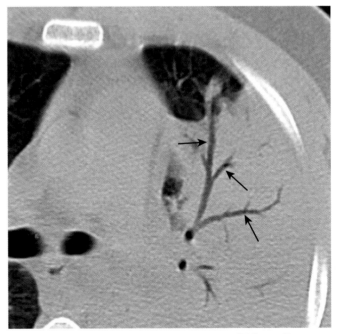

**Fig. 4.3 Air Bronchograms Demonstrated on CT Scan.** Numerous black, branching structures *(arrows)* represent air that is now visible inside the bronchi because the surrounding airspaces are filled with inflammatory exudate in this patient with an obstructive pneumonia from a bronchogenic carcinoma.

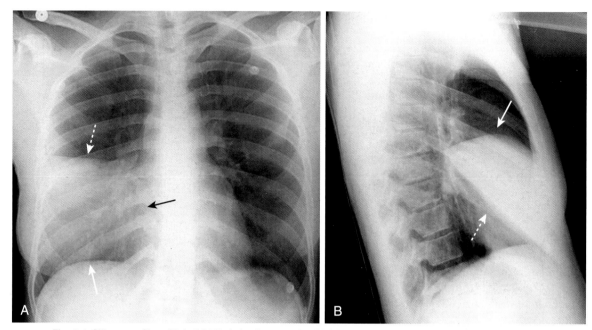

**Fig. 4.4** Silhouette Sign, Right Middle Lobe Pneumonia. (A) A homogeneous area of increased density is seen to the right of the heart. It obscures the right heart border *(black arrow)*. This is the **silhouette sign** and it establishes that the disease (1) is in contact with the right heart border (which lies anteriorly in the chest) and (2) that the disease is the same radiographic density as the heart (in this case, fluid or soft tissue). The disease does not obscure the right hemidiaphragm *(solid white arrow)*. It is also bounded superiorly by the minor (horizontal) fissure *(dashed arrow)*, placing it in the **right middle lobe**. (B) The area of the consolidation is indeed anterior, located in the right middle lobe, bounded by the major fissure below *(dashed arrow)* and the minor fissure above *(solid arrow)*.

- Airspace disease may also demonstrate the *silhouette sign* (Fig. 4.4).
  - The **silhouette sign** is most useful on conventional radiographs and occurs when two objects **of the same radiographic density** (e.g., water and soft tissue) **are in contact with each other, which results in the loss of the edge or margin between them.** The silhouette sign is a valuable tool for the localization of disease not only in the chest but in the analysis of imaging studies throughout the body.
- The characteristics of airspace disease are summarized in Box 4.2.

## SOME CAUSES OF AIRSPACE DISEASE

There are many causes of airspace disease, three of which will be highlighted here. Each is described in greater detail later in the text.
- **Pneumonia (see also Chapter 8)**
  - About 90% of the time, community-acquired lobar or segmental pneumonia is caused by *Streptococcus pneumoniae* (Fig. 4.5). Pneumonia usually manifests as patchy,

---

### BOX 4.2    Characteristics of Airspace Disease

- Produces opacities in the lung, which can be described as **fluffy, cloud-like, and hazy.**
- The **margins** of airspace disease are fuzzy and **indistinct.**
- The **opacities** tend to be **confluent**, merging into one another.
- **Air bronchograms** or the **silhouette sign** may be present.

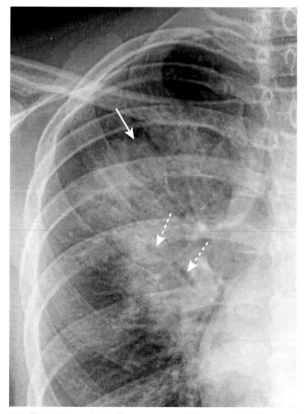

**Fig. 4.5** Right Upper Lobe Pneumococcal Pneumonia. Close-up view of the right upper lobe demonstrates fluffy airspace disease *(solid arrow)* with air bronchograms *(dashed arrows)*. This patient had *Streptococcus pneumoniae* cultured from the sputum.

segmental, or lobar airspace disease. Pneumonias may contain air bronchograms. **Clearing** usually occurs **in less than 10 days** (pneumococcal pneumonia may clear within 48 hours).

- **Pulmonary alveolar edema (see also Chapter 11)**
  - Acute, pulmonary alveolar edema classically produces **bilateral, perihilar airspace disease,** sometimes described as having a *bat-wing* or *angel-wing configuration* (see Fig. 4.1).
  - It is usually **bilateral** but may be **asymmetric.** Pulmonary edema, which is **cardiac** in origin, is frequently associated with **pleural effusions** and fluid that thickens the **major** and **minor fissures.**
  - Because pulmonary edema fluid fills not only the airspaces but the bronchi themselves, there are **usually no air bronchograms** seen in pulmonary alveolar edema. Classically, **pulmonary edema clears rapidly** after treatment (<48 hours).
- **Aspiration (see also Chapter 8)**
  - Aspiration tends to affect whatever part of the lung is **most dependent** at the time the patient aspirates and its manifestations depend on the substance(s) aspirated. For most bedridden patients, aspiration usually occurs into either the **lower lobes** or the **posterior portions of the upper lobes.**
  - Because of the course and caliber of the right main bronchus, **aspiration occurs more often in the right lower lobe** than the left lower lobe (Fig. 4.6).
  - Depending on what is aspirated and whether it becomes infected will determine the radiographic appearance of aspiration and how quickly the airspace disease resolves. **Aspiration** of bland **(neutralized)** gastric juice or **water usually clears rapidly** within 24 to 48 hours whereas aspiration that becomes **infected** can take **weeks** to resolve.

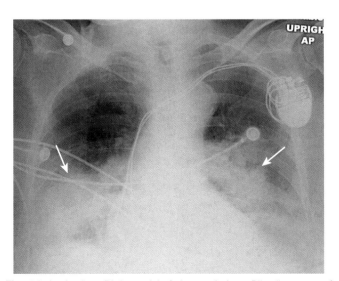

**Fig. 4.6 Aspiration, Right and Left Lower Lobes.** Bibasilar areas of increased density that are fluffy in appearance with indistinct margins are characteristic of airspace disease *(arrows).* The **bibasilar distribution** of this disease should raise the suspicion of aspiration as an etiology. This patient had a recent stroke and aspiration was demonstrated on a video swallowing study.

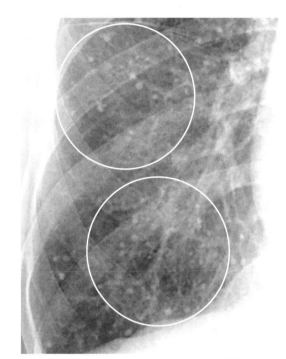

**Fig. 4.7 Varicella Pneumonia.** Innumerable calcified granulomas, which occur in the lung interstitium, are seen here as small, discrete nodules in the right lung *(circles).* This patient had a history of *varicella* (chickenpox) pneumonia years earlier. Varicella pneumonia heals with multiple small, calcified granulomas remaining.

## CHARACTERISTICS OF INTERSTITIAL LUNG DISEASE

- The lung's interstitium consists of **connective tissue, lymphatics, blood vessels, and bronchi.** These are the structures that surround and support the airspaces.
- Interstitial lung disease (sometimes referred to as **infiltrative lung disease**) produces what can be thought of as discrete **"particles"** of disease that develop in the abundant interstitial network of the lung.
- The characteristics of interstitial lung disease are summarized in Box 4.3.
- These "particles" of disease can be further characterized as having **three patterns of presentation** (Fig. 4.8):
  - **Reticular interstitial disease** appears as a network of **lines** (Fig. 4.8A).

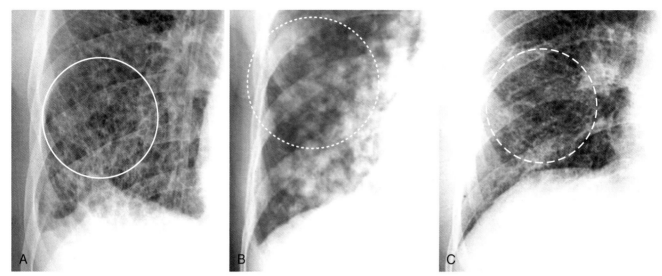

**Fig. 4.8 Three Patterns of Interstitial Lung Disease.** (A) The disease is primarily **reticular** in nature, consisting of crisscrossing lines (*circle*). This patient had advanced sarcoidosis. (B) The disease is predominantly **nodular** (*circle*). The patient was known to have thyroid carcinoma, and these nodules represent innumerable, small metastatic foci in the lungs. (C) **Reticulonodular** interstitial disease of the lung. Most interstitial diseases of the lung have a mixture of both a reticular (lines) and nodular (dots) pattern, as does this case, which is a close-up view of the right lower lobe in another patient with sarcoidosis (*circle*).

- **Nodular interstitial disease** appears as an assortment of **dots** (Fig. 4.8B).
- **Reticulonodular interstitial disease** contains **both** lines and dots (Fig. 4.8C).

> **! DIAGNOSTIC PITFALLS**
>
> - Sometimes, there is so much interstitial disease present that the overlapping elements of disease may **superimpose** and mimic airspace disease on conventional chest radiographs. Superimposition of all of the lung's content on radiographs may make the tiny packets of interstitial disease seem **coalescent** and appear more like airspace disease.
> - **Solution:** Look at the **periphery** of such confluent shadows in the lung to help in determining whether they are, in fact, caused by airspace disease or a superimposition of numerous reticular and nodular densities (Fig. 4.9). A CT scan of the chest will provide even better characterization of the disease.

## SOME CAUSES OF INTERSTITIAL LUNG DISEASE

- Just as with the airspace pattern, many diseases produce an interstitial pattern in the lung. Several will be discussed briefly here. They are roughly divided into those diseases that are predominantly *reticular* and those that are predominantly *nodular*.

> **» IMPORTANT POINTS**
>
> - Keep in mind that **many diseases have patterns that overlap and many interstitial lung diseases have mixtures of both reticular and nodular changes** (i.e., reticulonodular disease).

## Predominantly Reticular Interstitial Lung Diseases

- **Pulmonary interstitial edema**
  - Pulmonary interstitial edema can occur because of increased capillary **pressure** (congestive heart failure),

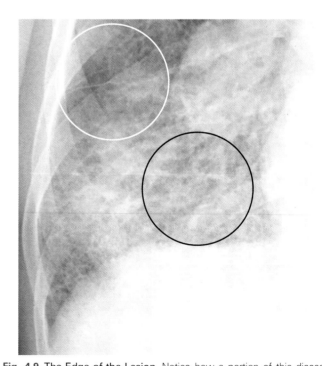

**Fig. 4.9 The Edge of the Lesion.** Notice how a portion of this disease appears confluent, like airspace disease, because of the superimposition of all of the tissues of the lung upon each other *(black circle)*. Always look at the peripheral margins of parenchymal lung disease to best determine the nature of the abnormality. At the periphery of this disease *(white circle)*, this is more clearly seen to be reticular and interstitial, not airspace disease.

increased capillary **permeability** (allergic reactions), or decreased fluid **absorption** (lymphangitic carcinomatosis from metastatic disease).

- Considered the precursor of pulmonary alveolar edema, pulmonary interstitial edema classically manifests **four key radiologic findings:** *fluid in the fissures* (major and minor), *peribronchial cuffing* (from fluid in the walls of bronchioles), *pleural effusions,* and *Kerley B lines* (Fig. 4.10).
- Classically, the patient may have **few physical findings** in the lungs (rales) even though their chest radiograph demonstrates considerable pulmonary interstitial edema, because almost all of the fluid is in the interstitium of the lung, rather than in the airspaces.
- With appropriate therapy, pulmonary interstitial edema usually clears rapidly (<48 hours).
- **Interstitial pneumonia**
  - There are many forms of interstitial pneumonia, the most common being *usual interstitial pneumonia.* Another form, called *nonspecific interstitial pneumonia,* is a pattern of disease that does not fall easily into any of the other categories.
  - **Usual interstitial pneumonia (UIP)**
    - UIP is sometimes used to mean *idiopathic interstitial fibrosis.* UIP is more **common in older men** and has associations with **cigarette smoking** and **gastroesophageal reflux.**
    - Chest radiographs may be **normal** in UIP. The earliest manifestation on chest radiographs consists of a **fine**

reticular pattern, particularly at the lung bases. The pattern then becomes coarser as the disease progresses and ends with a pattern that is called *honeycombing* (other diseases also produce honeycombing). There may also be **progressive volume loss.**

- Imaging diagnosis is made on CT scans of the chest where **honeycombing, subpleural reticular opacities,** and **traction bronchiectasis** are present, especially at the lung bases (Fig. 4.11).
- **Idiopathic pulmonary fibrosis** is considered the end-stage disease along the spectrum of these interstitial pneumonias.
- **Nonspecific interstitial pneumonia (NSIP)**
  - NSIP is a pattern of lung injury that is seen in a large percentage of patients with **connective tissue diseases,** such as **scleroderma,** who have pulmonary findings.
  - Patients with a pattern of NSIP, in general, have a **better prognosis** than patients with UIP.
  - Imaging diagnosis is made on CT scans of the chest where basilar *ground-glass opacities* are present, sometimes with **subpleural sparing** adding specificity to the diagnosis. **Traction bronchiectasis** is seen in advanced cases (Fig. 4.12).
- **Lymphangitic carcinomatosis (see "Metastases to the lung" in the next section)**

## Predominantly Nodular Interstitial Diseases

- **Bronchogenic carcinoma (see Chapter 10)**
  - There are four major cell types of bronchogenic carcinoma: **adenocarcinoma, squamous cell carcinoma, small cell carcinoma,** and **large cell carcinoma.**
  - Adenocarcinomas, in particular, can present as a **solitary peripheral pulmonary nodule.**

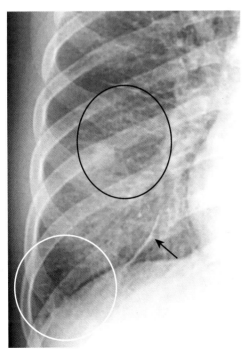

**Fig. 4.10** Pulmonary Interstitial Edema Secondary to Congestive Heart Failure. A close-up view of the right lung shows an accentuation of the pulmonary interstitial markings (*black circle*). (The nodular density in the circle is the superimposed nipple.) There are multiple Kerley B lines (*white circle*) representing fluid in thickened interlobular septa. Fluid is seen thickening the inferior accessory fissure (*arrow*).

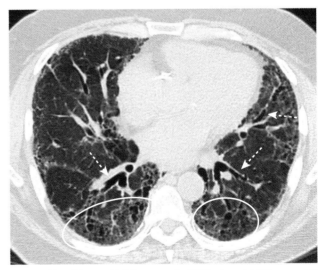

**Fig. 4.11** Usual Interstitial Pneumonia (UIP). An axial CT scan of the chest shows abnormalities at the lung bases, in a subpleural location, the typical distribution for UIP. There are small cystic spaces called *honeycombing* (*ovals*) with evidence of **bronchiectasis,** as manifest by thickened bronchial walls (*arrows*).

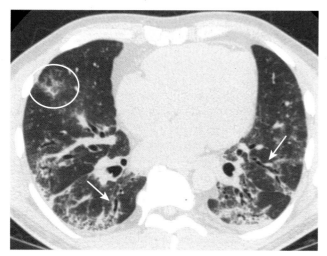

**Fig. 4.12** Nonspecific Interstitial Pneumonia (NSIP). A *ground-glass opacity* is seen in a subpleural location on the right (*circle*). Ground-glass opacities are nonspecific abnormal areas of the lung that have increased attenuation (are whiter) in which the vascular markings and bronchi mostly appear intact. They can be associated with both benign and malignant diseases. Also present is bronchiectasis in both lungs (*arrows*). The patient was known to have scleroderma.

- As a rule, on conventional chest radiographs, nodules or masses in the lung are more **discrete** than airspace disease, producing a relatively clear demarcation between the nodule and the surrounding normal lung tissue.
- CT scans may demonstrate **spiculation** or **irregularity** of the lung nodule itself that may not be apparent on conventional radiographs (Fig. 4.13).
- **Metastases to the lung** (Fig. 4.14)
  - Metastases to the lung can be divided into three categories depending on the pattern of disease demonstrated in the lung.

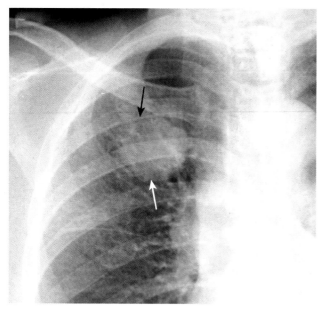

**Fig. 4.13** Adenocarcinoma, Right Upper Lobe. A mass is seen in the right upper lobe (*white arrow*). Its margin is slightly indistinct along the supero-lateral border (*black arrow*). CT scan of the chest confirmed the presence of the mass and also demonstrated paratracheal and right hilar adenopathy. The mass was biopsied and was an adenocarcinoma, primary to the lung.

- *Hematogenous metastases* arrive via the bloodstream and usually produce two or more **nodules** in the lungs that, when they achieve a large size, are sometimes called *cannonball metastases.* Primary tumors that classically produce nodular metastases in the lung include **breast, colorectal, renal cell, bladder and testicular, head and neck carcinomas, soft tissue sarcomas, and malignant melanoma** (Fig. 4.14A).

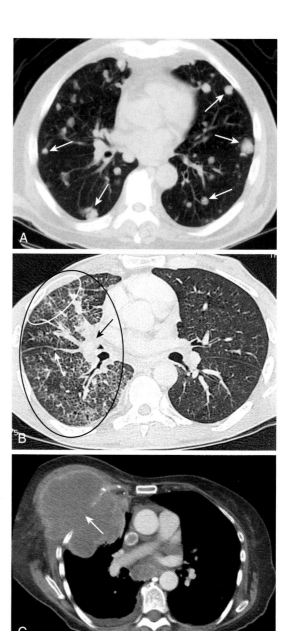

**Fig. 4.14** Metastases to the Lung, CT Scans. (A) There are multiple **discrete nodules of varying size** throughout both lungs (*arrows*). The diagnosis of exclusion is metastatic disease whenever multiple nodules are found in the lungs. In this case the metastases were from colon carcinoma. (B) The interstitial markings in the right lung are prominent (*black oval*) and there are thickened septal lines (*white oval*), fluid in the fissure (*white arrow*), and lymphadenopathy (*black arrow*) representing **lymphangitic carcinomatosis from a bronchogenic carcinoma.** (C) In this case, the lung cancer has invaded and grown through the chest wall (*arrow*) by direct extension.

- The second form of tumor dissemination is *lymphangitic spread.* The pathogenesis of lymphangitic spread to the lungs is somewhat controversial but most likely involves blood-borne spread to the pulmonary capillaries and then invasion of adjacent lymphatics. An alternative means of lymphangitic spread is obstruction of central lymphatics usually in the hila with retrograde dissemination through the lymphatics in the lung.
  - Regardless of the mode of transmission, lymphangitic spread to the lung tends to **resemble pulmonary interstitial edema from congestive heart failure** except, unlike congestive heart failure, it tends to be **localized to a single lung segment, lobe, or only one lung.**
  - Findings include **Kerley lines, fluid in the fissures, and pleural effusions** (Fig. 4.14B).
  - Primary tumors that classically produce the lymphangitic pattern of metastases in the lung include **breast, lung, stomach, pancreatic, and, infrequently, prostate carcinoma.**
- *Direct extension* is the least common form of tumor spread to the lungs because the **pleura is surprisingly resistant to the spread of malignancy** through direct violation of its layers. Direct extension would most likely produce a **localized subpleural mass** in the lung, frequently with **adjacent rib destruction** (Fig. 4.14C).

## Mixed Reticular and Nodular Interstitial Disease (Reticulonodular Disease)

- **Sarcoidosis**
  - In addition to the **bilateral hilar** and **right paratracheal adenopathy** characteristic of this disease, about half of patients with thoracic sarcoid also demonstrate **interstitial lung disease.** The interstitial lung disease is frequently a mixture of both **reticular** and **nodular** components.
  - The progression of disease in sarcoid tends to start with adenopathy (**Stage I**), proceed to a combination of both interstitial lung disease and adenopathy (**Stage II**) and then progress to a stage in which the adenopathy regresses while the interstitial lung disease remains (**Stage III**).
  - Pulmonary fibrosis is present in **Stage IV** disease.
  - Most patients with parenchymal lung disease from sarcoidosis will undergo complete resolution of the disease (Fig. 4.15).

## Mixed Airspace and Interstitial Disease

- Not all diseases obey the rule of producing **either** airspace **or** interstitial disease. Some produce a mixture of **both** at the same time or may initially present as airspace disease followed in time by interstitial disease. **Tuberculosis** is one such disease.

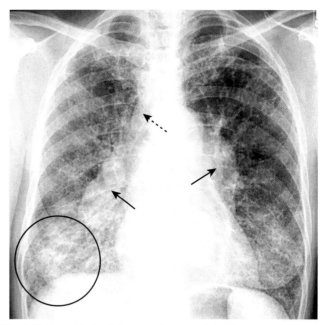

**Fig. 4.15** Sarcoidosis. A frontal radiograph of the chest reveals bilateral hilar (*solid black arrows*) and right paratracheal adenopathy (*dashed black arrow*), a classic distribution for the adenopathy in sarcoidosis. In addition, the patient has diffuse, bilateral interstitial lung disease (*circle*) that is **reticulonodular** in nature.

## Tuberculosis

- Up to a third of the world's population is believed to have been infected with *Mycobacterium tuberculosis* (TB). While the incidence of TB decreased in the United States, it has been increasing in developing countries. Most infections cause no symptoms but about 1 in 10 go on to active tuberculosis.

### Primary Pulmonary Tuberculosis

- Relatively few patients with primary TB have clinical manifestations. The **upper lobes** are affected slightly more than the lower. Classical manifestations include **lobar pneumonia** (Fig. 4.16), especially with associated **adenopathy,** unilateral **hilar or mediastinal adenopathy without parenchymal disease** (more common in children), and **large and typically asymptomatic pleural effusions** (more common in adults) (Fig. 4.17). **Cavitation is rare.**

### Postprimary Tuberculosis ("Reactivation TB")

- Most cases of TB in adults occur as reactivation of a primary focus of infection acquired in childhood. The infection is limited mainly to the **apical** and **posterior segments of the upper lobes** and the **superior segments of the lower lobes.** *Caseous necrosis* and the *tubercle* (accumulations of mononuclear macrophages, Langerhans giant cells surrounded by lymphocytes and fibroblasts) are the pathologic hallmarks of postprimary TB.
- **Healing** typically occurs with the development of **fibrosis** and **contraction.**

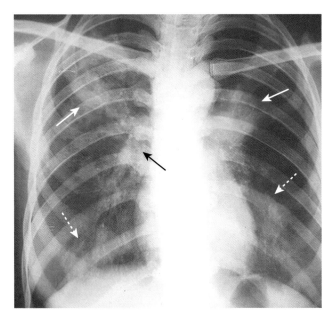

**Fig. 4.16** Primary Tuberculosis. There is prominence of the right hilum caused by adenopathy *(black arrow)*. Unilateral hilar adenopathy may be the only manifestation of primary infection with *Mycobacterium tuberculosis,* especially in children. When it produces pneumonia, primary TB affects the upper lobes *(solid white arrows)* slightly more than the lower *(dashed white arrows).*

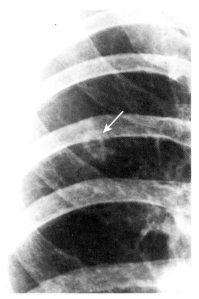

**Fig. 4.18** Postprimary Tuberculous Cavity. There is a thin-walled upper lobe cavity with no air-fluid level *(arrow)*. The characteristics are consistent with tuberculosis. In the presence of a cavity, activity is best excluded on a **clinical basis.** This patient had clinical findings of active tuberculosis.

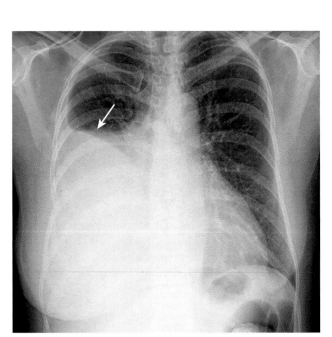

**Fig. 4.17** Tuberculous Effusion. A large, right pleural effusion is present *(arrow)*. Tuberculous effusions are **exudates** that can occur in either primary or postprimary forms of the disease but are **more common in the primary form.** They are usually **unilateral** and have a tendency to loculate (see **Chapter 7**). They may grow large, as in this case, while the patient is still relatively symptom-free.

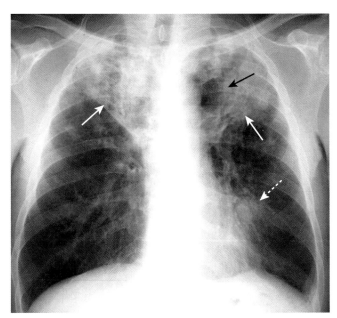

**Fig. 4.19** Postprimary TB with Transbronchial Spread. There is a pneumonia in both upper lobes *(solid white arrows)*. Numerous lucencies (cavities) are seen in the airspace disease in both upper lobes (especially, *black arrow* on the left). **A cavitary upper lobe pneumonia is presumptively TB,** until proven otherwise. In addition, there is airspace disease in the lingula *(dashed white arrow)*, another finding suggestive of TB, a disease which can spread via a **transbronchial route** to the opposite lower lobe or another lobe in the same lung.

### Patterns of Distribution of Postprimary Tuberculosis
- Bilateral upper lobe **cavitary disease** is very common. The cavity is usually **thin-walled, smooth on its inner margin, and contains no air-fluid level** (Fig. 4.18).

- Postprimary TB may also present as **pneumonia.**
- *Transbronchial spread* may occur—from one upper lobe to the **opposite** lower lobe or to another lobe in either lung (Fig. 4.19).

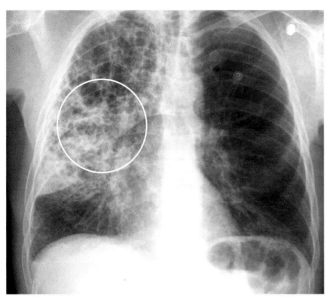

**Fig. 4.20 Tuberculous Bronchiectasis.** Bronchiectasis secondary to tuberculosis, both primary and postprimary, is relatively common. It may occur as a result of endobronchial infection or adjacent fibrosis *(traction bronchiectasis)*. The apical and posterior segments of the upper lobes are the most common sites. Multiple, small cystic structures creating an appearance that resembles a **honeycomb** may be seen *(circle)*.

- *Bronchiectasis*, usually asymptomatic, can develop (Fig. 4.20).
- *Bronchostenosis* may develop many years after the initial infection due to fibrosis and stricture leading to chronic lobar atelectasis (*middle lobe syndrome*).
- Solitary pulmonary nodules—the *tuberculoma*—may occur in either primary or postprimary disease. These are **round** or **oval** lesions frequently associated with small, discrete shadows in the immediate vicinity of the lesion called *satellite* lesions.
- Formation of a **pleural effusion** in **postprimary TB** almost always means direct spread of the disease into the pleural cavity and should be regarded as an *empyema*. This fluid accumulation carries a **graver prognosis** than the pleural effusion of the **primary form.**

*Miliary Tuberculosis*
- The onset of miliary TB is insidious. **Fever, chills, and night sweats are common.** It may take weeks between the time of dissemination and the radiographic appearance of disease. Miliary TB may occur as a manifestation of **either primary TB** or **postprimary TB**, although the clinical appearance of

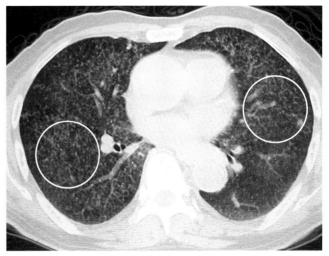

**Fig. 4.21 Miliary Tuberculosis.** There are innumerable small, round nodules present *(circles)* in this axial CT scan of the chest in a patient with miliary tuberculosis. At the start of the disease, the nodules are so small they are frequently difficult to detect on conventional radiographs.

miliary TB may not occur for many years after initial infection.
- When first visible, the miliary nodules **measure about 1 mm in size**; they can grow to 2 to 3 mm if left untreated. When treated, clearing is rapid. **Miliary TB seldom, if ever, heals with calcifications** (Fig. 4.21).
- Box 4.4 lists some causes of miliary lung disease.

## CASE QUIZ 4 ANSWER

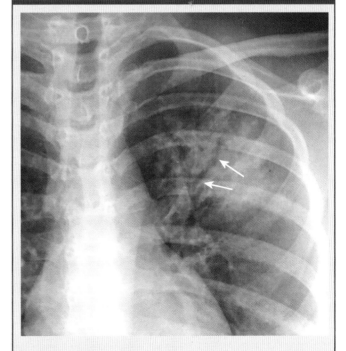

The fluffy, confluent density and the presence of air bronchograms *(arrows)* indicates this is airspace disease. Along with the history of fever, pneumonia would be the most likely diagnosis.

---

### BOX 4.4   Some Causes of Miliary Lung Disease

- Miliary nodules are usually 1 to 3 mm in size. Some of the more common causes are:
  - Miliary tuberculosis
  - Histoplasmosis
  - Sarcoidosis
  - Pneumoconiosis, especially silicosis

## TAKE HOME POINTS

- Parenchymal lung disease can be divided into **airspace (alveolar)** and **interstitial (infiltrative)** patterns.
- Recognizing the pattern of disease can help in reaching the correct diagnosis.
- Characteristics of **airspace disease** include fluffy, confluent densities that are indistinctly marginated and may demonstrate air bronchograms.
- An **air bronchogram** is typically a sign of airspace disease; it occurs when something other than air (e.g., inflammatory exudate or blood) surrounds the bronchus allowing the air inside the bronchus to become visible.
- When two objects of the **same** radiographic density are in **contact** with each other, the normal edge or margin between them will disappear. The loss of the margin between these two objects is called the **silhouette sign,** which is useful throughout radiology in identifying either the **location** or the **radiographic density** of the abnormality in question.
- Examples of airspace disease include pulmonary alveolar edema, pneumonia, and aspiration.
- Characteristics of **interstitial lung disease** include discrete "particles" or "packets" of disease with distinct margins that tend to occur in a pattern of **lines (reticular), dots (nodular),** or, very frequently, a combination of **lines and dots (reticulonodular).**
- Examples of interstitial lung disease include pulmonary interstitial edema, interstitial pneumonia, bronchogenic carcinoma, metastases to the lung, pulmonary fibrosis, and sarcoidosis.
- **Tuberculosis** is an example of a disease process that can demonstrate both airspace and interstitial lung patterns.

 Additional content is available online including chapters on Nuclear Medicine, Artificial Intelligence, Radiation Dose and Safety, an Early History of Radiology, and a compendium of 200 Diagnostic Radiology Signs.

# 5

# Recognizing the Causes of an Opacified Hemithorax

*William Herring, MD, FACR*

- There are three major causes of an opacified hemithorax (plus one other that is less common). They are:
  - **Atelectasis of the entire lung**
  - **A very large pleural effusion**
  - **Pneumonia of an entire lung**
  - And a fourth cause
    - **Pneumonectomy**—removal of an entire lung

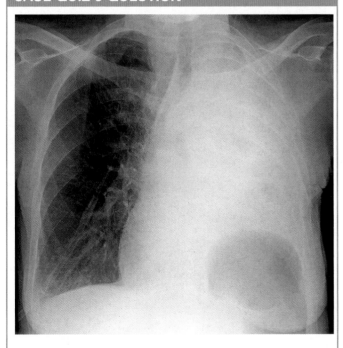

This 61-year-old heavy smoker presents with cough and shortness of breath. Is the most likely cause of her opacified hemithorax a large pleural effusion, pneumonia involving the entire lung, or atelectasis? The answer is at the end of this chapter.

## ATELECTASIS OF THE ENTIRE LUNG

- **Atelectasis of an entire lung** usually results from **complete obstruction of the right or left main bronchus.** With bronchial obstruction, no air can enter the lung. The remaining air in the lung is absorbed into the bloodstream through the pulmonary capillary system, leading to **loss of volume** of the affected lung.
- In adults, such atelectasis might be caused by an **obstructing neoplasm**, like a bronchogenic carcinoma. In younger individuals, **asthma** may produce **mucous plugs** that obstruct the bronchi. A **foreign body** may be aspirated (in children, peanuts are a frequent culprit) that also leads to bronchial obstruction. Critically ill patients also develop atelectasis from **mucous plugs.**
- In *obstructive atelectasis* (also called *resorptive atelectasis*), even though there is volume loss within the affected lung, **the visceral and parietal pleura almost never separate from each other.** That is an important fact about atelectasis and is sometimes confusing to beginners who try to picture **atelectasis** and a **pneumothorax** as both producing collapse of a lung without understanding why they look completely different radiographically (Fig. 5.1, Table 5.1).
  - Because the visceral and parietal pleura **do not separate** from each other in atelectasis, mobile structures in the thorax are "**pulled toward**" the side of the atelectasis producing a *shift* (movement) of these mobile thoracic structures **toward the side of opacification.**
  - The most visible mobile structures in the thorax are the **heart**, the **trachea**, and the **hemidiaphragms.** In **obstructive atelectasis**, one or all of these structures will **shift toward the side of opacification (toward side of volume loss)** (Fig. 5.2).
- Table 5.2 summarizes the movement of the mobile structures in the thorax in patients with obstructive atelectasis.

## MASSIVE PLEURAL EFFUSION

- If fluid, whether blood, an exudate, or a transudate, fills the pleural space so as to opacify almost the entire hemithorax, then the **fluid may act like a mass** compressing the underlying lung tissue. A pleural effusion compresses the lung beneath it, but that finding is usually not visible on conventional chest radiographs.

• Massive pleural effusions are frequently the result of malignancy, either in the form of a **bronchogenic carcinoma** or secondary to **metastases to the pleura** from a distant organ. Trauma can produce a **hemothorax,** and **tuberculosis** is notorious for causing large, clinically silent effusions (see Fig. 4.17). The effusions from **congestive heart failure,** while very common, are most often **bilateral** *(but asymmetric)* and they **rarely** grow large enough to **occupy an entire hemithorax.**

### TABLE 5.1　Pneumothorax Versus Obstructive Atelectasis

| Feature | Pneumothorax | Obstructive Atelectasis |
|---|---|---|
| **Pleural space** | Air in the pleural space **separates** the visceral from the parietal pleura. | The visceral and parietal pleura **do not separate** from each other. |
| **Density** | The pneumothorax itself will appear "black" (air density). The hemithorax may appear more lucent than normal. | Atelectasis is the absence of air in the lung. The hemithorax will appear more opaque ("whiter") than normal. |
| **Shift** | There is **never** a shift of the heart or trachea **toward** the side of a pneumothorax. | There is almost **always** a shift of the heart and trachea **toward** the side of the atelectasis. |

### TABLE 5.2　Recognizing a "Shift" in Atelectasis/Pneumonectomy

| Structure | Normal Position | Right-Sided Atelectasis or Pneumonectomy | Left-Sided Atelectasis or Pneumonectomy |
|---|---|---|---|
| **Heart** | Midline | Heart moves rightward; left heart border may come to lie near left side of spine | Heart moves leftward; right heart border overlaps the spine |
| **Trachea** | Midline | Shifts toward right | Shifts toward left |
| **Hemidiaphragm** | Right slightly higher than left | Right hemidiaphragm moves upward and may disappear (silhouette sign) | Left hemidiaphragm moves upward and may disappear (silhouette sign); shadow of stomach bubble may be elevated |

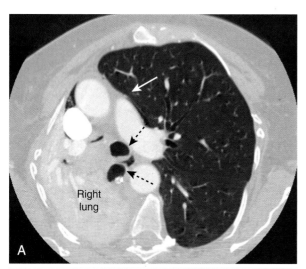

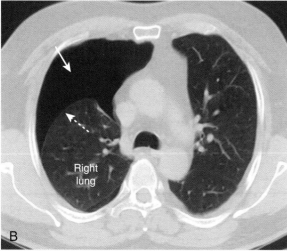

Fig. 5.1 Obstructive Atelectasis Versus a Pneumothorax: Two Different Causes of Lung Collapse and the Difference in Their Radiologic Appearance. (A) There is **atelectasis** of the entire right lung from an obstructing endobronchial lesion. The **visceral and parietal pleura remain in contact** with each other. Other mobile structures in the mediastinum, such as the trachea and right main bronchus *(black arrows),* shift toward the atelectasis. The left lung over-expands and crosses the midline *(white arrow).* (B) This patient has a large right-sided **pneumothorax**. Air *(solid white arrow)* interposes between the visceral *(dashed white arrow)* and parietal pleura (not visible), causing the lung to undergo passive atelectasis. Because there is no bronchial obstruction, the compressed right lung continues to be aerated. There is no shift of the mobile mediastinal structures toward the side of a pneumothorax.

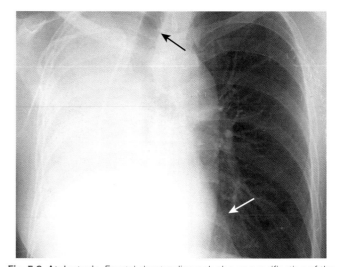

Fig. 5.2 Atelectasis. Frontal chest radiograph shows opacification of the entire right hemithorax. The trachea *(black arrow)* has moved rightward from the midline **toward** the side of the opacification. There is a shift of the heart toward the right *(white arrow).* These findings are characteristic of volume loss from atelectasis of the entire lung. The patient had an endobronchial metastasis from a known breast cancer.

## » IMPORTANT POINTS

When enough pleural fluid accumulates, the **large effusion "pushes" mobile structures away** and there is a shift of the heart and trachea **away from the side of opacification** (Fig. 5.3).

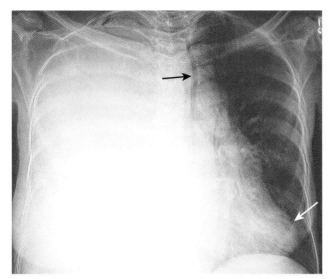

**Fig. 5.3** Large Pleural Effusion. There is complete opacification of the right hemithorax. The trachea is deviated to the left *(black arrow)* and the apex of the heart is also displaced to the left, close to the lateral chest wall *(white arrow)*. These findings are characteristic of a **large pleural effusion** that is producing a mass effect. Almost two liters of serosanguinous fluid were removed at thoracentesis. The fluid contained malignant cells from a primary bronchogenic carcinoma.

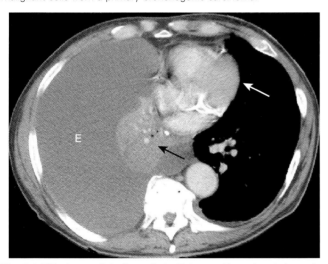

**Fig. 5.4** Effusion and Atelectasis in Balance. There is a balance between a large **pleural effusion** (E) and **atelectasis** of the right lung *(black arrow)* so that there is **no significant resultant shift** of the mobile midline structures. The heart essentially remains in its normal position *(white arrow)*. This combination of findings is highly suggestive of a central bronchogenic malignancy with a malignant effusion.

## ! DIAGNOSTIC PITFALLS

- At times, there may be a perfect **balance** between the **push** of a large malignant effusion and the **volume loss** caused by underlying obstructive atelectasis secondary to the malignancy itself.
- In an adult patient with an **opacified hemithorax, no air bronchograms** and **little or no shift** of the mobile thoracic structures, it is important to suspect an **obstructing bronchogenic carcinoma**, perhaps with metastases to the pleura. A CT scan of the chest will reveal the abnormalities (Fig. 5.4).

---

- Table 5.3 summarizes the movement of the mobile structures in the thorax in patients with a large pleural effusion.

## PNEUMONIA OF AN ENTIRE LUNG

- When pneumonia is the cause, inflammatory exudate fills the air spaces causing consolidation and opacification of the lung.
- The hemithorax becomes opaque because the lung no longer contains air, but there is neither a pull toward the side of the pneumonia by volume loss nor a push away from the side of the pneumonia by a large effusion. There is **no shift** of the heart or trachea (Fig. 5.5).
- Air bronchograms may be present.

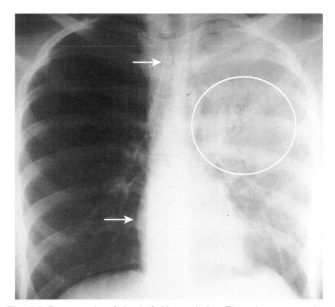

**Fig. 5.5** Pneumonia of the Left Upper Lobe. There is near-complete opacification of the left hemithorax with little **shift** of the trachea and no shift of the heart *(arrows)*. There are air bronchograms suggested within the upper area of opacification *(circle)*. These findings suggest a pneumonia rather than atelectasis or pleural effusion. The patient had *Streptococcus pneumoniae* in the sputum and improved quickly on antibiotics.

| TABLE 5.3 **Recognizing a "Shift" in Pleural Effusion** | | | |
|---|---|---|---|
| **Structure** | **Normal Position** | **Right-Sided Effusion** | **Left-Sided Effusion** |
| **Heart** | Midline | Heart moves leftward; apex may lie near the left lateral chest wall | Heart moves rightward; more of heart protrudes to right of spine |
| **Trachea** | Midline | Shifts toward left | Shifts toward right |
| **Hemidiaphragm** | Right higher than left | Right hemidiaphragm disappears on chest radiograph (silhouette sign) | Left hemidiaphragm disappears on chest radiograph (silhouette sign) |

| TABLE 5.4 | **Recognizing a "Shift" in Pneumonia** | | |
| --- | --- | --- | --- |
| **Structure** | **Normal Position** | **Right-Sided Pneumonia** | **Left-Sided Pneumonia** |
| Heart | Midline | There is usually no shift of the heart from its normal position | There is usually no shift of the heart from its normal position |
| Trachea | Midline | Midline | Midline |
| Hemidiaphragm | Right higher than left | Right hemidiaphragm may disappear on chest radiograph (silhouette sign) | Left hemidiaphragm may disappear on chest radiograph (silhouette sign) |

- Table 5.4 summarizes the movement of the mobile structures in the thorax in patients with pneumonia of the entire lung.

## POSTPNEUMONECTOMY

- *Pneumonectomy* means the removal of an entire lung.
- In order to perform this procedure, **either the 5th or 6th rib on the affected side is almost always removed.** In most cases, **metallic surgical clips will be visible in the region of the hilum** on the pneumonectomized side.
- For about 24 hours after the surgery, only air occupies the hemithorax from which the lung has been removed (Fig. 5.6).

- Over the course of the next 2 weeks, the hemithorax gradually **fills with fluid.**
- By about 4 months after surgery, the pneumonectomized hemithorax should be **completely opaque.**
- Eventually, **fibrous tissue forms in the pneumonectomized hemithorax** and in most patients the **entire hemithorax is forever completely opaque.** The heart and trachea shift **toward** the side of opacification.

> **! DIAGNOSTIC PITFALLS**
>
> - The chest x-ray may look identical to that of a patient with atelectasis of the entire lung. To tell the difference, look for the missing 5th or 6th rib and look for the surgical clips in the hilum to indicate a pneumonectomy has been performed (Fig. 5.7).

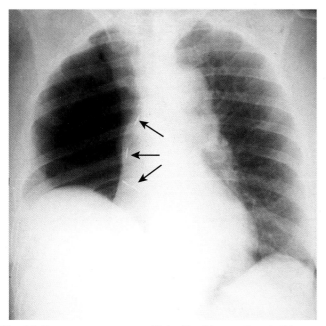

**Fig. 5.6 Postpneumonectomy, Right Hemithorax, Day 1.** This postoperative radiograph was obtained less than 24 hours after this patient underwent a pneumonectomy on the right side for a bronchogenic carcinoma. There are surgical clips in the region of the right hilum *(arrows)* and the right fifth rib has been surgically removed in order to perform the pneumonectomy. Over the next several weeks, the **right hemithorax will fill with fluid** followed by a gradual shift of the heart and mediastinal structures **toward** the side of the pneumonectomy.

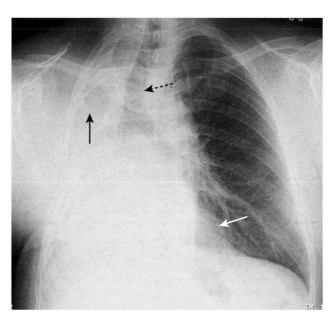

**Fig. 5.7 One Year After Pneumonectomy.** There is complete opacification of the right hemithorax. The right 5th rib *(solid black arrow)* is surgically absent. The heart *(solid white arrow)* and trachea *(dashed black arrow)* are deviated **toward** the side of opacification. These signs are characteristic of **volume loss.** The surgery had been performed 1 year earlier for a bronchogenic carcinoma. The fluid that gradually filled the right hemithorax immediately following the pneumonectomy has probably fibrosed leading to a permanent shift toward the pneumonectomized side.

## CASE QUIZ 5 ANSWER

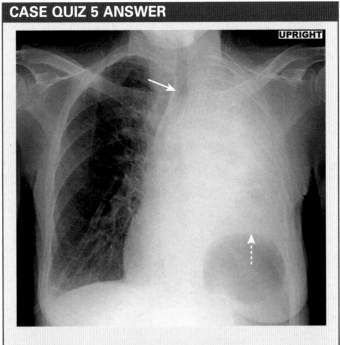

The entire left hemithorax is opacified while the trachea *(solid arrow)* is pulled slightly toward the left and the elevated stomach bubble *(dashed arrow)* is indirect evidence that the left hemidiaphragm is higher than normal. Both of these signs point toward atelectasis of the left lung. The patient had an obstructing bronchogenic carcinoma in the left main bronchus.

## TAKE HOME POINTS

- The differential possibilities for an opacified hemithorax should include **atelectasis** of the entire lung, a very large **pleural effusion, pneumonia of the entire lung, or postpneumonectomy.**
- The trachea, heart, and hemidiaphragms are mobile structures that have the capability of moving slightly *(shifting)* if there is either something pushing on them or something pulling them.
- With **atelectasis,** there is a shift **toward** the side of the opacified hemithorax because of volume loss in the affected lung.
- With a **large pleural effusion,** there is a shift **away** from the side of opacification because the large pleural effusion can act as if it were a mass.

- With **pneumonia** of most or the entire lung, there is usually **no shift**, but air bronchograms may be present.
- Occasionally, the shift of a malignant effusion may be balanced by the opposite shift of atelectasis caused by an underlying, obstructing bronchogenic carcinoma, so that the hemithorax will be completely opaque but there will be no shift of the midline structures.
- In the **postpneumonectomy** patient, there is eventually volume loss on the side from which the lung has been removed, and the clues to such surgery may include surgical **absence of the 5th or 6th rib** on the affected side or **metallic surgical clips** in the hilum.

 Additional content is available online including chapters on Nuclear Medicine, Artificial Intelligence, Radiation Dose and Safety, an Early History of Radiology, and a compendium of 200 Diagnostic Radiology Signs.

# 6

# Recognizing Atelectasis

*William Herring, MD, FACR*

## WHAT IS ATELECTASIS?

- Common to all forms of atelectasis is a **loss of volume in some or all of the lung, frequently** (but not always) **leading to increased density of the lung involved.**
  - The lung normally appears "black" on a chest radiograph because it contains air. When the air in all or part of the lung is absent because of resorption or compression as in atelectasis, that part of the lung usually becomes **whiter (more dense or more opaque).**

### CASE QUIZ 6 QUESTION

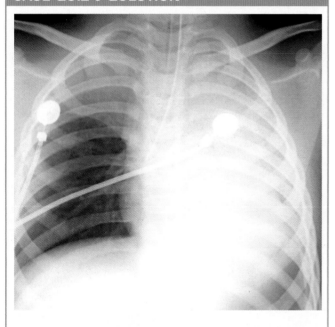

You are asked to check a radiograph obtained for post-insertion positioning of an endotracheal tube after it is placed in an infant. What is your assessment? The explanation is contained in this chapter and the answer appears at the end of the chapter.

## TYPES OF ATELECTASIS

- Atelectasis can be divided physiologically into *obstructive atelectasis* and *nonobstructive atelectasis.*
- **Obstructive atelectasis** is the form in which a lesion or object that obstructs a bronchus leads to subsequent resorption of air from the alveoli distal to the obstruction.
- **Nonobstructive atelectasis** can be caused by a loss of contact between the parietal and visceral pleurae, compression of the lung, loss of surfactant, and scarring.
- The types of atelectasis are summarized in Table 6.1.

### Obstructive Atelectasis

- Obstructive atelectasis is associated with the **resorption of air from the alveoli** through the pulmonary capillary bed **distal to an obstructing lesion** of the bronchial tree. The most common causes are shown in Table 6.2.
  - **The affected lobe or lung collapses** and becomes more opaque because it contains no air. The **collapse leads to volume loss** in the affected lobe or lung. Because the visceral and parietal pleurae invariably remain in contact with each other as the lung loses volume, this volume loss creates a *shift* of the slightly mobile structures of the thorax **toward** the area of **atelectasis.**
  - The rate at which air is absorbed and the lung collapses depends on its gas content when the bronchus is occluded and how rapidly the occlusion occurs. It takes about **18 to 24 hours for an entire lung to collapse** with the patient breathing room air **but less than an hour** with the patient breathing near 100% oxygen.
- Most of the **signs of obstructive atelectasis** are listed in Box 6.1.

### BOX 6.1 Signs of Obstructive Atelectasis

- Displacement of the major or minor fissure*
- Increased density of the atelectatic portion of lung
- Shift of the mobile structures in the thorax (i.e., the heart, trachea, and/or hemidiaphragms)
- *Compensatory overinflation of the unaffected segments, lobes, or lung

*Toward the atelectasis

## TABLE 6.1 Types of Atelectasis

| Type | Associated With | Remarks |
|---|---|---|
| **Obstructive Atelectasis** | | |
| **Obstructive atelectasis (resorptive atelectasis)** | Obstruction of a bronchus from malignancy, mucous plugging, foreign bodies, or external compression | Visceral and parietal pleura maintain contact with each other; "mobile" structures in the thorax are pulled toward the atelectasis |
| **Nonobstructive Atelectasis** | | |
| **Passive atelectasis** | Large pneumothorax, pleural effusion, or space-occupying lesion in the thorax; also seen at the lung base from a poor inspiration | Intervening air or fluid in the pleural space disrupts the normal contact between the parietal and visceral pleura; **compressive atelectasis** is a form of passive atelectasis |
| **Adhesive atelectasis** | Acute respiratory distress syndrome (ARDS) | Related to deactivation of surfactant |
| **Subsegmental atelectasis** | Splinting, especially in postoperative patients and those with pleuritic chest pain | May be related to deactivation of surfactant; does not usually lead to volume loss; disappears in days |
| **Cicatrization atelectasis** | Pulmonary diseases that heal with scarring, tuberculosis being most common | Fibrosis leads to a reduction in lung volume, most often in the upper lobes |

## TABLE 6.2 Most Common Causes of Obstructive Atelectasis

| Cause | Remarks |
|---|---|
| **Tumors** | Includes bronchogenic carcinoma (especially squamous cell), endobronchial metastases, carcinoid tumors |
| **Mucous plug** | Especially in bedridden individuals; postoperative patients; those with asthma, cystic fibrosis |
| **Foreign body aspiration** | Especially peanuts, small toys; following a traumatic intubation |

- Many of the signs of obstructive atelectasis are shown in a photographically manipulated composite image (Fig. 6.1). They include:
  - **Displacement (shift) of the interlobar fissures** (major and minor) **toward** the area of atelectasis.
  - **Increase in the density of the affected lung or lobe.**
  - **Displacement (shift) of the mobile structures of the thorax.** The **mobile structures** are those capable of slight movement due to changes in lung volume and include:
    - The **trachea**, which is normally **midline** in location, may shift **toward** the side of volume loss. There is normally a **slight rightward deviation** of a portion of the trachea at the site of the left-sided **aortic knob.**
    - The **right heart border** normally projects at least **1 cm to the right of the spine** on a nonrotated, frontal radiograph but with atelectasis, especially of either of the **lower lobes,** the heart may shift toward the side of the atelectasis. When the heart shifts toward the **right,** the left heart border may approach the spine. When the heart shifts toward the **left,** the right heart border may overlie the spine.
    - The **hemidiaphragms** may move in response to volume loss. The hemidiaphragm will be **silhouetted** by atelectasis of either lower lobe, but the position of the left hemidiaphragm may be inferred by noting elevation of the stomach bubble with an atelectatic left lung.

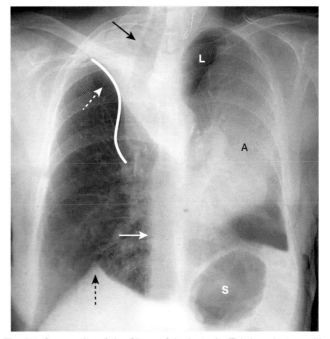

**Fig. 6.1** Composite of the Signs of Atelectasis. This is a photographic composite of many of the signs associated with obstructive atelectasis, all of which are described in the text. The signs shown could not be present all together in any given patient but each is a feature of atelectasis. They are: deviation of the trachea toward the side of volume loss *(solid black arrow);* shift of an interlobar fissure toward the volume loss *(dashed white arrow);* the ***Reverse S Sign of Golden*** *(curved line);* shift of the mobile mediastinal structures bringing the right heart border over the spine in left-sided atelectasis *(solid white arrow);* a ***juxtaphrenic peak*** *(dashed black arrow)* and elevation of the hemidiaphragm; the ***Luftsichel Sign*** of left upper lobe atelectasis (L); increased density of the affected lung or lobe (A); and elevation of the stomach bubble (S) and hemidiaphragm.

### ▶▶ IMPORTANT POINTS

- Normally, the **right hemidiaphragm is almost always higher than the left** by about half the distance of the interspace between two adjacent ribs. In about 10% of normal people, the left hemidiaphragm is higher than the right.

- **Overinflation of the unaffected ipsilateral lobes or the contralateral lung.** The greater the volume loss and the longer its presence, the more likely the lung on the side **opposite** the atelectasis or the **unaffected lobe(s) in the ipsilateral lung** will **overinflate** to compensate for the volume loss. This may be especially noticeable on the lateral projection by an **increase in the size of the retrosternal clear space** and on the frontal projection by **extension of the overinflated contralateral lung across the midline** (see Fig. 6.12B).

## Passive Atelectasis

- *Passive atelectasis* occurs either when there is **disruption of the contact** between the parietal and visceral pleurae, e.g., from a pleural effusion, pneumothorax, or thoracic mass (Fig. 6.2A), or by **hypoinflation** of the lungs due to a poor inspiration (Fig. 6.2B). The latter form of lung **compression** does not cause separation of the visceral and parietal pleura.
  - When caused by an obstructing bronchogenic carcinoma and associated with a large malignant effusion, atelectasis

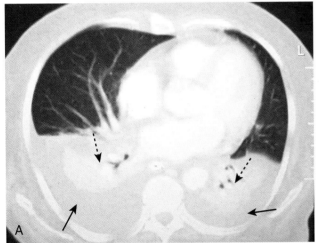

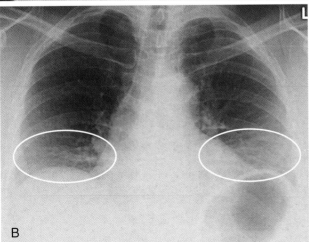

**Fig. 6.2** Compressive (Passive) Atelectasis. (A) Axial CT scan of the chest shows compressive atelectasis of both lower lobes *(dashed arrows)* by bilateral pleural effusions *(solid arrows)*. (B) Passive compression of the lung can occur from a poor inspiratory effort, which is manifest as patchy increased density at the lung bases *(ovals)*.

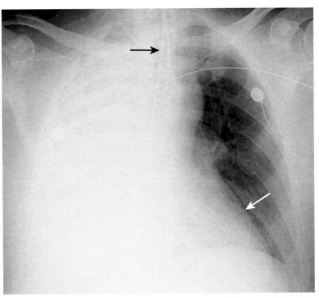

**Fig. 6.3** Atelectasis and Effusion in Balance, an Ominous Combination. There is complete opacification of the right hemithorax. There are neither air bronchograms to suggest pneumonia nor any shift of the trachea *(black arrow)* or heart *(white arrow)*. The absence of any shift suggests the possibility of atelectasis and pleural effusion in balance, a combination that should raise suspicion for a central bronchogenic carcinoma (producing obstructive atelectasis) with metastases (producing a large pleural effusion).

and pleural effusion combined may produce an **opacified hemithorax, no air bronchograms, and little or no shift of the mobile thoracic structures**, a combination suspicious for a thoracic malignancy (Fig. 6.3).

> **! DIAGNOSTIC PITFALLS**
>
> - Passive atelectasis secondary to a poor inspiratory effort may **mimic airspace disease** at the bases.
> - Consider passive atelectasis if the patient has taken **fewer than an eight posterior-rib** breath.
> - Check the lateral projection for confirmation of the presence of real airspace disease at the base.

> **▶ IMPORTANT POINTS**
>
> - This might be a good time to review the chart from **Chapter 5: Recognizing the Causes of an Opacified Hemithorax** (see Table 5.1) highlighting the markedly different appearances of a large pneumothorax versus atelectasis of the entire lung (see Fig. 5.1)

## Adhesive Atelectasis

- **Pulmonary surfactant** is produced by Type II pneumocytes and acts to reduce the surface tension of alveoli, decreasing their tendency to collapse. If there is a decrease or absence of surfactant, the alveoli collapse more easily, producing *adhesive atelectasis.*
- This form of atelectasis can be seen in *acute respiratory distress syndrome* (ARDS) (see Chapters 11 and 27) in both adults and neonates and has also been implicated in

the formation of linear densities at the lung bases called ***subsegmental atelectasis.***

## Subsegmental Atelectasis

- **Subsegmental atelectasis** (also called **discoid, plate-like,** or **linear atelectasis**) produces the least volume loss of any of the forms of atelectasis.
- Subsegmental atelectasis may occur because of surfactant defects and is observed mostly in patients who are ***splinting*** (i.e., not taking a deep breath), such as postoperative patients or patients with pleuritic chest pain.
- Subsegmental atelectasis produces **linear densities** of varying thickness usually **parallel to the diaphragm,** most commonly at the **lung bases.** It does not produce a sufficient amount of volume loss to cause a shift of the mobile thoracic structures (Fig. 6.4).
- It tends to clear rapidly with deep breathing.

> **❗ DIAGNOSTIC PITFALLS**
>
> - On a single study, without prior examinations for comparison, subsegmental atelectasis and **chronic, linear scarring can look identical.** Subsegmental atelectasis **typically disappears within a matter of days** with resumption of normal, deep breathing whereas **scarring remains.**

## Round (or Rounded) Atelectasis

- This form of what some consider as compressive atelectasis is **usually seen at the periphery of the lung base** and develops from a **combination of prior pleural disease** (e.g., asbestos exposure or tuberculosis) **and the formation of a pleural effusion that produces adjacent atelectasis.**
- When the pleural effusion recedes, it is believed that the underlying pleural disease leads to a portion of the **atelectatic lung becoming "trapped."**
- This produces a **mass-like lesion** that can be confused for a tumor, especially on chest x-rays.
- On a CT scan of the chest, the bronchovascular markings characteristically lead from the round atelectasis back to the hilum, producing a ***comet-tail appearance*** (Fig. 6.5).

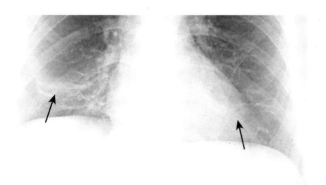

**Fig. 6.4 Subsegmental Atelectasis.** Close-up view of the lung bases demonstrates several linear densities extending across all segments of the lower lobes, paralleling the diaphragm *(arrows)*. This is a characteristic appearance of *subsegmental atelectasis*. The patient was postoperative from abdominal surgery and was unable to take a deep breath. The atelectasis disappeared within a few days after surgery.

## Scarring and Atelectasis (Cicatrization Atelectasis)

- ***Cicatrization (or cicatrizing) atelectasis*** is mainly the result of fibrosis and scar formation. The end result of the fibrosis leads to a reduction in lung volume.
- The most common cause of cicatrization atelectasis is tuberculosis. Tuberculosis frequently produces a **reticular pattern** in the **upper lobe** and is commonly associated with **pleural thickening** (Fig. 6.6).

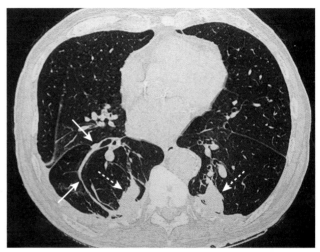

**Fig. 6.5 Round Atelectasis, Both Lower lobes.** There are pleural-based, mass-like densities in both lower lobes *(dashed arrows)*. On the right, there is a **comet-tail**-shaped bronchovascular marking *(solid arrows)* that emanates from the "mass" and extends back to the hilum. This combination of findings is characteristic of round atelectasis and should not be mistaken for a tumor.

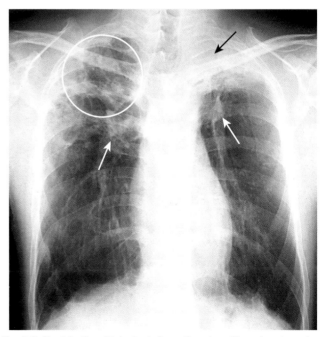

**Fig. 6.6 Cicatrization Atelectasis from Scarring.** There is volume loss in both upper lobes in this patient with chronic scarring from tuberculosis. Fibrotic stranding is seen in the right upper lobe *(circle)*, marked pleural thickening on the left *(black arrow)* and upward retraction of both hila *(white arrows)*.

- Other **granulomatous infections** such as histoplasmosis and diseases like silicosis, scleroderma, radiation pneumonitis (late stage), and idiopathic pulmonary fibrosis can also produce volume loss by means of scarring.

## Patterns of Collapse in Lobar Atelectasis

- Obstructive atelectasis produces **consistently recognizable patterns of collapse** depending on the location of the atelectatic lobe and the degree to which such factors as collateral airflow between lobes and obstructive pneumonia allow the affected lobe to collapse.
- In general, lobes collapse in a **fan-like** configuration with the **base** of the fan-shaped triangle **anchored at the pleural surface** and the **apex of the triangle anchored at the hilum.**
- Other, unaffected lobes may undergo compensatory hyperinflation in an attempt to "fill" the affected hemithorax and this hyperinflation may limit the amount of shift of the mobile chest structures.

> **! DIAGNOSTIC PITFALLS**
>
> - The **more atelectatic a lobe or segment** becomes (i.e., the smaller its volume), the **less visible** it is on the chest radiograph.
> - This can lead to the false assumption that improvement has occurred when, in fact, the atelectasis is worsening.
> - This can usually be resolved with a careful analysis of the study to check for the degree of displacement of the interlobar fissures or hemidiaphragms or with a CT scan of the chest.

- The patterns of lobar atelectasis are best described in conjunction with their respective images (Figs. 6.7–6.12).
- **Right upper lobe atelectasis** (Fig. 6.7)
  - If there is a large enough mass in the right hilum producing right upper lobe atelectasis, the combination of the **hilar mass** and the **upward shift of the minor fissure** produces a characteristic appearance on the frontal radiograph called the *S sign of Golden (or the Reverse S Sign of Golden)* (see Fig. 6.1).

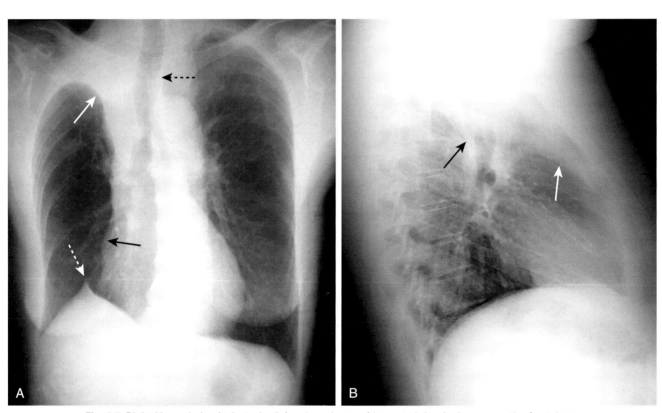

**Fig. 6.7 Right Upper Lobe Atelectasis.** A fan-shaped area of increased density is seen on the frontal projection (A) representing the airless right upper lobe. The minor fissure is displaced upward *(solid white arrow)*. The trachea is shifted to the right *(dashed black arrow)*. There is elevation of the right hemidiaphragm in a characteristic pattern called a ***juxtaphrenic peak*** *(dashed white arrow)*. The heart is shifted slightly to the right *(solid black arrow)*. (B) In a different patient with right upper lobe atelectasis, the lateral view demonstrates a similar wedge-shaped density near the apex of the lung. The minor fissure *(white arrow)* is pulled upward and the major fissure is pulled forward *(black arrow)*.

- **Left upper lobe atelectasis** (Fig. 6.8)
  - Compensatory **overinflation** of the **lower lobe** may cause the superior segment of the left lower lobe to extend to the apex of the thorax on the affected side producing a sickle-shaped lucency called the ***luftsichel sign*** (see Fig. 6.1).
- **Atelectasis of either lower lobe** (Fig. 6.9)

 **IMPORTANT POINTS**

- In the critically ill patient, atelectasis occurs most frequently in the **left lower lobe.** Always check the visibility of the left hemidiaphragm to be sure it is seen in its entire extent through the heart shadow since left lower lobe atelectasis can manifest by disappearance (silhouetting) of all or part of the left hemidiaphragm (see Fig. 6.9C).

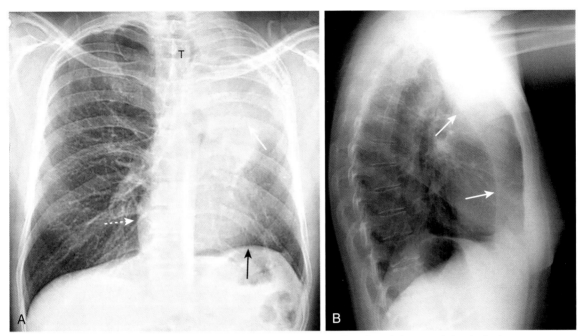

**Fig. 6.8 Left Upper Lobe Atelectasis.** (A) On the frontal projection, there is increased density in the upper lung field involving the left upper lobe *(solid white arrow)* representing the atelectatic left upper lobe. The trachea (T) and the heart border *(dashed white arrow)* are shifted slightly toward the left. Notice how the left hemidiaphragm *(black arrow)* has been pulled up higher than the right. (B) The lateral projection in another patient shows a band-like zone of increased density *(arrows)* representing the atelectatic left upper lobe sharply demarcated by the major fissure, which has been displaced anteriorly. Both patients had squamous cell carcinomas obstructing the left upper lobe bronchi.

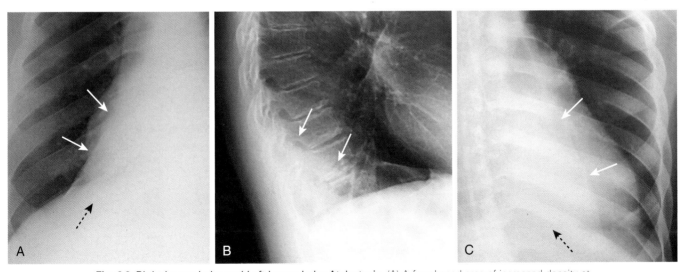

**Fig. 6.9 Right Lower Lobe and Left Lower Lobe Atelectasis.** (A) A fan-shaped area of increased density at the right lung base *(white arrows)* is sharply bound by the displaced major fissure representing the characteristic appearance of right lower lobe atelectasis. The medial portion of the right hemidiaphragm has been silhouetted by the airless lobe above it *(black arrow)*. (B) On the lateral view, the major fissure *(arrows)* is displaced posteriorly. The small triangular density in the posterior costophrenic sulcus is in the characteristic location for lower lobe atelectasis for **either** lower lobe. (C) In another patient, there is a fan-shaped, triangular density representing the left lower lobe bounded superiorly by the displaced major fissure *(white arrows)*. Notice how the unaerated lower lobe silhouettes the left hemidiaphragm *(black arrow)*.

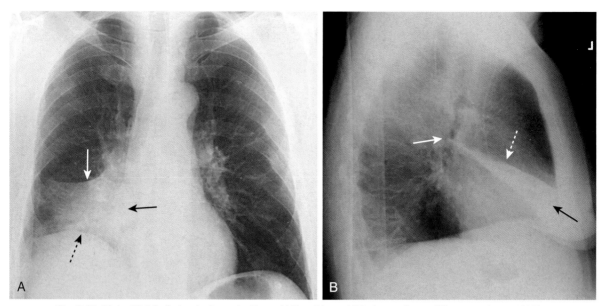

**Fig. 6.10** **Right Middle Lobe Atelectasis.** Frontal (A) and lateral (B) views of two different patients. (A) The triangular-shaped right middle lobe is increased in density with volume loss evident by downward displacement of the minor fissure *(white arrow)*. Where the dense middle lobe is in contact with the right heart, the border disappears *(solid black arrow)*, but since it is not in contact with the right hemidiaphragm, the hemidiaphragm is well seen *(dashed black arrow)*. (B) There is a triangular density with its base directed anteriorly *(black arrow)* and its apex at the hilum *(solid white arrow)*. The minor fissure is displaced downward *(dashed white arrow)*.

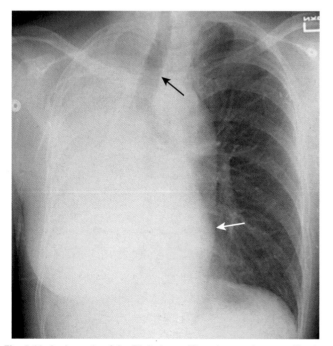

**Fig. 6.11** **Atelectasis of the Right Lung.** There is complete opacification of the right hemithorax with shift of the trachea *(black arrow)* toward the side of the atelectasis. The hemidiaphragm on the right side is silhouetted by the nonaerated lung above it. The left heart border is displaced far to the right and now almost overlaps the spine *(white arrow)*. This patient had an endobronchial metastasis in the right main bronchus from her left-sided breast cancer. Did you notice the left breast was surgically absent?

- **Right middle lobe atelectasis** (Fig. 6.10)
- **Atelectasis of the entire right lung** (Fig. 6.11) **or left lung** (Fig. 6.12)

## HOW ATELECTASIS RESOLVES

- Depending in part on the rapidity with which the segment, lobe, or lung became atelectatic, atelectasis has the capacity to **resolve within hours or last for many days once the obstruction has been removed.**
- Slowly resolving lobar or whole-lung atelectasis may manifest patchy areas of airspace disease surrounded by progressively increasing zones of aerated lung until the atelectasis has completely cleared.

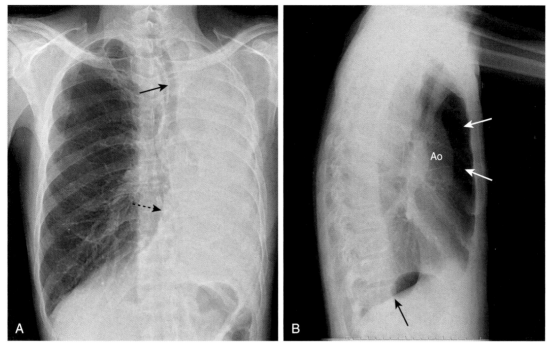

**Fig. 6.12 Atelectasis of the Left Lung.** (A) There is complete opacification of the left hemithorax with shift of the trachea *(solid black arrow)* to the left. The right heart border, which should project about a centimeter to the right of the spine, has been pulled over the spine *(dashed black arrow)*. The heart itself is not visible because it is no longer bordered by an air-filled lung. (B) The right lung is overaerated and extends across the midline *(white arrows)* interposing itself anterior to the aorta (Ao). Only the right hemidiaphragm is visible *(black arrow)* because there is no air in the lung above the left hemidiaphragm. The patient had an obstructing bronchogenic carcinoma in the left main bronchus.

## CASE QUIZ 6 ANSWER

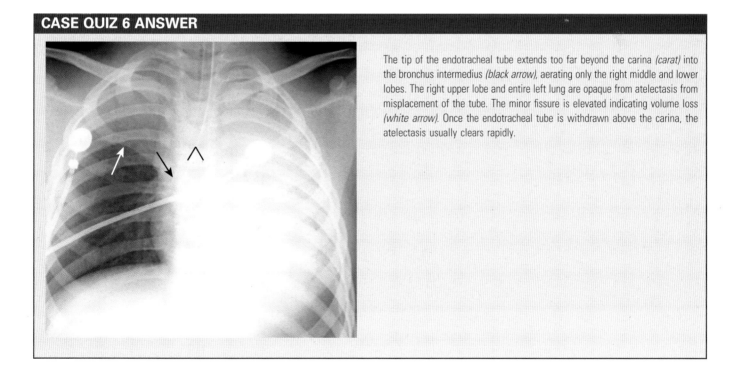

The tip of the endotracheal tube extends too far beyond the carina *(carat)* into the bronchus intermedius *(black arrow)*, aerating only the right middle and lower lobes. The right upper lobe and entire left lung are opaque from atelectasis from misplacement of the tube. The minor fissure is elevated indicating volume loss *(white arrow)*. Once the endotracheal tube is withdrawn above the carina, the atelectasis usually clears rapidly.

## TAKE HOME POINTS

- Common to all forms of atelectasis is **volume loss,** but the radiographic appearance of atelectasis will differ depending on the **type** of atelectasis.
- The three most commonly observed types of atelectasis are **subsegmental atelectasis** (also known as **discoid** or **plate-like atelectasis**), **compressive or passive atelectasis**, and **obstructive atelectasis.**
- **Subsegmental atelectasis** most often occurs in patients who are not taking a deep breath (splinting) and produces linear densities, usually at the lung bases.
- **Compressive atelectasis** occurs passively when the lung is collapsed from a large, adjacent pleural effusion, tumor, or pneumothorax. When the underlying abnormality is removed, the lung usually reexpands.
- **Round atelectasis** is a type of passive atelectasis in which the lung does not reexpand when a pleural effusion recedes, usually due to preexisting pleural disease. Round atelectasis may appear as a mass-like lesion on chest radiographs, mimicking a tumor.
- **Obstructive atelectasis** occurs distal to an occluding lesion of the bronchial tree because of reabsorption of the air in the distal airspaces via the pulmonary capillary bed.
- Obstructive atelectasis produces consistently recognizable **patterns** of collapse based on the assumptions that the visceral and parietal pleura invariably remain in contact with each other and every lobe of the lung is anchored at or near the hilum.
- **Signs of obstructive atelectasis** include displacement of the fissures, increased density of the affected lung, shift of the mobile structures of the thorax toward the atelectasis, and compensatory overinflation of the unaffected ipsilateral or contralateral lung.
- **Cicatrization atelectasis** is a loss of lung volume secondary to scarring, most often from TB and usually in the upper lobes.
- Atelectasis tends to resolve quickly if it occurs acutely; the more chronic the process, the longer it usually takes to resolve.

 Additional content is available online including chapters on Nuclear Medicine, Artificial Intelligence, Radiation Dose and Safety, an Early History of Radiology, and a compendium of 200 Diagnostic Radiology Signs.

# 7

# Recognizing a Pleural Effusion

*William Herring, MD, FACR*

## NORMAL ANATOMY AND PHYSIOLOGY OF THE PLEURAL SPACE

- **Normal anatomy**
    - The **parietal pleura lines the inside of the thoracic cage** and the **visceral pleura adheres to the surface of the lung** parenchyma including its interface with the mediastinum and diaphragm.
    - The **enfolds of the visceral pleura form the interlobar fissures**—the **major** (*oblique*) and **minor** (*horizontal*) on the right, only the major on the left. The space between the visceral and parietal pleura, i.e., the ***pleural space,*** is a **potential space** normally containing only **about 2 to 5 mL of pleural fluid** (see Fig. 2.1).

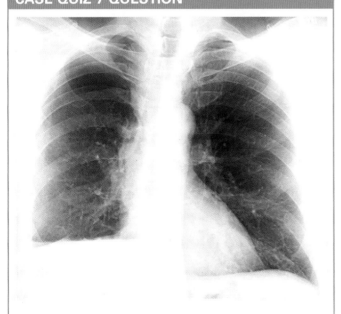

### CASE QUIZ 7 QUESTION

This 56-year-old male presented to the emergency department with shortness of breath after a motor vehicle collision. An upright chest x-ray was obtained. There is a serious injury that required immediate intervention suggested by a fundamental finding on this image. The answer is at the end of this chapter.

- **Normal physiology**
    - Normally, several hundred milliliters of pleural fluid are produced and reabsorbed each day. Fluid is **produced primarily at the parietal pleura** from the pulmonary capillary bed and is **resorbed at both the visceral pleura and by lymphatic drainage through the parietal pleura.**

## MODALITIES FOR DETECTING PLEURAL EFFUSIONS

- **Conventional radiography** is frequently the first step in detecting a pleural effusion. Other modalities used include **CT** and **ultrasound (US).** CT and US are both sensitive in detecting small amounts of fluid. CT is best in evaluating the disease underlying the effusion or in complete opacification of the hemithorax by effusion. Ultrasound can be especially helpful in guiding an intervention to remove the pleural fluid. The fundamental appearances of pleural effusion are similar regardless of the modality.

## CAUSES OF PLEURAL EFFUSIONS (TABLE 7.1)

- Fluid accumulates in the pleural space when the rate at which the fluid **forms** exceeds the rate by which it is **cleared.**
    - The **rate of formation** may be **increased** by:
        - **Increasing hydrostatic pressure,** as in left-heart failure.

| TABLE 7.1 Some Causes of Pleural Effusions | |
|---|---|
| **Cause** | **Examples** |
| **Excess formation of fluid** | Congestive heart failure <br> Hypoproteinemia <br> Parapneumonic effusions <br> Hypersensitivity reactions |
| **Decreased resorption of fluid** | Lymphangitic carcinomatosis <br> Elevated central venous pressure <br> Decreased intrapleural pressure |
| **Transport from peritoneal cavity** | Ascites |

- Decreasing colloid osmotic pressure, as in hypoproteinemia.
  - Increasing capillary permeability, as can occur in toxic disruption of the capillary membrane in pneumonia or hypersensitivity reactions.
- The rate of **resorption** can **decrease** by:
  - **Decreased absorption** of fluid **by lymphatics, either from lymphangitic carcinomatosis** or from **increased venous pressure,** which decreases the rate of fluid transport via the thoracic duct.
  - **Decreased pressure in the pleural space,** as in atelectasis of the lung due to bronchial obstruction.
- Pleural effusions can also form when there is **transport of peritoneal fluid from the abdominal cavity** through openings in the diaphragm or via lymphatics from a subdiaphragmatic process.

## TYPES OF PLEURAL EFFUSIONS

- Pleural effusions are divided into *transudates* or *exudates* depending primarily on their **protein content** and their **LDH (lactate dehydrogenase) concentrations. Transudates** typically have **lower protein** concentrations, **lower specific gravity,** and **lower LDH** concentrations than exudates.
- **Transudates** are usually bilateral and tend to form when there is **increased capillary hydrostatic pressure** or **decreased osmotic pressure.** Causes include:
  - **Congestive heart failure,** primarily left-heart failure, is the most common cause of a transudative pleural effusion.
  - **Hypoalbuminemia**
  - **Cirrhosis**
  - **Nephrotic syndrome**
- **Exudates** are usually unilateral and tend to be the result of inflammation, connective tissue disease, or malignancy.
  - **The most common cause of an exudative pleural effusion is malignancy.**
  - An *empyema* is an exudate containing pus.
  - In a *hemothorax,* the fluid has a hematocrit that is greater than 50% of the blood hematocrit.
  - A *chylothorax* contains increased triglycerides or cholesterol.

## SIDE-SPECIFICITY OF PLEURAL EFFUSIONS

- Certain diseases tend to produce **bilateral** pleural effusions, and some are more often unilateral.
- Diseases that usually produce **bilateral effusions:**
  - **Congestive heart failure** usually produces about the same amount of fluid in each hemithorax, sometimes slightly more on the right than the left side. If there are **markedly** different amounts of fluid in each hemithorax, suspect a **parapneumonic effusion** or **malignancy** on the side with the significantly greater volume of fluid.
  - **Lupus erythematosus** usually produces bilateral effusions, but when unilateral it is usually **left-sided.**

- Diseases that can produce **effusions on either side (but are usually unilateral):**
  - **Tuberculosis** and other exudative effusions associated with infectious agents, including viruses.
  - **Pulmonary thromboembolic disease**
  - **Trauma**
- Diseases that usually produce only **left-sided effusions:**
  - **Pancreatitis**
  - **Distal thoracic duct obstruction**
  - **Dressler syndrome** (Box 7.1, Fig. 7.1)
- Diseases that mostly produce only **right-sided effusions:**
  - **Abdominal disease related to the liver or ovaries.** Some ovarian tumors can be associated with a right pleural effusion and ascites (*Meigs syndrome*).
  - **Rheumatoid arthritis,** which can produce an effusion that remains unchanged for years.
  - **Proximal thoracic duct obstruction.**

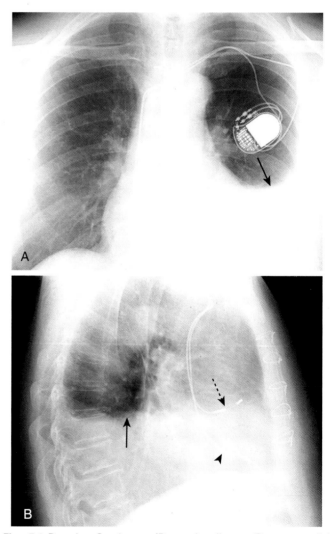

**Fig. 7.1** Dressler Syndrome (Postpericardiotomy/Postmyocardial Infarction Syndrome). (A) There is a left pleural effusion present *(solid arrows in A and B)*. This patient had coronary artery bypass surgery several weeks earlier. Incidentally, the patient has a dual-lead pacemaker in place and, on the lateral projection (B), the leads are seen in the region of the right atrium *(dashed arrow)* and right ventricle *(arrowhead)*.

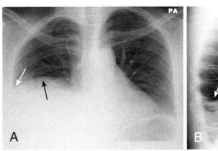
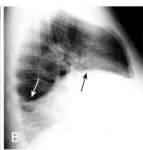

# RECOGNIZING THE DIFFERENT APPEARANCES OF PLEURAL EFFUSIONS

- Forces that influence the appearance of pleural fluid on a chest radiograph depend on the **position** of the patient, the force of **gravity**, the **amount** of fluid, and the degree of **elastic recoil** of the lung. The descriptions that follow, unless otherwise indicated, assume the patient is in the upright position.

## Subpulmonic Effusions

- It is believed that **almost all pleural effusions first collect in a subpulmonic location beneath the lung** between the parietal pleura lining the superior surface of the diaphragm and the visceral pleura lining the lower lobe.
- If the effusion remains entirely subpulmonic in location, it may be difficult to detect on conventional radiographs except for contour alterations in what appears to be the hemidiaphragm but is **actually** the interface between the pleural fluid and the base of the aerated lung.
- The different appearances of subpulmonic effusions are summarized in Table 7.2 and Figs. 7.2 and 7.3.

### ▶▶ IMPORTANT POINTS

- ***Subpulmonic*** does **not** mean ***loculated.***
- **Most subpulmonic effusions flow freely** as the patient changes position.

**Fig. 7.2 Right-sided Subpulmonic Effusion.** (A) In the frontal projection, the *apparent right hemidiaphragm* appears to be elevated *(black arrow).* The edge to which this arrow points represents the interface between the effusion and the base of the lung, not the actual hemidiaphragm, which has been rendered invisible by the pleural fluid that has accumulated above it. There is blunting of the right costophrenic sulcus (angle) *(white arrow).* (B) On the lateral projection, there is blunting of the posterior costophrenic sulcus *(white arrow).* The apparent hemidiaphragm is **rounded posteriorly** but then characteristically has a **flatter anterior** contour as the effusion interfaces with the major fissure on the right side *(black arrow).*

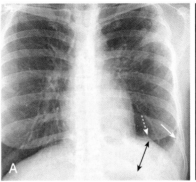
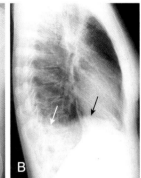

**Fig. 7.3 Left-sided Subpulmonic Effusion.** (A) In the frontal projection, there is more than 1 cm distance between the air in the stomach and the apparent left hemidiaphragm *(double black arrow).* The dashed white arrow represents the boundary between the aerated lung and the effusion. The actual hemidiaphragm is not visible. There is blunting of the costophrenic sulci *(solid white arrows)* on both projections. (B) On the lateral projection, the apparent hemidiaphragm flattens anteriorly as the effusion interfaces with the major fissure *(solid black arrow).*

## TABLE 7.2    Recognizing a Subpulmonic Effusion

| RIGHT-SIDED FINDINGS (FIG. 7.2) | | LEFT-SIDED FINDINGS (FIG. 7.3) | |
| --- | --- | --- | --- |
| **Frontal View** | **Lateral View** | **Frontal View** | **Lateral View** |
| The highest point of the **apparent hemidiaphragm**[a] is displaced more laterally than the highest point of a normal hemidiaphragm (which is usually in the middle). More difficult to recognize than left-sided subpulmonic effusions because the liver below is the same density as the pleural fluid above it. | Posteriorly, the **apparent hemidiaphragm**[a] has a curved arc but as it meets the junction with the major fissure, the apparent hemidiaphragm[a] assumes a flat edge that drops sharply to the anterior chest wall. | Increased distance between the stomach bubble and the **apparent left hemidiaphragm**[a] (should normally be only about 1 cm from top of stomach bubble to bottom of aerated left lower lobe). The highest point of the apparent hemidiaphragm[a] is displaced more laterally than the highest point of a normal hemidiaphragm. | Posteriorly, the **apparent hemidiaphragm**[a] has a curved arc, but as it meets the junction with the major fissure, the apparent hemidiaphragm[a] assumes a flat edge that drops sharply to the anterior chest wall. |

[a]**Apparent hemidiaphragm** is the term used because the shadow being cast is actually from the **subpulmonic fluid** interfacing with the base of the lung. The **actual hemidiaphragm** is **not visible**, silhouetted by the soft tissue in the abdomen below it and the pleural fluid above it.

## Blunting of the Costophrenic Angles

- As the subpulmonic effusion grows in size, it first fills and thus ***blunts*** the normally acute **posterior costophrenic sulcus**, visible on the lateral view of the chest. This occurs with approximately **75 mL of fluid** (Fig. 7.4).

- When the effusion reaches about 300 mL in size, it blunts the lateral costophrenic angle, visible on the frontal chest radiograph (Fig. 7.5).

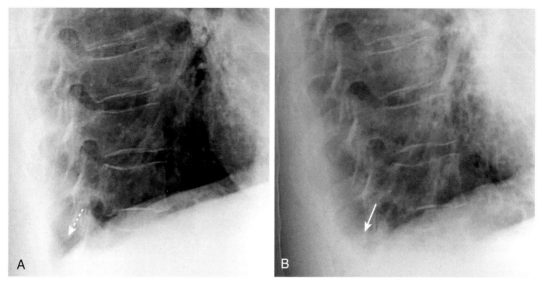

**Fig. 7.4 Normal and Blunted Posterior Costophrenic Sulci, Lateral Projection.** When approximately 75 mL of fluid has accumulated in the pleural space, the fluid will typically ascend in the thorax and blunt the posterior costophrenic sulcus first. (A) The normal, posterior costophrenic sulci, are acutely angled *(dashed arrow)*. (B) A few months later, during an episode of congestive heart failure, the same patient has small, bilateral pleural effusions as demonstrated by blunting of the same costophrenic sulci *(solid arrow)*.

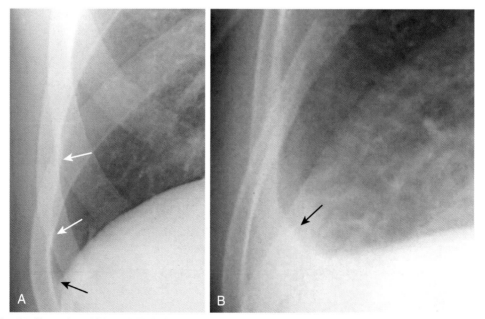

**Fig. 7.5 Normal and Blunted Right Lateral Costophrenic Sulcus.** (A) The hemidiaphragm usually makes a sharp and acute angle as it meets the lateral chest wall on the frontal projection to produce the lateral costophrenic sulcus *(black arrow)*. Notice how aerated lung normally extends to the inner margin of each of the ribs *(white arrows)*. (B) When an effusion reaches about 300 mL in volume, the lateral costophrenic sulcus loses its acute angulation and becomes ***blunted*** *(arrow)*.

## ! DIAGNOSTIC PITFALLS

- **Pleural thickening** caused by scarring can also produce blunting of the costophrenic angle. One helpful clue is that scarring sometimes creates a characteristic **ski-slope appearance**, unlike the meniscoid appearance of a pleural effusion (Fig. 7.6). Also, pleural thickening will not change in location with a change in patient position, as most effusions will.

## The Meniscus Sign

- Because of the natural elastic recoil of the lungs, **pleural fluid appears to rise higher along the lateral margin of the thorax than it does medially** in the frontal projection. This produces a characteristic *meniscoid* shape to the effusion, higher on the sides, lower in the middle (Fig. 7.7).

## ▶ IMPORTANT POINTS

- In the lateral projection, the fluid also assumes a U shape, usually ascending equally high both anteriorly and posteriorly.
- Identifying an abnormal thoracic density that demonstrates a **meniscoid shape** is strongly suggestive of a **pleural effusion.**

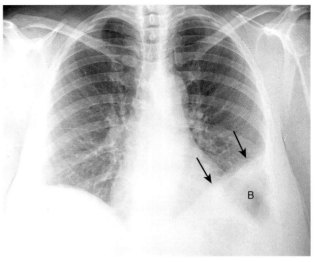

Fig. 7.6 Scarring Producing Blunting of the Left Costophrenic Sulcus. Scarring from such things as previous infection, hemorrhage, or surgery in the pleural space sometimes produces a characteristic *ski-slope appearance* of blunting *(arrows)*, unlike the **meniscoid** appearance of a pleural effusion. There is bowel gas (B) below the elevated left hemidiaphragm. This scarring would not change in appearance or location with a change in the patient's position, unlike a free-flowing pleural effusion.

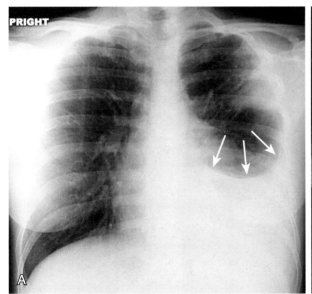 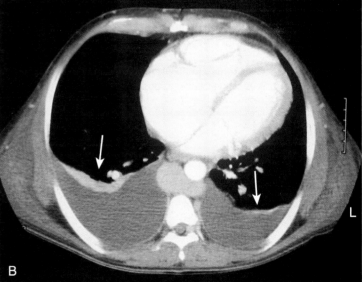

Fig. 7.7 Meniscus Sign, Pleural Effusion. (A) On the frontal projection in the upright position, an effusion typically produces a U-shaped density with the fluid rising higher along the edges than the center of the effusion *(arrows)* called the *meniscus sign.* (B) In a different patient, an axial CT scan with the patient in the supine position displays bilateral pleural effusions, each demonstrating a meniscoid shape *(arrows)*.

- **Effect of patient positioning on the appearance of pleural fluid:**
  - In the **upright position**, pleural fluid descends to the **base** of the thoracic cavity due to the force of gravity. In the **supine position**, the same free-flowing effusion will layer along the **posterior** pleural space and produce a homogeneous "haze" over the entire hemithorax when viewed *en face* on a chest x-ray (Fig. 7.8).
  - *Decubitus views,* infrequently used now, produce the same effect (Fig. 7.9).

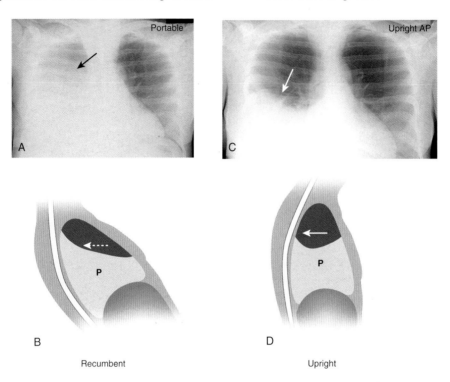

**Fig. 7.8 Effect of Patient Positioning on the Appearance of a Pleural Effusion.** (A) With the patient in the recumbent position, this right-sided effusion layers posteriorly and produces a "haze" over the entire hemithorax that is most dense at the base and less dense toward the apex of the lung *(arrow)*. (B) In this diagram of the recumbent position, the x-ray beam *(arrow)* traverses layering pleural fluid. (C) In the **same patient** x-rayed a few minutes later in a more upright position, pleural fluid *(arrow)* falls to the base of the pleural space due to the force of gravity. (D) The upright diagram shows how the x-ray beam traverses less fluid than before *(arrow)*. This simple alteration in **position** can produce the mistaken impression that the size of an effusion has changed even though the only change has been patient positioning. *P,* Pleural fluid.

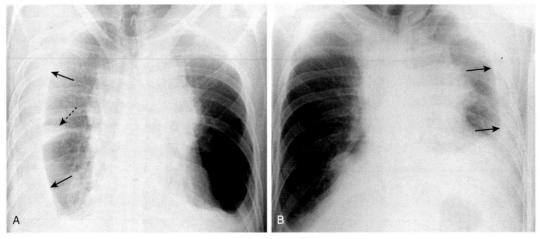

**Fig. 7.9 Decubitus Views of the Chest.** A decubitus view of the chest is obtained with the patient lying on either their right or left side with the x-ray beam directed parallel to the floor. It is used very infrequently now compared to CT for evaluation of the underlying lung. (A) A **right lateral decubitus** view of the chest is exposed with the patient lying on the right side where any free-flowing fluid in the right pleural space will form a band-like density *(solid arrows)*. The fluid also interposes between the folds of the minor fissure *(dashed arrow)*. (B) In a **left lateral decubitus** view of the chest, the patient lies on their left side and free fluid in the left pleural space layers along the dependent side *(arrows)*. (A) and (B) are the same patient who had bilateral pleural effusions from lymphoma.

- Depending on the patient's degree of recumbence, the upper lung fields may appear clearer (blacker) if the patient is more upright since the fluid settles to the base of the thorax or the upper lung fields may appear denser (whiter) as the patient becomes more supine and the effusion begins to **layer posteriorly.** This change in appearance can occur with the **same volume** of pleural fluid simply redistributed in the pleural space because of patient positioning (see Fig. 7.8). Ideally, each portable chest radiograph would be exposed with the patient in the same position.

## Opacified Hemithorax

- When the **hemithorax of an adult contains about 2 liters** of fluid, the **entire hemithorax will be opacified** (Fig. 7.10).
- As fluid fills the pleural space, the lung will undergo passive atelectasis (see Chapter 6).
- **Most effusions are sufficiently opaque** on conventional chest radiographs **so as to mask whatever disease may be present in the** underlying lung. **CT is the modality usually employed** to visualize the lung rendered impenetrable by an effusion (Fig. 7.11).
- **Large effusions** can have a mass-like effect and **displace the heart and trachea away** from the **side of opacification** (see Fig. 7.10).
- For more on the opacified hemithorax, go to Chapter 5.

## Loculated Effusions

- **Adhesions in the pleural space**, most often caused by old infection or hemothorax, **may limit the normal mobility of a pleural effusion**, so that it remains in the same location no matter what position the patient assumes. This produces a *loculated effusion.*
- **Imaging findings of loculated effusions:**
  - Loculated effusions **can be suspected when an effusion has an unusual shape or location in the thorax** (e.g., the effusion defies gravity by remaining at the nondependent part of the thorax when the patient is upright on a conventional radiograph or in the supine position on a CT scan of the chest) (Fig. 7.12).

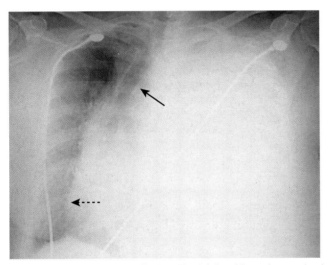

**Fig. 7.10 Large Left Pleural Effusion.** The left hemithorax is completely opacified and there is a shift of the mobile mediastinal structures such as the trachea *(solid arrow)* and the heart *(dashed arrow)* **away** from the side of opacification. This is characteristic of a large pleural effusion, which can act like a mass. This patient had a left-sided bronchogenic carcinoma.

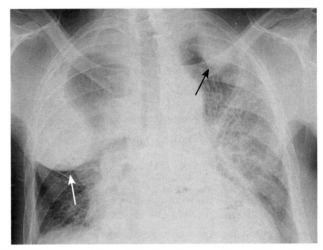

**Fig. 7.12 Loculated Pleural Effusions.** There are bilateral fluid collections *(arrows)* that have unusual shapes and seem to defy gravity, because they are trapped in the pleural space, usually by adhesions. Pleural-based metastases were accounting for the loculated fluid in this patient.

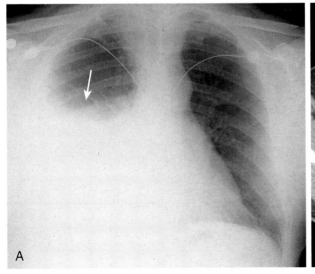

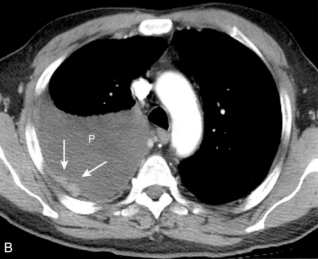

**Fig. 7.11 Pleural Metastases Seen on CT.** (A) The frontal chest radiograph displays a right pleural effusion *(arrow)*. It is impossible to see the underlaying lung. (B) An axial CT scan of the same patient demonstrates not only the pleural fluid (P) but nodularity of the pleural surface *(arrows)* representing metastatic implants secondary to a small cell carcinoma of the lung.

- **Loculation of pleural fluid has therapeutic importance** since such collections tend to be traversed by multiple adhesions, which make it difficult to drain the noncommunicating pockets of fluid with a single pleural drainage tube in the same way free-flowing effusions can be drained.
- For more on the use of **ultrasound in pleural effusions**, see Chapter 19.

## Fissural Pseudotumors

- *Pseudotumors* (also called *vanishing tumors*) are **sharply marginated collections of pleural fluid** contained either between the layers of an **interlobar pulmonary fissure** or in a subpleural location just beneath the fissure. They are **transudates,** which **almost always occur in patients with congestive heart failure (CHF).**
- The imaging findings of a pseudotumor are characteristic so that they should not be mistaken for an actual tumor (from which they derive their name).
  - They are **lenticular in shape**, most often occur in the **minor fissure (75%)**, and frequently have **pointed ends on each side** where they insinuate into the fissure, much like the shape of a **lemon.** They **do not tend to flow freely** with a change in patient positioning (Fig. 7.13).
- They **disappear when the underlying condition (usually CHF) is treated** but they **tend to recur in the same location** each time the patient's heart failure recurs.

## Laminar Effusions

- A laminar effusion (Fig. 7.14) is a form of pleural effusion in which the fluid assumes a **thin, band-like density paralleling the lateral chest wall, especially near the costophrenic angle.** The lateral costophrenic angle tends to maintain its

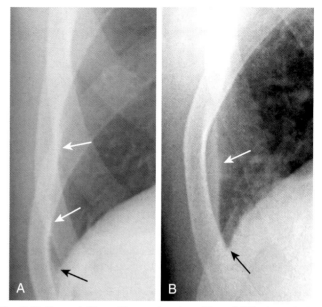

**Fig. 7.14 Normal Chest Versus Laminar Pleural Effusion.** (A) The normally aerated lung extends to the inner margin of each of the ribs *(white arrows)*. The costophrenic sulcus is sharp *(black arrow)*. (B) There is a thin band of increased density *(white arrow)* that extends superiorly from the lung base but does not appear to cause blunting of the costophrenic angle *(black arrow)*. This is the appearance of a ***laminar pleural effusion.*** This patient was in congestive heart failure.

acute angle with a laminar effusion, unlike the blunting that occurs with a usual pleural effusion.
- Laminar effusions are **almost always the result of** elevated left atrial pressure, as in **congestive heart failure** or secondary to **lymphangitic carcinomatosis. They are usually not free-flowing.**

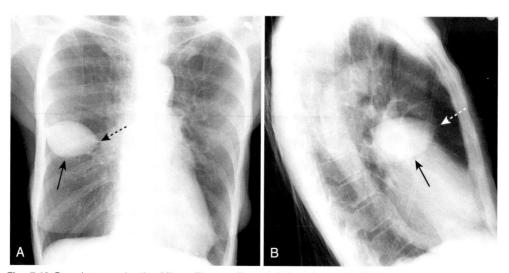

**Fig. 7.13 Pseudotumor in the Minor Fissure, Frontal (A) and Lateral (B) Projection.** (A) A sharply marginated collection of pleural fluid contained between the layers of the minor fissure produces a characteristic **lenticular shape** *(solid black arrows in A and B)* that frequently has pointed ends on each side where it insinuates into the fissure so that pseudotumors look like a ***lemon*** on frontal (A) or lateral (B) chest radiographs *(dashed black arrow on A and dashed white arrow on B)*. Pseudotumors always occur along the course of a fissure that, along with their shape, helps distinguish them from an actual tumor of the lung.

## Hydropneumothorax

- The presence of *both* abnormal amounts of **fluid** in the pleural space *and* **air** in the pleural space (pneumothorax) is called a *hydropneumothorax* (Fig. 7.15).
- Some of the more common causes of a hydropneumothorax are **trauma, surgery,** or a **recent thoracentesis to remove pleural fluid** in which air entered the pleural space.

- *Bronchopleural fistula,* an abnormal and relatively uncommon connection between the bronchial tree and the pleural space most often due to tumor, surgery, or infection, can also produce both air and fluid in the pleural space.
- CT is frequently necessary to distinguish between some presentations of **hydropneumothorax** and a large **lung abscess,** both of which may have a similar appearance on conventional chest radiographs.

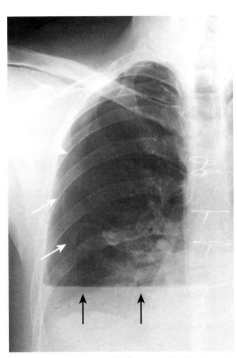

**Fig. 7.15** Hydropneumothorax. Unlike pleural effusions alone, whose meniscoid shape is governed by the elastic recoil of the lung, hydropneumothorax produces an **air-fluid level** marked by a straight edge and a sharp, air-over-fluid interface *(black arrows)* when the exposure is made with a horizontal x-ray beam. This person was stabbed in the right side and there is a moderately large pneumothorax as shown by the visceral pleural white line *(white arrows)*. Unlike CT, conventional radiography is unable to distinguish between blood and any other pleural fluid.

### CASE QUIZ 7 ANSWER

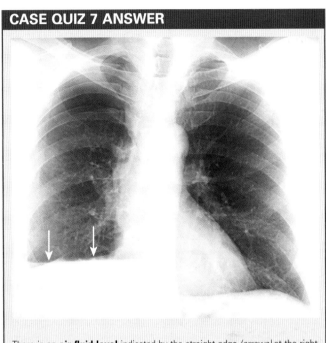

There is an **air-fluid level** indicated by the straight edge *(arrows)* at the right base, which is an indication that there is not only an abnormal amount of fluid in the pleural space but air as well—in this case a **hemopneumothorax** from a ruptured intercostal artery which required repair.

## TAKE HOME POINTS

- Pleural effusions collect in the **potential space** between the visceral and parietal pleura and are either **transudates** or **exudates,** depending primarily on their protein content and LDH concentration.
- Normally, a few milliliters of fluid are present in the pleural space; about **75 mL** are required to **blunt** the **posterior costophrenic sulcus** (seen on the lateral view) and about **200 to 300 mL** to **blunt** the **lateral costophrenic sulcus** (seen on the frontal view). Approximately **2 L** of fluid will cause opacification of the **entire hemithorax** in an adult.
- Whether an effusion is unilateral or bilateral, mostly right-sided or mostly left-sided, can be an important clue as to its etiology.
- Most pleural effusions begin their life collecting in the pleural space between the hemidiaphragm and the base of the lung; these are called **subpulmonic effusions.**
- As the amount of fluid increases, it forms a **meniscus** shape on the upright chest radiograph due to the natural elastic recoil properties of the lung.
- Very large pleural effusions may behave like a **mass** and produce a shift of the mobile mediastinal structures (e.g., the heart) **away** from the side of the effusion.

- In the absence of pleural adhesions, effusions will **flow freely** and change location with a change in the patient's position; with pleural adhesions (usually from old infection or hemothorax), the fluid may assume unusual appearances or occur in atypical locations. Such effusions are said to be **loculated.**
- A **pseudotumor** is a type of effusion that occurs in the fissures of the lung (mostly the minor fissure) and is most frequently secondary to CHF; it clears when the underlying heart failure is treated.
- **Laminar effusions** are best recognized at the lung base just above the costophrenic angles on the frontal projection and most often occur as a result of either CHF or lymphangitic carcinomatosis.
- A **hydropneumothorax** consists of both air and increased fluid in the pleural space and is recognizable on an upright view of the chest by a straight, air-fluid interface rather than the typical meniscus shape of pleural fluid alone.

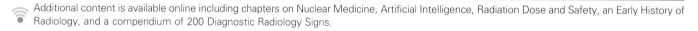

Additional content is available online including chapters on Nuclear Medicine, Artificial Intelligence, Radiation Dose and Safety, an Early History of Radiology, and a compendium of 200 Diagnostic Radiology Signs.

# 8

# Recognizing Pneumonia

*William Herring, MD, FACR*

## GENERAL CONSIDERATIONS

- Pneumonia can be defined as **consolidation of the lung produced by inflammatory exudate, usually as a result of an infectious agent.**
- **Most pneumonias produce airspace disease, either lobar or segmental.** Other pneumonias demonstrate **interstitial disease** and some produce findings in both the airspaces and the interstitium.

### CASE QUIZ 8 QUESTION

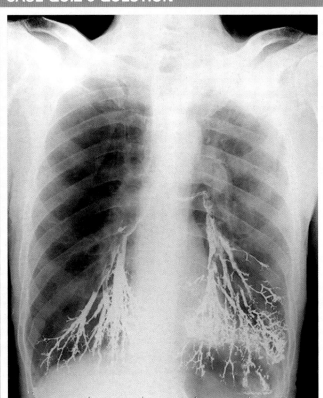

This is a chest x-ray immediately following a diagnostic test the patient was undergoing. While not a pneumonia, this case illustrates prior knowledge of the different radiographic densities and a mechanism for developing a pneumonia described in this chapter. What might explain this unusual appearance? The answer is at the end of the chapter.

- Most microorganisms that produce pneumonia are **spread to the lungs via the tracheobronchial tree, either through inhalation or aspiration** of the organisms. In some instances, microorganisms are spread via the bloodstream and in even fewer cases, by direct extension.
- Because many different microorganisms can produce similar imaging findings in the lungs, it is **difficult to identify with certainty the causative organism from the radiographic presentation alone.** However, **certain patterns** of disease **are very suggestive** of a particular causative organism (Table 8.1).
- Some use the term "infiltrate" synonymously with pneumonia, but many diseases, from amyloid to pulmonary fibrosis, can *infiltrate* the lung.

### TABLE 8.1 Patterns that Might Suggest a Causative Organism

| Pattern of Disease | Likely Causative Organism |
|---|---|
| Upper lobe cavitary pneumonia with spread to the opposite lower lobe | *Mycobacterium tuberculosis* (TB) |
| Upper lobe lobar pneumonia with bulging interlobar fissure | *Klebsiella pneumoniae* |
| Lower lobe cavitary pneumonia | *Pseudomonas aeruginosa* or anaerobic organisms *(Bacteroides)* |
| Perihilar interstitial disease or perihilar airspace disease | *Pneumocystis carinii (jirovecii)* |
| Thin-walled upper lobe cavity | *Coccidioides* (coccidiomycosis), TB |
| Airspace disease with effusion | *Streptococci, staphylococci*, TB |
| Diffuse nodules | *Histoplasma, Coccidioides, Mycobacterium tuberculosis* (histoplasmosis, coccidiomycosis, TB) |
| Soft-tissue, finger-like shadows in upper lobes | *Aspergillus* (allergic bronchopulmonary aspergillosis) |
| Solitary pulmonary nodule | *Cryptococcus* (cryptococcosis) |
| Spherical soft-tissue mass in a thin-walled upper lobe cavity | *Aspergillus* (aspergilloma) |
| Bilateral, peripheral, lower lobe ground-glass opacities | *SARS-CoV-2* (COVID-19) |

# GENERAL CHARACTERISTICS OF PNEUMONIA

- Because **pneumonia** fills the involved airspaces or interstitial tissues with some form of fluid or inflammatory exudate, pneumonias **appear denser (whiter) than the surrounding, normally aerated lung.**
- **Pneumonia may contain air bronchograms** if the bronchi themselves are not filled with inflammatory exudate or fluid (see Fig. 5.5).
  - Air bronchograms are **much more likely to be visible when the pneumonia involves the central portion** of the lung around the hilum. Near the periphery of the lung, the bronchi are usually too small to be visible (Fig. 8.1).
  - Remember that anything of fluid or soft-tissue density that replaces the normal gas in the airspaces may also produce this sign so an **air bronchogram is not specific for pneumonia** (see Chapter 4).
- Pneumonia that involves the airspaces **appears fluffy** and its **margins are indistinct.**
  - **Where pneumonia abuts a pleural surface,** such as an interlobar fissure or the chest wall, **it will be sharply marginated.**
- **Interstitial** pneumonia, on the other hand, may produce prominence of the connective tissues, vessels, and bronchi that make up the interstitium of the lung but also may spread to adjacent airways and resemble airspace disease.

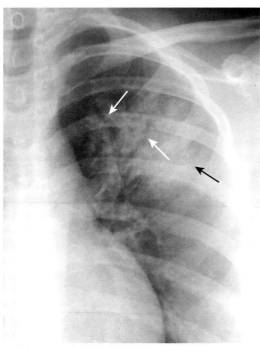

**Fig. 8.1 Left Upper Lobe Pneumonia.** There are several black, branching structures *(white arrows)* in this left upper lobe pneumonia that represent typical **air bronchograms** consistent with airspace disease. This patient had pneumococcal pneumonia. The disease is homogeneous in density, except for the presence of the air bronchograms. Because this is airspace disease, its outer edges are poorly marginated, indistinct, and fluffy *(black arrow)*.

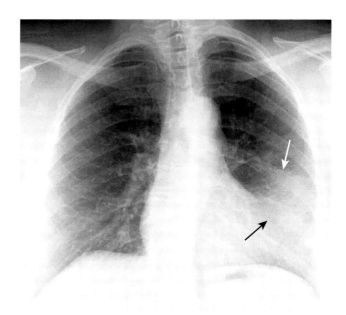

**Fig. 8.2 Lingular Pneumonia.** There is airspace disease in the lingula of the left upper lobe *(white arrow)*. The disease is of homogeneous density. Because the pneumonia and the heart are the same radiographic density, the border between them disappears **(silhouetted)** *(black arrow)*.

- Except for the presence of air bronchograms, airspace **pneumonia is usually homogeneous in density** (Fig. 8.2).
- In some types of pneumonia (i.e., bronchopneumonia), **the bronchi as well as the airspaces contain inflammatory exudate.** This can lead to **atelectasis associated with the pneumonia.**
- Box 8.1 summarizes the keys to recognizing pneumonia.

# PATTERNS OF PNEUMONIA

- Pneumonias may be distributed in the lung in several patterns described as *lobar, segmental, interstitial, round, and cavitary* (Table 8.2).
- Remember, these are terms that simply describe the distribution of the disease in the lungs; they aren't diagnostic of pneumonia because many other diseases can produce similar patterns in the lung.

---

### BOX 8.1   Recognizing a Pneumonia: Key Signs

- More **opaque** than surrounding normal lung.
- With airspace disease, the margins may be **fluffy** and **indistinct** except when they abut a pleural surface, like the interlobar fissures, where the margin will be sharp.
- Pneumonia tends to be **homogeneous** in density.
- They may contain **air bronchograms.**
- **Interstitial pneumonias** may produce reticular prominence in the lungs.
- Pneumonias may be associated with **atelectasis** in the affected portion of the lung.

## TABLE 8.2 Patterns of Appearance of Pneumonias

| Pattern | Characteristics |
| --- | --- |
| Lobar | Homogeneous consolidation of affected lobe frequently with air bronchograms |
| Segmental (bronchopneumonia) | Patchy airspace disease frequently involving several segments simultaneously; no air bronchogram; atelectasis may be associated |
| Interstitial | Reticular interstitial disease usually diffusely spread throughout the lungs early in the disease process; may progress to airspace disease |
| Round | Spherically shaped pneumonia usually seen in the lower lobes of children; may resemble a mass |
| Cavitary | Produced by numerous microorganisms, chief among them being *Mycobacterium tuberculosis* |

## Lobar Pneumonia

- The **prototypical lobar pneumonia is pneumococcal pneumonia** caused by *Streptococcus pneumoniae* (Fig. 8.3).
- Although we are calling it lobar pneumonia, the patient may present before the disease involves the entire lobe. In its most classical form, the disease fills most or all of a lobe of the lung.
- Because lobes are bound by interlobar fissures, **one or more of the margins of a lobar pneumonia may be sharply**

marginated. Where the disease is not bound by a fissure, it will have an **indistinct** and **irregular margin.**
- Lobar pneumonias almost always produce a *silhouette sign* where they come in contact with the heart, aorta, or diaphragm and they almost always contain *air bronchograms* if they involve the central portions of the lung.

## Segmental Pneumonia (Bronchopneumonia)

- The **prototypical bronchopneumonia is that caused by** *Staphylococcus aureus.* Many gram-negative bacteria, such as *Pseudomonas aeruginosa,* can produce the same picture.
- Bronchopneumonias are spread centrifugally via the tracheobronchial tree to **many foci in the lung at the same time.** Therefore **they frequently involve several segments** of the lung simultaneously.
- Because lung segments are not bound by fissures, all of the **margins of segmental pneumonias tend to be fluffy and indistinct** (Fig. 8.4).
- Unlike lobar pneumonia, **segmental bronchopneumonias produce exudate that fills the bronchi.** Therefore **air bronchograms are usually not present** and there is frequently some **volume loss (atelectasis)** associated with bronchopneumonia.

## Interstitial Pneumonia

- The **prototypes** for **interstitial pneumonia** are **viral pneumonia** and *Mycoplasma pneumoniae* as well as **Pneumocystis pneumonia** in patients with acquired immune deficiency syndrome (AIDS).
- Interstitial pneumonias tend to involve the airway **walls** and **alveolar septa** and may produce, especially early in their course, a **fine, reticular pattern** in the lungs.

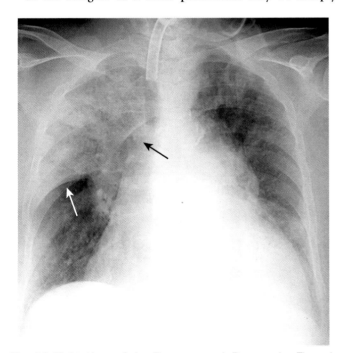

**Fig. 8.3 Right Upper Lobe Pneumococcal Pneumonia.** There is airspace disease in the right upper lobe that occupies the entire lobe. The inferior margin of the pneumonia is sharply marginated by the minor or horizontal fissure *(white arrow).* Where the disease contacts the ascending aorta *(black arrow),* the border of the aorta is silhouetted by the fluid density of the pneumonia.

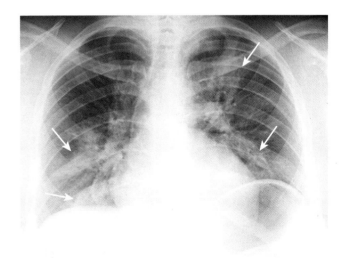

**Fig. 8.4 Staphylococcal Bronchopneumonia.** There are multiple, irregularly marginated patches of airspace disease in both lungs *(arrows).* This is a characteristic distribution and appearance of **bronchopneumonia.** Staphylococcal pneumonia is more common in children, hospitalized patients, and debilitated adults. It also can develop in young adults after a bout of influenza. Methicillin-resistant *Staphylococcus aureus* (MRSA) pneumonia may be particularly difficult to treat.

- Most **interstitial pneumonias eventually spread to the adjacent alveoli** and produce patchy or confluent airspace disease **making the original interstitial nature of the pneumonia impossible to recognize** radiographically.

> **IMPORTANT POINTS**
>
> - *Pneumocystis carinii (jirovecii)* **pneumonia (PCP)**
>   - PCP is the **most common** clinically recognized infection in patients with AIDS.
>   - It classically presents as a **perihilar, reticular interstitial pneumonia**, or as **airspace disease that may mimic the central distribution pattern of pulmonary edema** (Fig. 8.5).
>   - Other presentations, such as unilateral airspace disease or widespread, patchy airspace disease are less common.
>   - There are usually **no pleural effusions** and **no hilar adenopathy.**
>   - Opportunistic infections **usually occur with CD4 counts under 200** per cubic mL of blood.

## Round Pneumonia

- Some pneumonias, mostly in children, can assume a **spherical shape** on chest radiographs. These *round pneumonias* are almost always **posterior** in the lungs, usually **in the lower lobes.**
- Causative agents include *Haemophilus influenzae, Streptococcus,* and *Pneumococcus.*
- A round pneumonia could be confused with a tumor mass except that symptoms associated with infection usually accompany the pulmonary findings and lung tumors are uncommon in children (Fig. 8.6).

## Cavitary Pneumonia

- The prototypical organism producing cavitary pneumonia is *Mycobacterium tuberculosis.* Tuberculosis is discussed in Chapter 4.

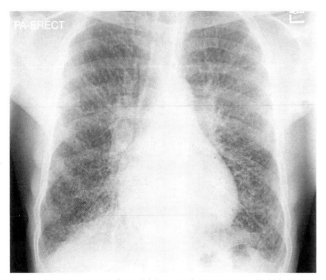

**Fig. 8.5** *Pneumocystis Carinii* (*Jirovecii*) Pneumonia (PCP). There is bilateral, diffuse **interstitial** lung disease that is primarily **reticular** in nature. Without the additional history that this patient had acquired immune deficiency syndrome (AIDS), this could be mistaken for pulmonary interstitial edema or for a chronic, fibrotic process such as sarcoidosis. There are, however, no pleural effusions present, as might be expected with pulmonary interstitial edema, and there is no evidence of hilar adenopathy, as might occur in sarcoid.

> **IMPORTANT POINTS**
>
> - **Cavitation is common in postprimary tuberculosis (reactivation tuberculosis) but rare in primary TB.** The cavities are usually located in the upper lobes, are bilateral and **thin-walled**, and have **a smooth inner margin** and **no air-fluid level** (Fig. 8.7).
> - **Transbronchial spread** (from one upper lobe to the opposite lower lobe, or to another lobe in the same lung) should make you think of infection with *Mycobacterium tuberculosis.*

- **Other infectious agents** that produce cavitary disease:
  - **Staphylococcal pneumonia** can cavitate and produce thin-walled *pneumatoceles.*
  - *Streptococcal* pneumonia, *Klebsiella* pneumonia, and *coccidiomycosis* can also produce cavitating pneumonias.

## Aspiration

- There are many causes of aspiration of foreign material into the tracheobronchial tree, among them neurologic disorders

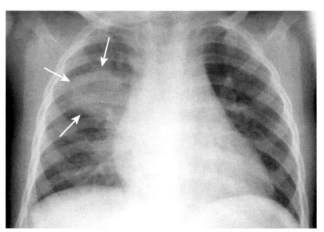

**Fig. 8.6** Round Pneumonia. There is a soft tissue density in the right mid-lung field that has a rounded appearance *(arrows)*. This is a 2-year-old who had a cough and fever. Round pneumonia is rare after the age of 12 years and tumors are rare in children, so the differential diagnosis favors pneumonia in someone of this age.

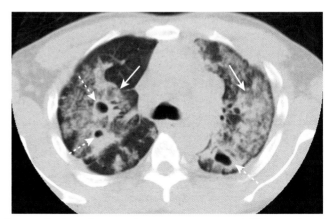

**Fig. 8.7** Cavitary Pneumonia. A nonenhanced axial CT image through the upper lobes demonstrates bilateral airspace disease *(solid arrows)* containing multiple lucencies representing cavities *(dashed arrows)*. The cavities contain no air-fluid levels. Upper lobe cavitary pneumonia is presumptively TB, until proven otherwise. This patient had postprimary tuberculosis (reactivation tuberculosis).

(stroke, traumatic brain injury), altered mental status (anesthesia, drug overdose), gastroesophageal reflux, and postoperative changes from head and neck surgery.

- **Acute aspiration** will produce radiographic findings of airspace disease. Its **location**, the **rapidity** with which it appears, and the group of patients **predisposed** to aspirate are clues to its etiology (Fig. 8.8).
- **Recognizing the different types of aspiration** (Table 8.3)
  - The clinical and radiologic course of aspiration depends on **what** was aspirated.
  - **Aspiration of bland (neutralized) gastric juices or water**
    - This is technically **not a pneumonia** because it does not involve an infectious agent, is handled by the lungs as if it were pulmonary edema fluid, and **classically remains for only a day or two before clearing** through resorption.
  - **Aspiration that produces pneumonia due to microorganisms in the lung**
    - Although **we routinely aspirate numerous microorganisms present in the normal oropharyngeal flora**, there are some patients in whom these microorganisms can develop into pneumonia, including those

who are immunocompromised, elderly, debilitated, or have underlying lung disease.
- **Pneumonia** caused by aspiration is usually due to **anaerobic organisms**, such as *Bacteroides*. These organisms produce **lower lobe airspace disease** that **frequently cavitates**. They may take **months to resolve**.
- **Aspiration of unneutralized stomach acid (*Mendelson syndrome*)**
  - When large quantities of unneutralized gastric acid are aspirated, **chemical pneumonitis develops**, producing dependent lobe airspace disease or diffuse **pulmonary edema**. The disease may appear quickly, within a few **hours** of the aspiration. Clearing may take **days or longer** and the chemical pneumonitis is prone to become **secondarily infected.**

## COVID-19

- Coronavirus disease 2019 *(COVID-19)* is the infectious disease caused by the severe acute respiratory syndrome coronavirus 2 *(SARS-CoV-2),* declared a pandemic by the World Health Organization in 2020.
- Many **symptomatic** patients demonstrate fever, cough, fatigue, smell and taste disturbances, and expectoration. Most patients experience mild to moderate respiratory distress but recover without requiring additional treatment.
- **Conventional chest x-rays** may show **patchy** or **diffuse airspace disease.** Pleural effusions are uncommon (Fig. 8.9).
- The most common **CT findings**, alone or in combination, are *ground-glass opacities*, frequently **bilateral**, **posterior**, and **lower lobe.** Sometimes, **vascular enlargement** is present. These findings are not specific for COVID-19. Those who do require a chest CT are most often examined **without intravenous contrast** (Fig. 8.10).

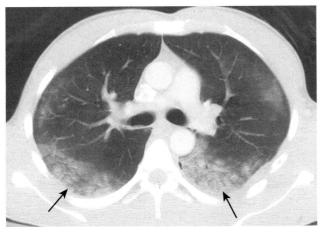

**Fig. 8.8 Aspiration, Both Lower Lobes.** Single, axial CT image of the lungs demonstrates bilateral lower lobe airspace disease *(arrows)* in a patient who had aspirated. Aspiration usually affects the most dependent portions of the lung. In the upright position, the lower lobes are affected. In the supine position, the superior segments of the lower lobes and the posterior segments of the upper lobes are most involved.

| TABLE 8.3 | Three Patterns of Acute Aspiration |
|---|---|
| **Pattern** | **Characteristics** |
| **Bland gastric acid or water** | Rapidly appearing and rapidly clearing airspace disease in dependent lobe(s); not a pneumonia |
| **Infected aspirate (aspiration pneumonia)** | Usually lower lobes; frequently cavitates and may take months to clear |
| **Unneutralized stomach acid (chemical pneumonitis)** | Almost immediate appearance of dependent airspace disease that frequently becomes secondarily infected |

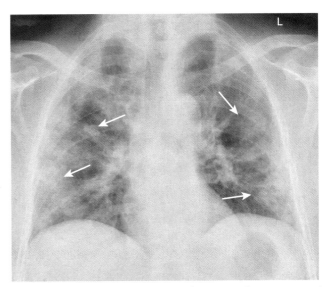

**Fig. 8.9 COVID-19 Chest Radiograph.** Chest x-ray in a symptomatic patient with SARS-CoV-2 infection shows bilateral, peripheral, somewhat nodular lung opacities *(arrows)* consistent with the disease, but similar in appearance to the pattern of many other coronaviruses such as severe acute respiratory distress coronavirus (SARS) and swine flu (H1N1).

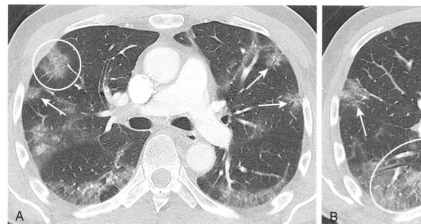
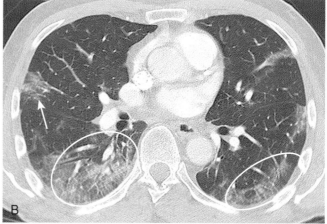

**Fig. 8.10** COVID-19 CT. Two images from the same patient with COVID-19. (A) There are peripheral ***ground-glass opacities*** *(arrows)* in the mid-lungs with their typical rounded morphology *(circle)*. Ground-glass densities on CT are areas of increased attenuation with preserved bronchial and vascular markings. They are a nonspecific sign. (B) A lower image demonstrates a pattern called ***crazy-paving*** *(ovals)* as well as peripheral ground-glass opacity *(arrow)*. Crazy-paving is a descriptive term applied to ground-glass opacities with a superimposed network of septal thickening seen on high-resolution chest CT.

- Clinically **asymptomatic** patients with known SARS-CoV-2 infection frequently have **normal chest CT** examination results. In one study, up to 18% of cases demonstrated normal chest x-rays or CT when early in the disease course. Once **symptomatic**, less than 10% of patients with COVID-19 have a **normal chest CT** examination.
- Chest imaging is advised to assess for COVID-19 progression in cases of clinical worsening, or cardiopulmonary complications such as ***acute respiratory distress syndrome (ARDS),*** pulmonary embolism, superimposed pneumonia, or heart failure.

## LOCALIZING PNEUMONIA

- Although it is true that an antibiotic will travel to every lobe of the lung without regard for which lobe actually harbors the pneumonia, determining the location of a pneumonia may provide clues to the **causative organism** (e.g., if in the upper lobes, think of TB) and the presence of **associated pathology** (e.g., if in lower lobes, think of recurrent aspiration) (see Table 8.1).
- **On conventional radiographs,** it is always **best to localize any disease by using two views taken at 90° to each other** (***orthogonal views***), like a frontal and lateral chest radiograph. CT will further localize and characterize the disease as well as demonstrate associated pathology, such as pleural effusions or cavities too small to see on conventional radiographs.
- Sometimes, only a frontal radiograph may be available, as with critically ill or debilitated patients who require a portable bedside examination. Nevertheless, it is still frequently **possible to localize the pneumonia using only the frontal radiograph** by analyzing which anatomic

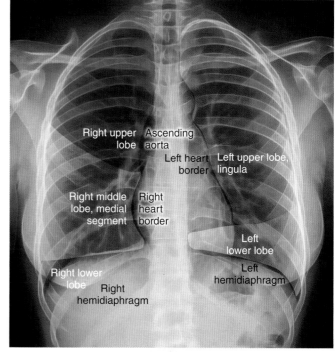

**Fig. 8.11** Localizing Airspace Disease on the Frontal Radiograph. Based on the availability of only a frontal chest x-ray, it is frequently possible to localize the lobe in which the airspace disease is present. This graphic shows which part of the heart, aorta, or hemidiaphragm may be silhouetted by contact with airspace disease in the contiguous lobe of the lung.

structure's margins are obscured by the disease (i.e., the **silhouette sign**) (Fig. 8.11).
- The **silhouette sign** (see also Characteristics of Airspace Disease in Chapter 4) states that if two objects of the **same** radiographic density **are in contact with** each other, then the **edge between them disappears** (see Fig. 8.2).

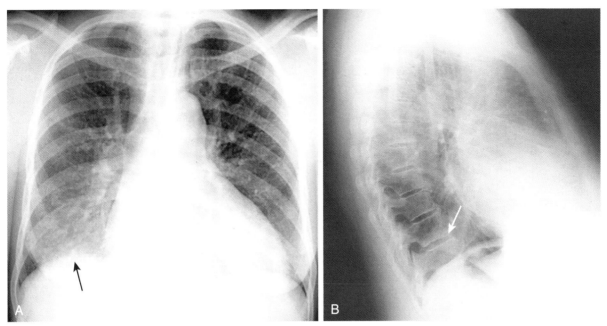

**Fig. 8.12 The Spine Sign.** A lateral view of the chest may sometimes suggest airspace disease that is not immediately apparent on the frontal film or confirm its presence, as in this case. (A) There is a suggestion of airspace disease in the right lower lobe on the frontal view *(arrow)* that is confirmed on the lateral view (B) by the pneumonia being superimposed on the lower spine *(arrow)*, making the spine appear "whiter" (denser) just above the diaphragm—the *spine sign* (see also Fig. 2.6).

- Another helpful localizing radiographic sign is the *spine sign* (Fig. 8.12)
  - On the lateral chest radiograph, the **thoracic spine normally appears to get darker (blacker) as you survey it from the shoulder girdle to the diaphragm.**
    - This is because the x-ray beam normally needs to penetrate more tissue (more bones and muscle) around the shoulders than it does just above the diaphragm, where it needs to pass through only the heart and aerated lungs.
  - **When disease** of soft tissue or fluid density **involves the posterior portion of the lower lobe,** more of the x-ray beam will be absorbed by the new, added density and **the spine will appear to become "whiter" (more opaque) just above the posterior costophrenic sulcus.**
    - This is called the *spine sign* and it provides another way to localize disease in the lungs.

⟫ **IMPORTANT POINTS**

- Lower lobe disease may **not** be apparent on the frontal projection if it lies **deep in the posterior costophrenic sulcus.** Therefore the spine sign may be the only indicator of the presence of lower lobe disease, like lower lobe pneumonia, which may be otherwise invisible on the frontal projection.

- Fig. 8.13 is a composite of the characteristic localizing appearances of lobar pneumonia as seen on a frontal chest radiograph.

## HOW PNEUMONIA RESOLVES

- Pneumonia can resolve in 2 to 3 days if the organism is sensitive to the antibiotic administered, especially pneumococcal pneumonia.
- **Most pneumonias typically resolve from within (*vacuolize*),** gradually disappearing in a patchy fashion over days or weeks (Fig. 8.14).

⟫ **IMPORTANT POINTS**

- If a pneumonia **does not** resolve in several weeks, consider the presence of an underlying **obstructing lesion**, such as a **neoplasm**, that is preventing adequate drainage from that portion of the lung.
- A CT scan of the chest may help to demonstrate the obstructing lesion.

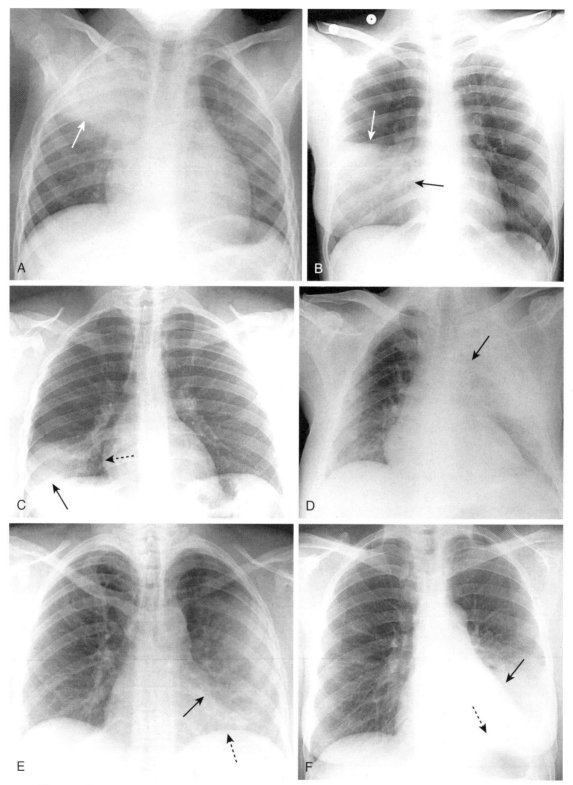

**Fig. 8.13** Composite Appearances of Lobar Pneumonias. (A) **Right upper lobe.** The disease obscures (silhouettes) the ascending aorta and produces a sharp margin where it abuts the minor fissure *(arrow).* (B) **Right middle lobe.** The disease silhouettes the right heart border *(black arrow)* and produces a sharp margin where it abuts the minor fissure *(white arrow).* (C) **Right lower lobe.** The disease silhouettes the right hemidiaphragm *(solid arrow)* but spares the right heart border *(dashed arrow).* (D) **Left upper lobe.** The disease obscures the aortic knob *(arrow).* (E) **Lingula.** The disease silhouettes the left heart border *(solid arrow)* but spares the left hemidiaphragm *(dashed arrow).* (F) **Left lower lobe.** The disease obscures the left hemidiaphragm *(dashed arrow)* but spares the left heart border *(solid arrow).*

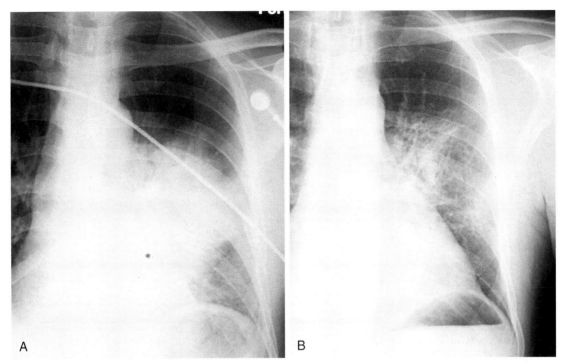

A   B

**Fig. 8.14 Resolving Pneumonia.** Pneumonia can resolve in several days if the organism is sensitive to the antibiotic administered, especially pneumococcal pneumonia. Most pneumonias, like that in the radiographs of the left lung taken 4 days apart (A) and (B), typically resolve from within **(vacuolize),** gradually disappearing in a patchy fashion over days or weeks.

## CASE QUIZ 8 ANSWER

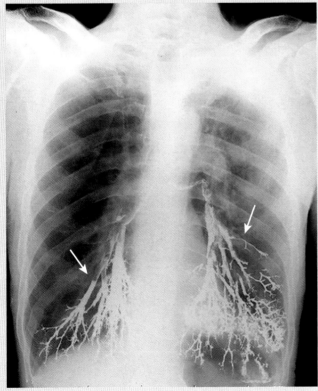

The patient aspirated liquid barium he was drinking while standing for an examination to study his swallowing function. Barium is inert and has a high density, which is why it is routinely used as a GI tract contrast agent. The barium was aspirated into the lungs and gravitated to the lower lobe bronchi. While striking in appearance, the barium will not itself cause pneumonia and will be reabsorbed over time. The patient was asymptomatic.

## TAKE HOME POINTS

- Pneumonia is more opaque than the surrounding normal lung and its margins may be **fluffy** and **indistinct** except for where it abuts a pleural margin; it tends to be **homogeneous** in density; it may contain **air bronchograms** and may be associated with **atelectasis.**

- Although there is considerable overlap in the patterns of pneumonia different organisms produce, there are some appearances that are highly suggestive of particular etiologies.

- **Lobar pneumonia** (prototype: pneumococcal pneumonia) tends to be homogeneous, occupies most or all of a lobe, has air bronchograms centrally, and produces the **silhouette sign.**

- **Segmental pneumonia** (prototype: staphylococcal pneumonia) tends to be multifocal, does not have air bronchograms, and can be associated with volume loss because the bronchi are also filled with inflammatory exudate.

- **Interstitial pneumonia** (prototype: viral pneumonia or PCP) tends to involve the airway walls and alveolar septa and may produce, especially early in its course, a fine, reticular pattern in the lungs; later in its course, it may produce airspace disease.

- **Round pneumonia** (prototype: haemophilus) usually occurs in **children** in the lower lobes **posteriorly** and can resemble a mass, the clue being that actual masses in children are uncommon.

- **Cavitary pneumonia** (prototype: tuberculosis) contains lucent cavities produced by lung necrosis as its hallmark; **postprimary tuberculosis** usually involves the upper lobes; it can spread via a transbronchial route that can infect the opposite lower lobe or another lobe in the same lung.

- **Aspiration** occurs in the most dependent portion of the lung at the time of the aspiration, usually the lower lobes or the posterior segments of the upper lobes; aspiration can be bland and clear quickly, can be infected and take months to clear, or be from a chemical pneumonitis that can take weeks to clear.

- Symptomatic **COVID-19** patients who undergo CT frequently show bilateral, peripheral ground-glass opacities, particularly at the bases.

- Pneumonia can be localized by using the **silhouette sign** and the **spine sign** as aids.

- Pneumonias frequently resolve in such a way that they contain patchy areas of newly aerated lung within the confines of the previous pneumonia **(vacuolization).**

 Additional content is available online including chapters on Nuclear Medicine, Artificial Intelligence, Radiation Dose and Safety, an Early History of Radiology, and a compendium of 200 Diagnostic Radiology Signs.

# 9

# Recognizing the Correct Placement of Lines and Tubes and Their Potential Complications: Critical Care Radiology

*William Herring, MD, FACR*

Patients in the critical or intensive care units (ICU) are monitored on a frequent basis with portable chest radiography both to check on the position of their multiple assistive devices and to assess their cardiopulmonary status.

## CASE QUIZ 9 QUESTION

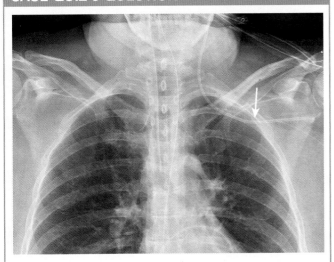

This patient just had a central venous catheter inserted on the left side in the subclavian vein *(arrow)* and you are asked to check this postinsertion radiograph to see if it is correctly positioned. What is your answer? The correct answer appears at the end of this chapter.

- Diseases commonly seen in critically ill patients are discussed in other chapters (Table 9.1).
- In this chapter, you'll get practical advice for evaluating the successful (or unsuccessful) insertion and ultimate position of multiple tubes, lines, catheters, and other supportive apparatus used in the ICU. **Information for even more devices can be found online** (e-Fig. 9.1 *to* e-Fig. 9.10).
- Almost always, a conventional radiograph is obtained **after** the insertion or attempted insertion of one of these devices to check on its position and to rule out any unintended consequences.
- Therefore **for each tube or device, you will learn:**

| TABLE 9.1 **Common Diseases in Critically Ill Patients** | |
|---|---|
| **Finding or Disease** | **Discussed in** |
| Acute respiratory distress syndrome | **Chapter 11** |
| Aspiration | **Chapter 8** |
| Atelectasis | **Chapter 6** |
| Congestive heart failure (pulmonary edema) | **Chapter 11** |
| Pleural effusion | **Chapter 7** |
| Pneumomediastinum | **Chapter 24** |

- **Why** they are used
- **Where** they belong when properly placed
- **How** such devices can be malpositioned and **what** complications may occur from the device (Box 9.1).

## ENDOTRACHEAL AND TRACHEOSTOMY TUBES

### Endotracheal Tubes (ETT)

- **Why they are used**
  - Assist ventilation
  - Isolate the trachea to permit control of the airway
  - Prevent gastric distension

### BOX 9.1 **Postprocedure Warning Signs**

- There are many complications besides malpositioning that can follow an invasive procedure, but a few are more **common** and should raise suspicion when they occur **immediately after** the procedure.
- For any tube, line, or device that either enters or passes through the **thorax**, be alert for postprocedure:
  - Appearance or increase in **pleural effusion**
  - **Pneumothorax**
  - **Pneumomediastinum**
  - **Widening** of the mediastinal shadow
- For any tube, line, or device inserted in the **abdomen**, be alert for postprocedure:
  - **Pneumoperitoneum**

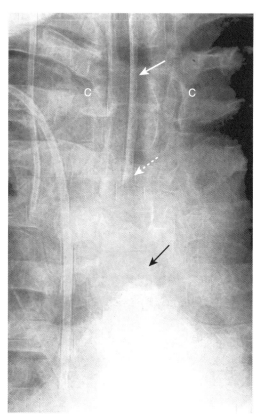

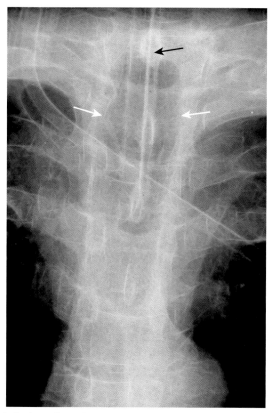

**Fig. 9.1 Endotracheal Tube in Satisfactory Position.** Endotracheal tubes have a radiopaque marker stripe *(solid white arrow)*. The tip is diagonally angled *(dashed white arrow)*. In adults, they usually have an inflatable cuff. Most endotracheal tubes are inserted via the oral, rather than the nasal, route. With the patient's head in the neutral position, the tip of ETT should be roughly half the distance between the medial ends of clavicles (C) and the carina *(black arrow)*.

**Fig. 9.2 Endotracheal Tube with Cuff Overinflated.** This overinflated balloon *(white arrows)* of the endotracheal tube *(black arrow)* is wider than the diameter of the trachea. The cuff should not distend the trachea. Prolonged compression on the tracheal wall by an overinflated cuff can result in necrosis of the wall and tracheal stenosis.

- • Provide a direct route for suctioning
- • Administer medications
- • **Correct placement of an ETT**
  - • Endotracheal tubes are usually **wide-bore tubes** (about 1 cm) with a **radio-opaque marker stripe** and **no side-holes. The tip is frequently diagonally shaped.**
  - • With the patient's head in the **neutral** position (i.e., bottom of mandible is at the level of C5-C6), the **tip of the ETT should be about 3 to 5 cm from the carina** or roughly **half the distance between the medial ends of clavicles and the carina** (Fig. 9.1).
  - • Ideally the **diameter of the endotracheal tube should be one-half to two-thirds the width of trachea.** An inflated cuff (balloon), if present, may fill—but shouldn't distend—the lumen of the trachea (Fig. 9.2).

> ▶▶ **IMPORTANT POINTS**
>
> - • **How to find the location of the carina on a frontal chest radiograph**
>   - • Follow the **right** or **left** main bronchus backward until either meets the opposite main bronchus.
>   - • Alternatively, the carina projects over the **T5, T6, or T7** vertebral bodies in 95% of people.

- • **Movement of tip with flexion and extension**
  - • Neck **flexion** may cause **2 cm of descent** of the tube tip. This is why the tip should be 3 to 5 cm above the carina.
  - • Neck **extension** from neutral **may cause 2 cm of ascent** of the tip.
  - • There is a silly, but helpful, rhyming sentence to help remember the direction of movement of the tip of an ETT with movement of the head: "The tip of the **hose** (i.e., ETT) follows the tip of the **nose.**"
- • **Incorrect positioning and complications of an ETT**
  - • **Most common malposition:** because of the shallower angle and wider diameter of the **right main bronchus** or bronchus intermedius, the **tip of the ETT will tend to slide into the right-sided bronchial tree** preferentially to the left.
    - • This can lead to **atelectasis** (especially of the nonaerated right upper lobe and left lung) (see Case Quiz 6).
    - • Intubation of the right main bronchus could also lead to a **right-sided tension pneumothorax.**
  - • Inadvertent esophageal intubation will produce a dilated stomach.

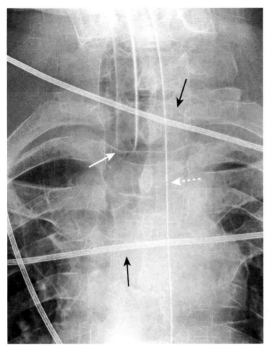

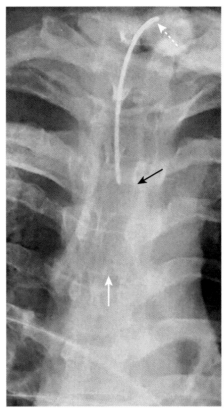

**Fig. 9.3 Endotracheal Tube Too High.** The tip of the tube *(solid white arrow)* should not be placed in or near the larynx or pharynx as the balloon cuff can produce damage to these structures if it remains in this position. High placement can also predispose to aspiration. This patient also has an NGT *(dashed white arrow)* and several overlying cardiac monitor leads *(black arrows)*. Patients in a critical care environment frequently have multiple overlying tubes and lines that can complicate interpretation.

**Fig. 9.4 Tracheostomy Tube in Correct Position.** The tip *(black arrow)* is about halfway between the stoma in which the tracheostomy tube was inserted *(dashed white arrow)* and the carina *(solid white arrow)*. This is usually around the level of T3. The tip of a tracheostomy tube is not affected by flexion and extension of the neck.

- The tip of the tube should not be positioned in the larynx or pharynx as damage to the vocal cords can occur (Fig. 9.3).

## Tracheostomy Tubes
- **Why they are used**
  - In patients with airway obstruction at or above level of larynx
  - In respiratory failure requiring long-term intubation (>21 days)
  - For airway obstruction during sleep apnea
  - When there is paralysis of the muscles that affect swallowing or respiration
- **Correct placement of a tracheostomy tube** (Fig. 9.4)
  - The **tip** should be **about halfway between the stoma** in which the tracheostomy tube was inserted **and the carina.** The carina is usually around the **level of T3.**
  - Unlike an ETT, the placement of the tip of a tracheostomy tube is not affected by flexion and extension of the head.
  - **The width of the tracheostomy tube should be about two-thirds the width of trachea.**
- **Incorrect placement and complications of a tracheostomy tube**

- Immediately after insertion look for signs of inadvertent **perforation of the trachea** such as pneumomediastinum, pneumothorax, and subcutaneous emphysema.
- If the tracheostomy tube is equipped with a **cuff,** the cuff should generally be inflated to a diameter that **fills,** but **does not distend, the normal tracheal contour.**
- **Long-term complication of tracheostomies:**
  - **Tracheal stenosis is the most common late-occurring complication** of a tracheostomy tube and can occur at the entrance stoma, level of the cuff, or at the tip of tube, but is **most common at the stoma.**

## INTRAVASCULAR CATHETERS
### Central Venous (Pressure) Catheters (CVC, CVP)
- **Why they are used**
  - For venous access to instill chemotherapeutic and hyperosmolar agents not suitable for peripheral venous administration
  - Measurement of central venous pressure
  - To maintain and monitor intravascular blood volume
- **Correct placement of central venous catheters**
  - **Central venous catheters** have a **small diameter (3 mm)** and are **uniformly opaque without a marker stripe.**

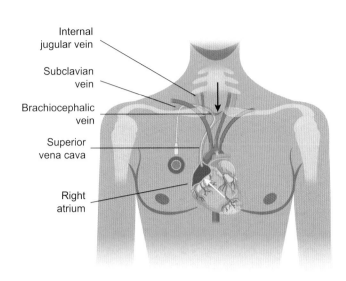

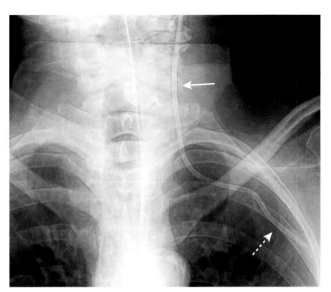

Fig. 9.7 Central Venous Catheter Malpositioned in Internal Jugular Vein. Central venous catheters, especially those placed by the subclavian route *(dashed arrow)*, can be malpositioned. They are most often malpositioned with their tips in the right atrium or the internal jugular vein, as in this case *(solid arrow)*. The catheter was removed and repositioned.

Fig. 9.5 Central Venous Catheter (CVC). CVCs are usually inserted either by the **subclavian vein** or **internal jugular vein** route. The internal jugular veins join the subclavian veins to form the **brachiocephalic (innominate) veins** that, in turn, drain into the **superior vena cava**. The junctions of the subclavian and brachiocephalic veins generally occur **posterior** to the **medial** end of the clavicle *(black arrow)* where the path of the catheter should begin **descending lateral to the right side of the spine. The tip should lie in the superior vena cava at its junction with the right atrium** *(white arrow)*. The junction of the superior vena cava and the right atrium usually lies at the level of 5th or 6th thoracic vertebral body or about two vertebral bodies **below** the level of the carina.

- Their correct placement is shown in Fig. 9.5 and Fig. 9.6.
- **Incorrect placement and complications of central venous catheters**
- Central venous catheters are **most often malpositioned with their tips in the right atrium or internal jugular vein** (Fig. 9.7). In the right atrium, they can produce **cardiac arrhythmias.** When central venous catheters are malpositioned, they may provide **inaccurate central venous pressure readings.**

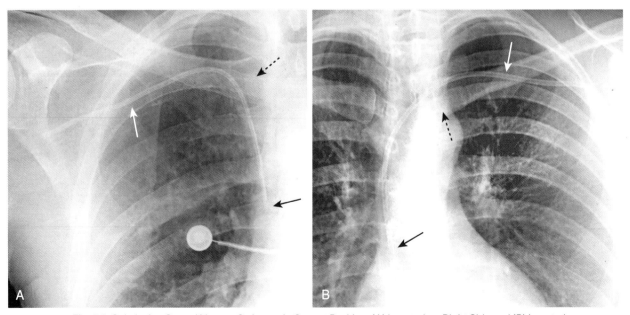

Fig. 9.6 Subclavian Central Venous Catheters in Correct Position, (A) Inserted on Right Side and (B) Inserted on Left. In both patients, there is a central venous catheter in place inserted via the subclavian vein *(solid white arrows)*. Each catheter passes under the medial ends of the clavicles *(dashed black arrows)* before descending to the right of the spine with their tips at the superior vena cava/right atrial junction *(solid black arrows)*.

- **Pneumothorax** can occur in up to 5% of CVC insertions, more often with the subclavian approach than the internal jugular route.
- **All bends in the catheter should be smooth curves. Occasionally CVCs may perforate the vein** and lie outside of the blood vessel. Look for **sharp bends/kinks** in the catheter as a clue to a potential **perforation.**
- Sometimes, they may be **inadvertently inserted in the subclavian artery** rather than the subclavian vein. Suspect **arterial placement** if the **blood return is pulsatile** upon placement and the course of the catheter **follows the aortic arch** or **fails to descend to the right of the spine** (Fig. 9.8).

> ## ▶▶ IMPORTANT POINTS
>
> - **Two or more attempts at inserting a CVC**
>   - A frontal chest radiograph is obtained following placement of a CVC. **Should initial placement fail,** it is customary to **obtain a chest radiograph before trying insertion on the other side** to avoid the possibility of producing bilateral pneumothoraces.

## Peripherally Inserted Central Catheters (PICC)

- **Why they are used**
  - For long-term venous access (months)
    - To administer medications such as chemotherapy or antibiotics
  - For frequent blood sampling
    - Because of their small size, they can be introduced via an antecubital vein
- **Correct placement of peripherally inserted central catheters**
  - The **tip** should lie **within** the **superior vena cava** but may be placed in an axillary vein. Because the lines are so

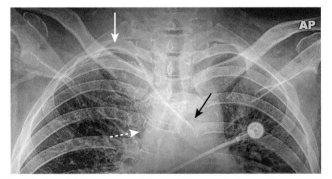

**Fig. 9.8 Arterial Placement of Central Venous Catheter.** Note that this catheter, inadvertently inserted into the subclavian artery *(solid white arrow)*, does **not** begin descending on the right side of the spine *(dashed white arrow)* as it should and its tip *(black arrow)* crosses the midline and overlies the aorta, away from the location of the superior vena cava.

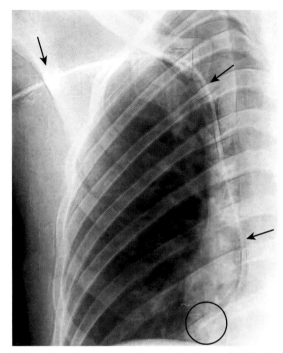

**Fig. 9.9 Peripherally Inserted Central Catheter (PICC) in Right Atrium.** A PICC *(arrows)* is inserted in the upper forearm or lower arm and fed through the axillary vein to the superior vena cava (SVC) or junction between the SVC and right atrium. In this case the tip extends to the region of the right atrium *(circle).*

small, they may be difficult to visualize radiographically (Fig. 9.9).
- **Incorrect placement and complications of peripherally inserted central catheters**
  - Tips may become **malpositioned** over time, rather than on initial insertion.
  - **Thrombosis** of the line may occur because of its small lumen size.

## Pulmonary Artery Catheters (Swan-Ganz Catheters)

- **Why they are used**
  - Monitor hemodynamic status of critically ill patients
  - Help in differentiating cardiac from noncardiac pulmonary edema
- **Correct placement of pulmonary artery catheters (also known as *pulmonary capillary wedge pressure catheters*)**
  - Pulmonary artery catheters **have the same appearance as central venous catheters but are longer.**
  - Inserted via the subclavian vein or internal jugular vein, their tips are floated out into the proximal right or proximal left pulmonary artery. The **tip of the pulmonary**

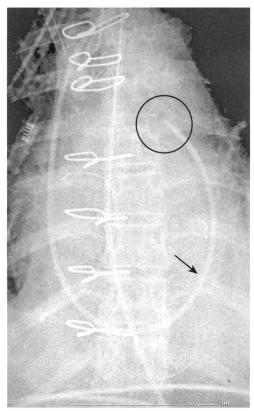

**Fig. 9.10** Pulmonary Artery (Swan-Ganz) Catheter in Correct Position. A pulmonary artery catheter *(arrow)* is a multilumen catheter that has the same appearance as a central venous line but its tip *(circle)* is "floated" out into the pulmonary artery through inflation of a small balloon at the tip. If the tip is "wedged" in a small pulmonary vessel, a measurement called **pulmonary capillary wedge pressure** can be made. In the presence of a normal mitral valve, this measurement reflects left atrial pressure.

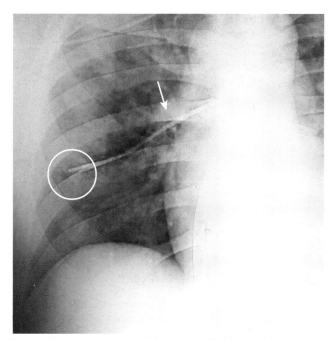

**Fig. 9.11** Pulmonary Artery Catheter with Tip Too Peripheral. The tip of this pulmonary artery catheter *(circle)* is located near the periphery of the right lung, too far from the right pulmonary artery *(arrow)*. The tip of this catheter should lie within 2 cm of the hilar shadow. The catheter was withdrawn because the tip in this location increases the risk of a complication, such as **pulmonary infarction** or **pseudoaneurysm** formation.

- **The catheter tip should not lie in a distal branch of a pulmonary artery** as this increases the risk of complication (Fig. 9.11).

## Multiple Lumen Catheters (Hemodialysis Catheters)

- **Why they are used**
  - Hemodialysis
  - Simultaneous ports for administration of medication and blood sampling
- **Correct placement of multiple lumen catheters for hemodialysis**
  - These are **large-bore catheters** that are **typically marked with a central stripe.**
  - There are many variations in design among different commercial brands but all have at least two lumens arranged coaxially inside a single catheter sheath with the goal to **minimize the amount of recirculation** that occurs between the two internal ports.
  - The **"arterial" port** from which blood is **withdrawn** from the patient is **proximal to the "venous" port** through which blood is **returned** to the patient to minimize recirculation of blood. Some catheters are designed as two, separate single-lumen catheters with one catheter tip in

---

artery catheter should be no more than about 2 cm from the hila (Fig. 9.10).
- A balloon at the catheter's tip is temporarily inflated only when pressure measurements are made and should then be deflated.
- **Incorrect placement and complications of pulmonary artery catheters**
  - Serious complications are **uncommon.**
  - The most common significant complication is **pulmonary infarction** from occlusion of a pulmonary artery by the catheter itself or from emboli arising from catheter.
  - Catheter tips peripherally located in the lung may produce a localized, confined blood vessel perforation *(pseudoaneurysm)* in the lung that can be recognized by sudden appearance of **consolidation** or a **mass** that forms at the **site of the catheter tip** in a critical care patient who also develops hemoptysis.

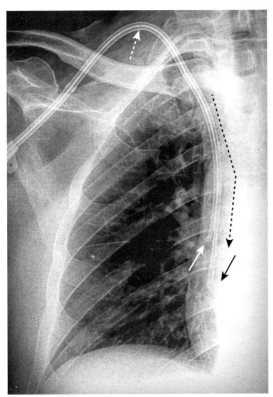

**Fig. 9.12 Double Lumen Hemodialysis Catheter in Correct Position.** These large-bore catheters with at least two lumens are typically marked with a central stripe *(dashed white arrow)*. Since the direction of blood flow is as indicated by the dashed black arrow, in order to minimize immediate recirculation the tip from which blood is **withdrawn** from the patient *(solid white arrow)* is more **proximal** than the tip through which blood is **returned** to the patient *(black arrow)*.

the superior vena cava and the other catheter tip in the right atrium (Fig. 9.12).
- The **right internal jugular** route is **most often used for access** and has the lowest incidence of clotting.
- **Incorrect placement and complications of multiple lumen catheters**
  - **Immediate complications** can include **pneumothorax** or **malposition** or **perforation** of the tip.
  - **Long-term complications** include **infection** and **thrombosis** of the vein containing the catheter or **occlusion** of the catheter itself.

# PLEURAL DRAINAGE TUBES

- **Why they are used**
  - To remove either air or abnormal collections of fluid from the pleural space
- **Correct placement of pleural drainage tubes**
  - Chest tubes are **wide-bore tubes** with a **radio-opaque stripe** used as a marker. The marker stripe is **discontinuous** at the site of a **side-hole.**
  - Ideal positioning is **anterosuperior for evacuating a pneumothorax** and **posteroinferior for draining an effusion**, but chest tubes usually work well no matter where positioned (Fig. 9.13).

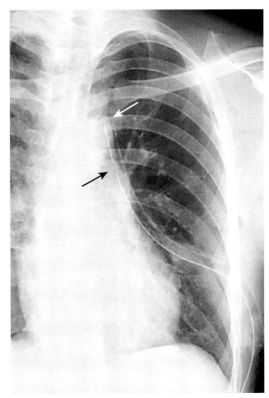

**Fig. 9.13 Chest Tube in Correct Position.** The chest tube has a side-hole *(black arrow)*. The white arrow points to the tip of the tube. Chest tubes are inserted in an intercostal space as close to the superior rib margin as possible because the intercostal nerves and blood vessels course along the lower margin of each rib. This tube was inserted for a pneumothorax, which has been evacuated.

- **None of the side-holes should lie outside of the thoracic wall.** If the side-hole extends outside of the chest wall, this can produce an *air-leak* leading to both inadequate drainage and subcutaneous emphysema (Fig. 9.14).

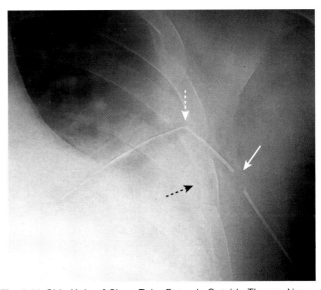

**Fig. 9.14 Side-Hole of Chest Tube Extends Outside Thorax.** None of the side-holes of a chest tube *(solid white arrow)* should lie **outside** the rib cage *(dashed black arrow)* as this one does. This can produce an *air-leak* leading to persistence of the underlying problem, in this case a pleural effusion. This tube is also **kinked** as it enters the chest *(dashed white arrow)*, which may further reduce its drainage efficiency.

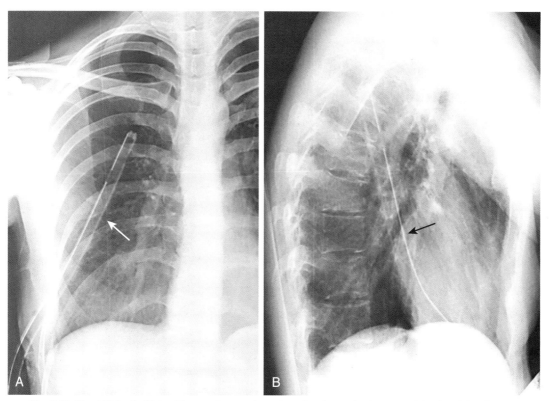

**Fig. 9.15 Chest Tube in Major Fissure.** Suspect insertion of a chest tube into one of the interlobar fissures when the tube is oriented along the course of the fissure. This tube lies within the right major fissure [*white arrow on the frontal view* (A) *and black arrow on the lateral view* (B)]. Malpositions like this can lead to inefficient drainage.

- **Incorrect placement and complications of pleural drainage tubes**
  - Most malpositions cause **inadequate drainage** rather than serious complication. This includes malpositions in which the tube is inadvertently placed in the major fissure (Fig. 9.15).
  - **Serious complications are uncommon** and include:
    - **Bleeding secondary to laceration of intercostal artery**
    - **Laceration of liver or spleen on insertion**
    - **Rapid reexpansion of a collapsed lung** caused either by a large pneumothorax or a large pleural effusion may lead to unilateral, ***reexpansion pulmonary edema.***

# CARDIAC DEVICES

## Pacemakers
- **Why they are used**
  - Used for cardiac conduction abnormalities
  - Certain conditions refractory to medical treatment (e.g., congestive heart failure)
- **Correct placement of cardiac pacemakers**
  - All pacemakers consist of a ***pulse generator*** usually implanted subcutaneously in the left anterior chest wall and **at least one lead** *(electrode)* inserted percutaneously, most often via the subclavian vein.

⟫ **IMPORTANT POINTS**

- The **tip of one lead is almost always located in the apex of the right ventricle.** Remember that **in the frontal projection, the apex of the right ventricle lies to the left of the spine** and on the lateral film the **apex of the right ventricle is anterior** (Fig. 9.16).

- Some pacemakers have two leads (usually their tips are in the right atrium and right ventricle) while others may have three leads (with their tips usually in the right atrium, right ventricle, and coronary sinus).
- **All leads should have gentle curves.** There should be no sharp kinks in the electrodes.
- **Incorrect placement and complications of cardiac pacemakers**
  - **Pneumothoraces** are infrequent complications of either pacemaker or automatic implantable cardiac defibrillator (AICD) insertion.
  - **Fracture of the leads** may occur at any of three places: the generator itself, the site of venous access, or the tip of the lead. Breaks in the lead can be **recognized by discontinuity in the wire lead** itself (Fig. 9.17).
  - **Leads can perforate the heart** producing cardiac tamponade. **Look for sharp bends** in leads secondary to perforation of a blood vessel.

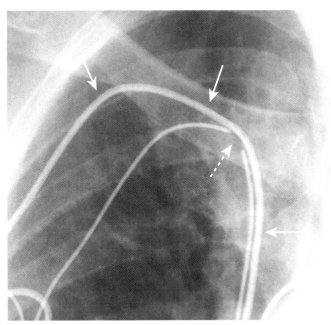

**Fig. 9.17 Fractured Pacemaker Lead.** Fractures of pacemaker or automatic implantable cardiac defibrillator (AICD) leads may occur at any of three places. In this patient, the break *(dashed arrow)* occurred at the point of insertion into the subclavian vein. The broken lead had been discovered earlier and a second, intact lead is already in place *(solid arrows)*.

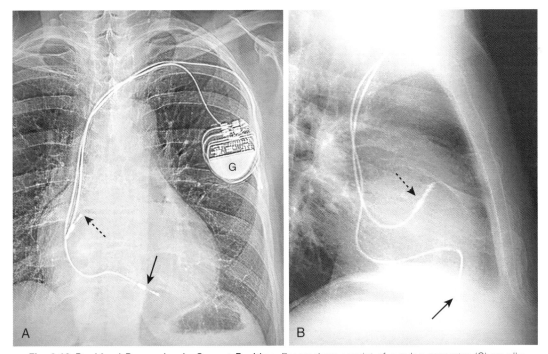

**Fig. 9.16 Dual-lead Pacemaker in Correct Position.** Pacemakers consist of a pulse generator (G) usually implanted in the left chest wall and one or more electrode leads inserted via the subclavian vein. This patient has a **dual-lead** pacemaker. One of the leads is in the apex of the right ventricle *[solid arrow in (A) and (B)]* while the other lead is in the right atrium *[dashed arrow in (A) and (B)]*. Notice that the right ventricular lead *(solid black arrows)* normally projects to the left of the midline (A) and anteriorly (B), and the right atrial lead typically curls upward in (A) and (B).

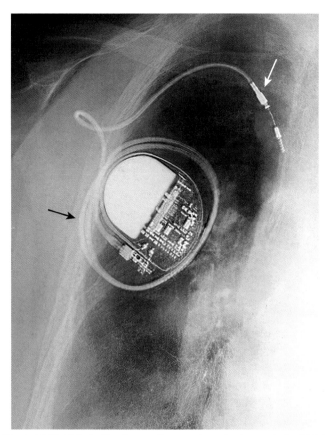

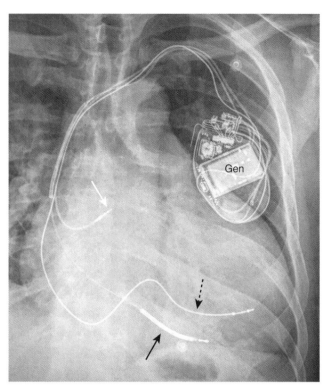

**Fig. 9.18** Twiddler's Syndrome. Some patients inadvertently "twiddle" with their subcutaneous pulse generator and, if the subcutaneous tissue allows, may rotate the generator repeatedly on its own axis over time, curling the lead(s) around the device *(black arrow)*. This can retract the tip of the electrode from the inner wall of the right ventricle, rendering the pacemaker useless. This lead has retracted to the superior vena cava *(white arrow)*. "Twiddling" can also affect an AICD or chest infusion port.

**Fig. 9.19** Automatic Implantable Cardiac Defibrillator (AICD). The generator (Gen) for an AICD is placed in the subcutaneous tissue of the anterior chest wall (pectoral area). AICDs have a thicker segment which is part of the defibrillation coil or coils *(solid white and black arrows)*. The electrodes are fed through the superior vena cava with their tips in the right atrium *(solid white arrow)* and the apex of the right ventricle *(solid black arrow)*. This AICD has a third lead that entered the coronary sinus *(dashed black arrow)*.

- Leads may retract from normal contact with the ventricular wall because the patient twists or *twiddles* the pacemaker generator under the skin, unknowingly winding the leads around the generator and causing retraction of the tips *(Twiddler's syndrome)* (Fig. 9.18) or from subcutaneous migration of the pacer.
- Leads may be **ectopically placed,** e.g., in the hepatic vein.

## Automatic Implantable Cardiac Defibrillators (AICD)

- **Why they are used**
  - To prevent sudden death, usually from tachyarrhythmias like ventricular fibrillation or ventricular tachycardia
- **Correct placement of automatic implantable cardiac defibrillators**
  - AICDs can usually be **differentiated from pacemakers by the wider and more opaque segment of at least one of the electrodes** (Fig. 9.19). One electrode is usually

placed in the superior vena cava or brachiocephalic vein. If another electrode is used, its tip is placed in the apex of the right ventricle.
  - **All bends in the leads should be smooth curves,** not sharp kinks.
- **Incorrect placement and complications of automatic implantable cardiac defibrillators**
  - Leads may **migrate** and become dislodged
  - Leads may **fracture**

## Intra-aortic Balloon Pump (IABP)

- **Why they are used**
  - To improve cardiac output and improve perfusion of the coronary arteries following surgery or in patients with cardiogenic shock or refractory ventricular failure.
  - Placed in the proximal **descending** thoracic aorta, a long, cylindrical **balloon** is **inflated** in **diastole**, increasing blood flow to the coronary arteries, and is **deflated** in **systole**, which reduces the cardiac afterload.
- **Correct placement of intra-aortic balloon pumps**

- The tip can be identified by a small, linear metallic marker (Fig. 9.20). The tip should lie distal to the origin of the left subclavian artery so as not to occlude it.

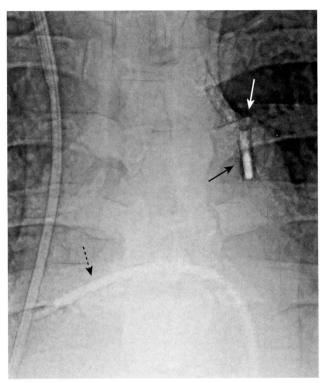

**Fig. 9.20 Intra-aortic Balloon Pump (IABP).** Inserted via the femoral artery, a long "hot dog–shaped" balloon is rhythmically inflated during early diastole and deflated during early systole. The tip can be identified by a small, linear metallic marker in the region of the descending thoracic aorta *(solid black arrow)*. The tip should lie distal to origin of the left subclavian artery so as not to occlude it. This is usually about 2 cm from the **top of the aortic arch** *(solid white arrow)*. There is also a Swan-Ganz catheter in place in the right pulmonary artery *(dashed black arrow)*.

- The metallic marker may point slightly toward the right in the region of aortic arch.
- When inflated, the sausage-shaped balloon may be visualized as an air-containing structure in the descending thoracic aorta.
- **Incorrect placement and complications of intra-aortic balloon pumps**
  - If the catheter is **too proximal**, the inflated balloon may **occlude the great vessels** leading to stroke.
  - If the balloon is **too distal**, the device has **decreased effectiveness.**
  - Aortic dissection and arterial perforation may occur infrequently.

# GASTROINTESTINAL TUBES

## Nasogastric Tubes (NGT)

- **Why they are used**
  - Short-term feeding
  - Gastric sampling and decompression through suction
  - Administering medication
- **Correct placement of nasogastric tubes**
  - Nasogastric tubes are **wide tubes** (about 1 cm) marked with a **radio-opaque stripe** that is **discontinuous** at a **side-hole,** usually about **10 cm from the tip.**
  - **The tip and any side-holes** of the tube should **extend about 10 cm into the stomach beyond the esophagogastric (EG) junction** to prevent aspiration after administration of a feeding into the esophagus (Fig. 9.21).

> **▶ IMPORTANT POINTS**
>
> - **How to recognize the location of the EG junction**
>   - The **EG junction** is usually **located** near the **junction of the left hemidiaphragm** and the **left side** of the **thoracic spine** (see Fig. 9.21A).

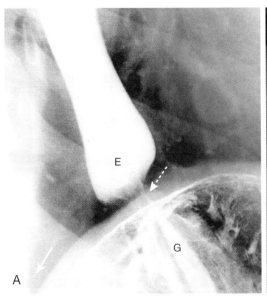

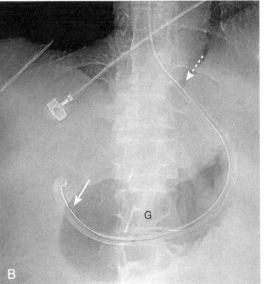

**Fig. 9.21 Normal Esophagogastric Junction; Nasogastric Tube in Stomach.** (A) This is a close-up view of the left lower thorax from an upper gastrointestinal series to illustrate the close proximity of the esophagogastric (EG) junction *(dashed arrow)* to the junction of the left hemidiaphragm and the spine *(solid arrow),* thus allowing the diaphragmatic junction to serve as a landmark for the position of the EG junction. (B) In a different patient, an NGT enters the stomach at the EG junction *(dashed arrow)* and extends around the greater curvature of the stomach almost to the pylorus. The "break" in the marker stripe *(solid arrow)* marks the location of the side-hole, about 10 cm from the tip. *E,* Esophagus; *G,* stomach.

- **Incorrect placement and complications of nasogastric tubes**
  - The **nasogastric tube is the most commonly malpositioned of all tubes and lines.**
    - **Coiling of the NG tube in the esophagus is the most common malposition.**
    - It may be **inadvertently inserted into the trachea** and enter a bronchus (Fig. 9.22).
    - **Perforation** caused by an NG tube is **rare** but, when it occurs, it usually occurs in the cervical esophagus.
    - A long-term, indwelling NG tube **can lead to gastroesophageal reflux** that may, in turn, produce **esophagitis** and **stricture**.
  - Always obtain a confirmatory radiograph before feeding the patient or administering any medication through the tube.

## Feeding Tubes (Dobbhoff Tubes)

- **Why they are used**
  - Used for nutrition

- **Correct placement of feeding tubes**
  - The ideal position of the **tip of the feeding tube is considered to be postpyloric, i.e., in the duodenum or jejunum,** the rationale being to reduce risk of aspiration after feeding (Fig. 9.23). In fact, placement in the stomach is very common.
  - The tip of a feeding tube is recognizable by a weighted, metallic, linear density attached to the tip.
  - Did you know that the Dobbhoff tube was not named after a person called "Dobbhoff?" The tube is named after two physicians, Drs. Dobbie and Hoffmeister.
- **Incorrect placement and complications of feeding tubes**
  - Placement in the **trachea** rather than the esophagus may lead to the tip entering the **lung.** Always obtain a confirmatory radiograph before feeding the patient (Fig. 9.24).
  - **Perforation of the esophagus by the guidewire** is an uncommon complication.
    - Once the guidewire is removed, it is not reinserted.

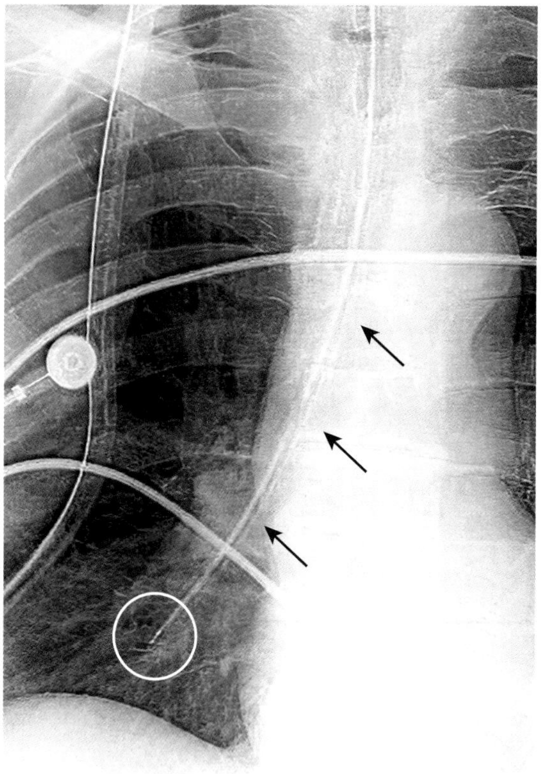

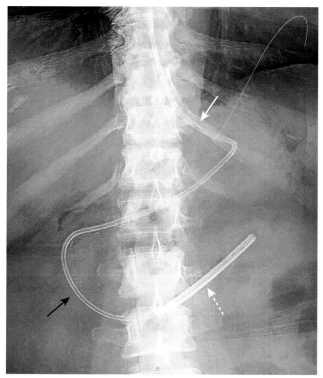

**Fig. 9.22 Nasogastric Tube in Right Lower Lobe Bronchus.** In this patient, the nasogastric tube *(arrows)* lies in the trachea instead of the esophagus and its tip extends to the right lower lobe of the lung *(circle)*. A radiograph to confirm positioning of a nasogastric tube is obtained before using it for feeding.

**Fig. 9.23 Feeding Tube in Duodenum.** The tip is usually recognizable by a weighted, metallic end *(dashed arrow)*. This feeding tube enters the stomach *(solid white arrow)*, courses around the duodenal sweep *(solid black arrow)*, and ends at the junction between the fourth portion of the duodenum and the jejunum.

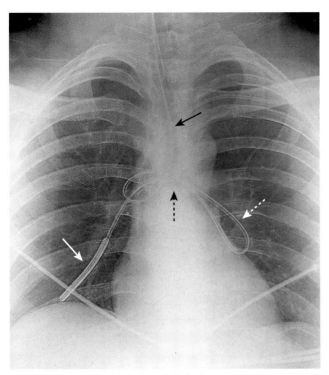

Fig. 9.24 Feeding Tube in Left and Right Lower Lobe Bronchi. In this case the feeding tube inadvertently entered the trachea *(solid black arrow)* and was advanced so that it looped back and forth from the left lower lobe bronchus *(dashed white arrow)* across the carina *(dashed black arrow)* to end in the right lower lobe bronchus *(solid white arrow)*.

## CASE QUIZ 9 ANSWER

The central venous catheter *(solid white arrow)* is malpositioned. Instead of its tip crossing the midline and descending behind the right clavicular head into the superior vena cava, it has wandered off into the left internal jugular vein *(black arrow)*. Also, the tip of the endotracheal tube *(dashed white arrow)* is less than 2 cm from the carina and should be withdrawn slightly.

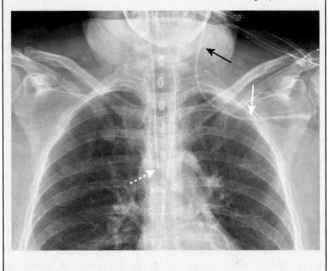

## 🏠 TAKE HOME POINTS

**Tube or Line\*: Desired position**

**Endotracheal tube (ETT):** Tip 3 to 5 cm from carina; usually, half the distance between the medial clavicles and carina

**Tracheostomy tube tip:** Halfway between stoma and carina

**Central venous catheter (CVC):** Tip in superior vena cava

**Peripherally inserted central catheter (PICC):** Tip in superior vena cava

**Swan-Ganz catheter:** Tip in proximal right or left pulmonary artery, within 2 cm from hilum

**Double lumen (hemodialysis) catheters:** Tips in either superior vena cava or right atrium (or both) depending on type of catheter

**Pleural drainage tube:** Anterosuperior for pneumothorax; posteroinferior for pleural effusion

**Pacemaker:** Tip at apex of right ventricle; other lead(s) in right atrium and/or coronary sinus

**Automatic implantable cardiac defibrillator (AICD):** One lead in superior vena cava; other lead(s) in right ventricle and/or coronary sinus

**Intra-aortic balloon pump (IABP):** Tip about 2 cm from top of aortic arch in descending thoracic aorta

**Nasogastric tube (NGT):** Tip in stomach, 10 cm from esophagogastric junction

**Feeding tube (Dobbhoff):** Tip ideally in the duodenum, but more frequently in stomach

\*Additional devices discussed online include: valve replacements, left ventricular assist devices, the Impella pump, left atrial occlusion clips, implantable loop recorders, coronary artery stents, tissue expanders, and percutaneous endoscopic gastrostomy tubes. See e-Fig. 9.1 to e-Fig. 9.10.
🛜 Additional content is available online including chapters on Nuclear Medicine, Artificial Intelligence, Radiation Dose and Safety, an Early History of Radiology, and a compendium of 200 Diagnostic Radiology Signs.

# 10

# Recognizing Other Diseases of the Chest

*William Herring, MD, FACR*

In this chapter, you will learn how to recognize mediastinal masses, benign and malignant pulmonary neoplasms, pulmonary thromboembolic disease, and selected airway diseases.

**CASE QUIZ 10 QUESTION**

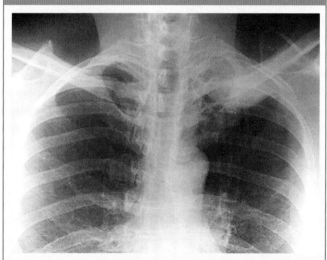

This is a view of the lung apices in a 73-year-old male with shoulder pain, a drooping eyelid, and constricted pupil on one side. You can deduce which side from the x-ray. What is the most likely diagnosis from the clinical history and this chest radiograph? See the correct answer at the end of this chapter.

- Several chest abnormalities are discussed in other chapters (Table 10.1).
- A discussion of all of the diseases imaged in the chest fills multivolume textbooks so we will concentrate on mediastinal masses and work our way outward to some of the most common lung diseases.

## MEDIASTINAL MASSES

- The mediastinum is an area whose **lateral margins are defined by the medial borders of each lung,** whose **anterior margin** is the **sternum and anterior chest** wall, and whose **posterior margin is the spine,** usually including the paravertebral gutters.
- The mediastinum has been arbitrarily subdivided into **three compartments** based on the **lateral chest x-ray:** the *anterior, middle, and posterior* compartments and each contains

its favorite set of diseases. The *superior mediastinum,* roughly the area above the plane of the aortic arch, is a division that is now usually combined with one of the other three compartments mentioned previously (Fig. 10.1).

| TABLE 10.1 Chest Abnormalities Discussed Elsewhere in This Text | |
|---|---|
| **Topic** | **Appears in** |
| Atelectasis | **Chapter 6** |
| Pleural effusion | **Chapter 7** |
| Pneumonia | **Chapter 8** |
| Pneumothorax, pneumomediastinum, and pneumopericardium | **Chapter 24** |
| Cardiac and thoracic aortic abnormalities | **Chapter 11** |
| Chest trauma | **Chapter 24** |

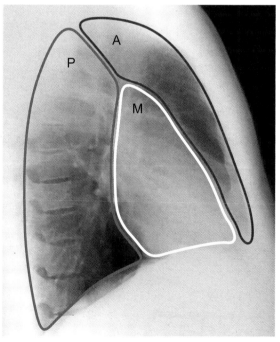

**Fig. 10.1 The Mediastinal Compartments.** Based on the chest radiograph, the anterior mediastinum extends from the back of the sternum to the anterior border of the heart and great vessels (A). The middle mediastinum extends from the anterior border of the heart and aorta to the posterior border of the heart and origins of the great vessels (M). The posterior mediastinum extends from the posterior border of the heart to the anterior border of the vertebral column (P). For most purposes, the posterior mediastinum also includes the paravertebral gutters.

- A newer classification, based primarily on CT, defines virtually the same three compartments mentioned previously but names them the *prevascular, visceral,* and *paravertebral* compartments. The new system was designed to be a universal classification system accepted by all specialties and based on **cross-sectional imaging** rather than chest radiography. For the purposes of this text, we will use the terms anterior, middle, and posterior mediastinum.

> ### ! DIAGNOSTIC PITFALLS
>
> - Since these compartments have no true anatomic boundaries, **diseases from one compartment may extend into another compartment.**
> - When a mediastinal abnormality becomes widespread or a mediastinal mass becomes quite large, it is often impossible to determine which compartment was its site of origin.

- **Differentiating a mediastinal mass from a parenchymal lung mass on frontal and lateral chest** radiographs can be difficult. Some helpful clues include:
  - If a **mass is completely surrounded by lung tissue on both the frontal and lateral projections, it lies within the lung,** not the mediastinum.
  - In general, **the margin of a mediastinal mass is sharper** than a mass originating in the lung.
  - Mediastinal masses frequently **displace, compress, or obstruct** other mediastinal structures (e.g., the trachea or esophagus).
- Ultimately, **CT imaging** of the chest is **more accurate** in determining the location and nature of a mediastinal mass than conventional radiographs.

## ANTERIOR MEDIASTINAL MASSES

- The **anterior mediastinum** is the compartment that extends from the **back of the sternum** to the **anterior border of the heart and great vessels.** In the newer classification, the term anterior mediastinum is replaced by the term **prevascular compartment** but contains almost the same elements.
- There is a **differential diagnosis for anterior mediastinal masses** that most often includes:
  - Substernal **thyroid masses**
  - **Lymphoma**
  - **Thymoma,** and
  - **Teratoma**
  - As a helpful way of remembering these four diseases, lymphoma is referred to as "Terrible lymphoma" in this list so that all of the diseases "start" with the letter "T" (Table 10.2).

### Thyroid Masses

- In **everyday practice, enlarged substernal thyroids** are the **most frequently encountered anterior mediastinal mass.**

### TABLE 10.2  Anterior Mediastinal Masses ("Four T's")

| Mass | What to Look for |
|------|------------------|
| **Thyroid goiter** | The only anterior mediastinal mass that routinely deviates the trachea |
| **Lymphoma (lymphadenopathy)** | Lobulated, polycyclic mass; frequently asymmetric; may occur in any compartment of the mediastinum |
| **Thymoma** | Look for a well-marginated mass that may be associated with myasthenia gravis |
| **Teratoma** | Well-marginated mass that may contain fat and calcium visible on CT scans |

The vast majority of these masses are *multinodular goiters* and the mass is called a *substernal goiter, substernal thyroid,* or *substernal thyroid goiter.*
- Multinodular goiters usually present as a mass in the neck, mostly in females. After a few decades, most patients with a multinodular goiter will develop hyperthyroidism. It is uncommon for them to be malignant.
- Substernal goiters characteristically displace the trachea either to the left or right **above the level of the aortic arch,** a tendency the other anterior mediastinal masses do not typically demonstrate.

> ### » IMPORTANT POINTS
>
> - Classically, **substernal goiters do not extend below the top of the aortic arch** (Fig. 10.2).
> - You should **think of an enlarged substernal thyroid** whenever you see **an anterior mediastinal mass that displaces the trachea.**

- On occasion, the isthmus or lower pole of either lobe of the thyroid may enlarge but project **downward** into the upper

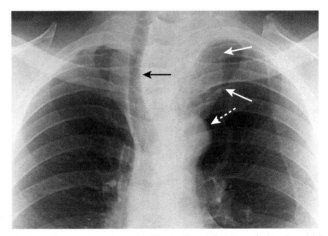

**Fig. 10.2 Substernal Thyroid Mass.** The left lobe of the thyroid is enlarged and projects downward into the upper thorax *(solid white arrows)* displacing the trachea to the right *(black arrow).* Note the mass does not extend below the top of the aortic arch *(dashed arrow).*

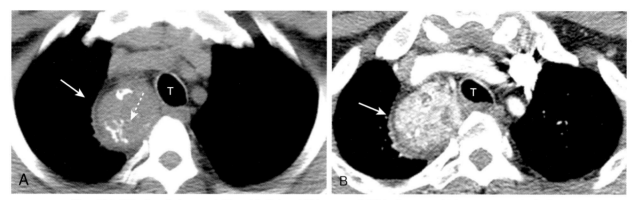

**Fig. 10.3** CT of a Substernal Thyroid Goiter Without and With Contrast Enhancement. (A) Before administration of intravenous contrast, this substernal thyroid mass *(solid white arrow)* is seen to be well-defined and contains coarse calcifications *(dashed white arrow)*. (B) After contrast administration and at the same level as before, the goiter avidly enhances with intravenous contrast, with a mottled appearance *(solid white arrow)*. This mass is displacing the trachea (T) slightly to the left.

thorax rather than **anteriorly** into the neck. About three out of four thyroid masses extend anterior to the trachea; the remaining 25% (almost all of which are right-sided) descend posterior to the trachea.

- Radioisotope **thyroid scans are the study of first choice** in confirming the diagnosis of a substernal thyroid as virtually all of them will display some uptake of the radioactive tracer that can be imaged and recorded with a special camera (see **e-Appendix A. Nuclear Medicine: Understanding the Principles and Recognizing the Basics**).

- **On CT,** substernal thyroid masses are part of and **contiguous with the thyroid gland,** frequently **contain calcification,** and **avidly take up intravenous contrast** but **with a mottled, inhomogeneous appearance** (Fig. 10.3).

## Lymphoma

- **Lymphadenopathy,** whether from lymphoma, metastatic carcinoma, sarcoid, or tuberculosis, is the most common cause of mediastinal masses overall.
- **Anterior mediastinal lymphadenopathy is most common in Hodgkin lymphoma, especially the nodular sclerosing variety.** Hodgkin lymphoma is a malignancy of the lymph nodes, more common in females, which most often presents with painless, enlarged lymph nodes in the neck.
- Unlike teratomas and thymomas, which are presumed to expand outward from a single abnormal cell, lymphomatous masses are frequently composed of several contiguously enlarged lymph nodes. As such, **lymphadenopathy frequently presents with a border that is lobulated** or **polycyclic in contour** due to the conglomeration of enlarged nodes that make up the mass.

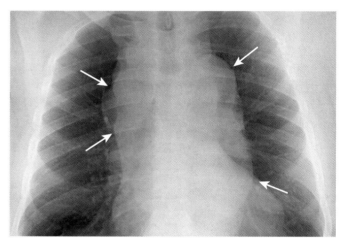

**Fig. 10.4** Mediastinal Adenopathy from Hodgkin Lymphoma. Lymphadenopathy frequently presents with a lobulated or polycyclic border due to the conglomeration of enlarged nodes that produce the mass *(arrows)*. Hodgkin lymphoma is usually confined to nodes above the diaphragm. Pain in the affected lymph nodes after alcohol consumption is a classical but uncommon sign of the disease.

> ### ⯈⯈ IMPORTANT POINTS
>
> - On chest radiographs, this lobulation **may help differentiate lymphadenopathy from other mediastinal masses** that may demonstrate a smoother contour.

- **Mediastinal lymphadenopathy** in **Hodgkin lymphoma** is usually **bilateral and asymmetric** (Fig. 10.4). In addition, asymmetric **hilar adenopathy** is associated with mediastinal adenopathy in many patients with Hodgkin lymphoma.

- In general, **mediastinal lymph nodes that exceed about 1 cm** measured along their **short axis** on CT scans of the mediastinum are **considered to be enlarged.**
- Lymphoma will **produce multiple, lobulated soft-tissue masses** or one **large, soft-tissue mass** from lymph node aggregation.
- The **mass is usually homogeneous** in density on CT (Fig. 10.5) but **may be heterogeneous** when it achieves a sufficient size to undergo **necrosis** (areas of lower attenuation, i.e., blacker) or **hemorrhage** (areas of higher attenuation, i.e., whiter).
- Some findings of lymphoma may **mimic** those of **sarcoidosis** since both produce thoracic adenopathy. Table 10.3 contains several key points to differentiate the two diseases.

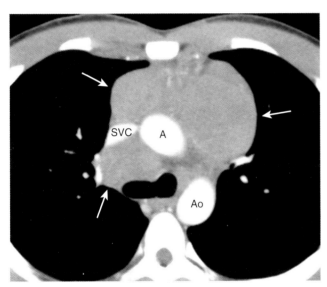

**Fig. 10.5 Anterior Mediastinal Adenopathy in Hodgkin Lymphoma.** On CT, lymphadenopathy will produce multiple, lobulated soft-tissue masses or a large soft-tissue mass from lymph node aggregation *(arrows)*. The mass is usually homogeneous in density, as in this case. The superior vena cava (SVC) is compressed, but not occluded, by the nodes. *A,* Ascending aorta; *Ao,* descending aorta.

## Thymic Masses

- **Normal thymic tissue can be visible on CT throughout life**, although the gland begins to **involute after age 20.**
- **Thymomas** are neoplasms of thymic epithelium and lymphocytes. They occur most often in **middle-aged adults**, generally at an **older** age than those with **teratomas.** Most thymomas are **benign.**

> ### ▶▶ IMPORTANT POINTS
>
> - Thymomas are **associated with myasthenia gravis about 35% of the time** they are present.
> - Conversely, about **15% of patients with** clinical **myasthenia gravis will** be found to **have a thymoma.**
> - The importance of identifying a thymoma in patients with myasthenia gravis lies in the more **favorable prognosis** for patients with myasthenia **after thymectomy.**

- On **CT scans, thymomas** classically present as a **smooth or lobulated mass** that arises near the **junction of the heart and great vessels** and which, like a teratoma, **may contain calcification** (Fig. 10.6).
- Other lesions that can produce enlargement of the thymus are rare and include thymic cysts, thymic hyperplasia, thymic lymphoma, carcinoma, or lipoma.

| TABLE 10.3 **Sarcoidosis vs. Lymphoma** | |
| --- | --- |
| **Sarcoid** | **Lymphoma** |
| Bilateral hilar and right paratracheal adenopathy are the classic combination | More often dominated by mediastinal adenopathy, but is associated with asymmetric hilar enlargement |
| Enlarged bronchopulmonary nodes are more peripheral | Enlarged hilar nodes are more central |
| Pleural effusion in about 5% | Pleural effusion more common, in about 30% |
| Anterior mediastinal adenopathy is uncommon | Anterior mediastinal adenopathy is common |

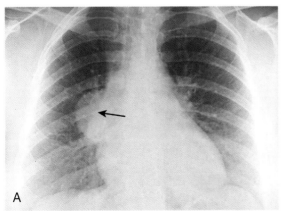

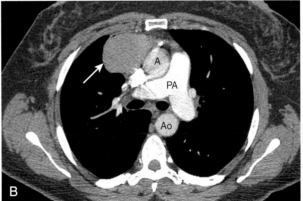

**Fig. 10.6 Thymoma, Chest Radiograph and CT Scan.** (A) The chest radiograph shows a smoothly marginated anterior mediastinal mass *(arrow)*. (B) Contrast-enhanced CT scan confirms the anterior mediastinal location and homogeneous density of the mass *(arrow)*. The patient had myasthenia gravis and improved following resection of the thymoma. *A,* Ascending aorta; *Ao,* descending aorta; *PA,* main pulmonary artery.

## Teratoma

- Teratomas are **germinal tumors** that typically **contain all three germ layers** (ectoderm, mesoderm, and endoderm). Most teratomas are benign and occur earlier in life than thymomas. Usually **asymptomatic** and discovered serendipitously, about **30% of mediastinal teratomas are malignant** and have a poor prognosis.
- The most common variety of teratoma is **cystic**, produces a **well-marginated mass** near the origin of the great vessels, and characteristically **contains fat, cartilage, and possibly bone on CT examination** (Fig. 10.7).

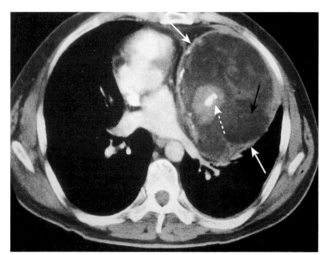

**Fig. 10.7 Mediastinal Teratoma.** This well-marginated, cystic teratoma arises near the origin of the great vessels. On CT, they characteristically contain fat *(black arrow)*, cartilage, and sometimes bone *(dashed white arrow)*. They are usually benign, well-encapsulated with an enhancing rim, as in this case *(solid white arrows)*. Treatment is surgical excision.

## MIDDLE MEDIASTINAL MASSES

- The **middle mediastinum** is the compartment that extends from the **anterior border of the heart and aorta** to the **posterior border of the heart** and contains the **heart**, the **origins of the great vessels, trachea,** and **main bronchi** along with **lymph nodes** (see Fig. 10.1). In the newer CT classification, the term **middle mediastinum** is replaced by the term *visceral compartment* and it extends farther posteriorly to include part of the mediastinum overlying the vertebral column.
- **Lymphadenopathy produces the most common mass in this compartment.** While Hodgkin lymphoma is the most likely cause of mediastinal adenopathy, other malignancies and several benign diseases can produce such findings.
  - Other malignancies that produce mediastinal lymphadenopathy include **small cell lung carcinoma** and **metastatic disease** such as from primary **breast carcinoma** (Fig. 10.8).
  - Benign causes of mediastinal lymphadenopathy include **infectious mononucleosis** and **tuberculosis,** the latter usually producing **unilateral mediastinal adenopathy.**

## POSTERIOR MEDIASTINAL MASSES

- The **posterior mediastinum** is the compartment that extends from the **posterior border of the heart** to the **anterior border of the vertebral column.** For imaging purposes, however, it is **considered to extend to either side of the spine into the paravertebral gutters** (see Fig. 10.1).
- The posterior mediastinum contains the **descending aorta, esophagus, lymph nodes,** is the site of masses representing **extramedullary hematopoiesis,** and, most importantly, is the home of **tumors of neural origin.** In the newer classification, the term posterior mediastinum is replaced by the term *paravertebral compartment* and contains almost exclusively neurogenic lesions.

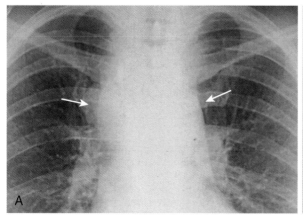 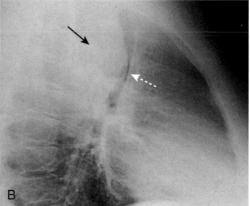

**Fig. 10.8 Middle Mediastinal Lymphadenopathy.** Mediastinal adenopathy may be "reactive" (e.g., tuberculosis), malignant (e.g., lymphoma, small cell lung carcinoma, and metastatic disease), or even occur with autoimmune diseases like systemic lupus erythematosus. This patient has a mediastinal mass demonstrated on both the frontal (A) *(arrows)* and lateral (B) views *(black arrow)*. The mass is pushing the trachea forward on the lateral view *(white arrow)*. The biopsied lymph nodes in this patient demonstrated small cell carcinoma of the lung.

## Neurogenic Tumors

- Although neurogenic tumors produce the largest percentage of posterior mediastinal masses, none of these lesions is particularly common. Neurogenic tumors include such entities as **neurofibroma, Schwannoma, ganglioneuroma,** and **neuroblastoma.**
- *Nerve sheath tumors (Schwannoma)* are the **most common** and are almost always **benign.** They usually affect persons 20 to 50 years of age and, since they are slow growing, may produce no symptoms until late in their course.
- Neoplasms that arise from nerve elements **other than the sheath,** like *ganglioneuromas* and *neuroblastoma,* are usually malignant.
- **Neurogenic tumors** will produce a soft-tissue **mass, usually sharply marginated,** in the paravertebral gutter (Fig. 10.9).

Both benign and malignant tumors **may erode adjacent ribs.** They may **enlarge neural foramina** producing *dumbbell*-shaped lesions that arise from the spinal canal but project through the neural foramen into the mediastinum (Fig. 10.10A).

- **Neurofibromas** most often occur as an **isolated tumor** arising from the Schwann cell of the nerve sheath **or as part of a syndrome** called *neurofibromatosis, type 1 (NF1).* As part of the latter, they are a component of a neurocutaneous bone dysplasia that can cause numerous abnormalities including **subcutaneous nodules, erosion of adjacent bone (*rib notching*), scalloping** of the posterior aspect of the vertebral bodies (Fig. 10.10B), **absence of the sphenoid wings,** *pseudarthroses,* and **sharp-angled kyphoscoliosis** at the thoracolumbar junction.

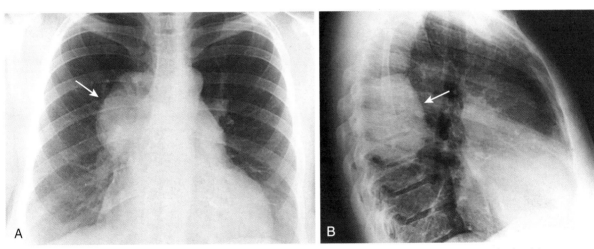

**Fig. 10.9 Neurofibromatosis.** There is a large, posterior mediastinal neurofibroma *(arrows)* seen in the right, paravertebral gutter on the frontal (A) and lateral (B) views. This patient had the syndrome of *neurofibromatosis, type 1 (NF1).*

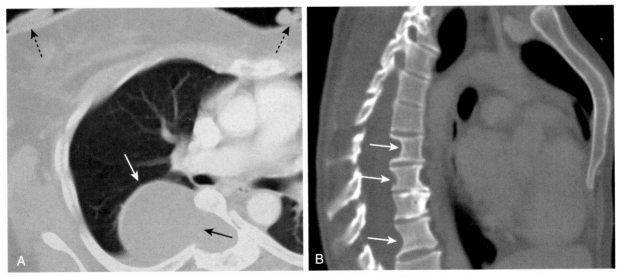

**Fig. 10.10 Dumbbell-shaped Neurofibroma and Posterior Scalloping.** (A) This patient demonstrates a large neurofibroma that is enlarging the neural foramen, eroding half of the vertebral body *(solid black arrow)*, and producing a dumbbell-shaped lesion that arises from the spinal canal but projects through the foramen into the mediastinum *(white arrow)*. Several cutaneous neurofibromas are visible on the skin surface *(dashed black arrows)* (B) In another patient, there is *scalloping* of the posterior vertebral bodies *(arrows)*, especially in the thoracic spine as shown in this sagittal CT. This is produced by diverticula of the thecal sac caused by dysplasia of the meninges that leads to erosion of adjacent bone through the pulsations transmitted via the spinal fluid.

## SOLITARY NODULE/MASS IN THE LUNG

- **The difference between a *nodule* and a *mass* is size:** in general, under 3 cm it is usually called a *nodule* and over 3 cm a *mass.*
- Much has been written about the workup of a patient in whom a single nodular density is discovered in the lung on imaging of the thorax, i.e., the *solitary pulmonary nodule (SPN).* It is estimated that as many as 50% of smokers have a nodule discovered by chest CT, yet a tiny percentage of small nodules show any malignant tendencies (growth or metastases) when followed for years.
- In evaluating a solitary pulmonary nodule, the **critical question** to be answered is: **is the nodule most likely benign or most likely malignant?** If most likely benign, it can be watched in follow-up whereas, if most likely malignant, it will almost certainly be managed aggressively

with therapies that themselves carry some risk of morbidity and mortality.
- The answer to the question of benign versus malignant will depend on many factors including the availability of **prior imaging studies** that **can help greatly in establishing stability of a lesion over time** (Fig. 10.11).
- Many nodules are discovered **incidentally** during CT imaging of the lung for an unrelated disease or CT imaging of another body part that contains part of the lungs (e.g., an abdominal CT that includes the lung bases). It is estimated about 1.5 million incidental, solitary pulmonary nodules are found each year in the United States, a number that has been increasing.
- Based on their **appearance on CT**, small nodules have been divided into those with a *solid* appearance versus those with a *subsolid* appearance. The CT appearance of nodules aids in

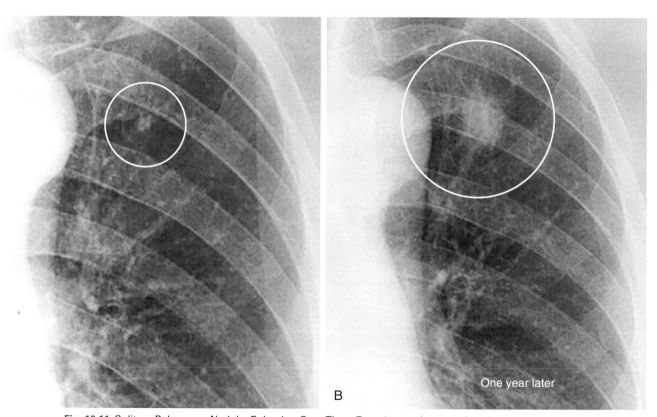

A                                                                                    B

**Fig. 10.11 Solitary Pulmonary Nodule, Enlarging Over Time.** Two close-up images taken 1 year apart are shown. (A) A small nodular density is present in the left upper lobe *(circle)* on an image obtained for comparison when image (B) was acquired 1 year later, by which time the nodule has clearly increased in size and shows an irregular outer margin, suggestive of malignancy *(circle).* Biopsy of the lesion demonstrated adenocarcinoma.

the clinical and radiologic management of their significance and follow-up (Fig. 10.12).

- **Subsolid nodules** are further divided into those that are **purely ground-glass nodules** and those that are **partly solid and partly ground-glass.**
- A *ground-glass nodule* is an area of increased attenuation (whiter) on CT in which the vascular and bronchial markings are **preserved** within the nodule, rather than obliterated by the nodule. Subsolid nodules are important because, when persistent, they may represent **adenocarcinoma** or its precursors (see Fig. 10.11).

- In 2017, an international society of chest radiologists (Fleischner Society) revised a previous set of evidence-based criteria establishing guidelines for the follow-up of **noncalcified nodules** found **incidentally** during **CT** in **adults** over 35 years of age. Their recommendations are shown in Table 10.4.
  - In summary, the new guidelines suggest a less-needed follow-up than previously for many stable, incidental

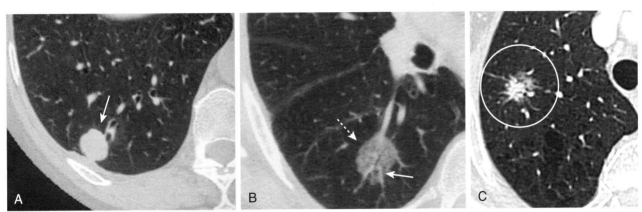

**Fig. 10.12 Solitary Pulmonary Nodules, CT Patterns.** Based on their appearance on CT, small nodules are divided into those with a **solid appearance** (A) *(arrow)* versus those with a **subsolid appearance. Subsolid nodules** are further divided into those that are **purely ground-glass nodules** (B) *(dashed arrow)* and those that are **partly solid and partly ground-glass** (C) *(circle)*. Note that the vascular markings are still visible in a ground-glass nodule (B) *(solid arrow)*. The malignancy rate for subsolid nodules is higher than that of solid nodules and the malignancy rate for partly solid nodules is higher than the rate for pure ground-glass nodules.

## TABLE 10.4 Fleischner Society Criteria for Follow-up of Incidental, Noncalcified Solitary Pulmonary Nodules

### Single Solid[a] Nodules

| Nodule Size (mm) | Less than 6 mm (<6 mm) | 6–8 mm | Greater than 8 mm (>8 mm) |
|---|---|---|---|
| **Low risk patients[b]** | No routine follow-up | CT at 6–12 months; then consider CT at 18–24 months | Consider CT at 3 months, PET/CT, or tissue sampling |
| **High risk patients[c]** | Optional CT at 12 months | CT at 6–12 months; then CT at 18–24 months | Consider CT at 3 months, PET/CT, or tissue sampling |

### Single Subsolid[d] Nodules

| Nodule Size (mm) | Less than 6 mm | ≥6 mm |
|---|---|---|
| Ground-glass[e] | No routine follow-up | CT at 6–12 months to confirm persistence; then CT every 2 years until 5 years |
| Partly solid | No routine follow-up | CT at 3–6 months to confirm persistence. If unchanged and solid component remains <6 mm, annual CT should be performed for 5 years. |

[a]**Solid nodules** are <3 cm well-circumscribed areas of increased attenuation (whiter) on CT that are homogeneous in appearance (see Fig. 10.12A).
[b]**Low risk patients:** Younger age, minimal or no smoking history, regular margin to nodule, location of nodule in an area **other** than upper lobe.
[c]**High risk patients:** Older age, heavy smoker, upper lobe location, irregular or spiculated nodule margins.
[d]**Subsolid nodules** are <3 cm well-circumscribed areas of increased attenuation that are either **purely ground-glass** nodules (see Fig. 10.12B) in appearance or **partly ground-glass and partly solid** nodules (see Fig. 10.12C).
[e]**Ground-glass nodules** are <3 cm well-circumscribed areas of greater attenuation on CT in which the bronchial and vascular markings are preserved rather than obliterated (see Fig. 10.12B).
*CT,* Computed tomography; *PET,* positron emission tomography.
From MacMahon H, Naidich DP, Goo JM, et al. Guidelines for management of incidental pulmonary nodules detected on CT images: From the Fleischner Society 2017. *Radiology* 2017;284:228–243.

solitary pulmonary nodules. Those that are **solid** and **unchanged** on serial CTs over a **2-year** period, or **subsolid** and **unchanged** over a **5-year** period, are likely benign and **do not need further diagnostic evaluation.**

## Signs of a Benign Versus Malignant Solitary Pulmonary Nodule

- **Size of the lesion.** Nodules less than 6 mm rarely show malignant behavior. Masses **larger than 5 cm have a 95% chance of malignancy** (Fig. 10.13).
- **Calcification.** The presence of calcification is usually determined by CT. **Lesions containing central, laminar, or diffuse patterns of calcification are invariably benign** (Fig. 10.14).
- **Margin.** Lobulation, spiculation, and shagginess all suggest malignancy (see Fig. 10.13).
- **Change in size over time.** Requires a previous study or sufficient confidence so as to obtain a follow-up study that will provide a basis of comparison of size over time.
  - **Malignancies** tend to **increase in size at a rate that is not so brief as to suggest an inflammatory etiology** (i.e., changes in weeks) **nor so prolonged as to suggest benignity** (i.e., no change over 2 years) (see Fig. 10.11).
    - Large cell carcinomas, as a cell type, grow the most rapidly.
    - Squamous cell carcinomas and small cell carcinomas tend to grow slightly less rapidly.
    - **Adenocarcinomas** grow the **most slowly.**

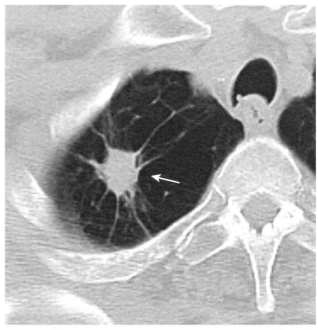

**Fig. 10.13 Right Upper Lobe Bronchogenic Carcinoma.** There is a large spiculated mass in the right upper lobe *(arrow)*. The relatively large size and irregular margins of this mass are consistent with a bronchogenic carcinoma. A percutaneous biopsy revealed an adenocarcinoma of the lung.

---

> ▶▶ **IMPORTANT POINTS**
>
> - **Presence of clinical symptoms as sign of malignancy.** When there are clinical signs or symptoms present (e.g., hemoptysis, weight loss, hoarseness), the chance that a pulmonary nodule is malignant increases.
> - Solitary pulmonary nodules that are surgically removed from those who showed **clinical signs or symptoms** and imaging findings that suggested malignancy are **malignant about 50% of the time in men over the age of 50.**

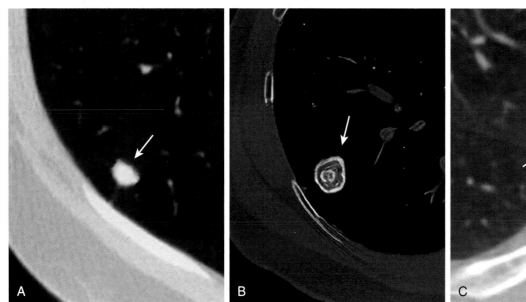

**Fig. 10.14 Calcified Granulomas.** When a pulmonary nodule is heavily calcified, it is almost always benign. (A) **Homogeneous calcification** *(arrow)* is common in tuberculous granulomas that are frequent sequelae of prior, usually subclinical tuberculous infection. (B) **Laminated calcification** *(arrow)* may also be seen in tuberculous granulomas and are signatures of a benign nodule. (C) **Target calcification** or central calcification *(black arrow)* can be seen in histoplasmomas *(white arrow)* and is diagnostic. CT can be used to differentiate between a calcified and a noncalcified pulmonary nodule with greater sensitivity than conventional radiographs.

- **Positron emission tomographic scans (PET scans)** can also help in differentiating benign from malignant nodules and provide insight into the site of any metastatic disease. Using a glucose analog (**fluorodeoxyglucose or FDG**), the test is based on the enhanced glucose metabolism and uptake of lung cancer cells. Usually, the nodules must be >1 cm in size for accurate characterization as being *PET-avid* (i.e., most likely malignant) (see **e-Appendix A. Nuclear Medicine: Understanding the Principles and Recognizing the Basics**).

## Benign Causes of Solitary Pulmonary Nodules

- **Granulomas.** Tuberculosis and histoplasmosis usually produce calcified nodules <1 cm in size, although tuberculomas and histoplasmomas can reach up to 4 cm.
  - **When calcified, they are clearly benign. Tuberculous** granulomas are usually **homogeneously calcified. Histoplasmomas** may have a laminated calcification or may contain a **central** or *target* **calcification**, which is diagnostic (see Fig. 10.14).

- **Hamartomas.** These are peripherally located lung tumors of **disorganized lung tissue** that characteristically **contain fat and calcification** on CT scan. The **classical calcification** of a hamartoma is called *popcorn calcification* (Fig. 10.15).
- Other, uncommon benign lesions that can produce solitary pulmonary nodules include rheumatoid nodules, fungal diseases like nocardiosis, arteriovenous malformations, and granulomatosis with polyangiitis (Wegener granulomatosis).

## BRONCHOGENIC CARCINOMA

- In the United States **lung cancer is the most common fatal malignancy in men** and the **second most common in women** (next to breast cancer).
- The **number** of nodules in the lung can help direct the workup. **Primary lung cancer** usually presents as a **solitary nodule or mass** while **metastatic disease** to the lung from another organ characteristically produces **multiple nodules/ masses.**

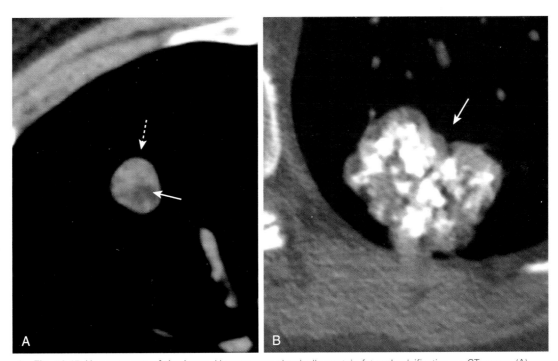

**Fig. 10.15 Hamartomas of the Lung.** Hamartomas classically contain fat and calcification on CT scans. (A) This smoothly marginated lung nodule *(dashed arrow)* contains fat *(solid arrow)* on CT, a clue that this is a hamartoma. (B) This large and heavily calcified lesion contains amorphous calcification likened to **popcorn** in appearance *(arrow)*. Since you are about halfway through this chapter, now might be a good time to reward yourself with a treat of some real popcorn (if you can).

## TABLE 10.5   Carcinoma of the Lung: Cell Types

| Cell Type and Clinical Manifestations | Graphic Representation | Cell Type and Clinical Manifestations | Graphic Representation |
|---|---|---|---|
| **Squamous Cell Carcinoma**<br>• Primarily central in location<br>• Arise in segmental or lobar bronchi<br>• Invariably produce bronchial obstruction leading to obstructive pneumonitis or atelectasis<br>• Tend to grow rapidly | | **Small Cell, Including Oat Cell Carcinoma**<br>• Primarily central in location<br>• Many contain neurosecretory granules that lead to an association of small cell carcinoma with paraneoplastic syndromes, such as Cushing syndrome, inappropriate secretion of antidiuretic hormone | |
| **Adenocarcinoma**<br>• Primarily peripheral in location<br>• Usually solitary except in the case of diffuse adenocarcinoma, which can present as multiple nodules<br>• Slowest growing | | **Large Cell Carcinoma**<br>• Diagnosis of exclusion for lesions that are non-small cell, and not squamous or adenocarcinoma<br>• Larger peripheral lesions<br>• Grow extremely rapidly | |

- Table 10.5 summarizes the classical manifestations and growth tendencies of the four **types** of bronchogenic carcinoma by cell type.
- **Recognizing a bronchogenic carcinoma**
  - They may be recognized by visualization of the **tumor itself**: i.e., a **nodule/mass in the lung** (see Figs. 10.12 and 10.13).
  - They may be suspected by recognizing the **effects of bronchial obstruction**: i.e., **pneumonitis** and/or **atelectasis**.
  - They may be suspected by recognizing the results of either their **direct extension or metastatic spread** to the lung, ribs, or to other organs.

## Bronchogenic Carcinomas Presenting as a Nodule/Mass in the Lung

- These are most often **adenocarcinomas.**
- The nodule/mass may have **irregular** and **spiculated margins** (see Fig. 10.14).
- The mass **may cavitate**, more often if it is of **squamous cell** origin (although cavitation also occurs with adenocarcinoma), usually producing a **relatively thick-walled** cavity with a **nodular and irregular inner margin** (Fig. 10.16).

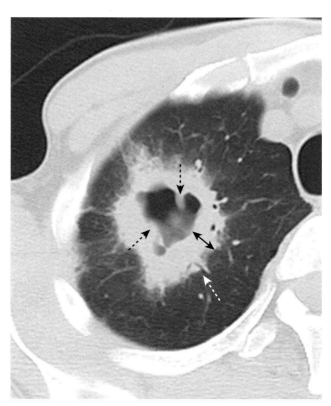

**Fig. 10.16 Cavitary Bronchogenic Carcinoma.** There is a large, cavitating neoplasm in the right upper lobe with a thick wall *(double black arrow)*, spiculated outer margin *(dashed white arrow)*, and a nodular internal margin *(dashed black arrows)*. Lung cancers can cavitate due to degeneration of the tumor itself or they can obstruct a bronchus leading to a more distal pneumonia that then cavitates. This was a squamous cell carcinoma.

## Bronchogenic Carcinoma Presenting with Bronchial Obstruction

- **Bronchial obstruction is most often caused by a squamous cell carcinoma.** Endobronchial lesions produce varying degrees of bronchial obstruction that can lead to pneumonitis or atelectasis.
  - **Obstructive pneumonitis and atelectasis** (see Fig. 6.11).
    - It is called *pneumonitis* because the obstructed lung is consolidated but frequently not infected (though it can be).
    - **Atelectasis** secondary to an endobronchial, obstructing lesion features the usual shifts of the fissures or mobile mediastinal structures **toward** the side of the atelectasis (see Chapter 6) as well as occasional visualization of the obstructing mass itself.

## Bronchogenic Carcinoma Presenting with Direct Extension or Metastatic Lesions

- **Rib destruction by direct extension.** *Pancoast tumor* is the eponym for a tumor arising from the superior sulcus of the lung, frequently producing destruction of one or more of the first three ribs on the affected side (Fig. 10.17 and Box 10.1).
- **Hilar adenopathy.** Usually unilateral on the same side as the tumor (Fig. 10.18).

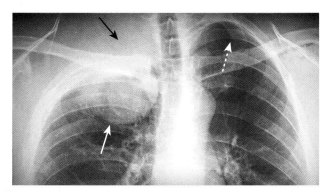

**Fig. 10.17 Pancoast Tumor, Right Upper Lobe.** A large soft-tissue mass is seen in the apex of the right lung *(solid white arrow)*. It is associated with rib destruction *(black arrow)*. On the normal left side, note the ribs are intact *(dashed white arrow)*. The finding of an apical soft-tissue mass with associated rib destruction is classical for a **Pancoast (superior sulcus) tumor**. The patient had swelling of the face from obstruction of the superior vena cava.

### BOX 10.1 Pancoast Tumor: Apical Lung Cancer (see Fig. 10.17)

- Manifests as a soft-tissue mass in the apex of the lung
- Most often adenocarcinoma or squamous cell carcinoma
- Frequently produces adjacent rib destruction
- May invade brachial plexus or cause Horner syndrome on affected side
- On the right side, it may produce superior vena caval obstruction

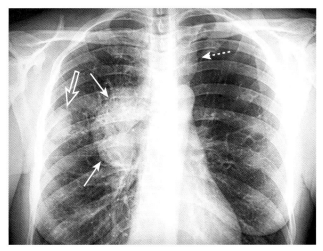

**Fig. 10.18 Bronchogenic Carcinoma with Hilar and Mediastinal Adenopathy.** There is a peripheral lung mass *(open arrow)* with evidence of ipsilateral hilar and mediastinal adenopathy *(solid arrows)* and contralateral mediastinal adenopathy *(dashed arrow)*. Spread to the mediastinal nodes on the side opposite the tumor tends to worsen prognosis for lung cancers. This was an adenocarcinoma of the lung.

- **Mediastinal adenopathy.** May be the sole manifestation of a small cell carcinoma, the peripheral lung nodule itself being invisible (see Fig. 10.8).
- **Other nodules in the lung.** One of the manifestations of adenocarcinoma primary to the lung itself may be multiple nodules throughout both lungs and, as such, may mimic metastatic disease.
- **Pleural effusion.** Frequently, there is associated lymphangitic carcinomatosis in the lung when there is a pleural effusion.
- **Metastases to bones.** These tend to be mixed osteolytic and osteoblastic.

## METASTATIC NEOPLASMS IN THE LUNG

### Multiple Nodules

- Multiple nodules in the lung are most often metastatic lesions that have traveled through the bloodstream from a distant primary *(hematogenous spread)*. Multiple metastatic nodules are **usually of slightly differing sizes** indicating tumor embolization that occurred at different times.
- The nodules are **frequently sharply marginated**, varying in size from **micronodular** (see Fig. 4.8B) to *cannonball* **masses**.
- For all practical purposes it is **impossible to determine the primary site** by the **appearance of the metastatic nodules**, i.e., all metastatic nodules appear similar.

### ▶▶ IMPORTANT POINTS

- Tissue sampling, whether by bronchoscopic or percutaneous biopsy, is the best means of determining the organ of origin of the metastatic nodule.

- Table 10.6 summarizes the primary malignancies most likely to metastasize to the lung hematogenously.

## Lymphangitic Carcinomatosis (Lymphangitic Spread of Carcinoma)

- With lymphangitic carcinomatosis, the tumor grows in and obstructs lymphatics in the lung producing a pattern that is **radiologically similar to pulmonary interstitial edema** from heart failure including **Kerley B lines, thickening of the fissures,** and **pleural effusions.**

> ## ▶▶ IMPORTANT POINTS
>
> - The findings **may be unilateral** or may **involve only one lobe,** a pattern that should alert you to suspect the possibility of lymphangitic carcinomatosis rather than congestive heart failure, which is usually bilateral (Fig. 10.19).

### TABLE 10.6 Some Common Primary Sites of Metastatic Lung Nodules

| Males | Females |
|---|---|
| Colorectal carcinoma | Breast cancer |
| Renal cell carcinoma | Colorectal carcinoma |
| Head and neck tumors | Renal cell carcinoma |
| Testicular and bladder carcinoma | Cervical or endometrial carcinoma |
| Malignant melanoma | Malignant melanoma |
| Sarcomas | Sarcomas |

- The **most common primary malignancies to produce lymphangitic carcinomatosis** are those that arise in or around the thorax: **breast, lung, and pancreatic carcinoma.**

## PULMONARY THROMBOEMBOLIC DISEASE (PE)

- Over **90% of pulmonary emboli develop from thrombi in the deep veins of the leg**, especially above the level of the popliteal veins. They are usually a **complication of surgery** or **prolonged bed rest** or **cancer.** Because of the **dual** circulation of the lungs (pulmonary and bronchial), **most pulmonary emboli do not result in infarction.**
- Although conventional chest radiographs **are** frequently abnormal in patients with PE, they mostly demonstrate nonspecific findings like **subsegmental atelectasis, small pleural effusions,** or **elevation of the hemidiaphragm. Conventional chest radiography** has a **high false-negative rate in detecting PE.**
- Chest radiographs **infrequently** manifest one of the "classic" findings for **pulmonary embolism,** which can include:
  - Wedge-shaped peripheral airspace disease (*Hampton hump*) (Fig. 10.20).
  - Focally absent or decreased pulmonary vasculature (*Westermark sign*) (see **e-Appendix F. Diagnostic Radiology Signs).**

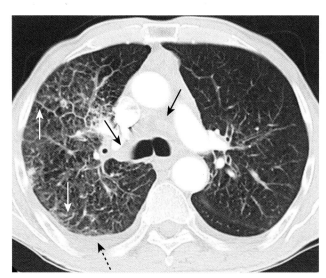

**Fig. 10.19 Bronchogenic Carcinoma with Lymphangitic Carcinomatosis.** There is extensive hilar and mediastinal adenopathy *(solid black arrows)* from a carcinoma of the lung. The interstitial markings are prominent in the right lung compared with the left and there are thickened interlobular septa (Kerley B lines) present *(white arrows)* along with a right pleural effusion *(dashed black arrow).* Adenocarcinomas are the most common cause of lymphangitic carcinomatosis. Tumor cells can usually be found in the lymphatics and pleural fluid.

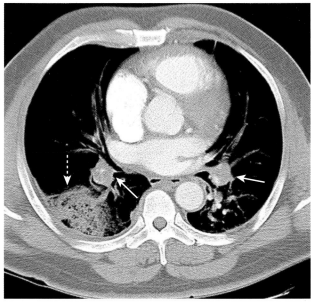

**Fig. 10.20 Hampton Hump.** A wedge-shaped, peripheral airspace density is present *(dashed arrow)* and associated with filling defects in both the left and right pulmonary arteries *(solid arrows)* representing blood clots. The wedge-shaped infarct is called a **Hampton hump.** Without the associated emboli being present, the peripheral airspace disease could have a differential diagnosis that includes pneumonia, lung contusion, or aspiration.

- **A prominent central pulmonary artery** *(knuckle sign)* (see e-Appendix F. Diagnostic Radiology Signs).

> ▶ **IMPORTANT POINTS**
>
> - If the chest radiograph is normal, a nuclear medicine ventilation-perfusion scan (V/Q scan) may be diagnostic. If, however, the chest radiograph is abnormal, CT is usually performed.

- **CT pulmonary angiography (CT-PA)** is made possible by the **fast data acquisition** of **spiral CT** scanners (one breath hold) combined with **thin slices** and **rapid bolus intravenous injection of iodinated contrast** that produce maximal opacification of the pulmonary arteries with little or no motion artifact.
- Another benefit of CT-PA studies is the ability to acquire images of the veins of the pelvis and legs by obtaining slightly delayed images following the pulmonary arterial phase of the study. In this way, **a deep venous thrombus** may be detected even if the pulmonary angiogram is nondiagnostic.
- CT-PA has a sensitivity **in excess of 90%** and has replaced the use of V/Q scans in patients with **chronic obstructive pulmonary disease** or a **positive chest radiograph** in whom a V/Q scan is known to be less sensitive.

- On CT-PA, acute **pulmonary emboli** appear as **partial or complete filling defects centrally located** within the **contrast-enhanced** lumina of the **pulmonary arteries** (Fig. 10.21).
- CT-PA has the **additional benefit** of **demonstrating other diseases** that may be present, like pneumonia, even if the study is negative for pulmonary embolism. CT-PA is also part of the diagnostic imaging examination called the ***triple rule-out*** in which patients presenting with **chest pain** can be simultaneously evaluated for **coronary artery disease, aortic dissection,** and **pulmonary embolism.**

## CHRONIC OBSTRUCTIVE PULMONARY DISEASE

- Chronic obstructive pulmonary disease (COPD) is defined as a disease **of airflow obstruction due to** *chronic bronchitis* **or** *emphysema.*
- **Chronic bronchitis** is defined **clinically** by **productive cough** whereas **emphysema** is defined **pathologically** by the presence of **permanent and abnormal enlargement and destruction of the air spaces distal to the terminal bronchioles.**

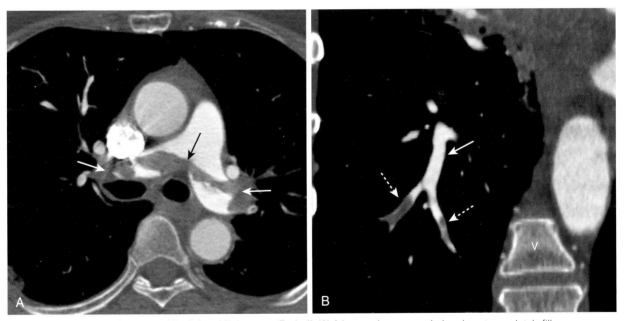

**Fig. 10.21 Saddle and Peripheral Pulmonary Emboli.** (A) A large pulmonary embolus almost completely fills both the left and right pulmonary arteries *(arrows)* in this contrast-enhanced CT. This is called a ***saddle embolus*** because it straddles several major pulmonary arteries. (B) Small, central filling defects *(dashed arrows)* are seen in a more peripheral pulmonary artery *(solid arrow)*. This pulmonary artery seems to be floating disconnected in the lung because the plane of this particular image does not display its connection to the pulmonary artery.

- On conventional radiographs, **the most reliable finding of COPD is hyperinflation,** including **flattening of the diaphragm,** especially on the **lateral** exposure (Fig. 10.22). Other findings may include an **increase** in the **retrosternal clear space, hyperlucency** of the lungs with fewer than normal vascular markings visible, and **prominence of the pulmonary arteries** from pulmonary arterial hypertension.
- **With CT, findings of COPD** may include **focal areas of low density** in which the cystic areas lack visible walls except where bounded by interlobular septa. CT is helpful in evaluating the extent of emphysematous disease and in planning for surgical procedures designed to remove bullae to reduce lung volume.
- **Emphysema has three pathologic patterns visible on CT:**
  - *Centriacinar (centrilobular) emphysema* features focal destruction limited to the respiratory bronchioles and the central portions of the acinus. It is **associated with cigarette smoking** and is most severe in the **upper lobes** (Fig. 10.23A).
  - *Panacinar (panlobular) emphysema* involves the entire alveolus distal to the terminal bronchiole. It is most

severe in the **lower lung zones** and generally develops in patients with homozygous *alpha 1-antitrypsin deficiency* (Fig. 10.23B).
- *Paraseptal emphysema* involves distal airway structures, alveolar ducts, and sacs. Localized to fibrous septa or to the pleura, it can lead to formation of bullae, which **may cause pneumothorax.** It is not associated with airflow obstruction (Fig. 10.23C).

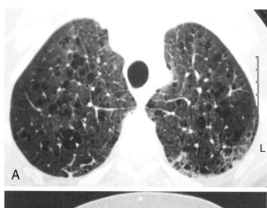

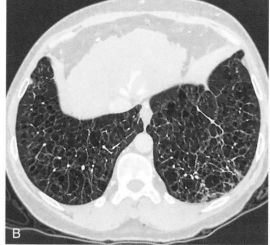

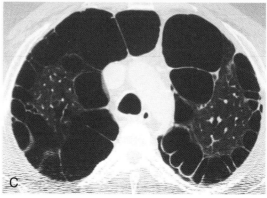

**Fig. 10.23** Types of Emphysema. (A) *Centriacinar (centrilobular) emphysema* is the most common type and is most severe in the upper lobes. It has a strong association with cigarette smoking. (B) *Panlobular (panacinar) emphysema* is most severe in the lower lung zones and generally develops in patients with homozygous alpha1-antitrypsin deficiency, although it can also be seen in smokers and the elderly. (C) *Paraseptal emphysema* tends to occur around the septae of the lungs or subpleural surfaces and may lead to pneumothorax.

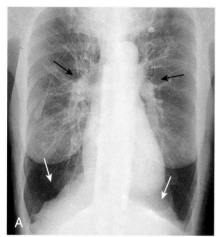

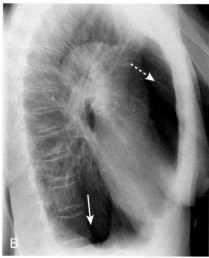

**Fig. 10.22** Emphysema, Conventional Radiography. On conventional radiographs, the imaging findings of chronic obstructive pulmonary disease are hyperinflation, including flattening of the diaphragm *(white arrows)*, increase in the size of the retrosternal clear space *(dashed arrow)*, hyperlucency of the lungs with decreased vascular markings, and enlargement of the pulmonary arteries secondary to pulmonary arterial hypertension *(black arrows)*.

## BULLAE, CYSTS, AND CAVITIES

- Bullae (singular: bulla), cysts, and cavities are all **air-containing lesions in the lung** of differing **size, location,** and **wall composition.**
- Almost any of these lesions can contain **fluid** instead of, or in addition to, air.
- Fluid usually develops as a result of **infection, hemorrhage,** or **liquefaction necrosis.**
- When these lesions are **completely filled with fluid,** they **will appear uniform in density** on conventional radiographs and CT scans, but they will typically demonstrate a **low CT number** that will differentiate them from a truly solid tumor.
- When they contain some fluid and some air, they will manifest an **air-fluid level** on a conventional radiograph (exposed with a horizontal x-ray beam) (Fig. 10.24) or on CT scans.

### Bullae

- Bullae measure **more than 1 cm** in size. They are usually **associated with emphysema.** They occur in the **lung parenchyma** and have a **very thin wall** (<1 mm) that is frequently **only partially visible** on conventional radiography but well seen on CT. On **conventional radiographs** their **presence is often inferred** by a localized paucity of lung markings (Fig. 10.25).
- They can **grow to fill the entire hemithorax** and compress the lung to such an extent on the affected side that the lung seems to disappear *(vanishing lung syndrome) (see e-Appendix F. Diagnostic Radiology Signs).*

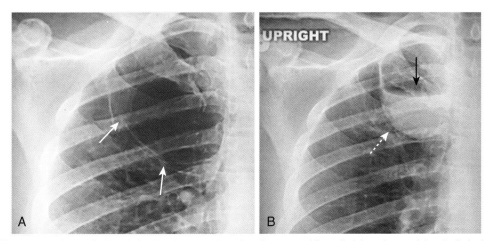

**Fig. 10.24 Infected Bulla.** (A) In this close-up, there is at least one thin-walled, but air-containing, bulla in the right upper lobe *(arrows)*. (B) Several weeks later, the bulla appears smaller *(white arrow)* but now contains both fluid and air *(black arrow)*. Bullae typically occur at the lung apex and are usually asymptomatic in and of themselves. Patients with infected bullae tend to be less sick than those with a lung abscess, which an infected bulla can mimic.

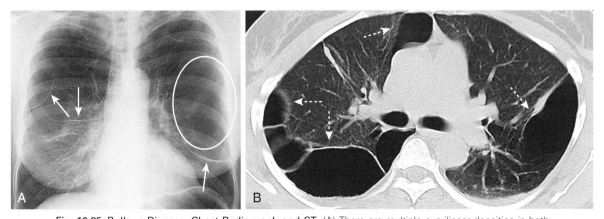

**Fig. 10.25 Bullous Disease, Chest Radiograph and CT.** (A) There are multiple curvilinear densities in both lungs representing the walls of bullae *(arrows)*. A paucity of lung markings is seen in the left mid lung *(oval)* consistent with bullous disease. (B) Multiple, thin-walled bullae are demonstrated by CT *(arrows)*. Characteristically, they contain no blood vessels but there may be septae that appear to traverse the bulla. Bullae may slowly increase in size and are associated with pneumothorax. If large and compromising the remainder of normal lung, they can be surgically resected.

- **Blebs** are **very small** bullae that usually form in the visceral pleura, mostly at the lung **apex.** They may be seen by CT but are too small to be visible on chest radiographs. They are thought to be associated with spontaneous pneumothoraces.

## Cysts

- Lung **cysts** are either **congenital** or **acquired.** They can occur in either the **lung parenchyma** or the **mediastinum.** They have a **thin wall** that is usually thicker than that of a bulla (**<3 mm**).
  - *Pneumatoceles* represent acquired **thin-walled cysts** that usually develop after a lung infection caused by such organisms as *Staphylococcus* or *Pneumocystis* (Fig. 10.26).

## Cavities

- Cavities can **vary in size** from a few millimeters to many centimeters. They occur in the **lung parenchyma** and usually result from a process that produces **necrosis** of the central portion of the lesion.
- Cavities usually have the **thickest wall** of any of these air-containing lesions **with a wall thickness from 3 mm to several cm** (see Fig. 10.16).
- Differentiation between three of the most frequent causes of cavities (carcinoma, tuberculosis, and pyogenic abscess) is summarized in Table 10.7.

## BRONCHIECTASIS

- Bronchiectasis is defined as **localized irreversible dilatation of part of the bronchial tree.** Although it can be associated with many other diseases, it is **usually caused by necrotizing bacterial infections** like those of *Staphylococcus* and *Klebsiella* and it usually affects the lower lobes.
- Bronchiectasis may also occur with cystic fibrosis, primary ciliary dyskinesia (**Kartagener syndrome**), allergic bronchopulmonary aspergillosis, and **Swyer-James syndrome** (unilateral hyperlucent lung).
- Clinically, **chronic productive cough** frequently associated with **hemoptysis** are the major symptoms.

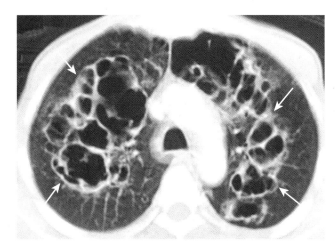

**Fig. 10.26 Cysts (Pneumatoceles) in Pneumocystis Pneumonia (PCP).** Cysts are visible on chest radiographs in 10% of patients with PCP and far more frequently with CT scans (up to 1 in 3 patients). They may occur in the acute or in the postinfective phase of the disease. They have a predilection for the upper lobes and are commonly multiple *(arrows).* Their etiology is unclear.

### TABLE 10.7 Differentiating Three Cavitating Lung Lesions

| Lesion | Thickness of the Cavity Wall | Inner Margin of Cavity |
| --- | --- | --- |
| **Bronchogenic carcinoma** (Fig. 10.27A) | Thick[a] | Nodular |
| **Tuberculosis** (Fig. 10.27B) | Thin | Smooth |
| **Lung abscess** (Fig. 10.27C) | Thick | Smooth |

[a]Thick = more than 5 mm; thin = less than 5 mm.

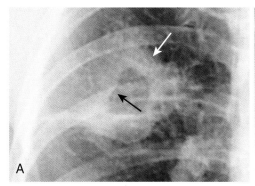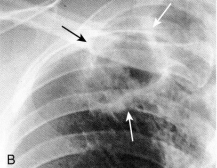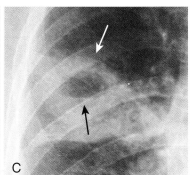

A    B    C

**Fig. 10.27 Cavitary Lesions of the Lung.** Three of the most common cavitary lesions of the lung can frequently be differentiated from each other by noting the **thickness** of the **wall** of the cavity and the **smoothness** or nodularity of its **inner margin.** (A) Squamous cell bronchogenic **carcinoma** characteristically produces a cavity with a thick wall *(white arrow)* and a nodular interior margin *(black arrow);* (B) **Tuberculosis** usually produces a relatively thin-walled, upper lobe cavity with a smooth inner margin *(arrows).* (C) A **lung abscess** typically demonstrates a thickened wall *(white arrow)* that, in this case, has a cavity with a smooth inner margin and an air-fluid level *(black arrow).*

- **Conventional radiographs** may demonstrate findings suggestive of the disease but are **usually not specific.**
  - Findings include parallel-line opacities (***tram-tracks***) due to thickened, dilated bronchial walls, **cystic lesions** as large as 2 cm in diameter due to cystic bronchiectasis, and **tubular densities** from fluid-filled bronchi (Fig. 10.28).
- **CT is the study of choice for diagnosing bronchiectasis.**
  - The hallmark lesion on CT is the ***signet ring sign*** in which the **bronchus**, frequently with a thickened wall, **becomes larger than its associated pulmonary artery,** which is the opposite of the normal relationship between the two. The bronchus may also show a failure to taper normally (Fig. 10.29).

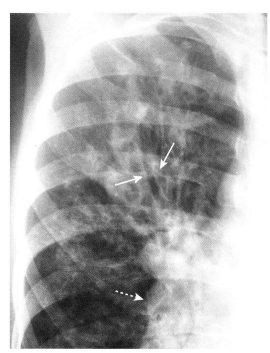

**Fig. 10.28 Bronchiectasis in Cystic Fibrosis.** Conventional radiographs may demonstrate parallel-line opacities called ***tram-tracks*** due to thickened walls of dilated bronchi *(solid arrows)*. Progressive, bilateral upper lobe bronchiectasis in children is highly suggestive of cystic fibrosis, an autosomal recessive disease secondary to dysfunction of exocrine glands. The hila may be prominent from either hilar adenopathy or pulmonary arterial hypertension *(dashed arrow)*.

**CASE QUIZ 10 ANSWER**

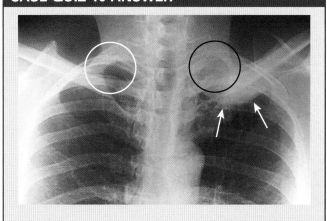

There is a soft-tissue mass in the left lung apex *(arrows)* associated with destruction of the left 2nd and 3rd ribs *(black circle)* consistent with a **Pancoast tumor** of the lung. (Compare the ribs in the black circle with the normal ribs in the white circle). The ocular findings can be explained by involvement of the cervical sympathetic chain (Horner syndrome) and the shoulder pain from invasion of the brachial plexus. In general, Pancoast tumors have a relatively poor prognosis in part because of their proximity to such critical structures.

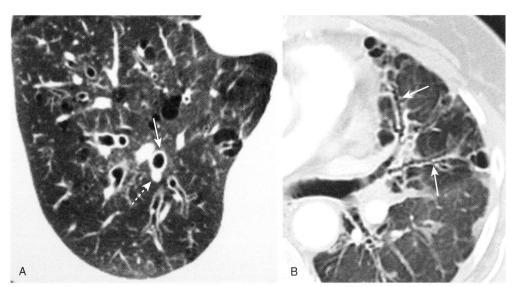

A          B

**Fig. 10.29 Bronchiectasis, CT.** (A) The key sign in bronchiectasis is the ***signet ring sign*** in which the bronchus with a thickened wall *(solid arrow)* becomes larger than its associated pulmonary artery *(dashed arrow)*. (B) The bronchi may also show ***tram-tracking,*** thickened walls, and a failure to taper normally *(arrows)*. An absence of the normal tapering of the bronchi is one of the most sensitive signs on CT. Cylindrical or tubular bronchiectasis, such as this, is the least severe of several types of bronchiectasis.

## TAKE HOME POINTS

- The mediastinum lies in the central portion of the thorax between the two lungs; it is arbitrarily divided into an **anterior, middle, and posterior** compartment based on the chest x-ray. A classification based on cross-sectional imaging divides the mediastinum into **prevascular, visceral, and paravertebral** compartments.

- Masses in the **anterior mediastinum** include substernal thyroid goiters, lymphoma, thymoma, and teratoma.

- The **middle mediastinum** is home primarily to lymphadenopathy from lymphoma and metastatic disease, such as from small cell carcinoma of the lung.

- The **posterior mediastinum** is the location of neurogenic tumors that originate either from the nerve sheath (mostly benign) or tissues other than the sheath (mostly malignant).

- Incidental **solitary pulmonary nodules (SPNs)** less than 6 mm in size are rarely malignant; in those in whom clinical or imaging findings suggest malignancy, about 50% over the age of 50 are malignant. The key question is to determine whether a nodule is most likely benign or most likely malignant in any given individual.

- Criteria on which an evaluation of benignity can be made include absolute **size** of the nodule upon discovery, presence of **calcification** within it, the **margin** of the nodule, and **change** in the size of the nodule over time.

- Evidence-based criteria have been developed to help determine the frequency and method of follow-up of the increasing number of solitary pulmonary nodules found **incidentally** on CT scans so as to optimize the role for further diagnostic interventions.

- **Bronchogenic carcinomas** can present in three ways: visualization of the tumor itself; recognition of the effects of bronchial obstruction, such as pneumonitis and/or atelectasis; or by identification of either their direct extension or metastatic spread to the chest or to distant organs.

- Bronchogenic carcinomas presenting as a solitary nodule/mass in the lung are most often **adenocarcinomas;** adenocarcinomas of the lung may sometimes present with multiple nodules, mimicking metastatic disease.

- Bronchogenic carcinoma presenting with bronchial obstruction is most often caused by **squamous cell carcinoma**, which is also the cell type most likely to cavitate.

- **Small cell carcinomas** are highly aggressive, centrally located, peribronchial tumors, the majority of which have already metastasized at the time of initial presentation; they can be associated with paraneoplastic syndromes such as inappropriate secretion of antidiuretic hormone and Cushing syndrome.

- Multiple nodules in the lung are most often **metastatic** lesions that have traveled through the bloodstream from a distant primary tumor (**hematogenous spread**); common sites of primaries for such metastases include colorectal, breast, renal cell, head and neck, bladder, uterine and cervical carcinomas, soft-tissue sarcomas, and melanoma.

- In **lymphangitic carcinomatosis,** a tumor grows in and obstructs lymphatics in the lung, producing a pattern that is radiologically similar to pulmonary interstitial edema from heart failure; primaries that metastasize to the lung in this fashion include breast, lung, and pancreatic cancer.

- Conventional radiography has a high false-negative rate in pulmonary thromboembolic disease because demonstration of "classical" findings such as a Hampton hump, Westermark sign, and knuckle sign is infrequent.

- **CT pulmonary angiography** is now widely used for the diagnosis of pulmonary embolism producing images of the pulmonary arteries with little or no motion artifact.

- **Chronic obstructive pulmonary disease** consists of emphysema and chronic bronchitis; of the two, chronic bronchitis is a clinical diagnosis, whereas emphysema is defined pathologically and has findings that can be seen on both conventional radiographs and CT scans.

- **Bullae, cysts, and cavities** are all air-containing lesions in the lung that differ in size, location, and wall composition; bullae, cysts, and cavities are seen on CT and may also be visible on conventional radiographs.

- Although **bronchiectasis** may be seen on conventional radiographs, CT is the study of choice; CT may demonstrate the **signet ring sign, tram-tracks,** cystic lesions, or tubular densities.

Additional content is available online including chapters on Nuclear Medicine, Artificial Intelligence, Radiation Dose and Safety, an Early History of Radiology, and a compendium of 200 Diagnostic Radiology Signs.

# 11

# Recognizing Adult Heart Disease

*William Herring, MD, FACR*

This chapter will discuss how to assess heart size, then describe the normal and abnormal contours of the heart on the frontal radiograph and, finally, illustrate some imaging findings in common cardiac diseases.

## CASE QUIZ 11 QUESTION

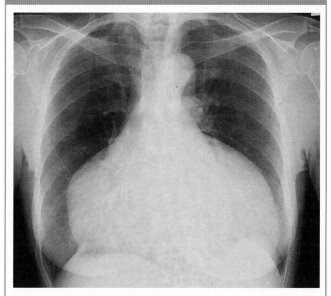

This 47-year-old female with a history of systemic lupus erythematosus presented with chest discomfort and muffled heart sounds. What is the most likely diagnosis based on the appearance of this chest radiograph? See the answer at the end of this chapter.

## RECOGNIZING AN ENLARGED CARDIAC SILHOUETTE

- The cardiac silhouette ("heart shadow") can appear enlarged on conventional radiographs for three main reasons (arranged in the order in which they will be discussed, not by frequency of occurrence):
  - **Pericardial effusion,** which can mimic the appearance of cardiomegaly on conventional radiographs.

- **Extracardiac** factors that produce apparent cardiac enlargement.
- And most importantly, true cardiac enlargement *(cardiomegaly).*

### Pericardial Effusion

- There are normally 15 to 50 cc of fluid in the pericardial space between the parietal and visceral pericardial layers. Abnormal accumulations of fluid begin in the **dependent portions of the pericardial space** that, in the supine position, is **posterior to the left ventricle** (Fig. 11.1A). As the pericardial effusion increases in size, it tends to accumulate more **along the right heart border** until it fills the pericardial space and **encircles the heart** (Fig. 11.1B).
- CT scans can demonstrate small pericardial effusions, although pericardial ultrasonography is usually the imaging study of first choice. Conventional radiographs are poor at defining a pericardial effusion.
- Some of the **causes** of pericardial effusions are outlined in Box 11.1.

### Extracardiac Causes of Apparent Cardiac Enlargement

- Sometimes, there is an **extracardiac** cause of *apparent* cardiac enlargement on conventional radiography that may cause the cardiothoracic ratio (see Fig. 3.1) to appear greater than 50%, **while the heart itself may actually be normal in size.**
- The extracardiac causes of apparent cardiomegaly are outlined in Table 11.1. **Magnification** of the heart produced by projection, usually on an antero-posterior (AP), supine, **portable chest examination,** is the most common cause of apparent cardiomegaly.

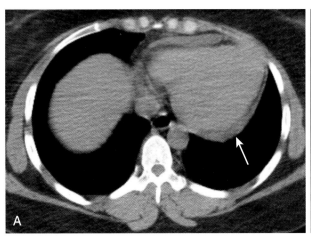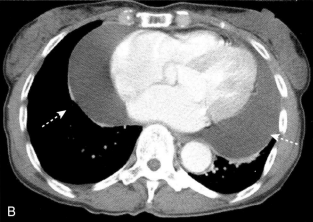

**Fig. 11.1 Pericardial Effusions, Small and Large.** (A) There is fluid in the pericardial space posterior to the heart *(arrow)* in this unenhanced CT of the lower chest. (B) In another patient, after intravenous contrast opacifies the heart, a larger pericardial effusion is seen to surround the heart *(arrows)*. Conventional chest radiographs may show an enlarged cardiac silhouette but cannot differentiate the soft-tissue density of the heart from the fluid density of the effusion.

## TABLE 11.1 Extracardiac Causes of Apparent Cardiomegaly

| Cause | Reason for Enlarged Appearance |
|---|---|
| AP portable supine chest is the most common cause | Magnification due to AP projection |
| Suboptimal inspiration | In expiration, the diaphragm moves upward and compresses the heart, making the heart appear larger than it would be in full inspiration. If there are eight to nine posterior ribs visible on the frontal chest radiograph, then the inspiration is adequate. |
| Obesity, pregnancy, ascites | These conditions may prevent an adequate inspiration. |
| **Pectus excavatum deformity,** a congenital deformity of the lowermost section of the sternum, causing it to bow inward and compress the heart | The heart is compressed between the sternum and the spine. |
| Rotation | Especially when it occurs to the patient's left, rotation may make the heart appear larger (see Fig. 2.2C–H). |
| Pericardial effusion | Other imaging modalities (most commonly ultrasound), CT, or electrocardiographic findings will help to identify pericardial fluid. |

*AP,* Anteroposterior; *CT,* computed tomography.

## TABLE 11.2 Recognizing Cardiomegaly on an AP Chest Radiograph

| Appearance of Heart on AP Study | Likely "Actual" Heart Size |
|---|---|
| **Borderline enlarged** | Normal size |
| **Significantly enlarged** | Enlarged |
| **Touching, or almost touching, the left lateral chest wall** | Definitely enlarged |

## Identifying Cardiac Enlargement on an AP Chest Radiograph

- So, is it possible to estimate the size of the heart on a portable chest radiograph? The answer is "yes." A good rule of thumb: If the heart appears enlarged on a **well-inspired, portable chest radiograph**, it probably is enlarged (Table 11.2 and Fig. 11.2).

## Recognizing Cardiomegaly on the Lateral Chest Radiograph

- Generally speaking, evaluation of cardiac size using conventional radiography is best made on the frontal chest radiograph. To evaluate for the presence of enlargement of the cardiac silhouette in the lateral projection, **look at the space posterior to the heart and anterior to the spine at the level of the diaphragm.** In a normal person, the **cardiac silhouette will usually not extend posteriorly and project over the spine** (Fig. 11.3A).

- As the **cardiac silhouette enlarges**, whether that enlargement is due to cardiomegaly or pericardial effusion, the **posterior border of the heart may extend to, or overlap, the anterior border of the thoracic spine.** This can be useful as a confirmatory sign of an enlarged cardiac silhouette (Fig. 11.3B).

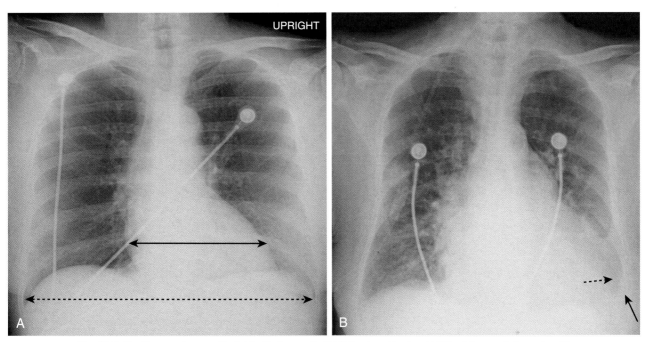

**Fig. 11.2 Cardiomegaly on a Portable Radiograph.** (A) If the heart is about 50% of the cardiothoracic ratio (ratio of length of the *solid double arrow* to *dashed double arrow*), then the heart is not enlarged. (B) If the heart *(dashed arrow)* is near or touching the lateral chest wall *(solid arrow)* then the heart is enlarged.

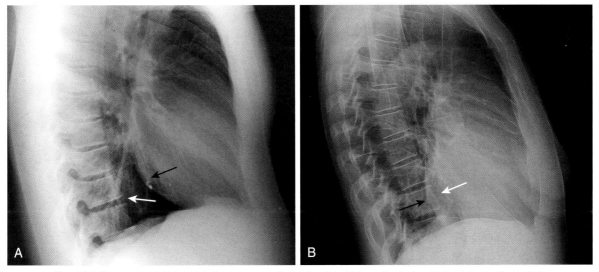

**Fig. 11.3 Normal and Enlarged Appearance of the Cardiac Silhouette in the Lateral Projection.** (A) In most normal patients, the posterior border of the heart *(black arrow)* does not overlap the thoracic spine *(white arrow)*. (B) In this patient with cardiomegaly, the posterior border of the heart *(black arrow)* overlaps the thoracic spine *(white arrow)*. The lateral projection can be used as a helpful confirmatory sign of enlargement of the cardiac silhouette.

# RECOGNIZING COMMON CARDIAC DISEASES

- In this section, several diseases will be discussed in more detail. Most of them produce abnormalities in size and contour of the heart or great vessels. For a **systematic approach** to recognizing the cardiac contour abnormalities on chest radiographs in adults, see **e-Appendix B. The ABCs of Heart Disease**. The diseases to be discussed here are:
- Congestive heart failure and pulmonary edema
- Cardiogenic versus noncardiogenic pulmonary edema
- Hypertensive cardiovascular disease
- Mitral stenosis
- Pulmonary arterial hypertension
- Aortic stenosis
- Cardiomyopathy
- Thoracic aortic aneurysm and aortic dissection
- Coronary artery disease

## Congestive Heart Failure

- The incidence of congestive heart failure (CHF) has grown rapidly over the last two decades so that CHF is one of the most common diagnoses in hospitalized patients over the age of 65.
- **Causes of congestive heart failure**
  - In the United States, the **two most common causes of CHF** are **coronary artery** disease and **hypertension**.
  - Other causes of CHF:
    - **Cardiomyopathy**, such as from long-standing alcohol abuse
    - **Cardiac valvular lesions** like aortic stenosis and mitral stenosis
    - **Arrhythmias**
    - **Hyperthyroidism**
    - **Severe anemia**
    - **Left-to-right shunts**
- Typically, **congestive heart failure** presents with **one of two radiographic patterns:** *pulmonary interstitial edema* or *pulmonary alveolar edema.* Not every feature of each pattern is always present and there is often overlap between the two patterns.

### Pulmonary Interstitial Edema

- There are **four key radiographic signs of pulmonary interstitial edema:**
  - **Thickening of the interlobular septa**
  - **Peribronchial cuffing**
  - **Fluid in the fissures**
  - **Pleural effusions**

### Thickening of the Interlobular Septa: Kerley B Lines

- The interlobular septae are not detectable on a normal chest radiograph but can become visible if they accumulate

excessive fluid, usually at a pulmonary (venous) capillary wedge pressure of about **15 mm Hg.** The thickened septae are called *septal lines* or *Kerley B lines* (named after Peter James Kerley, an Irish neurologist and radiologist).

- **Recognizing Kerley B lines**
  - Kerley B lines actually do exist. They will be visible on a frontal radiograph usually **at the lung bases,** at or **near the costophrenic angles.**
  - They are **very short** (1−2 cm long), **very thin** (about 1 mm), and **horizontal in orientation,** which means they are **perpendicular to the pleural surface.**
  - They **usually extend to and abut the pleural surface** (Fig. 11.4).
  - After repeated episodes of pulmonary interstitial edema, the **septal lines may fibrose** and therefore **remain, even after all other signs of pulmonary interstitial edema clear.** These are called *chronic Kerley B lines* and they may be present even if the patient is not clinically in congestive failure.
- **Kerley A lines**
  - Kerley was busy naming other lines seen in congestive heart failure besides the "B" line.
  - **Kerley A** lines appear when connective tissue around the bronchovascular sheaths in the lung distends with fluid. **Kerley A lines extend from the hila for several**

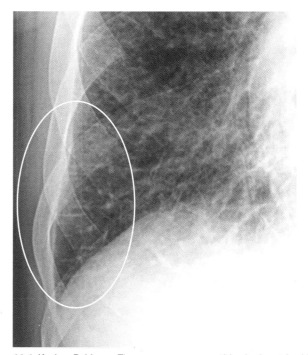

**Fig. 11.4 Kerley B Lines.** There are numerous, thin, horizontal white lines at the lung base abutting the pleural surface *(oval)*. Interlobular septae are not visible on a normal chest radiograph.

centimeters but **do not reach the periphery of the lung** like Kerley B lines (Fig. 11.5).

- Once he started, Kerley apparently had trouble stopping and he also described "C" lines, but there is some doubt that they exist as separate entities.

## Peribronchial Cuffing

- In adults, bronchi may **normally** be visible on-end (*en face*) in the region of the hila but the bronchial walls are usually so thin they are **not visible** more peripherally in the lung.

- When fluid accumulates in the interstitial tissue around and in the wall of a bronchus, such as occurs in congestive heart failure, the **bronchial wall becomes thicker and may appear as a ring-like density that can be seen on-end** in radiographs *(peribronchial cuffing).*

- When seen on-end, **peribronchial cuffing** appears as numerous, small, ring-like shadows that look like little *doughnuts* (Fig. 11.6).

## Fluid in the Fissures

- The **major** (or oblique) and **minor** (or horizontal) **fissures may be visible normally** but are almost never thicker than a line you could draw with the **point of a sharpened pencil** (Fig. 11.7A).

- **Fluid can collect between the two layers of visceral pleura that form the fissures or in the subpleural space,** between the visceral pleura and the lung parenchyma. This **fluid** distends the fissure and makes it **thicker,** more **irregular in contour,** and therefore **more visible** than normal (Fig. 11.7B).

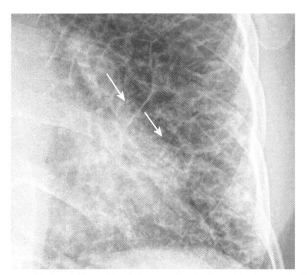

**Fig. 11.5  Kerley A Lines.** The A lines are interlacing white lines radiating from the hila *(arrows)* but not reaching the chest wall. They are longer than Kerley B lines. A network of Kerley lines is produced in the lungs in patients with congestive heart failure producing the "prominence of the pulmonary interstitial markings" described in that disease.

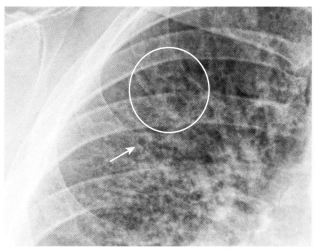

**Fig. 11.6 Peribronchial Cuffing.** When fluid accumulates in the interstitial tissue around and in the wall of a bronchus as it does in CHF, the normally invisible bronchial wall becomes thicker and can appear as ring-like densities when seen on-end *(arrow* and *circle).* Peribronchial cuffing may not always produce perfectly round circles.

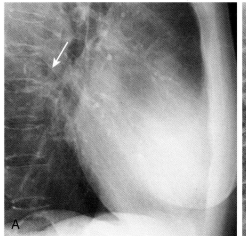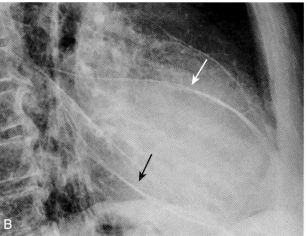

**Fig. 11.7 Normal Fissures and Fluid in the Fissures.** (A) If you are unable to see the fissures on this normal lateral radiograph, it is because they are frequently invisible. A small portion of the upper major fissure may barely be seen *(arrow).* (B) When fluid collects in the major *(black arrow)* and minor *(white arrow)* fissures, they become thicker and more irregular in their appearance. When the patient's heart failure clears, the fissures will return to their normal appearance, but after repeated and prolonged bouts of failure, fibrosis may result in permanent thickening of the fissures.

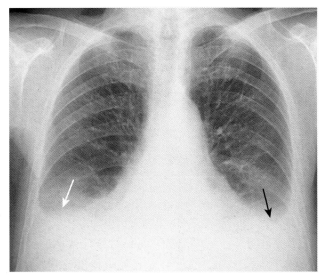

**Fig. 11.8 Pleural Effusions in Congestive Heart Failure.** There are bilateral pleural effusions *(arrows)*. It is common for the right pleural effusion in CHF *(white arrow)* to be slightly larger than the left *(black arrow)*. It is uncommon in CHF to have a large left pleural effusion alone, a finding that might prompt investigation of another cause for the effusion such as a malignancy or TB. This patient had congestive heart failure.

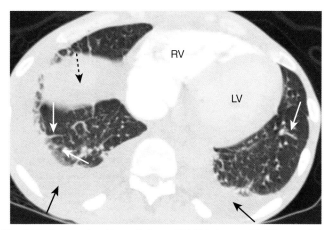

**Fig. 11.9 Congestive Heart Failure, CT.** This is an axial CT scan of the chest following intravenous injection of contrast. Note that the right heart is opacified but the contrast has not yet passed through the lungs a sufficient number of times to fully opacify the left heart. There are bilateral pleural effusions present and they layer posteriorly because the patient is being scanned supine *(solid black arrows)*. Fluid has insinuated itself into the fissure *(dashed black arrow)*. The thickened interlobular septae *(solid white arrows)* are Kerley B lines. *LV,* Left ventricle; *RV,* right ventricle.

## Pleural Effusion

- As a result of either increased production or decreased absorption of pleural fluid, fluid in excess of the normal 2 to 5 mL can collect in the pleural space, typically at a pulmonary capillary wedge pressure of about **20 mm Hg.**
- **Pleural effusions accompanying congestive heart failure are usually bilateral**, but can be asymmetric (Fig. 11.8).
  - When **unilateral**, they are **almost always right-sided.**

> ⟫ **IMPORTANT POINTS**
>
> - About 15% of the time, pleural effusions from CHF can be unilateral and on the left but if you see a unilateral left pleural effusion, you should think of causes other than CHF, like metastases, tuberculosis, or pulmonary thromboembolic disease.

- At times, pleural fluid accumulates in the form of a *laminar effusion* in which the fluid assumes a **thin, band-like density along the lateral chest wall, beginning near the costophrenic sulcus,** but often preserving the sulcus itself (see Fig. 7.14).
- For more about pleural effusions, see **Chapter 7-Recognizing a Pleural Effusion.**
- All of these findings can be seen on CT as well as conventional radiographs (Fig. 11.9).
- The key findings of **pulmonary interstitial edema** are summarized in Box 11.2.

## Pulmonary Alveolar Edema

- When the **pulmonary venous pressure is sufficiently elevated (about 25 mm Hg), fluid spills out of the**

> **BOX 11.2 Four Key Findings of Pulmonary Interstitial Edema**
>
> - Thickening of the interlobular septae, **Kerley B lines**, and fluid in the central connective tissue of the lungs, **Kerley A lines**
> - **Peribronchial cuffing:** fluid-thickened bronchial walls visualized on-end
> - **Fluid in the fissures:** opacification and thickening of the interlobar fissures
> - **Pleural effusion:** usually bilateral but, when unilateral, usually right-sided

**interstitial tissues** of the lung **into the airspaces.** This results in *pulmonary alveolar edema* (most often shortened to *pulmonary edema* without including "alveolar").

- The **radiographic findings** of **pulmonary alveolar edema are:**
  - **Fluffy, indistinct patchy airspace densities that are frequently centrally located.** The outer-third of the lung may be spared and the lower lung zones tend to be more affected than the upper. This produces the *bat-wing, angel-wing, or butterfly* configuration of pulmonary edema (Fig. 11.10).
  - **Pleural effusions** and **fluid in the fissures** are also commonly found in pulmonary alveolar edema on a cardiogenic basis.
- The key findings of **pulmonary alveolar edema** are summarized in Box 11.3.
- **What about cardiomegaly and cephalization?**
  - While most patients with congestive heart failure have an enlarged heart, most patients with an enlarged heart

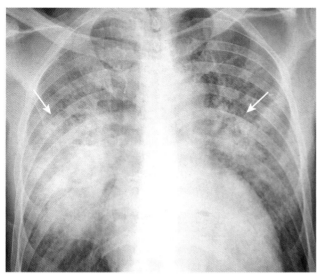

**Fig. 11.10 Bat-Wing Pattern of Pulmonary Edema.** Central airspace disease that spares the lung periphery is called a ***bat-wing (angel-wing)*** or ***butterfly*** pattern *(arrows)* and, while it may not be the most common manifestation of pulmonary edema, it is suggestive of that disease versus other airspace diseases such as pneumonia. The bat-wing pattern is seen in rapidly developing cardiac failure such as massive myocardial infarction and papillary muscle rupture. The patient had suffered an acute myocardial infarction.

---

### BOX 11.3 **Key Findings in Pulmonary Alveolar Edema**

- Fluffy, indistinct, patchy airspace densities
- ***Bat-wing*** or ***butterfly*** configuration frequently sparing the outer third of lungs
- Pleural effusions are usually present when the edema is cardiogenic in origin

---

are not in congestive heart failure. In any individual, **cardiomegaly itself is not a particularly sensitive indicator for the presence or absence of congestive heart failure.**

- *Cephalization,* defined as redistribution of flow in the lungs such that the upper lobe pulmonary vasculature becomes larger than the lower lobe vessels, **is difficult to identify for most beginners** and is meaningful only if you are certain the patient was **upright** at the time of the chest exposure. Since many or most patients suspected of having CHF are imaged supine, the sign is not very useful.
- **How pulmonary edema resolves**
  - Pulmonary edema generally is both **abrupt in onset** and **quick to clear**—typically in a matter of a few hours to a few days (Fig. 11.11).
  - Resolution frequently begins peripherally and moves centrally. Radiologic resolution may lag behind clinical improvement, especially if the patient has large pleural effusions that may last long after other radiographic signs have cleared.

## Noncardiogenic Pulmonary Edema

- Although congestive heart failure accounts for the majority of the cases of pulmonary edema (*i.e., cardiogenic pulmonary edema*), there are other, **noncardiogenic causes of pulmonary edema.**
- Among the causes of noncardiogenic pulmonary edema is a diverse group of diseases including:

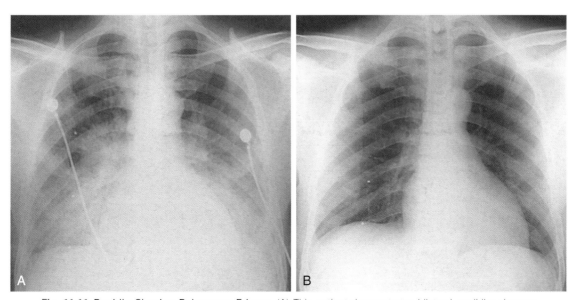

**Fig. 11.11 Rapidly Clearing Pulmonary Edema.** (A) This patient demonstrates bilateral, perihilar airspace disease consistent with pulmonary edema. (B) Four days later, the lungs are clear. Patients with acute respiratory distress syndrome (ARDS) are not likely to clear this quickly, nor are patients who have coexisting diseases such as renal or hepatic failure or superimposed pneumonia.

- **Increased capillary permeability** — includes all of the various causes of *acute (adult) respiratory distress syndrome* or *ARDS* such as:
  - Sepsis
  - Uremia
  - Disseminated intravascular coagulopathy
  - Smoke inhalation
  - Near-drowning
- **Volume overload**
- **Lymphangitic carcinomatosis**
- Other causes of noncardiogenic pulmonary edema may include:
  - **High-altitude pulmonary edema**
  - **Neurogenic pulmonary edema**
  - **Reexpansion pulmonary edema** (Fig. 11.12)
  - **Heroin or other drug overdoses, e.g., crack cocaine**

## Noncardiogenic Pulmonary Edema: Imaging Findings

- **Acute respiratory distress syndrome (ARDS) represents one form of noncardiogenic pulmonary edema** (Fig. 11.13).
  - Characteristically, **patients with ARDS are radiographically normal for 24 to 36 hours** after the initial insult, which could range from a direct effect on the lungs (aspiration of gastric contents) to a systemic cause (sepsis).
  - Then, pulmonary abnormalities become evident in the form of **pulmonary interstitial edema** or **patchy airspace disease** or in the typical pattern of bilateral **pulmonary alveolar edema.**
  - Clinically, the **patient demonstrates severe hypoxia, cyanosis, tachypnea, and dyspnea.**
  - Typically, the findings of ARDS stabilize after 5 to 7 days and begin improving in about 2 weeks. Complete clearing, when it occurs, may take months.

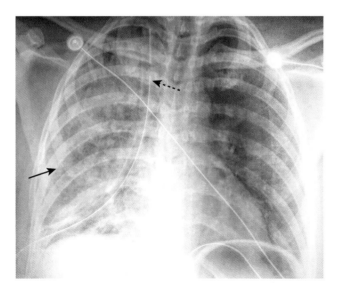

**Fig. 11.12 Reexpansion Pulmonary Edema.** Unilateral airspace disease affects the entire right lung *(solid arrow)*. In addition, a chest tube *(dashed arrow)* is seen on the same side. Reexpansion pulmonary edema results from the overly rapid expansion of a lung that has typically been chronically collapsed by pneumothorax or a large pleural effusion (as had been the case in this patient). Its exact cause is not known. Other causes of unilateral pulmonary edema can include either an abnormality on the same side as the pulmonary edema (e.g., prolonged positioning with the affected side dependent) or an abnormality on the opposite side (e.g., a large pulmonary embolus occluding flow to the opposite lung).

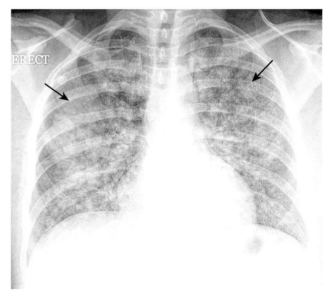

**Fig. 11.13 Acute Respiratory Distress Syndrome.** Even though this airspace disease has a central distribution similar to cardiogenic pulmonary edema *(arrows)*, there is no pleural fluid, fluid in the fissures, or cardiomegaly. The patient had inhaled crack cocaine. The lungs are the principal organs affected by crack cocaine use. Onset of pulmonary edema usually occurs after inhalation of a large dose. Black sputum is characteristic of crack cocaine smoking, from the carbonaceous residue that occurs from the process used to produce the inhaled product.

- In the later stages of ARDS, a **reticular interstitial lung pattern may develop,** although the majority of patients who survive tend to have little impairment of lung function.

## Differentiating Cardiac from Noncardiac Pulmonary Edema

### ▶▶ IMPORTANT POINTS

- The **patterns of cardiac (cardiogenic) and noncardiac (non-cardiogenic) pulmonary edema overlap considerably** and the patient's **history** and **clinical** picture are keys to establishing the most likely cause of pulmonary edema.

- In general, **noncardiogenic pulmonary edema** is:
  - **Less likely** to demonstrate **pleural effusions** and **Kerley B lines than cardiogenic pulmonary edema.**
  - **More likely** to demonstrate a **normal pulmonary capillary wedge pressure (PCWP)** of less than 12 mm Hg **than cardiogenic pulmonary edema.**
  - **More likely** to be associated with a **normal-sized heart** (see Fig. 11.13).
  - The key differences between cardiogenic and noncardiogenic pulmonary edema are summarized in Table 11.3.

| TABLE 11.3 **Cardiogenic Versus Noncardiogenic Pulmonary Edema** | | |
| --- | --- | --- |
| Imaging Finding | Cardiogenic | Noncardiogenic |
| **Pleural effusions** | Common | Infrequent |
| **Kerley B lines** | Common | Infrequent |
| **Heart size** | Frequently enlarged | May be normal |
| **Pulmonary capillary wedge pressure** | Elevated | Normal |

## Hypertensive Cardiovascular Disease

- Most of the time (90%), hypertension is **_essential hypertension_** with no identifiable cause. Heart failure, coronary artery disease, and cardiac arrhythmias are common complications of hypertension.
- Systemic hypertension can lead to left ventricular hypertrophy in about 20% of patients and more than twice as often if the patient is obese. Left ventricular hypertrophy occurs at the expense of the lumen, the wall becoming thicker while the lumen becomes smaller. Therefore, **the heart is usually normal or slightly increased in size** early in the disease, especially on conventional radiographs. It is not until the muscle begins to decompensate that the heart increases dramatically in size (Fig. 11.14).

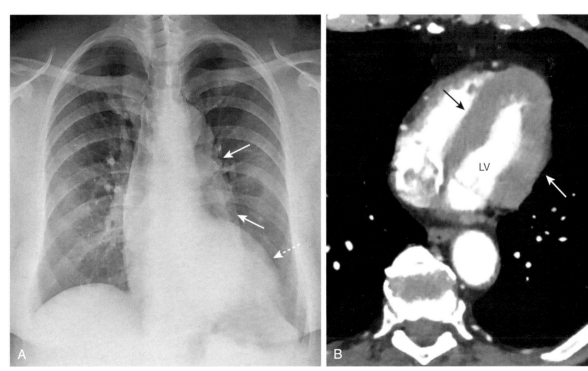

**Fig. 11.14 Hypertensive Cardiovascular Disease.** (A) The aorta itself is **_uncoiled_** (solid arrows) due to increased systemic blood pressure (see also Fig. 3.3). The left ventricle (dashed arrow) appears enlarged and a contrast-enhanced CT scan through the heart (B) demonstrates marked concentric hypertrophy of the left ventricular wall (arrows) that has occurred at the expense of the lumen (LV).

- **The aorta**, under increased systemic pressure, pivots outward around two anchor points: the **aortic valve** and the **aortic hiatus** in the diaphragm so that it **gradually** *uncoils,* becoming more prominent in **both** its **ascending** and **descending** portions (see Fig. 3.3).
- Prolonged systemic hypertension may eventually lead to congestive heart failure.

## Mitral Stenosis

- In developed nations, the incidence of mitral stenosis from rheumatic heart disease has declined markedly but it is still seen in the elderly and in younger individuals from developing countries. The **most common symptoms** are from **left heart failure:** dyspnea on exertion, orthopnea, and paroxysmal nocturnal dyspnea.
- Mitral stenosis leads to obstruction to the outflow of blood from the left atrium and usually becomes symptomatic when the **valve area falls below one-third** of its normal size. As the left atrial pressure builds, the left atrium enlarges and the increased pulmonary venous pressure *(i.e., pulmonary venous hypertension)* is reflected retrograde into the pulmonary circulation (Fig. 11.15).
- Upper lobe vessels become as large as, or more prominent than, lower lobe vessels *(cephalization).* Pulmonary venous hypertension eventually leads to congestive heart failure. With prolonged elevation of pulmonary venous pressure, there may be physical changes in the pulmonary vasculature leading to escalating *pulmonary vascular resistance* requiring ever-increasing levels of pulmonary **arterial** pressure.
- Eventually there is *pulmonary arterial hypertension* and right-sided heart failure (Fig. 11.16).

## Pulmonary Arterial Hypertension

- The normal mean pulmonary artery pressure is about 15 mm Hg. Pulmonary arterial hypertension may be *idiopathic (primary)* or *secondary* to another disease, frequently emphysema. Mitral stenosis is another cause of secondary pulmonary arterial hypertension.
- With **primary** pulmonary hypertension, the leading cause of death is **progressive right heart failure.** Secondary pulmonary hypertension shares comorbidities with the diseases that cause it, such as emphysema, recurrent thromboembolic disease, mitral stenosis, and congestive heart failure.
- The **imaging hallmark of pulmonary arterial hypertension** is a discrepancy in size between the central pulmonary vasculature (i.e., the main, right, and left pulmonary arteries are **large**) and the peripheral pulmonary vasculature. This discrepancy has been called *pruning.*
- On CT scans, the **main pulmonary artery is normally about the same diameter as the ascending aorta** but in

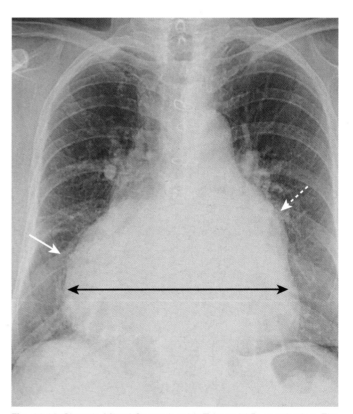

**Fig. 11.16 Chronic Mitral Stenosis with Tricuspid Regurgitation.** The heart is enlarged *(double black arrow).* The left atrium and left atrial appendage are markedly enlarged *(dashed white arrow).* Because of increased pulmonary vascular resistance and subsequent pulmonary arterial hypertension, the right heart has developed tricuspid regurgitation with marked enlargement of the right atrium *(solid white arrow).*

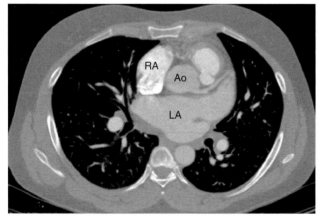

**Fig. 11.15 Mitral Stenosis.** This is a contrast-enhanced axial CT image through the heart. The left atrium (LA) is enlarged in this patient because of a stenotic mitral valve. Eventually, the increase in left atrial pressure is transmitted backward through the pulmonary venous and then pulmonary arterial circulations. *Ao,* Aorta; *RA,* right atrium.

**pulmonary arterial hypertension** the main pulmonary artery is usually larger than the aorta and **greater than 3 cm** in size (Fig. 11.17).

## Aortic Stenosis

- The classic triad of clinical symptoms in aortic stenosis is **chest pain**, symptoms related to **heart failure,** and **syncope.**

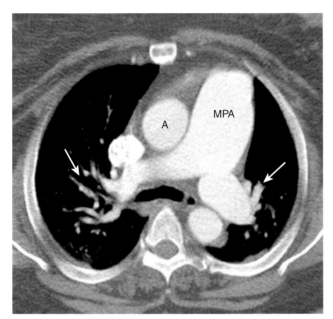

**Fig. 11.17 Pulmonary Arterial Hypertension.** Normally, the main pulmonary artery (MPA) is about the same diameter as the ascending aorta (A). In this patient, with pulmonary arterial hypertension, the MPA is much larger than the aorta. There is also a rapid attenuation in the size of the pulmonary arteries *(arrows)* called **pruning,** another feature of pulmonary arterial hypertension. This patient had a history of chronic pulmonary thromboembolic disease.

- Aortic stenosis may be secondary to a **congenital bicuspid aortic valve**, from **degeneration of a tricuspid valve** or, less frequently now, **rheumatic heart disease.**
- Because there is obstruction to left ventricular outflow from aortic stenosis and because the ventricles respond to obstruction by undergoing hypertrophy of their walls, the heart is usually normal in size **early** in the course of the disease.
- The **ascending aorta** may be unusually prominent because of *poststenotic dilatation,* a hallmark of a significantly stenotic lesion in any major artery in which, because of *eddy currents* and *turbulent flow,* there is increased intraluminal pressure for several centimeters **distal** to a partially obstructing lesion (Fig. 11.18A).
- **Calcification** of the aortic valve is easily seen on CT and has been shown to be predictive of increased likelihood of aortic stenosis and mortality from cardiovascular disease (Fig. 11.18B).
- Eventually, when the heart begins to decompensate it will become **enlarged** and congestive heart failure may ensue.

## Cardiomyopathy

- Although *cardiomyopathy* had been previously defined to include myocardial disease secondary to known cardiovascular disorders (such as ischemic heart disease or valvular disease), most current definitions of cardiomyopathy exclude such cardiovascular causes. Cardiomyopathy is a myocardial disorder in which the heart muscle is structurally and functionally abnormal. The three major forms are discussed below.

### Dilated Cardiomyopathy

- *Dilated cardiomyopathy* is, by definition, a condition in which there is **increased systolic and diastolic volume of the ventricles** associated with a **decreased ejection fraction (<40%).** It is the **most common** form of **cardiomyopathy** (90%).

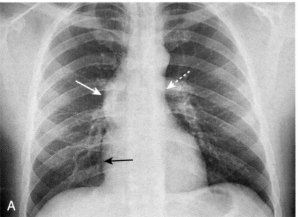
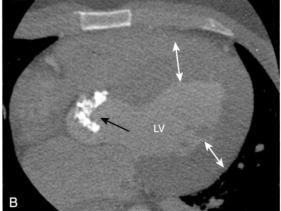

**Fig. 11.18 Aortic Stenosis.** (A) There is **poststenotic dilatation** isolated to the ascending aorta *(solid white arrow).* The ascending aorta should normally not project farther to the right than the right heart border *(black arrow).* Notice that the heart is not enlarged overall and the descending aorta *(dashed white arrow)* is normal in appearance. (B) This unenhanced axial CT scan of the heart shows dense calcification of the aortic valve *(black arrow)* and a markedly thickened left ventricular wall *(double white arrows)* from hypertrophy. *LV,* Left ventricular lumen.

- Most cases are *idiopathic (primary)* but others can be *secondary* to diseases such as myocarditis, collagen vascular disease, and alcohol abuse.
- **Decreased contractility** and **ventricular dilatation** are **hallmarks** so it is usually characterized by an **enlarged heart**, frequently associated with the imaging signs of **congestive heart failure** (Fig. 11.19).
- The diagnosis can usually be made by echocardiography following the initial chest radiograph, in concert with the clinical findings.
- **MRI** can provide the most accurate and reproducible findings for this disease. Using ECG-gated, cine-magnetic resonance angiography (MRA), **cardiac ejection fraction** and **cardiac dimensions** can be accurately assessed.
- **Radionuclide ventriculography** using small quantities of intravenously injected radioisotope can also determine ejection fraction.

## Hypertrophic Cardiomyopathy (HCM)

- *Hypertrophic cardiomyopathy (HCM)* can be familial in 50% of cases, typically inherited in an autosomal-dominant manner with variable penetrance. It is the leading cause of **sudden cardiac death** in preadolescent and adolescent children and has been implicated in the unexpected, sudden deaths from ventricular arrythmias of both amateur and professional athletes. Its major abnormality is **asymmetric** or **concentric thickening of the left ventricular myocardium** (Fig. 11.20).

- In most patients who present clinically, it can be associated with **obstruction** to **left ventricular outflow** (also called *hypertrophic obstructive cardiomyopathy* or *HOCM*) that may be caused by *systolic anterior motion (SAM)* of the anterior **mitral valve leaflet.**
  - *Systolic anterior motion* of the mitral valve refers to a **paradoxical motion** of the anterior (and sometimes posterior) mitral valve leaflet **toward the left ventricular outflow tract** obstructing egress from the left ventricle to the aorta during systole.
- HCM may be diagnosed with echocardiography or ECG-gated MRI of the heart in which hypertrophy of the left ventricular wall is demonstrated. **Asymmetric hypertrophy of the ventricular septum** *(ASH)* may be present but hypertrophy of any part of the left ventricular wall, whether concentric or asymmetric, may be noted.

## Restrictive Cardiomyopathy

- *Restrictive cardiomyopathy* is the least common form of the three types of cardiomyopathies described here. It is characterized by **increased stiffness** of the **myocardium,** which **decreases ventricular filling** during diastole and subsequently reduces cardiac output.

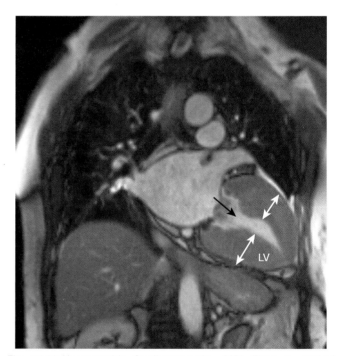

**Fig. 11.20 Hypertrophic Cardiomyopathy, MRI.** There is marked thickening of the left ventricular myocardium (LV) *(double white arrows)* in this coronal reconstruction of a bright blood *(black arrow)* cardiac magnetic resonance image. Overall mortality rates from the disease have been declining and it is consistent with normal longevity in the majority of patients. Whereas most patients with HCM are asymptomatic, the first clinical manifestation of the disease in some individuals can be a sudden catastrophic cardiac event, most likely from ventricular tachycardia or fibrillation. *(Courtesy Adam Guttentag, MD, Vanderbilt University Department of Radiology, Nashville, Tenn.)*

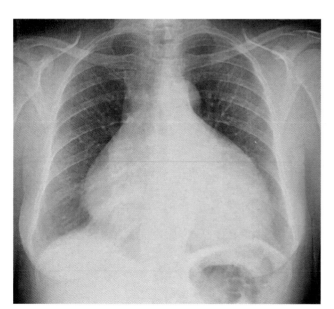

**Fig. 11.19 Dilated Alcoholic Cardiomyopathy.** Cardiomyopathies comprise a diverse group of diseases that affect the heart muscle. In this patient with dilated cardiomyopathy, the cardiac silhouette is markedly enlarged, primarily as a result of biventricular enlargement. The shape of the heart resembles that seen with a pericardial effusion. The patient had a long history of alcohol abuse. Dilated cardiomyopathy is frequently associated with congestive heart failure.

- It can be **idiopathic** but is usually secondary to an **infiltrative process** in the myocardium from such diseases as **amyloid, sarcoidosis, auto-immune disease, and prior chest radiation.** The predominant presenting symptoms are related to **congestive heart failure.**
- In restrictive cardiomyopathy, the **heart is usually not enlarged.** There are pulmonary changes of **congestive heart failure.**

> ### ▶▶ IMPORTANT POINTS
>
> - Restrictive **cardiomyopathy** is **clinically** similar to *constrictive pericarditis*, but differentiation between the two is important in that **constrictive pericarditis** is **surgically curable**, while **restrictive cardiomyopathy** has a relatively **poor prognosis.**
> - The key difference is that the **pericardium** is **thickened** in **constrictive pericarditis** while it is **normal** in **restrictive cardiomyopathy.**
> - MRI can demonstrate the thickness of the pericardium. The pericardium will be **normal** in **restrictive cardiomyopathy** so if the pericardium is normal in thickness (<4 mm), **constrictive pericarditis** can effectively be **excluded.** The pericardium is **thickened** in **constrictive pericarditis.** Therefore, if there is thickening of the pericardium with pericardial calcification (better seen on CT) **restrictive cardiomyopathy** can be **excluded** (Fig. 11.21).

## Aortic Aneurysms

- Aneurysms are **defined as enlargement of a vessel greater than 50% of its original size. Atherosclerosis** is the **most common cause** of a descending thoracic aortic aneurysm.

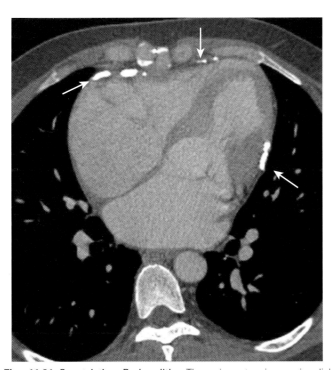

**Fig. 11.21 Constrictive Pericarditis.** There is extensive pericardial calcification *(arrows)*, most likely postinflammatory in etiology in this patient. Although **restrictive cardiomyopathy** and **constrictive pericarditis** can have identical clinical findings, the presence of pericardial calcifications **excludes** restrictive cardiomyopathy. If indicated, pericardiectomy holds the potential for cure for constrictive pericarditis.

The majority of patients with aortic aneurysms are also hypertensive.
- Most patients with aortic aneurysms are **asymptomatic** and the aneurysm is discovered **serendipitously.** When an aneurysm of the descending thoracic aorta expands, it may cause pain which classically, but not always, radiates to the back.
- As measured on CT or MRI scans, the **ascending aorta is usually <3.5 cm** in diameter and the **descending aorta is <3 cm.**
- An **aneurysm** of the thoracic aorta is usually defined as a **persistent enlargement of >4 cm.**
- In general, **aneurysms of 5 to 6 cm are at risk to rupture** and will require surgical intervention. The **rate of growth** of an aneurysm is also important in determining the need for surgical intervention and repair. Annual aneurysm growth rates should be <1 cm/year or elective resection may be considered.

### Recognizing a Thoracic Aortic Aneurysm

- The **appearance** of a thoracic aortic aneurysm on chest radiographs **will depend,** in part, **from which portion of the thoracic aorta it arises.** Aneurysms of the **ascending aorta** may extend **anteriorly** and to the **right.** Aneurysms of the **aortic arch** may produce a **middle mediastinal mass.** Aneurysms of the **descending aorta** project **posteriorly, laterally,** and to the **left** (Fig. 11.22).
- **Contrast-enhanced CT** is the modality **most often used** to diagnose a thoracic aortic aneurysm. MRI is also excellent at demonstrating aneurysms but is usually less available and more expensive.
- Aneurysms can appear as *fusiform* (**long**) or *saccular* (**globular**) in shape.

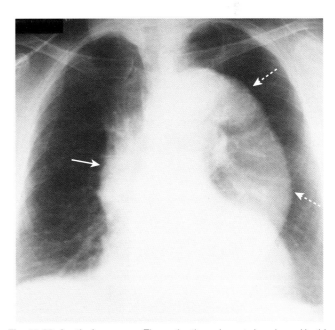

**Fig. 11.22 Aortic Aneurysm.** The entire thoracic aorta is enlarged in this 67-year-old man. The ascending aorta is abnormally prominent *(solid arrow)*. The descending thoracic aorta should normally parallel and almost disappear with the thoracic spine; as it becomes larger, it swings farther away from the spine, as in this case *(dashed arrows)*.

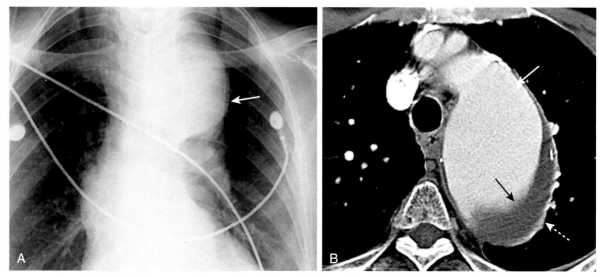

**Fig. 11.23 Aortic Aneurysm, Conventional Chest Radiograph and CT.** (A) Close-up view of a frontal radiograph of the chest demonstrates a large mediastinal soft-tissue mass *(arrow)*. This soft-tissue density represents a large aneurysm of the proximal descending aorta seen also on the CT scan (B). The aneurysm measured 6.7 cm, which placed it at significant risk for rupture. Calcification in the wall of an aneurysm is common *(dashed white arrow)*. Contrast material mixes with blood flowing in the lumen of the aorta *(solid white arrow)*, but the flowing blood is separated from the intimal calcification by a considerable amount of noncontrast-containing thrombus adherent to the wall *(black arrow)*.

- Their anatomy will be **more readily delineated on CT studies** using iodinated contrast material injected intravenously as a bolus, but they may be visible on noncontrast (unenhanced) studies as well. Often, both unenhanced and contrast-enhanced CT studies are obtained to fully evaluate the aneurysm and its contained clot.
- Frequently **calcification is seen in the intima,** which may be **separated** from the **contrast-filled lumen by varying amounts of clot** (Fig. 11.23).

## Thoracic Aortic Dissection

- **Aortic dissections most often originate in the ascending aorta** (classified as *Stanford type A)* or may involve only the **descending aorta** *(Stanford type B).*
- They result from a tear that allows blood to dissect in the wall for varying lengths of the aorta, usually along the media.
- In general, patients with **aortic dissection** have a **history of hypertension** and may have an **underlying condition that can predispose to dissection,** such as cystic medial degeneration, atherosclerosis, Marfan syndrome, Ehlers-Danlos syndrome, trauma, syphilis, or crack cocaine abuse.
- In many patients, **abrupt onset of ripping or tearing chest pain,** which is **maximal at its time of onset,** is the classical history.
- **Conventional radiographs** are **not significantly sensitive to be diagnostically reliable,** but they may **point to the diagnosis** when several imaging findings occur together, especially in the proper clinical setting. The findings are:
  - "Widening of the mediastinum" is a **poor means of establishing the diagnosis** because (a) it is commonly over-interpreted on portable supine radiographs, whereas

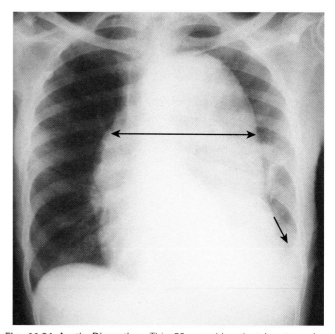

**Fig. 11.24 Aortic Dissection.** This 60-year-old patient has two signs suggestive of an aortic dissection: an indisputable widening of the mediastinum *(double arrow)* and a left pleural effusion *(arrow)*. He also had ripping chest pain. That combination should alert you to the presence of an aortic dissection. The diagnosis was confirmed by CT examination.

on the other hand, (b) it occurs in only about 1 in 4 cases of aortic dissection.
- **Left pleural effusion** (which **frequently represents a transudate** caused by pleural irritation, although transient hemorrhage from the aorta can also produce a hemothorax) (Fig. 11.24).

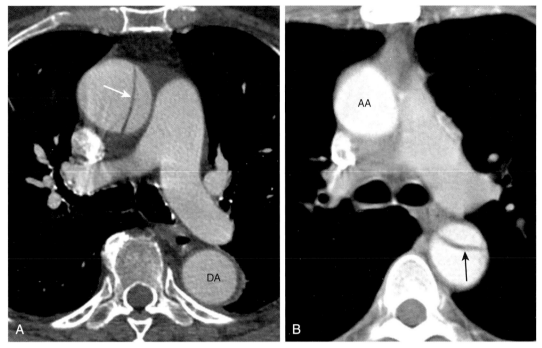

**Fig. 11.25** Aortic Dissections, Types A and B. (A) An intimal flap is seen to traverse the ascending aorta *(arrow)*. This is a Stanford type A dissection because of its involvement of the ascending aorta. (B) In another patient, there is a normal-appearing ascending aorta (AA) while there is an intimal flap noted traversing the descending aorta *(arrow)*. An ***intimal flap*** is the characteristic lesion of an aortic dissection. The smaller lumen is usually the **true** (original) lumen and the larger, **false** lumen is actually a channel that has been produced by blood dissecting through the media. *DA,* Descending aorta.

- **Left apical pleural cap** of fluid or blood
- **Loss of the normal shadow of the aortic knob**
- **Increased deviation of the trachea or esophagus to the right**
- Either MRI or contrast-enhanced CT have, in various studies, been shown to be equally as sensitive and specific for aortic dissection, so the imaging modality used will depend in part on the patient's hemodynamic stability and the availability of resources. Transesophageal ultrasound is also used to establish the diagnosis.

> **》 IMPORTANT POINTS**
>
> - On both **MRI and CT**, the **diagnosis rests on identification** of the ***intimal flap*** that separates the ***true*** **(original)** from the ***false lumen*** (i.e., the canal created by the dissection) (Fig. 11.25).

- In general, **type A (ascending aortic) dissections are treated surgically** whereas **type B (descending aortic dissections) are treated medically.**

## Coronary Artery Disease

- Coronary artery disease is the **leading cause of death worldwide.**
- The coronary artery lumen becomes narrowed by varying amounts of atheromatous plaque. Calcium may deposit in the muscular layers of the artery's walls. Vulnerable plaque

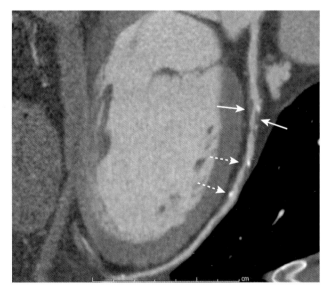

**Fig. 11.26** Cardiac CT, Coronary Artery Stenosis and Calcification. Contrast fills the lumen of the left anterior descending coronary artery except where atheromatous plaque *(solid arrows)* narrows the lumen by about 70%, a significant stenosis. Rupture of this soft plaque, hemorrhage, or clot formation can further narrow or completely occlude the lumen. There are also calcified plaques present *(dashed arrows)*.

may rupture, there may be vasospasm or there may be emboli that produce enough stenosis to lead to ***ischemia*** and possibly ***infarction*** of cardiac muscle (Fig. 11.26).

- MRI, CT, and nuclear medicine studies can be used in the evaluation of coronary artery disease.
  - MRI can demonstrate **postinfarct scar formation** and **myocardial contractility.** Ventricular **function** can be quantitatively assessed.
  - Cardiac CT is used for imaging of the coronary arteries. It has a **very high negative predictive value**—a negative test virtually rules out coronary artery disease. One of the major drawbacks in the use of cardiac CT angiography had been the relatively high x-ray dose delivered, but changes in equipment and new algorithms are reducing this dose considerably. Cardiac CT angiography requires injection of iodinated contrast material (Video 11.1).
  - CT may also be used in asymptomatic patients for *calcium scoring* in which the calcium found in the coronary arteries is used as a marker for coronary artery disease. The amount of calcium detected on a cardiac CT scan, and calculated by computer, can be a helpful **prognostic** tool. The findings on cardiac CT are expressed as a **calcium score,** the higher the score the more extensive the evidence for CAD and the higher the potential mortality from a cardiovascular event. Calcium scoring is performed without intravenous contrast (see Fig. 3.11).
  - CT can also demonstrate complications of myocardial infarction such as ventricular aneurysms and intracardiac clots.
- **Single photon emission computed tomography (SPECT)** is an imaging technique that blends the intravascular injection of a **radioactive isotope** with acquisition of images using a rotating nuclear gamma camera capable of three-dimensional localization of disease. Stress and resting myocardial perfusion images using SPECT imaging can demonstrate areas of **ischemia**, especially compared with the same study done at rest. Nuclear medicine studies can also estimate left ventricular function (see **e-Appendix A. Nuclear Medicine: Understanding the Principles and Recognizing the Basics**).
- For detecting coronary artery stenosis, coronary angiography remains the gold standard (see Video 3.1).

**CASE QUIZ 11 ANSWER**

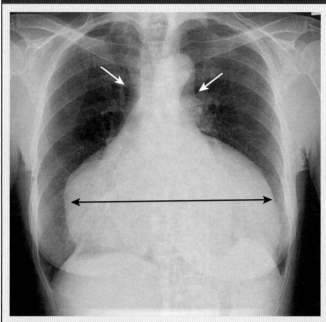

The cardiac silhouette is highly suggestive of the *flask-shape* or *water bottle* appearance seen in pericardial effusions. This patient had a very large pericardial effusion secondary to her known lupus. Note how the cardiac silhouette has increased in size disproportionately wider inferiorly *(double black arrow)* than superiorly *(white arrows),* another suggestive finding of a large pericardial effusion.

## ⌂ TAKE HOME POINTS

- In adults, a quick assessment of heart size can be made using the *cardiothoracic ratio,* which is the ratio of the widest transverse diameter of the heart compared with the widest internal diameter of the rib cage. In normal adults, the cardiothoracic ratio is usually less than 50%.
- **Extracardiac causes** can make the heart appear to be enlarged, even if it is actually normal, including anteroposterior (AP) portable studies, factors that inhibit a deep inspiration, abnormalities of the bony thorax, and the presence of a pericardial effusion.
- The heart will appear slightly **larger on an AP projection** than a PA (posteroanterior) projection of the chest because the heart is closer to the imaging surface on a PA exposure.
- On the lateral projection, the heart usually does not extend posteriorly to overlap the spine unless it is enlarged or there is a pericardial effusion.
- Two major patterns of congestive heart failure are pulmonary interstitial and pulmonary alveolar edema.
- The four key findings of **pulmonary interstitial edema** are thickening of the interlobular septa, peribronchial cuffing, fluid in the fissures, and pleural effusions.
- The key findings in **pulmonary alveolar edema** are fluffy, indistinct, patchy airspace densities; bat-wing or butterfly pattern of disease that frequently spares the outer third of lungs; and pleural effusions, especially with cardiogenic pulmonary edema.
- Causes of pulmonary edema can be divided into two major categories: cardiogenic and noncardiogenic causes.
- **Cardiogenic pulmonary edema** is more likely to have pleural effusions and Kerley B lines, cardiomegaly, and an elevated pulmonary capillary wedge pressure than noncardiogenic pulmonary edema.
- The **noncardiogenic causes of pulmonary edema** are a diverse group of diseases that include uremia, disseminated intravascular coagulopathy, smoke inhalation, near-drowning, and volume overload.

- **Acute respiratory distress syndrome** (ARDS) can be considered a subset of noncardiogenic pulmonary edema in which the clinical picture is one of severe hypoxia, cyanosis, tachypnea, and dyspnea.
- **Essential hypertension** is a common disease that can lead to congestive heart failure, coronary artery disease, and cardiac arrhythmias.
- **Mitral stenosis** has become less common with antibiotic treatment of rheumatic fever, but can lead to left and then right heart failure through chronic elevation of the pulmonary venous and arterial pressures with increased pulmonary vascular resistance.
- **Pulmonary arterial hypertension** may either be idiopathic (primary) or secondary to emphysema or recurrent thromboembolic disease. It produces *pruning* of the pulmonary vasculature and might be suspected when the main pulmonary artery achieves a diameter of 3 cm or more on CT or MRI.
- **Aortic stenosis** in the elderly is most often secondary to degeneration of a tricuspid aortic valve and can lead to angina, syncope, and/or congestive heart failure. The ascending aorta may be prominent from *poststenotic dilatation.*
- **Cardiomyopathies** are divided into several categories with dilated, hypertrophic, and restrictive forms being the most common. Restrictive cardiomyopathy must be differentiated from constrictive pericarditis with which it shares its clinical findings.
- **Aortic aneurysms** can be saccular, fusiform, or can dissect. Most thoracic aortic dissections begin in the ascending aorta (Stanford type A) and are treated surgically.
- **Coronary artery disease** is the leading cause of death worldwide and it, or its sequelae, can be imaged using a variety of techniques including CT, MRI, and SPECT.

 Additional content is available online including chapters on Nuclear Medicine, Artificial Intelligence, Radiation Dose and Safety, an Early History of Radiology, and a compendium of 200 Diagnostic Radiology Signs.

# 12

# Recognizing the Normal Abdomen and Pelvis: Conventional Radiographs

*William Herring, MD, FACR*

While imaging of the abdomen is now largely performed utilizing CT, ultrasound, or MRI, many patients still have conventional radiographs ("plain films") of the abdomen as a **first step** before other imaging studies are performed or as a method of **following-up** on findings demonstrated by other modalities. Many of the principles that guide the interpretation of conventional radiographs also apply to the modalities of CT, MRI, and ultrasound.

## CASE QUIZ 12 QUESTION

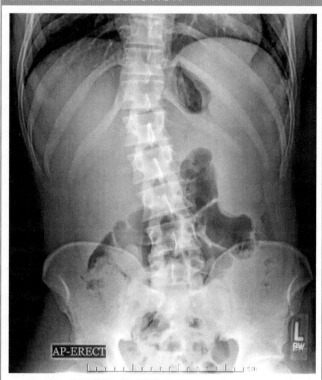

AP-ERECT

This is a 45-year-old male with a known history of leukemia. Conventional radiographs of the abdomen were obtained for abdominal discomfort and the upright abdominal view is shown. Palpation of the abdomen was abnormal. What abnormalities does this radiograph suggest? See the answer at the end of this chapter.

- In order to recognize *abnormal* findings on conventional radiographs of the abdomen, you must familiarize yourself with the appearance of *normal* first.

## WHAT TO LOOK FOR

- **First**, look at the **overall gas pattern.**
  - You are looking for the **overall** pattern, so don't spend too much time trying to identify every bubble of bowel gas you see.
- **Second,** check to see if there is **extraluminal air.**
- **Third,** look for **abnormal abdominal calcifications.**
- **Fourth,** look for any **soft-tissue masses.**

### Normal Bowel Gas Pattern

- Virtually all gas in the bowel comes from swallowed air. Only a fraction comes from the bacterial fermentation of food. For the purposes of this chapter, the terms **gas** and **air** are used interchangeably to refer to the contents of the bowel.
- Loops of bowel that contain a sufficient amount of air to fill the lumen completely are said to be **distended. Distension** of bowel is **normal.**
- Loops of bowel that are filled beyond their normal size are said to be **dilated. Dilatation** of the bowel is **abnormal.**
- **Stomach**
  - There is almost **always air in the stomach,** unless:
    - The patient has recently vomited, or
    - There is a nasogastric tube in the stomach and the tube is attached to suction.

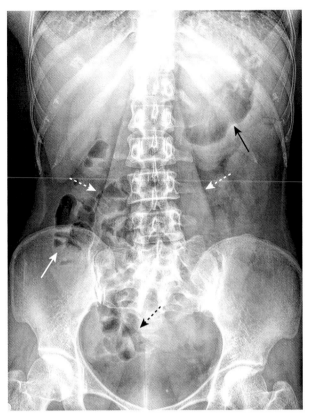

**Fig. 12.1 Normal Supine Abdomen.** This is the **scout** film of the abdomen, the supine view that gives you a general idea of the bowel gas pattern and allows you to search for abnormal calcifications and detect organomegaly. There is usually air in the stomach *(solid black arrow)* in about two or three loops of nondilated small bowel *(solid white arrow)* and in the rectosigmoid *(dashed black arrow)*. Depending on the amount of fat around the visceral structures, their outlines may be partially visible on conventional radiographs such as the psoas muscles in this image *(dashed white arrows)*.

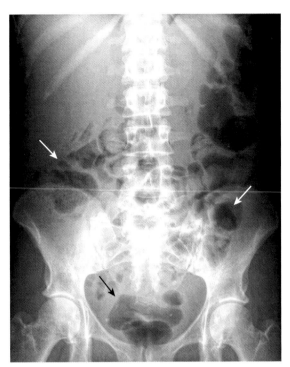

**Fig. 12.2 Normal Prone Abdomen.** In the prone position, the ascending and descending colon *(white arrows)* as well as the rectosigmoid (all posterior structures) are the highest parts of the large bowel and thus most likely to fill with air. There is air in the "S"-shaped rectosigmoid *(black arrow)*.

- **Small bowel**
  - There is usually a small amount of **air in about two or three loops of nondilated small bowel** (Fig. 12.1).
  - The **normal diameter of small bowel is less than 2.5 cm,** which is about 1 inch or the diameter of one United States quarter.
- **Large bowel**
  - There is **almost always air in the rectum or sigmoid.** There may be **varying amounts of gas** in the remainder of the **colon** (Fig. 12.2).
  - Use this rule to decide whether the **large bowel** is dilated or not:
    - **The large bowel can normally distend to about the same size as it does on a barium enema examination.** To give you an idea of how large that is, look at Fig. 12.3.
    - Stool is recognizable by the **multiple, small bubbles of gas** present within a semisolid appearing soft-tissue

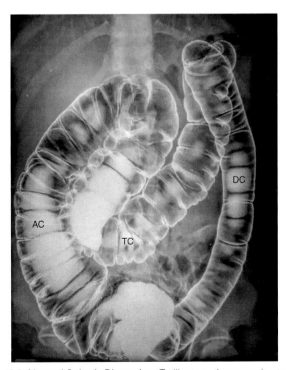

**Fig. 12.3 Normal Colonic Distension.** To illustrate the approximate size the normal colon may attain on a plain film, the colon shown is from an air-contrast barium enema. On a conventional radiograph, the entire colon would not contain this volume of air. This patient has had a ***double-contrast barium enema*** examination in which both air and barium were instilled as contrast agents. The combination allows for excellent visualization of the mucosal surface of the colon. *AC,* Ascending colon; *DC,* descending colon; *TC,* transverse colon.

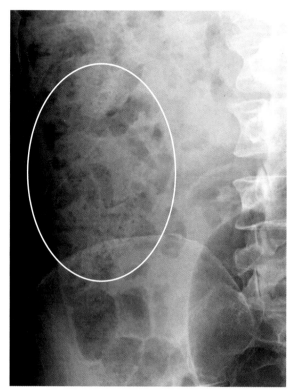

**Fig. 12.4 Appearance of Stool.** Stool contains numerous small bubbles of gas mixed within soft-tissue density *(oval)* as seen here in the ascending colon. Stool marks the location of the large bowel and can help in identification of individual loops of bowel on conventional radiographs.

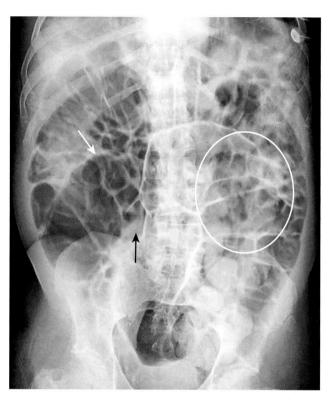

**Fig. 12.5 Aerophagia.** Virtually all bowel gas comes from swallowed air. Swallowing large quantities of air may produce a picture called ***aerophagia,*** characterized by numerous irregularly shaped, air-containing loops of bowel *(circle and arrows).* The bowel loops are distended and overlapping but not dilated.

mass. Recognizing the appearance of stool will help in localizing the large bowel (Fig. 12.4).

---

**⏵⏵ | IMPORTANT POINTS**

- Individuals who swallow excessive quantities of air may develop ***aerophagia,*** accompanied by belching, bloating, and abdominal distension. A gas pattern characterized by numerous **polygonal-shaped**, air-containing loops of bowel, none of which is dilated, may be seen (Fig. 12.5).

---

## Normal Gastrointestinal Tract Air-Fluid Levels

- **Stomach**
  - There is almost always **air and fluid** in the stomach so there is **almost always an air-fluid level visible in the stomach** on either an upright abdomen, a study done with the patient in the decubitus position, or an upright chest radiograph.
    - **To see an air-fluid level**, the path of the **x-ray beam must be directed horizontally**—parallel to the floor.
- **Small bowel**
  - **Two or three air-fluid levels** in small bowel may be seen normally on an upright or decubitus view of the abdomen.
- **Large bowel**
  - The large bowel functions, in part, to remove fluid so **there are usually no** or **very few air-fluid levels in the colon** (Fig. 12.6).

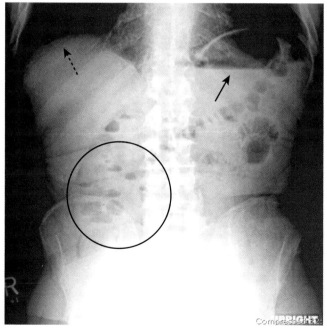

**Fig. 12.6 Normal Air-Fluid Levels, Upright Abdomen.** There are two things to look for on an upright view of the abdomen: **air-fluid levels** and **free intraperitoneal air**. Normally, there is an air-fluid level in the stomach *(solid arrow).* There may be short, air-fluid levels in a few nondilated loops of small bowel *(circle).* There are usually very few or no air-fluid levels in the colon. Free air, were it present, would be visible just below the right hemidiaphragm *(dashed arrow)* and would be easier to recognize on the right than the left.

| Organ | Normally Contains Gas | Normally Has Air/Fluid Levels |
|---|---|---|
| **TABLE 12.1   Normal Distribution of Gas and Fluid in the Abdomen** | | |
| **Stomach** | Yes | Yes |
| **Small bowel** | Yes, 2–3 loops | Yes |
| **Large bowel** | Yes, especially rectosigmoid | No |

▶▶ **IMPORTANT POINTS**

- There may be many air-fluid levels present in the colon if the patient has had a recent enema or if the patient is taking medication with a strong anticholinergic, antiperistaltic effect.

- The normal distribution of bowel gas and fluid is summarized in Table 12.1.

## Differentiating Large from Small Bowel

- **Recognizing large bowel**
  - **Large bowel is peripherally placed** around the perimeter of the abdominal cavity except for the right upper quadrant, which is occupied by the liver (Fig. 12.7).
  - *Haustral markings* usually do not extend completely across the large bowel from one wall to the other. If they should connect one wall with another, **haustral markings are spaced more widely apart** than the valvulae conniventes of the small bowel (Fig. 12.8).

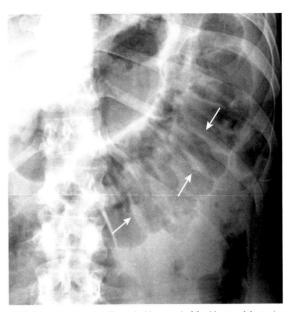

**Fig. 12.8 Normal Large Bowel Haustral Markings.** Most haustral markings in the colon do not traverse the entire lumen and therefore do not extend from one wall to the opposite wall *(arrows)*. This is unlike the appearance of the **valvulae conniventes** in the small bowel that do appear to traverse the entire lumen. The haustral markings are also spaced more widely apart than the valvulae of the small bowel (see Fig. 12.9).

- **Recognizing small bowel**
  - **Small bowel is centrally placed** in the abdomen. **Valvulae markings typically extend across the lumen** of small bowel from one wall to the other. The **valvulae are spaced much closer together** than the haustra of the large bowel (Fig. 12.9).

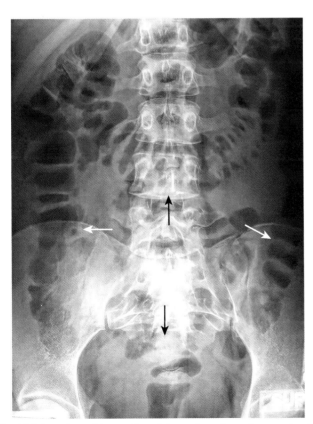

**Fig. 12.7 Location of Large Bowel.** Large bowel usually occupies the periphery of the abdomen. The small bowel is located more centrally. Here, large bowel *(arrows)* contains a normal amount of air.

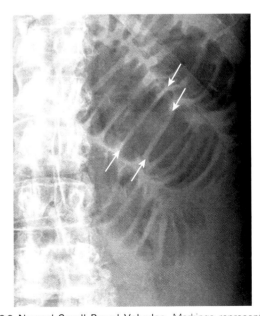

**Fig. 12.9 Normal Small Bowel Valvulae.** Markings representing the valvulae conniventes usually traverse the full width of the lumen of the small bowel, from one wall to the other. In addition, the valvulae are spaced closer together than the haustra of the large bowel, even when the small bowel is dilated. The arrows point to two valvulae that traverse the entire lumen in this close-up of dilated small bowel.

- Small bowel can achieve a maximally dilated diameter of **about 5 cm.** Large bowel can dilate to several times that size.

## ACUTE ABDOMINAL SERIES

- Almost every Department of Radiology has a series of radiographic images (i.e., a protocol) that is routinely obtained in patients who have acute abdominal pain. These series are sometimes called *obstruction series* or *complete abdominal series* or *acute abdominal series* or something similar. We will call such a combination of views an **acute abdominal series.**
- The views that make up such a series will vary not only between facilities but also based on each patient's ability to accommodate to the positioning needed to obtain the views. In general, views may include:
  - A **supine view** of the abdomen is almost always obtained (sometimes called a *flat plate* or *KUB* [for kidneys, ureters, and bladder]).
  - A **prone** or **lateral rectum view** is the most variable as to whether it is acquired.
  - An **upright view (or left lateral decubitus view)** may depend on the patient's condition.
  - A frontal **chest x-ray** (upright or supine) may also be included.
- Table 12.2 summarizes **what to look for on each of the views** of an acute abdominal series.

### Supine View (Scout Film) (See Fig. 12.1)

- **Why it is important**
  - For the **overall appearance of the bowel gas pattern**, its general location, volume, and configuration is **more important** than identifying every small bubble of air on the radiograph.
  - In identifying the **presence or absence of calcifications.**
  - For identifying the **presence of soft-tissue masses.**
- **How it is acquired**
  - The patient lies on their back on the x-ray table or stretcher, and the x-ray beam is directed vertically downward (Fig. 12.10).
- **Substitute view**

- There is really no other view that substitutes for a supine view of the abdomen. Virtually all patients, regardless of their condition, can tolerate this part of the examination.

### Prone View

- **Why it is important**
  - **For identifying gas in the rectum and/or sigmoid**
    - Since the rectum and sigmoid are the **highest points of the large bowel** with the person lying prone on the x-ray table, air will rise into the rectosigmoid.
      - Almost no air is introduced into the rectosigmoid during the course of a routine rectal examination.
  - **For identifying gas in the ascending and descending colon**
    - Since these two parts of the large bowel, besides the rectosigmoid, are posteriorly positioned, air should also collect in them when the patient is lying prone (see Fig. 12.2).
- **How it is acquired**
  - The patient lies on their abdomen on the x-ray table or stretcher and the x-ray beam is directed vertically downward (Fig. 12.11).

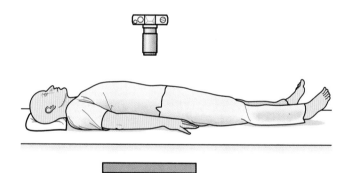

**Fig. 12.10 Positioning for Supine View of the Abdomen.** The patient lies on their back on the x-ray table or stretcher. The x-ray beam is directed vertically downward. The camera icon represents the x-ray tube, which would actually be positioned about 40 inches above the **cassette**, represented by the gray rectangle under the table.

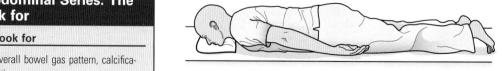

**Fig. 12.11 Positioning for Prone View of the Abdomen.** The patient lies on their abdomen on the x-ray table or stretcher and the x-ray beam is directed vertically downward. Once again, the camera icon represents the x-ray tube, positioned about 40 inches above the cassette, represented by the gray rectangle under the patient.

| TABLE 12.2 **Acute Abdominal Series: The Views and What to Look for** | |
| --- | --- |
| View | Look for |
| **Supine abdomen** | Overall bowel gas pattern, calcifications, masses |
| **Prone abdomen or lateral rectum** | Gas in the rectosigmoid |
| **Upright abdomen** | Free air, air-fluid levels in the bowel |
| **Upright chest** | Free air, pneumonia, pleural effusions |

- **Substitute view**
  - Frequently, patients are **unable to lie prone** because of their physical condition (e.g., recent surgery or severe abdominal pain).
  - These patients can turn on their **left side** and have a **lateral view of the rectum** exposed with a **vertical beam** to substitute for the prone radiograph (Fig. 12.12). The lateral view of the rectum will usually demonstrate the presence or absence of air in the rectum and/or sigmoid (Fig. 12.13).

> ## ▶▶ IMPORTANT POINTS
>
> - **Why rectal air is important to identify**
>   - As we shall see in Chapter 14, for a period of time **after** the bowel becomes mechanically obstructed, continued peristalsis will function to eliminate any gas **distal** to the point of obstruction. The rectum, a structure that is distal to virtually every possible point of a bowel obstruction, should be evacuated of its gas. The **absence of gas** in the rectum could, therefore, be an important clue to the **presence of a mechanical bowel obstruction.**

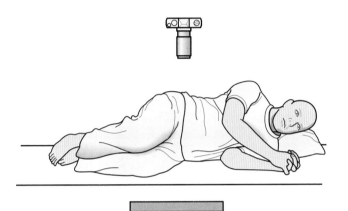

**Fig. 12.12 Positioning for the Lateral Rectum View.** Patients who cannot lie prone can usually turn on their left side to have a lateral view of the rectum exposed with a vertical beam. This substitutes for a prone view of the abdomen.

## Upright View of Abdomen

- **Why it is important**
  - For detecting **free air in the peritoneal cavity** (i.e., extraluminal air).
  - For identifying **air-fluid levels within the bowel lumen** (see Fig. 12.6).
- **How it is acquired**
  - The patient stands or sits up and the exposure is made with the **x-ray beam directed horizontally**, parallel to the plane of the floor (Fig. 12.14).
- **Substitute view**
  - Frequently, patients with the signs and symptoms of an acute abdomen cannot tolerate standing or sitting up for an upright view of their abdomen.
  - In such cases, a **left lateral decubitus view** of the abdomen can be substituted for the upright radiograph. For a left lateral decubitus view, the **patient lies on their left side on the x-ray table.** This is done so that any *extraluminal (free) air* will distribute itself at the

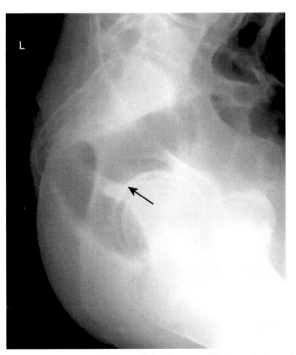

**Fig. 12.13 Normal Lateral View of the Rectum.** The lateral view of the rectum will usually demonstrate the presence *(arrow)* or absence of air in the rectum and/or sigmoid. This, as discussed in Chapter 14, can be helpful at times in suggesting mechanical obstruction of the bowel.

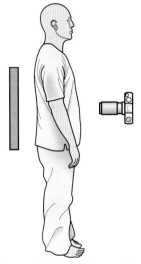

**Fig. 12.14 Positioning of Patient for an Upright View of the Abdomen.** The patient stands or sits upright and the x-ray beam is directed horizontally, parallel to the plane of the floor for this view. The x-ray tube represented by the camera icon is again positioned about 40 inches from the cassette, represented by the gray rectangle behind the patient.

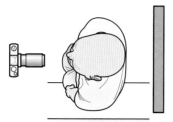

**Fig. 12.15** Positioning of the Patient for a Left Lateral Decubitus View of the Abdomen. Patients who cannot tolerate an upright view of their abdomen can have a left lateral decubitus view as a substitute. The patient lies on his or her left side on the examining table; the x-ray tube is usually positioned anteriorly *(camera icon)* and the cassette *(gray rectangle)* is placed in back of the patient. The x-ray beam is directed horizontally, parallel to the floor at a distance of about 40 inches from the patient.

**highest part of the abdominal cavity,** which will be on the patient's **right** side (Fig. 12.15).

- **Free air should be easily visible** over the **outside edge of the liver** where there is normally no bowel gas present (Figs. 12.16AB).
  - If, on the other hand, a right lateral decubitus view was obtained, any free air, if present, would rise to the left side of the abdomen. The left side of the abdomen is the normal location of the stomach bubble as well as gas in the splenic flexure of the colon, either of which could be mistaken for free air.
- In order **to see the free air, the x-ray beam must be directed horizontally,** parallel to the floor, when a decubitus view is obtained.

### BOX 12.1   To See an Air-fluid Level on Conventional Radiographs, You Must Have

- Air
- Fluid
- A horizontal x-ray beam (parallel to the plane of the floor)

- Air-fluid interfaces **cannot** be visualized on conventional radiographs taken with a vertical x-ray beam, e.g., supine studies.

- Box 12.1 summarizes the elements that must be present to be able to visualize air-fluid levels in the abdomen.

### Upright (or Supine) View of Chest

- **Why it is important**
  - For detecting **free air beneath the diaphragm.**
  - For visualizing **pneumonia at the lung bases,** which might mimic the symptoms of an acute abdomen.
  - For finding **pleural effusions,** which could be secondary to an intraabdominal process and help identify its presence.
    - **Pancreatitis,** for example, **may be associated with a left pleural effusion.**
    - Some **ovarian tumors** may occasionally be associated with **right-sided or bilateral pleural effusions.**
    - An abscess beneath the right hemidiaphragm *(subphrenic abscess)* **may be associated with a right pleural effusion.**
    - See Chapter 7 for more on the laterality of pleural effusions.
- **How it is acquired**

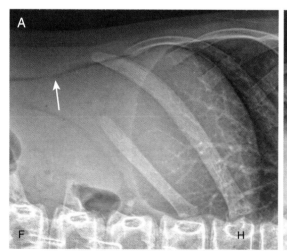
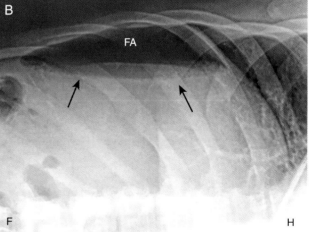

**Fig. 12.16** Normal Left Lateral Decubitus View of the Abdomen and Free Air. (A) With the patient lying on the examining table with their left side down, an exposure is made with a horizontal x-ray beam (parallel to the floor), so that any **free air** will distribute itself at the highest part of the abdominal cavity, above the liver on the patient's right side. There is no free air in this patient. There is, however, a normal lucency *(arrow)* that points to the ***properitoneal fat stripe.*** (B) In another patient, this one with a perforated ulcer, free air (FA) is visible as a black crescent over the outside edge of the liver along with an **air-fluid level** from free fluid and air in the peritoneal cavity *(arrows)*. F, Direction of patients' feet; H, direction of patients' head.

- The **patient stands** or **sits up** and an exposure of the thorax is made using a **horizontal x-ray beam** (Fig. 12.17).
- **Substitute view for an upright chest x-ray**
  - If the patient cannot tolerate standing for an upright view of their chest, **a supine view of the chest may be obtained** with the patient lying on the stretcher or x-ray table.
  - For a supine view, the x-ray beam is directed **vertically downward** and **free air, especially small amounts, may not be visible.**

## EXTRALUMINAL AIR

- Extraluminal air is abnormal and discussed in **Chapter 15**.

## CALCIFICATIONS

### Recognizing Abnormal Calcifications and Their Causes

- Abnormal abdominal calcifications are discussed in **Chapter 16**.
- There are two common **nonpathologic calcifications** that should not be confused with abnormal calcifications of the abdomen.
  - *Phleboliths* are small, rounded calcifications that represent calcified venous thrombi that occur with increasing age, most often in the pelvic veins of women. They classically have a **lucent center** that helps to differentiate them from ureteral calculi with which phleboliths can be confused (Fig. 12.18).

- **Calcification of the rib cartilages** occurs with advancing age and, while not a true abdominal calcification, can sometimes be confused for renal or biliary calculi when these rib calcifications overlie the kidney or region of the gallbladder. Calcified cartilage tends to have an **amorphous, speckled appearance,** and the calcified cartilage will occur in an arc corresponding to that of the anterior rib cartilage as it sweeps back toward its articulation with the sternum (Fig. 12.19).

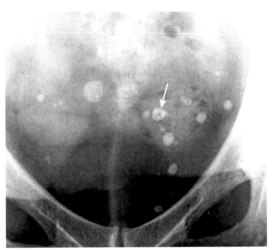

**Fig. 12.18 Phleboliths.** Phleboliths are calcifications most often found in the pelvis in women with increasing age. They classically have a lucent center *(arrow)*. They are almost always incidental and nonpathologic, but they can prove challenging diagnostically because their location and appearance are similar to ureteral calculi.

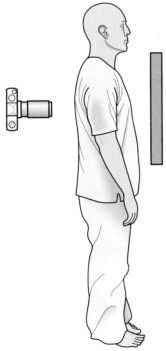

**Fig. 12.17 Positioning of Patient for an Upright Chest Radiograph.** The patient sits upright or stands with their anterior chest wall closest to the cassette. The x-ray beam passes horizontally so that any free air in the abdomen would rise to a position under the diaphragm and be visible.

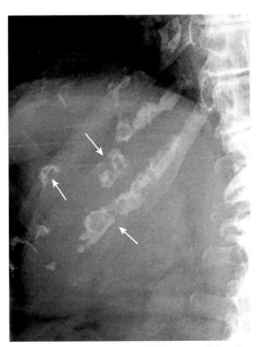

**Fig. 12.19 Calcified Rib Cartilages.** Calcification of the rib cartilages *(arrows)* appears to be a physiologic process that is more common in females and rare under the age of 35. It has been postulated that it may be a response to strains imposed by muscular activity. A difference in the pattern of calcification between males and females has been used by forensic pathologists to identify gender in postmortem examinations.

# RECOGNIZING ORGANOMEGALY

- **Conventional radiographic evaluation of soft-tissue structures in the abdomen** (such as the liver, spleen, kidneys, gallbladder, urinary bladder, or soft-tissue masses like tumors or abscesses) **is limited** because these structures are **soft-tissue densities** and they are **surrounded by other soft tissues or fluid** of similar density. Only a **difference in density** between two adjacent structures **will render their outlines visible** on conventional radiographs.
- Still, conventional radiographs are easy to obtain and frequently the first study ordered in a patient with abdominal symptoms.

> **IMPORTANT POINTS**
>
> - There are **two fundamental ways of recognizing the presence** and **estimating the size of soft-tissue masses or organs** on conventional radiographs of the abdomen:
>   - The first is by **direct visualization of the mass and its borders,** which can only occur if it is surrounded by something of a different density other than the mass, like that of **fat** or **free air.**
>   - The second is to recognize **indirect evidence of the mass** or enlarged visceral organ by **recognizing pathologic displacement of air-filled loops of bowel** from their expected locations.

## Liver

- **Normal**
  - The liver normally displaces all bowel gas from the right upper quadrant.
  - Occasionally, a **tongue-like projection of the right lobe** of the liver may extend to the iliac crest, **especially in females.** This is called a *Riedel lobe* and is normal (Fig. 12.20).
- **Enlarged liver**
  - **An enlarged liver might be suggested** from conventional radiographs if there is displacement of all bowel from the right upper quadrant **down to the iliac crest** and **across the midline** (Fig. 12.21). **Conventional radiographs are poor for estimating the size of the liver.** Imaging evaluation of liver size is best made using CT, MRI, or ultrasound.

## Spleen

- **Normal**
  - The adult **spleen is about 12 cm in length** and **usually does not project below the 12th posterior rib.** As a general rule, the **spleen is about as large as the left kidney.**
- **Enlarged spleen**
  - As an aid in identifying splenomegaly, keep in mind that the normal position of the **stomach bubble** (i.e., air in the gastric fundus) **is nestled beneath the highest part of the left hemidiaphragm** about midway between the abdominal wall and the spine (see Fig. 12.1).

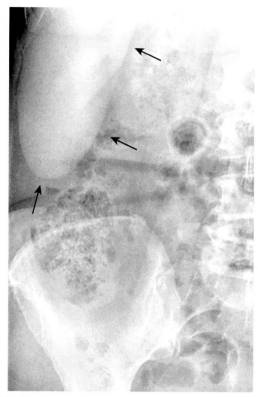

**Fig. 12.20 Riedel Lobe of the Liver.** A normal anatomic variant, particularly found in females, is this tongue-like, inferior projection of the right lobe of the liver *(arrows)*. It can mimic a palpable liver mass.

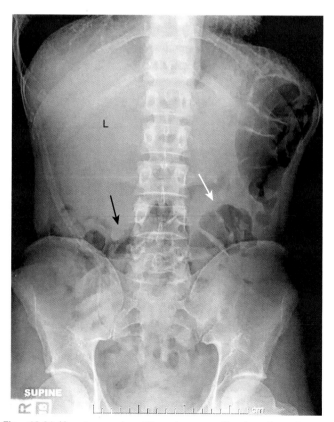

**Fig. 12.21 Hepatomegaly.** Although conventional radiographs are notoriously poor for evaluating liver size, sometimes the liver can become so enlarged it will be obvious even on plain films. If the liver (L) displaces all bowel loops from the right upper quadrant down to the pelvis *(arrows)*, then hepatomegaly is highly suggested, such as in this patient with cirrhosis.

- If the spleen projects well **below the 12th posterior rib** and/or **displaces the stomach bubble** toward or across the midline, the spleen is probably enlarged (Fig. 12.22).

## Kidneys

- **Normal**
  - Portions of the kidney outlines may be visible on conventional radiographs if there is an adequate amount of perirenal fat present.
  - The **kidney length is approximately the height of four lumbar vertebral bodies** or about **10 to 14 cm in size in an adult.**

- The liver depresses the right kidney so that the **right kidney is usually lower in the abdomen than the left kidney** (Fig. 12.23).
- The left **kidney is roughly the same length as the spleen.**
- **Enlarged kidney**
  - Usually only extremely enlarged kidneys or very large renal masses will be recognizable on conventional radiographs by displacement of bowel gas (Fig. 12.24).

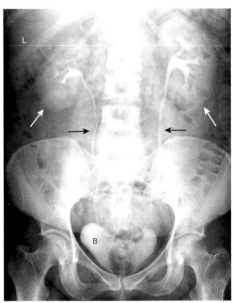

**Fig. 12.23 Position of the Kidneys.** This is one image from an *intravenous urogram* (also called an *intravenous pyelogram* or *IVP*) in which the patient received an intravenous injection of iodinated contrast that was then excreted by the kidneys. It was a routine study used extensively in the 20th century but is now mostly replaced by CT and US. Both kidney outlines *(white arrows)*, ureters *(black arrows)*, and urinary bladder (B) can be seen. The liver (L) normally depresses the right kidney more inferiorly than the left kidney.

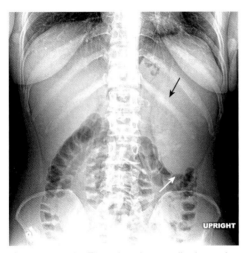

**Fig. 12.22 Splenomegaly.** The spleen is normally about 12 cm in length and usually does not project below the 12th posterior rib. If the spleen *(white arrow)* projects well below the 12th posterior rib *(black arrow)* and/or displaces the normally left-sided stomach bubble toward or across the midline, the spleen is probably enlarged, as it is in this patient with leukemia.

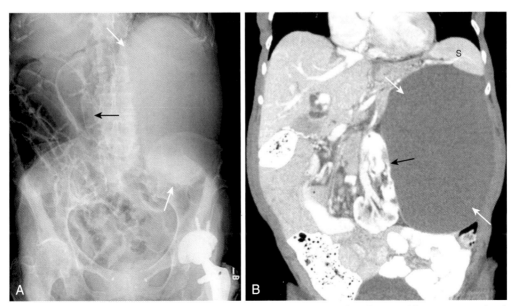

**Fig. 12.24 Enlarged Kidney.** Soft-tissue masses or organomegaly can be diagnosed from a conventional radiograph either by visualizing the **edge of the mass** if there is fat or air surrounding it or by **displacement of bowel.** (A) On the conventional radiograph, there is a soft-tissue density in the left upper quadrant *(white arrows)* that is displacing bowel to the right *(black arrow)*. (B) A coronal reformatted CT scan of the same patient demonstrates a large renal cyst *(white arrows)* arising from the compressed left kidney *(black arrow)*, displacing it and the adjacent bowel. The spleen (S) is also being compressed by the cyst.

## Urinary Bladder

- **Normal**
  - The bladder is frequently surrounded by **enough extravesical fat that at least the dome is visible** in most individuals. The bladder is an oval structure with its long axis parallel to the long axis of the pelvis and the **base of the bladder positioned just above the top of the symphysis pubis.**
  - The urinary bladder is about the size of a small cantaloupe when distended and about the size of a lemon when contracted (Fig. 12.25).
- **Enlarged urinary bladder**
  - Bladder enlargement is usually recognized by displacement of bowel upward and out of the pelvis by a mass of soft-tissue density. Bladder outlet obstruction is much more common in men from enlargement of the prostate, so that a pelvic soft-tissue mass is more likely to be a dilated bladder in a male than a female (Fig. 12.26A).

## Uterus

- **Normal**
  - The uterus usually sits atop the dome of the bladder. There is frequently a lucency produced by fat between the top of the bladder and the bottom of the uterus. The **normal uterus is about 8 cm by 4 cm by 6 cm.**
- **Enlarged uterus**
  - **Ultrasound** is the **best** tool for **evaluating the size of the uterus and ovaries.**
  - **Occasionally uterine enlargement**, when marked, **may be visible** on **conventional radiographs** (Fig. 12.26B).

## Psoas Muscles

- One or both of the psoas muscles may be visible if there is adequate extraperitoneal fat surrounding them. Inability to visualize one or both psoas muscles is not a reliable indicator of retroperitoneal disease (see Fig. 12.1).

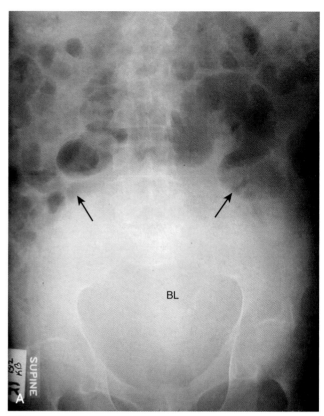

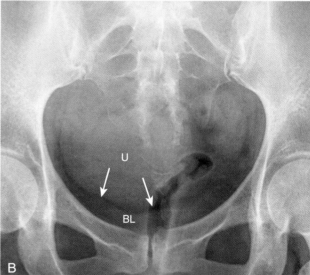

**Fig. 12.26 Distended Urinary Bladder and Enlarged Uterus.** (A) The distended bladder (BL) is visualized as a soft-tissue mass that ascends from the pelvis into the lower abdomen, displacing the bowel into the mid-abdomen *(arrows)*. This was a 72-year-old man with bladder outlet obstruction from benign prostatic hypertrophy. (B) In a different patient, the uterus (U) is slightly enlarged. It can be distinguished from the bladder because there is a fat plane *(arrows)* between the uterus and the urinary bladder (BL) below it.

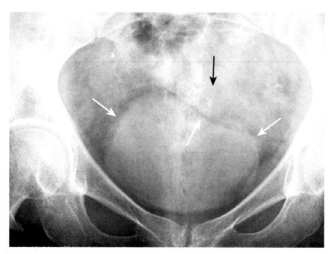

**Fig. 12.25 Normal Urinary Bladder.** Close-up of the pelvis demonstrates the outline of the urinary bladder made visible by perivesical fat *(white arrows)*. In males, the sigmoid colon usually occupies the space just above the bladder *(black arrow)* while in females, the soft tissue above the bladder may be either the uterus or sigmoid colon.

## CASE QUIZ 12 ANSWER

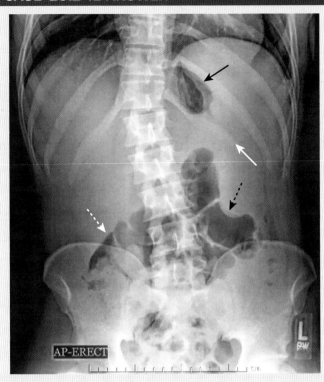

The bowel gas pattern suggests **hepatosplenomegaly**, consistent with the patient's known diagnosis of leukemia. An enlarged spleen displaces the stomach bubble toward the midline *(solid black arrow)*. The splenic flexure is also depressed downward *(dashed black arrow)* by the enlarged spleen and projects below the 12th rib *(solid white arrow)*. In addition an enlarged liver depresses the hepatic flexure of the colon downward almost to the pelvis *(dashed white arrow)*. Bowel displacement can suggest organomegaly.

## TAKE HOME POINTS

- Evaluation of the abdomen should focus on four main areas: the gas pattern, free air, soft-tissue masses or organomegaly, and abnormal calcifications.
- Normally, air is present in the stomach and colon, especially the rectosigmoid, whereas a small amount of air (two to three loops) may normally be seen in the small bowel.
- Normally, an air-fluid level is seen in the stomach; there may be two to three air-fluid levels in nondilated small bowel, but usually no air-fluid level is visible in the colon.
- An **acute abdominal series** may consist of: a supine abdomen, prone abdomen (or its substitute, which is a lateral rectum view), upright abdomen (or its substitute, which is a left lateral decubitus view), and an upright chest (or its substitute, which is a supine chest).

- The **supine view** of the abdomen is the general scout view for the bowel gas pattern and is useful for identifying calcifications and for detecting organomegaly or soft-tissue masses.
- The **prone view** allows air to be seen in the rectosigmoid, which is important in the identification of mechanical obstruction of the bowel.
- The **upright abdomen** may demonstrate air-fluid levels in the bowel or free intraperitoneal air.
- The **upright chest radiograph** may demonstrate free air beneath the diaphragm, pleural effusion (which may provide a clue as to the presence and the nature of intraabdominal pathology), or pneumonia (which can mimic an acute abdomen).
- CT, US, and MRI have essentially replaced conventional radiography in the assessment of organomegaly or abdominal soft-tissue masses.

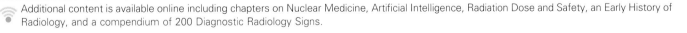

Additional content is available online including chapters on Nuclear Medicine, Artificial Intelligence, Radiation Dose and Safety, an Early History of Radiology, and a compendium of 200 Diagnostic Radiology Signs.

# 13

# Recognizing the Normal Abdomen and Pelvis: Computed Tomography

*William Herring, MD, FACR*

## INTRODUCTION TO ABDOMINAL AND PELVIC CT

It is estimated that around 90 million CT scans of all kinds were performed in the United States in 2019. Almost 10% of all visits to the emergency department are for abdominal pain of a nontraumatic nature. Many of those patients undergo a CT scan of the abdomen and pelvis performed to detect or clarify their clinical findings. Since the advent of CT, exploratory surgery has become rare and the need for emergency surgery has dramatically decreased.

### CASE QUIZ 13 QUESTION

This is a text-only question. A 66-year-old male presents with what may be a pulsatile abdominal mass. What imaging examination would be the most appropriate as an initial screening study?
1. MRI of the abdomen
2. Conventional radiograph of the abdomen
3. Abdominal angiogram
4. Ultrasound of the abdomen
   See the correct answer at the end of this chapter.

- As with all imaging studies, one of the guiding principles in CT scanning of the abdomen and pelvis is to maximize the differences in density between tissues to best demonstrate their unique anatomy. Toward that end, abdominal CT studies make extensive use of **intravenous** and **oral contrast** agents.

## INTRAVENOUS CONTRAST IN CT SCANNING

- CT scans **can be performed with and/or without the intravenous administration of iodinated contrast** material but, **in general, they yield more diagnostic information** that is more easily detectable **when intravenous contrast can be used.** CT scans done with **intravenous contrast** are called *contrast enhanced* or simply *enhanced*. Typically, the radiologist will choose the scanning parameters to optimize the CT study for the patient's particular clinical issues. For example, different rates of contrast administration and timing of the scan will allow diagnostic enhancement of hepatic vessels versus the liver parenchyma.

- Although it might sound like a great idea to give everyone contrast, keep in mind that **iodinated contrast** can have **adverse effects** and produce **serious reactions** in **susceptible individuals** (Box 13.1).

### BOX 13.1  Contrast Reactions

- Intravenous contrast materials available today are **nonionic, low-osmolar solutions containing a high concentration of iodine** that circulate through the bloodstream, opacify those tissues and organs with high blood flow, are absorbed by x-rays (and therefore appear "whiter" on images), and are finally excreted in the urine by the kidneys.
- In some patients who have compromised renal function suggested by an estimated glomerular filtration rate (eGFR) less than 30 mL/min/1.73 m$^2$ or a serum creatinine 1.5 mg/dL or higher who are not undergoing maintenance dialysis, prophylaxis with intravenous normal saline may reduce the risk for contrast-associated acute kidney injury in such patients. Although usually reversible, in a small number of patients with underlying renal insufficiency, renal dysfunction may permanently worsen.
- Iodinated contrast agents can sometimes produce **mild side effects** including a feeling of warmth, nausea and vomiting, and local irritation (itching and hives) at the site of injection. These side effects usually require no treatment. Occasional idiosyncratic, allergic-like reactions may also include itching, hives, and laryngeal irritation.
- Asthmatics and those with a history of severe allergies or prior reactions to intravenous contrast have a higher likelihood of contrast reactions (but still very low overall) and may benefit from steroids, diphenhydramine (Benadryl®), and cimetidine (e.g., Tagamet®) administered prior to and/or after injection. Prior shellfish allergy bears absolutely NO relationship to iodinated contrast reactions.
- In about 0.01 to 0.04% of all patients, **severe and idiosyncratic reactions** to contrast can occur that can produce intense bronchospasm, laryngeal edema, circulatory collapse, and, very rarely, death (1 in 200,000 to 300,000).
- In patients with a history of intravenous contrast reactions, **oral contrast** can be safely administered without the need for premedication.

# ORAL CONTRAST IN CT SCANNING

- For abdominal and pelvic CT imaging, **oral contrast** may also be administered to define the bowel, although its use has diminished as the quality of CT images has improved. Oral contrast is usually **not employed in chest CT scanning** unless there is a particular question concerning the esophagus.
- Orally administered contrast, frequently given in doses divided over time to allow earlier contrast to reach the colon while later contrast opacifies the stomach, is utilized for many abdominal CT scans except those performed for **trauma**, the *stone search* **study**, and studies specifically directed toward evaluating vascular structures like the **aorta.**
- One of two different types of oral contrast may be used. The most widely used is a dilute solution of **barium sulfate**, the same contrast agent employed in upper gastrointestinal studies and barium enemas. If there is concern for bowel perforation and the possibility that contrast may exit from the lumen of the bowel, an iodine-based, water-soluble contrast is sometimes used (e.g., **Gastrografin**®). Contrast may also be introduced rectally to opacify the distal colon more quickly than it would take for orally administered contrast to reach the large bowel or through a Foley catheter to quickly opacify the urinary bladder.
- You will probably not be required to make the decision of when or if to use contrast as **the radiologist will usually tailor the examination to best answer the clinical question being asked.** That means it is **always important** to provide as much clinical information as possible when requesting a study.
- Table 13.1 summarizes, in general, **when intravenous and oral contrast are utilized** for particular problems.
- Table 13.2 outlines some of the common **patient preparations** that are generally suggested for a variety of imaging studies. Preparation instructions may vary depending on

## TABLE 13.1 CT Scans: When Contrast Is Used

| IV Contrast Used | IV Contrast Usually Not Used |
|---|---|
| **Chest** | |
| CT-pulmonary angiogram *(CT-PA)* for pulmonary embolism | Evaluation of diffuse infiltrative lung diseases using HRCT |
| Evaluation of the mediastinum or hila for mass or adenopathy | Confirmation of the presence of a lung nodule suspected from conventional radiographs |
| Detect aortic aneurysm or dissection | Detect pneumothorax/pneumomediastinum |
| Evaluation of blunt or penetrating trauma | Calcium scoring for the coronary arteries |
| Characterization of pleural disease (metastases, empyema) | Known allergies to contrast or renal failure |
| CT densitometry of pulmonary masses | |
| Evaluation of the coronary arteries | |
| **IV Contrast Used** | **IV Contrast Usually Not Used** |
| **Abdomen and Pelvis** | |
| Evaluate for the presence of and/or to characterize a mass and to stage or follow-up malignancies | CT colonography, unless staging a suspected cancer detected by colonoscopy |
| Trauma | Search for a ureteral calculus |
| Abdominal pain (e.g., appendicitis) | |
| Detect aortic aneurysm or dissection | |
| **WHEN ORAL CONTRAST IS USED** | |
| Most cases of nontraumatic abdominal pain | |
| Inflammatory bowel disease | |
| Abdominal or pelvic abscess | |
| Locate the site of bowel perforation, including fistulae | |

*HRCT,* High-resolution computed tomography; *IV,* intravenous.

## TABLE 13.2 Preparations for Imaging Studies

| Study | Before Order Is Placed | Before Start of the Study | After Study Is Done |
|---|---|---|---|
| **CT** | | | |
| **Head CT** with or without contrast | Solicit history of previous contrast reaction | Assessment of renal function may be needed before contrast injections | Nothing |
| **Body CT without contrast** | Nothing | No preparation needed | Nothing |
| **Body CT with** oral **contrast** and/or IV contrast | Solicit history of previous contrast reaction | Assessment of renal function may be needed before contrast injections; oral contrast is given just before study | Nothing |

*Continued*

## TABLE 13.2 Preparations for Imaging Studies—cont'd

| Study | Before Order Is Placed | Before Start of the Study | After Study Is Done |
|---|---|---|---|
| **US** | | | |
| **Upper abdomen**, general survey study: aorta, gall bladder, inferior vena cava, liver, pancreas, renal stenosis, retroperitoneal, spleen | Nothing | Nothing to eat or drink for several hours prior to examination | Nothing |
| **Renal or kidney** | Nothing | Patient may be asked to drink a prescribed amount of water to distend bladder 1–2 hours before procedure; patient should not empty bladder | Nothing |
| **Male or female pelvis** or lower abdomen; obstetric/gynecologic US | Nothing | Patient may be asked to drink a prescribed amount of water to distend bladder 1–2 hours before procedure; patient should not empty bladder | Nothing |
| **Renal transplant**, thyroid, and vascular studies | Nothing | No preparation needed | Nothing |
| **MRI** | | | |
| **Without contrast** | Solicit history of working with metal, grinding, welding, or possible metal in eyes (patient may need an orbital x-ray); solicit history of pacemaker, aneurysm clips, neural stimulators, IUD, permanent makeup, cochlear implants, artificial heart valves, pregnancy, metallic fragments, claustrophobia | No preparation needed | Nothing |
| **With contrast** | Solicit history of working with metal, grinding, welding, or possible metal in eyes (patient may need an orbital x-ray); solicit history of pacemaker, aneurysm clips, neural stimulators, IUD, permanent makeup; cochlear implants, artificial heart valves, pregnancy, metallic fragments, claustrophobia | Assessment of renal function may be needed before contrast injections | Nothing |
| **Barium Study** | | | |
| **Esophagram** or video fluoroscopic swallowing examination | Nothing | No preparation needed | Nothing |
| **Upper gastrointestinal series**/small bowel series | Nothing | Nothing to eat or drink for several hours prior to study | Nothing |
| **Barium enema**; virtual colonography | Nothing | Bowel preparation to cleanse colon before study may consist of oral laxatives, suppositories, fluids | Mild laxative if desired |
| **Mammography** | | | |
| **Mammogram** | Nothing | Patient should not use any deodorant, perfume, powder, ointment, or any other skin products on chest, breast, or under arms on the day of appointment | Nothing |
| **Nuclear Medicine** | | | |
| **Thyroid** uptake and scan | No intravenous, iodinated contrast studies within previous 4–8 weeks | Stop thyroid medications or foods high in iodine content | Nothing |
| **Bone density** | Is the patient pregnant? | No contrast or barium studies for 48 hours prior to the procedure. No food restriction | Nothing |
| **Bone scan** | Is the patient pregnant? | No food restriction | Nothing |
| **Cardiac** treadmill and pharmacologic stress test | Is the patient pregnant? | Nothing to eat or drink for several hours prior to the examination; no caffeine several hours prior to the examination | Nothing |

the facility and individual patient needs. In general, a patient is permitted to take their oral medications with a small sip of water, even when instructions are nothing to eat or drink before the study.

# ABDOMINAL CT: GENERAL CONSIDERATIONS

- Conventional radiography, ultrasonography, CT, and MRI can all be utilized in the imaging evaluation of abdominal abnormalities.
- Each has advantages and disadvantages inherent to its own particular technology and the choice of modality is frequently based on the patient's clinical condition (Table 13.3).
- While advances in CT imaging have resulted in better diagnostic studies, they may have come with an unintended consequence: potentially higher **radiation dose.** The radiation dose delivered by CT studies is dependent on many factors including the type of equipment, the energy of the x-rays used to produce the images, and the size of the patient.
- Ongoing research has involved the potential use of dual energy sources for CT scanning in certain situations that would allow for post-processing subtraction of the iodinated contrast to produce sets of both contrast and virtual noncontrast images with one scan, thus reducing the need to scan the patient twice. Dose-reducing measures are being employed including the use of optimized CT settings, reduction in the x-ray energy used, limiting the number of repeat scans, and assuring—through appropriate consultation—that the **benefits** derived from obtaining the study **outweigh** any potential **risks** of the radiation exposure.

> ### ▶▶ IMPORTANT POINTS
>
> - **History** and **physical examination** continue to be an essential part of evaluating abdominal abnormalities not only to suggest an etiology but in helping to determine which, if any, imaging studies will provide the best yield in establishing the correct diagnosis.

# ABDOMINAL CT: BY ORGAN

## Liver

- By convention, **CT scans**, like most other radiologic studies, **are viewed** with the **patient's right on your left and the patient's left on your right.** If the patient is scanned in the supine position, as most usually are, the **top** of each image is **anterior** and the **bottom** of each image is **posterior.**
- The liver receives its blood **supply** from both **hepatic arteries** and **portal veins** and **drains** to the inferior vena cava via the **hepatic veins.** The normal liver parenchyma is supplied 80% by the portal vein and 20% by the hepatic artery, so it will enhance mostly in the portal venous phase.
- The liver is **morphologically** divided into **right, left, and caudate lobes** based on its external appearance.

## TABLE 13.3 Imaging of the Abdomen and Pelvis Modalities Compared

| Uses | Advantages | Disadvantages |
|---|---|---|
| **Conventional Radiography** | | |
| Primarily used for screening in cases of abdominal pain | Readily available Relatively low cost Can be done portable Patients tolerate procedure well | Has lower sensitivity Uses ionizing radiation |
| **Ultrasonography (US)** | | |
| Primary imaging mode for gallbladder and biliary tree Screening for aortic aneurysm Identification of vascular abnormalities and flow Detection of ascites Primary imaging mode for the female pelvis | Readily available Relatively low cost Uses no ionizing radiation Patients tolerate procedure well Can be portable (point-of-care studies) | Operator dependent More difficult to interpret |
| **Computed Tomography** | | |
| Diagnostic modality of choice for most abdominal abnormalities, including trauma | Usually available Lower cost than MRI High spatial-resolution and image reconstruction Evaluates multiple organ systems simultaneously | Higher cost than US Uses ionizing radiation Possible inability to use intravenous contrast in patients with compromised renal function Possibility of contrast reactions Patient weight and size may affect scanning |
| **Magnetic Resonance Imaging (MRI)** | | |
| Problem-solving for difficult diagnoses Extension of known disease into surrounding soft tissues (staging) Vascular anatomy | High soft-tissue contrast No ionizing radiation No iodinated contrast Image reconstruction in any plane | Usually highest cost of imaging modalities Limited availability Longer scan times Claustrophobia, patient weight, and size may preclude study Monitoring issues in acutely ill patients Incompatible with certain medical devices or foreign bodies in patient |

- The larger **right lobe** is subdivided into **two segments:** the *anterior* and *posterior.* The **left lobe** is subdivided into **two segments:** the *medial* and *lateral.*
- A prominent, fat-filled fissure that contains the *falciform ligament* and *ligamentum teres* (formerly the umbilical

vein) separates the **medial and lateral segments** of the **left lobe** of the liver (Fig. 13.1).

- This anatomic division is not very useful for hepatic surgery since the **vascular distribution of the liver defines its anatomy** and the vascular anatomy is what directs the surgical approach to liver lesions.
  - The liver is **functionally** divided into **eight independently functioning segments** (also sometimes called *sectors*), each of which has its own branch of the portal vein, hepatic artery, bile duct, and venous drainage via the hepatic vein.
  - These functional segments can be identified utilizing cross-sectional imaging such as CT or MRI to localize visible disease to specific segments.
  - The most commonly used functional classification is named after French surgeon and anatomist Claude **Couinaud** and its importance for hepatic surgery is that it allows resection of one or more diseased segments while sparing the remaining normal segments (Fig. 13.2).
- The outer surface of the liver is normally smooth. The normal liver usually appears homogeneous in density on CT, and its attenuation should always be **denser than or equal to the density of the spleen on noncontrast scans.**
- The adult liver usually measures **15 cm or less on coronal scans at its maximum height.** Care must be taken not to measure the length at the site of a Riedel lobe of the liver, a normal inferior projection from the right lobe seen mainly in females (see Fig. 12.20). The liver's greatest **transverse measurement is 20 to 26 cm.**
- The diaphragmatic surface of the liver is affixed by connective tissue to a triangular section of the undersurface of the diaphragm, termed the ***bare area*** (Fig. 13.3). This will have importance later in differentiating ascites from pleural effusion (Chapter 17).
- **Liver volume** can be calculated using CT (as well as US and MRI). The volume of the liver will vary by gender and by

patient weight. The adult liver volume is about 1500 cm$^3$. Liver volume determinations may be used for liver resection, transplantation, and in evaluating the progression of various diseases, such as alcohol-related liver disease.

## Spleen

- On early contrast-enhanced scans, the spleen may be inhomogeneous in its attenuation, a finding that should disappear over the course of the next several minutes.

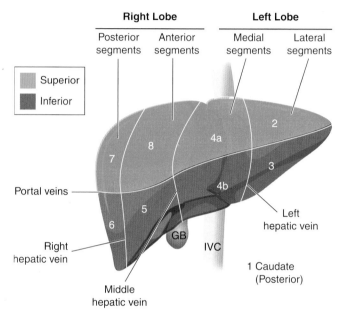

**Fig. 13.2 Functional Classification of Liver Segments.** This is the Couinaud classification of liver segments, which divides the liver into eight functionally independent segments (as numbered) facilitating surgical removal of one or more segments while allowing normal segments to remain. The ***superior*** and ***inferior*** group of segments are served by branches of the portal veins. They are further subdivided by the right, middle, and left hepatic veins into ***posterior, anterior, medial,*** and ***lateral*** segments. So, for example, segment 8 is called the anterior superior segment. Segment 1 (the caudate lobe) is located posteriorly. *GB,* Gallbladder; *IVC,* inferior vena cava.

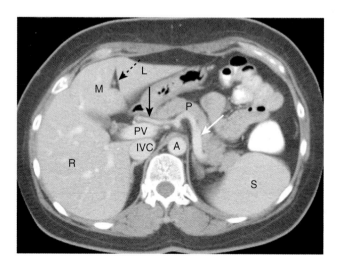

**Fig. 13.1 Normal Liver Anatomy.** The ligamentum teres *(dashed black arrow)* divides the left lobe of the liver into a medial (M) and lateral segment (L) with the larger right lobe (R) lying more posterior. The portal vein (PV) lies just posterior to the hepatic artery *(solid black arrow).* The splenic artery *(white arrow)* follows the path of the pancreas (P) toward the spleen (S). The inferior vena cava (IVC) lies to the right of the aorta (A).

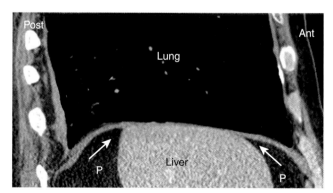

**Fig. 13.3 "Bare Area" of the Liver.** The ***bare area*** of the liver *(arrows)* has no **peritoneal covering but is affixed directly to the undersurface of the diaphragm.** As such, it is impossible for ascitic fluid in the peritoneal cavity (P) to insert itself between the liver and the lung, which will be important for differentiating **pleural effusion** from **ascites** on axial CT (see Chapter 17). *Ant,* Anterior; *Post,* posterior.

- The **normal** adult spleen may have **lobulations,** not to be confused with lacerations. The splenic artery and vein enter and exit at the hilum of the spleen.
- The spleen is usually **about 12 cm long, does not project** substantially below the margin of the **12th rib,** and is about the **same size as the left kidney.**

## Pancreas

- The pancreas is a retroperitoneal organ oriented obliquely so that the entire organ is not seen on any one axial image of the upper abdomen (Fig. 13.4).
- The pancreatic duct may be visible and measures 3 to 4 mm in diameter.
- The **head** of the pancreas measures **3 cm** in maximum dimension, the **body 2.5 cm,** and the **tail 2 cm.** The gland is about **12 to 15 cm in length.** As a person ages, the gland may undergo fatty infiltration giving it a "feathery" appearance (Fig. 13.5).

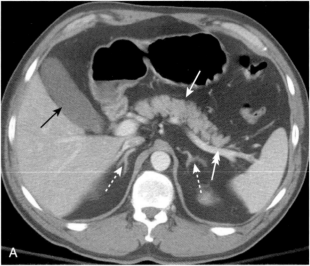

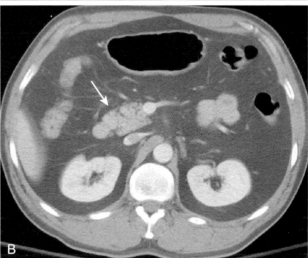

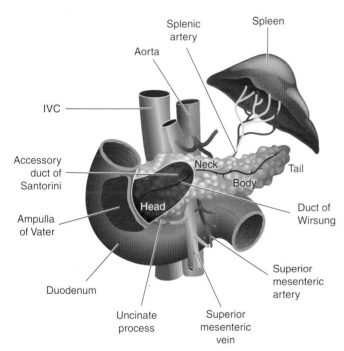

**Fig. 13.4 Pancreatic Anatomy.** The **tail** of the pancreas is usually the most superior part of the organ, lying in the hilum of the spleen. The **body** lies more inferiorly and the **neck** rests anterior to the superior mesenteric vessels. The **head** of the pancreas is nestled in the duodenal loop. The **uncinate process** is part of the head, variable in size, and curves around the superior mesenteric vein. The **splenic vein** (not shown) courses along the posterior border of the pancreas draining into the **superior mesenteric vein,** and the **splenic artery** runs along the superior border of the pancreas from the celiac axis to the spleen. The **main pancreatic duct (of Wirsung)** empties into the duodenum at the **ampulla.** There is sometimes an **accessory pancreatic duct of Santorini.** *IVC,* Inferior vena cava.

**Fig. 13.5 Normal Pancreas, CT.** (A) The body of the pancreas *(solid white arrow)* and splenic artery *(double white arrow)* are shown. Additionally well seen are both adrenal glands *(dashed white arrows)* and gallbladder *(solid black arrow).* (B) Normal head of pancreas *(arrow).* Because of its oblique orientation, the entire pancreas is not visualized on a single axial image of the abdomen.

## Kidneys

- The kidneys are retroperitoneal organs, encircled by varying amounts of fat and enclosed within a fibrous capsule.
- They are surrounded by the *perirenal space* that, in turn, is delimited by the **anterior and posterior renal fasciae.** Certain fascial attachments, muscles, and other organs define a series of spaces that produce predictable patterns of abnormality when those spaces are filled with fluid, pus, blood, or air.
- In adults, the **left kidney** is **minimally larger** than the **right,** each kidney being about **11 cm** in size or about the **same size** as the **spleen.**
- The **right renal artery** passes **posterior** to the inferior vena cava (IVC). The **renal veins** lie **anterior to the arteries;** the

longer left renal vein passes anterior to the aorta before draining into the inferior vena cava (Fig. 13.6).

- The **renal hilum** contains the renal pelvis and the renal artery and vein. The **upper poles** of the kidneys are more posterior than the lower poles and are tilted medially toward the spine.

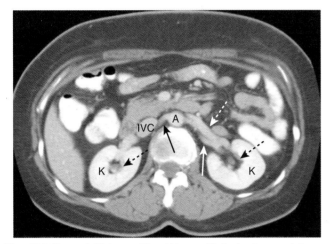

**Fig. 13.6 Normal Kidneys.** The kidneys (K) lie in the renal fossae bilaterally. The normal renal sinus, containing fat, occupies the central portion of the kidneys *(dashed black arrows)*. The right renal artery *(solid black arrow)* runs posterior to the inferior vena cava (IVC). The left renal vein *(dashed white arrow)* here lies anterior to the left renal artery *(solid white arrow)*. A, Abdominal aorta.

- Dedicated renal CT scans frequently use a precontrast view of the kidneys followed by a series of images obtained at timed intervals after the injection of intravenous contrast *(multiphasic study)* (Fig. 13.7).
- So long as they are functioning properly, the **kidneys are the major route** for excretion of **iodinated contrast** material. They should therefore **enhance** whenever intravenous contrast is administered. Over time, the urine will become more opacified, increasing significantly from its normal water density, sometimes requiring delayed imaging of the urinary tract.
- If the kidneys are not functioning properly, contrast is excreted through alternative pathways (e.g., bile, bowel), a process called *vicarious excretion* of contrast.

## Small and Large Bowel

- **Opacification** and **distension** of the bowel lumen are helpful for proper evaluation of the bowel wall regardless of the modality used to evaluate it. Wall thickness may seem artificially increased if the bowel is collapsed.
- The **small bowel** is usually **2.5 cm** or less in **diameter** with a **wall thickness** usually less than **3 mm**. Adjacent loops of small bowel are usually in contact with each other, depending in part on the amount of intraperitoneal fat present.
- The **colonic wall** is usually **less than 3 mm** thick with the colon **distended** and **less than 5 mm** with the colon **collapsed**. The **cecum** is recognizable by the presence of the terminal ileum and ileocecal valve. The positions of

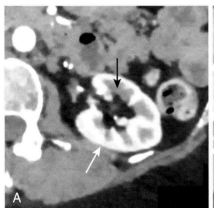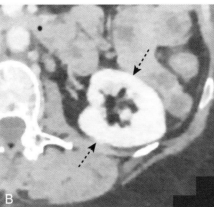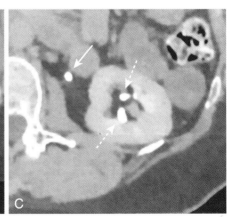

**Fig. 13.7 Multiphasic CT, Normal Left Kidney.** (A) The *corticomedullary phase* occurs about 30 to 70 seconds after the start of IV contrast injection and shows the corticomedullary junction between the outer, brighter cortex *(white arrow)* and the inner, less dense medulla *(black arrow)*. This phase can provide information about the renal vasculature and renal perfusion. (B) The *nephrographic phase* occurs about 80 to 100 seconds after injection and demonstrates homogeneous opacification of the kidney *(arrows)*. It is useful in evaluating the renal parenchyma, especially for renal neoplasms, as well as scarring and inflammatory disease. (C) The *excretory phase* is obtained about 5 to 10 minutes postinjection and may show urothelial abnormalities like tumors, papillary necrosis, and ureteral stricture. The intrarenal collecting system *(dashed arrows)* and ureter *(solid arrow)* are now opacified.

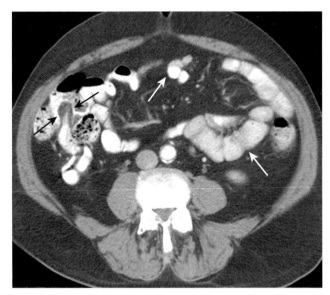

**Fig. 13.8 Normal Small Bowel.** Contrast fills a nondilated lumen (less than 2.5 cm). The small bowel wall is so thin that it is normally almost invisible *(white arrows)*. The terminal ileum can be recognized by the fat-containing "lips" of the ileocecal valve *(black arrows)* outlined with orally administered contrast in the lumen.

the transverse and sigmoid segments of the colon are variable, depending on their degree of redundancy (Fig. 13.8).

## Urinary Bladder

- The bladder is an **extraperitoneal organ**, the extraperitoneal space being continuous with the retroperitoneum. The **dome of the bladder** is covered by the **inferior reflection of the peritoneum.**
- The bladder's location in **males** is superior to the prostate gland and anterior to the rectum. In **females,** the bladder is anterior to the vagina and anteroinferior to the uterus. The ureters enter the posterolateral aspect of the bladder at the trigone.
- The **bladder wall measures 5 mm or less with the bladder distended.**
- The bladder is **best evaluated when distended** with either urine or urine-containing contrast but the **bladder wall is usually visible** whether or not intravenous contrast has been administered (Fig. 13.9).

**CASE QUIZ 13 ANSWER**

**Abdominal aortic ultrasound (#4)** is the initial imaging modality of choice when a pulsatile abdominal mass is present and an abdominal aortic aneurysm is suspected. In patients who may not be well-suited for a US (e.g., morbidly obese) a noncontrast CT may be substituted. For definitive diagnosis and imaging prior to intervention, CT-angiography or MR-angiography are recommended. For more clinical/imaging scenarios like these, see **What to Order When** online.

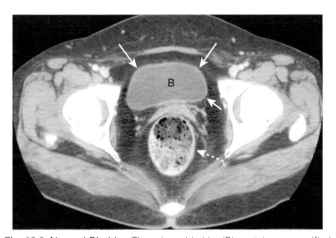

**Fig. 13.9 Normal Bladder.** The urinary bladder (B) contains unopacified urine in this early image of a contrast-enhanced CT scan of the pelvis. The bladder wall *(solid arrows)* is thin and of equal thickness around the circumference of the bladder. The rectum lies posterior to the bladder *(dashed arrow)*.

## TAKE HOME POINTS

- Computed tomography studies make extensive use of intravenous and oral contrast agents to maximize the differences in density between structures so as to best demonstrate their anatomy.
- In general, intravenous contrast-enhanced CT scans yield more diagnostic information, which is more easily recognizable when contrast can be used.
- Iodinated contrast agents may occasionally produce **side effects,** such as warmth or nausea and vomiting; rarely idiosyncratic **allergic-like reactions** occur, leading to more severe symptoms and death.
- Oral and/or rectal contrast may be used to define the bowel and help in differentiating bowel from adjacent lymph nodes or pathologic, fluid-containing lesions.
- In a number of clinical settings, either iodinated and/or oral contrast improve the diagnostic accuracy of CT scanning. Imaging studies are usually tailored by the radiologist based on the clinical problem.

- It is essential to provide an **appropriate history** to help in determining which, if any, imaging study will provide the best yield in establishing the correct diagnosis.
- Advances in CT imaging have resulted in better diagnostic studies, but they may carry the potential for a **higher radiation dose.** Dose-reducing measures are being employed to assure that the benefits derived from obtaining a study outweigh any potential risks of the radiation exposure.
- Some of the common patient preparations that are used for a variety of imaging studies are outlined.
- The advantages and disadvantages of the major imaging modalities in the abdomen are compared.
- The normal CT appearances of the liver, spleen, pancreas, kidneys, bowel, and bladder are described.

 Additional content is available online including chapters on Nuclear Medicine, Artificial Intelligence, Radiation Dose and Safety, an Early History of Radiology, and a compendium of 200 Diagnostic Radiology Signs.

# 14

# Recognizing Bowel Obstruction and Ileus

*William Herring, MD, FACR*

In Chapters 12 and 13, we discussed how to recognize the normal intestinal gas pattern on conventional radiographs and computed tomography (CT). In this chapter, you will learn how to recognize and categorize the four most common abnormal bowel gas patterns and their causes. These abnormal patterns of bowel gas will appear the same whether imaged initially by conventional radiography or by CT scanning. CT is superior in revealing the location, degree, and cause of an obstruction and in demonstrating any signs of reduced bowel viability.

### CASE QUIZ 14 QUESTION

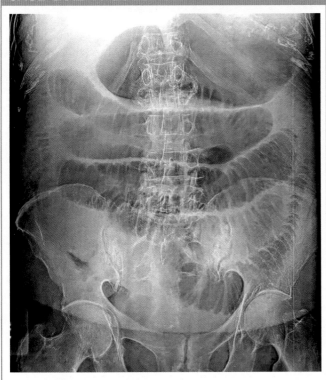

This is a supine view of the abdomen in a 57-year-old who has been having crampy abdominal pain for several hours. What diagnosis does this appearance suggest? See the correct answer at the end of this chapter.

- Abnormalities of bowel function are suggested by the history and clinical findings.
- The key questions in assessing bowel obstruction on imaging studies are:
  - Are there **dilated loops of small and/or large bowel?**
  - On CT, is there a **transition point?**
  - On plain films, is there **air in the rectum or sigmoid?**

## ABNORMAL GAS PATTERNS

- Abnormal intestinal gas patterns can be divided into two main categories, each of which can be subdivided into two subcategories (Box 14.1).
- *Functional ileus* is one main category in which it is presumed that **one or more loops of bowel lose their ability to propagate the peristaltic waves of the bowel,** usually because of some **local irritation or inflammation,** leading to impaired propulsion of bowel contents proximal to the affected loop(s).
- There are **two kinds** of **functional ileus.**
  - *Localized ileus* affects only **one or two loops,** usually of **small bowel** (*also called sentinel loops*).
  - *Generalized adynamic ileus* affects **many loops of large and small bowel,** and frequently the stomach as well.
- *Mechanical obstruction* is the other main category of abnormal bowel gas pattern. With mechanical obstruction, a **physical, organic, obstructing lesion prevents the passage of intestinal content** past the point of either the small or large bowel blockage.
- There are **two kinds** of **mechanical obstruction.**
  - **Small bowel obstruction** (SBO)
  - **Large bowel obstruction** (LBO)

### BOX 14.1 Abnormal Bowel Gas Patterns

| Functional Ileus | Mechanical Obstruction |
|---|---|
| • Localized ileus (sentinel loops) | • Small bowel obstruction (SBO) |
| • Generalized adynamic ileus | • Large bowel obstruction (LBO) |

# LAWS OF THE GUT

## ⟫ IMPORTANT POINTS

- The bowel reacts to a mechanical obstruction in more-or-less predictable ways.
- After the obstruction occurs, **peristalsis continues** (except in the loop of bowel involved in a functional ileus) in an attempt to propel intestinal contents through the bowel.
- Loops **proximal** to the **obstruction** soon become **dilated with swallowed air and/or secreted fluid.**
  - This can occur within a few hours of a complete small bowel obstruction.
- Loops **distal** to an **obstruction** will eventually become **decompressed or airless,** as their contents are evacuated.
- In a mechanical obstruction, **the loop(s) that will become the most dilated** will either be the **loop of bowel** with the **largest resting diameter before** the onset of the obstruction (usually the **cecum** in the large bowel), or the **loop(s) of bowel** just **proximal** to the **obstruction.**
- The *transition point,* the **site of obstruction,** and the location where the bowel changes in caliber from dilated to collapsed may be visible on CT.

- Most patients with a mechanical obstruction will present with some form of **abdominal pain, abdominal distension,** and **constipation.** Patients may present with vomiting **early** in the course of a **proximal small bowel obstruction and later** in the course of the illness if it is **a distal small bowel obstruction.**
- **Prolonged obstruction** with persistently elevated intraluminal pressures can lead to vascular compromise, **necrosis,** and **perforation** in the affected loop of bowel. At this point, bowel sounds may become **hypoactive** or **absent.**
  - We'll look at each of the four abnormal bowel gas patterns in detail (Table 14.1).

### TABLE 14.1 Abnormal Gas Patterns: Summary

| | Air in Rectum or Sigmoid | Air in Small Bowel | Air in Large Bowel |
|---|---|---|---|
| **Normal** | Yes | Yes, 1—2 loops | Rectum and/or sigmoid |
| **Localized ileus** | Yes | 2—3 dilated loops | Rectum and/or sigmoid |
| **Generalized ileus** | Yes | Multiple dilated loops | Yes, dilated |
| **Small bowel obstruction (SBO)** | No | Multiple dilated loops | No |
| **Large bowel obstruction (LBO)** | No | None, unless ileocecal valve is incompetent | Yes, dilated |

- For each of the four abnormal gas patterns, we will examine their **pathophysiology,** most likely **causes,** key **imaging features,** and **diagnostic pitfalls.**

# FUNCTIONAL ILEUS: LOCALIZED

- **Pathophysiology**
  - **Focal irritation** of a loop or loops of bowel **occurs most often from inflammation of an adjacent visceral organ** (e.g., pancreatitis may affect bowel loops in the left upper quadrant, diverticulitis in the left lower quadrant).
  - The **loop(s) affected** are almost always loops of **small bowel** and, because they **herald the presence of other underlying pathology,** they are called *sentinel loops.*
  - The **irritation causes these loops to lose their normal function and become aperistaltic,** which in turn leads to **dilatation** of these loops.
  - Because a **functional ileus does not produce the degree of obstruction that a mechanical obstruction does,** some gas continues to pass through the defunctionalized bowel past the point of the localized ileus.
  - **Air** usually reaches and **is visible in the rectum or sigmoid** on conventional radiographs.
- **Causes of a localized ileus**
  - The **dilated loops of bowel tend to occur** in the **same anatomic area** as the **inflammatory or irritative process** of the adjacent abdominal organ, although this may not always be the case.
  - From conventional radiographs the exact cause of the functional ileus can only be inferred by its location. On CT scans of the abdomen, however, the **cause** of the localized ileus is frequently identifiable.
  - Table 14.2 summarizes **sites of a localized ileus** and their **most common cause.**
- **Key imaging features of a localized ileus**
  - On conventional radiographs, there are **one or two** *persistently dilated* loops of small bowel.
    - *Persistently* means that these **same loops remain dilated** on **multiple views** of the abdomen (supine, prone, upright abdomen) or on **serial studies** done over the course of time.
    - *Dilated* means the small bowel loops are **persistently larger than 2.5 cm.** Small bowel loops involved in a **functional ileus** usually **do not dilate as greatly as** those that are **mechanically obstructed.**

### TABLE 14.2 Causes of a Localized Ileus

| Site of Dilated Loops | Cause(s) |
|---|---|
| **Right upper quadrant (RUQ)** | Cholecystitis |
| **Left upper quadrant (LUQ)** | Pancreatitis |
| **Right lower quadrant (RLQ)** | Appendicitis |
| **Left lower quadrant (LLQ)** | Diverticulitis |
| **Mid-abdomen** | Ulcer or kidney/ureteral calculus |

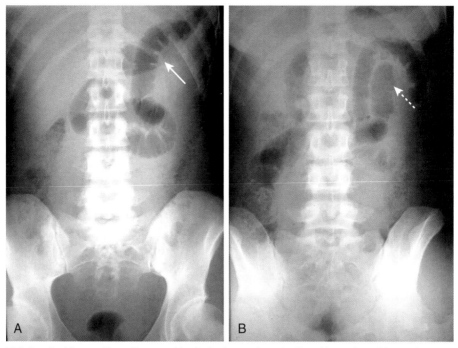

**Fig. 14.1 Sentinel Loops From Pancreatitis.** A single, persistently dilated loop of small bowel is seen in the left upper quadrant on both the supine (A) *(arrow)* and prone (B) *(arrow)* radiographs of the abdomen representing a sentinel loop or **localized ileus.** A localized ileus is called a **sentinel loop** because it often signals the presence of an adjacent irritative or inflammatory process. This patient had acute pancreatitis.

- Infrequently, the sentinel loop may be **large bowel,** rather than small bowel. This can especially occur in the **cecum,** with diseases such as appendicitis.
- **Air-fluid levels are frequently** seen in **sentinel loops.**
- There is usually **gas in the rectum or sigmoid** in a localized ileus (Fig. 14.1).

---

### ! DIAGNOSTIC PITFALLS

- **Differentiating a localized ileus from an early SBO**
  - A **localized ileus may resemble an** *early* mechanical **SBO** (i.e., there may be a few dilated loops of small bowel with air in the colon in both). *Early* means the **patient has had symptoms for a day or two.** Patients who have had obstructive symptoms for a week or more usually no longer demonstrate imaging findings of an "early" obstruction.
  - A combination of the clinical and laboratory findings and CT scanning of the abdomen that demonstrates the underlying pathology should help differentiate localized ileus from small bowel obstruction (Fig. 14.2).

## FUNCTIONAL ILEUS: GENERALIZED

- **Pathophysiology**
  - In a generalized adynamic ileus, the **entire bowel is aperistaltic or hypoperistaltic.** Swallowed **air dilates** and **fluid fills most loops of both small and large bowel.**

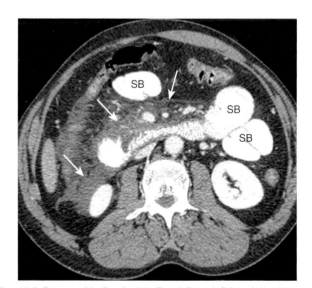

**Fig. 14.2 Pancreatitis Producing Focal Bowel Dilatation.** While the cause of a sentinel loop can usually only be inferred from conventional radiographs, CT scans can demonstrate the underlying abnormality producing the bowel irritation. In this contrast-enhanced axial CT scan of the upper abdomen with oral contrast, the pancreas is inflamed, enlarged, and edematous and there is haziness of the peri-pancreatic fat *(arrows).* The inflammation can affect peristalsis in adjacent loops of small bowel (SB) and lead to dilatation of the loops.

| TABLE 14.3 Causes of a Generalized Adynamic Ileus | |
|---|---|
| **Cause** | **Remarks** |
| **Postoperative** | Usually abdominal surgery |
| **Electrolyte imbalance** | Especially diabetics in ketoacidosis |

- A **generalized adynamic ileus is almost always the result of abdominal or pelvic surgery** in which the bowel is manipulated during the surgery.
- **Causes of a generalized adynamic ileus** are summarized in Table 14.3.
- **Key imaging features of a generalized adynamic ileus**
  - The **entire bowel is usually air-containing and dilated,** both large and small bowel. The stomach may be dilated as well.
  - The absence of peristalsis and the continued production of intestinal secretions usually produce **many long air-fluid levels in the bowel.**
  - Because this is not a mechanical obstruction, there usually is **gas in the rectum or sigmoid. No transition point** is identified on CT of the abdomen (Fig. 14.3).

- Bowel sounds are frequently absent or hypoactive.
- **Differentiating other causes of dilated bowel**
  - Patients do not present to the emergency department with a generalized adynamic ileus unless they are 1 or 2 days postoperative (abdominal or gynecologic surgery) or they have a severe electrolyte imbalance (e.g., hypokalemia).
  - Many patients who have either **colonic pseudoobstruction** (see the end of this chapter) or **aerophagia** may be mistakenly thought to have a generalized ileus on abdominal radiographs.

## MECHANICAL OBSTRUCTION: SMALL BOWEL

- **Pathophysiology**
  - A lesion, either inside or outside of the small bowel, obstructs the lumen.
  - If the obstruction is **complete** and if enough time has elapsed since the onset of symptoms, **there is usually no air in the rectum or sigmoid.**

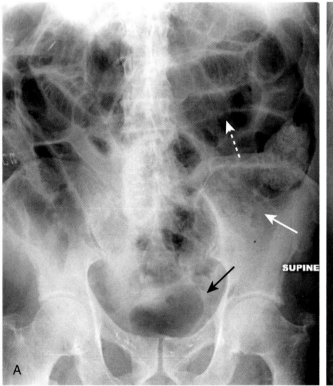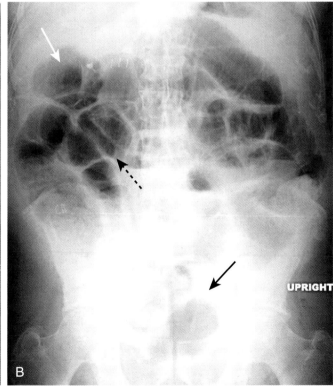

**Fig. 14.3 Generalized Adynamic Ileus, Supine (A) and Upright Abdomen (B).** In both images, there are dilated loops of large *(solid white arrows)* and small bowel *(dashed white and black arrows)* with gas seen down to and including the rectum *(solid black arrows).* The patient had absent bowel sounds and had undergone colon surgery the day before.

## ▶▶ IMPORTANT POINTS

- Over time, **from the point of obstruction** *backward,* the **small bowel dilates** from continuously swallowed air and from intestinal fluid that is still produced by the stomach, pancreatic, biliary systems, and small bowel.
- **Peristalsis continues and may increase** in an effort to overcome the obstruction.
- This can lead to **high-pitched, hyperactive bowel sounds.**
- As time passes, the peristaltic waves **empty the small bowel along with the colon** of their contents **from the point of obstruction** *forward.*

---

- **Causes of a mechanical small bowel obstruction** are summarized in Table 14.4, Fig. 14.4.
- **Key imaging features of mechanical small bowel obstruction**
  - On conventional radiographs, **there are multiple dilated loops** (>2.5 cm) **of small bowel** proximal to the point of the obstruction.
    - As they begin to dilate, **small bowel loops** may appear to **stack up** on one another, forming a *step-ladder appearance*, usually beginning in the left upper quadrant and proceeding, depending on how distal the

### TABLE 14.4  Causes of a Mechanical Small Bowel Obstruction

| Cause | Remarks |
|---|---|
| **Postsurgical adhesions** | Most common cause of a small bowel obstruction; most frequent following appendectomy, colorectal surgery, and pelvic surgery; **transition point** may be seen on small bowel CT. |
| **Malignancy** | Primary malignancies of the small bowel are rare; secondary tumors, such as gastric and colonic carcinomas and ovarian cancers, may compromise the lumen of the small bowel. |
| **Hernia** | An inguinal hernia may be visible on conventional radiographs if air-containing loops of bowel are seen over the obturator foramen; most hernias are easily seen on CT (Fig. 14.4). |
| **Gallstone ileus** | May be visible on conventional radiographs or CT if air is seen in the biliary tree and (rarely) a gallstone is present in distal loops of small bowel (see Chapter 15). |
| **Intussusception** | Ileocolic intussusception, the most common form, produces SBO. |
| **Inflammatory bowel disease** | Thickening of the bowel wall may occur with compromise of the lumen in patients with Crohn disease, most likely in the terminal ileum. |

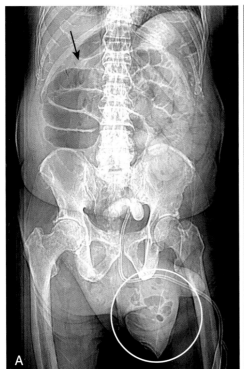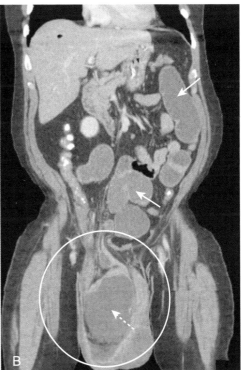

**Fig. 14.4 Small Bowel Obstruction From Inguinal Hernia.** (A) The scout image from a CT scan of the abdomen reveals dilated loops of small bowel *(arrow)* caused by a left inguinal hernia *(circle)*. Loops of bowel should normally not be present in the scrotum. (B) Coronal-reformatted CT scan on another patient shows multiple fluid-filled and dilated loops of small bowel *(solid arrows)* from an inguinal hernia *(white circle)* containing another dilated loop of small bowel *(dashed arrow)*.

small bowel obstruction is, to the right lower quadrant (Fig. 14.5).

- Generally speaking, **the more proximal the small bowel obstruction** (e.g., proximal jejunum), **the fewer dilated loops** there will be; the **more distal the obstruction** (e.g., at the ileocecal valve), the **greater the number of dilated small bowel loops.**

> ## » IMPORTANT POINTS
>
> - In a mechanical small bowel obstruction there should always be a **disproportionate dilatation of small bowel compared with the collapsed large bowel** (Fig. 14.6).

- On upright or decubitus radiographs, there will usually be **numerous air-fluid levels in the small bowel** proximal to the obstruction.
- If enough time has elapsed to decompress and empty the bowel distal to the point of obstruction, **there will be little or no gas in the colon, especially the rectum.**

- **The CT findings of a small bowel obstruction:**
  - **Fluid-filled and dilated loops of small bowel** (>2.5 cm in diameter) proximal to the point of obstruction.
  - Identification of a *transition point,* which is where the **bowel changes caliber** from **dilated to normal** indicating the site of the obstruction. In the absence of identifying a

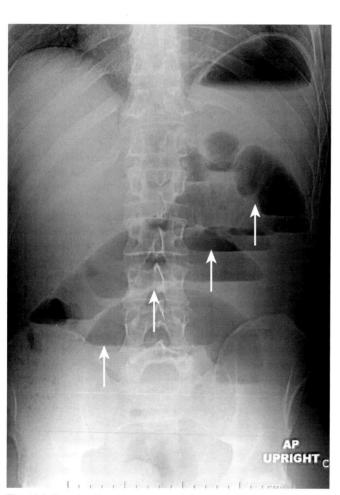

**Fig. 14.5 Step-Ladder Appearance of Obstructed Small Bowel.** This sign may be seen on upright, abdominal views in patients with a mechanical SBO due to the arrangement of fluid-filled and dilated small bowel loops in a step-wise configuration following the position of the jejunum in the left upper quadrant to the ileum in the right lower quadrant *(arrows).* This was a distal small bowel obstruction caused by a carcinoma of the colon that obstructed the ileocecal valve.

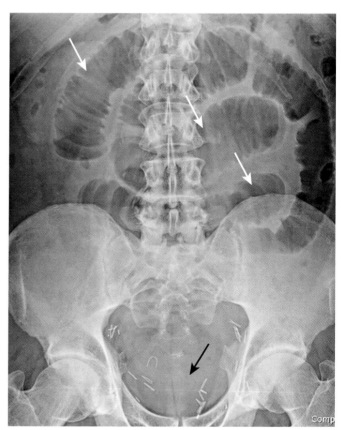

**Fig. 14.6 Mechanical Small Bowel Obstruction.** There are multiple dilated loops of small bowel *(white arrows)* with no gas in the rectosigmoid *(black arrow)* consistent with a mechanical small bowel obstruction. The obstruction was secondary to adhesions.

## ⚠ DIAGNOSTIC PITFALLS

- **Differentiating a *partial* SBO from a *functional (localized) adynamic ileus***
  - An **intermittent** (also known as a ***partial*** or ***incomplete***), mechanical small bowel obstruction is one that **allows some gas to pass the point of obstruction**, at least at times, and can lead to a confusing picture because gas may pass into the colon long after the large bowel would be expected to be devoid of such gas. **Partial or incomplete small bowel obstruction** occurs **more often in patients** in whom **adhesions** are the etiology (Fig. 14.7).
  - CT with oral contrast should be able to demonstrate a partial small bowel obstruction by locating the transition point or, alternatively, identify the abnormality producing the sentinel loops (Fig. 14.8).

## ⏩ IMPORTANT POINTS

- **CT is the most sensitive study** for diagnosing the site and cause of a mechanical small bowel obstruction.
  - CT scans for bowel obstruction can be performed with or without oral contrast, the latter utilizing the fluid already present in the bowel as a form of contrast. Current guidelines have moved away from using orally administered contrast in suspected small bowel obstruction.
  - **Intravenous contrast** is used to detect **complications** of bowel obstruction, such as **ischemia** and **strangulation.**

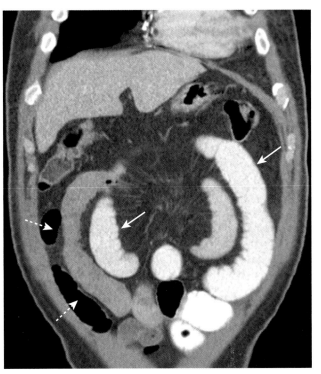

**Fig. 14.8 Partial Small Bowel Obstruction.** Coronal-reformatted CT scan with oral contrast shows dilated and contrast-containing loops of small bowel *(solid arrows)*. Although there is still air in the collapsed colon *(dashed arrows)*, the disproportionate dilatation of small bowel identifies this as a small bowel obstruction.

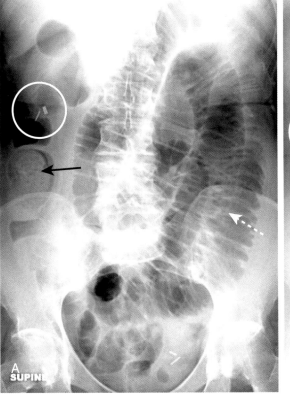
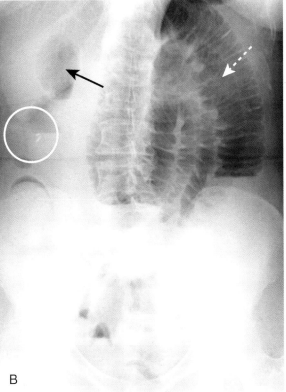

**Fig. 14.7 Partial Small Bowel Obstruction, Supine (A) and Upright (B).** The important observation is that even though there is air in the large bowel *(solid black arrows)*, the small bowel is **disproportionately dilated** in both views *(white arrows)* compared to the large bowel, a finding consistent with small bowel obstruction. Small bowel obstructions are more common in patients with adhesions from previous surgery as indicated by the surgical clips *(circles)* in this patient.

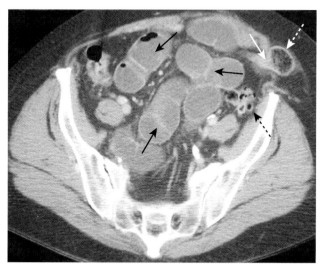

**Fig. 14.9** Small Bowel Obstruction Caused by a Spigelian Hernia. A Spigelian hernia is one that occurs at the lateral edge of the rectus abdominis muscle at the semilunar line. This patient has a **transition point** *(solid white arrow)* as the small bowel enters the hernia *(dashed white arrow)*. More proximally, there are multiple dilated loops of small bowel *(solid black arrows)* indicating obstruction. The colon lies beyond the point of obstruction and is collapsed *(dashed black arrow)*.

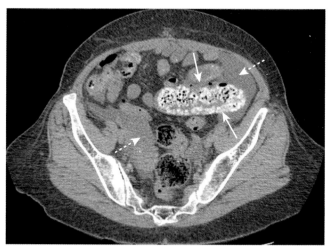

**Fig. 14.11** Small Bowel Feces Sign. There is air mixed with debris and old oral contrast in a dilated loop of small bowel *(solid arrows)*. There are proximal fluid-containing, dilated loops of small bowel *(dashed arrows)*. The patient had a CT scan with oral contrast several days earlier for abdominal pain and returned for this noncontrast scan when symptoms persisted. Intestinal debris and fluid may accumulate in the loop found just proximal to a small bowel obstruction and present with this finding that resembles fecal material in the colon.

mass or other obstructive cause at the transition point, the cause is almost certainly **adhesions** (Fig. 14.9).

- **Collapsed small bowel and/or colon distal to the point of obstruction** (Fig. 14.10)
- *Small bowel feces sign.* Proximal to the transition point of a small bowel obstruction, intestinal debris and fluid may accumulate producing the appearance of fecal material in the small bowel. This is a sign of SBO (Fig. 14.11).

- *Closed-loop obstruction* occurs when **two points** of the **same loop** of bowel are **obstructed** at a **single location.** The closed loop usually remains dilated and may form a U- or C-shaped structure. Most closed-loop obstructions are caused by adhesions (Fig. 14.12). In the small bowel, a closed-loop obstruction carries a higher risk of **strangulation** of the bowel. In the large bowel, a closed-loop obstruction is called a *volvulus.*

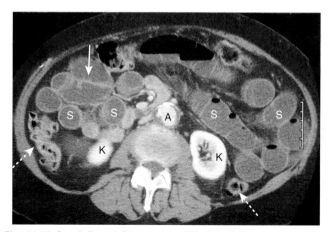

**Fig. 14.10** Small Bowel Obstruction, CT with IV Contrast. There are multiple dilated and fluid-filled loops of small bowel (*S* marks selected loops) while the colon is collapsed *(dashed arrows)*, indicating a small bowel obstruction. The bowel wall is not thickened and normally enhances with intravenous contrast that we know the patient received from the enhanced appearance of the aorta (A) and kidneys (K). **Absence** of bowel wall enhancement is useful for assessing SBO complications, such as ischemia and strangulation.

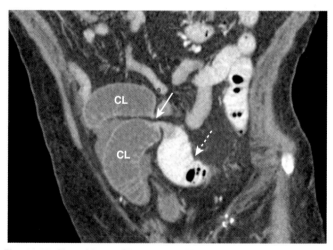

**Fig. 14.12** Closed-Loop Obstruction, CT Lower Abdomen. A loop of small bowel (CL) is obstructed twice at the same point of a twist *(solid arrow)* producing a closed loop. No oral contrast enters the closed loop but is present in a more proximal loop of small bowel *(dashed arrow)*. Closed-loop obstructions are important because of their higher incidence of bowel necrosis from strangulation of the bowel.

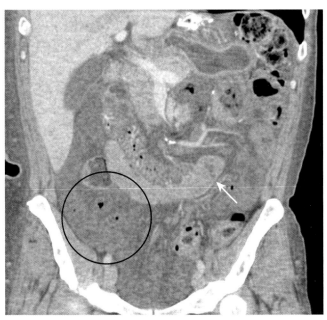

**Fig. 14.13** Bowel Necrosis, Contrast-Enhanced CT. A dilated loop of small bowel demonstrates faint but normal enhancement of the wall *(arrow)* on this coronal reformat of a contrast-enhanced CT, while more distal, dilated loops of small bowel show no wall enhancement *(circle)*. The bowel wall should normally enhance with IV contrast (see Fig. 14.10). The lack of enhancement is an indication of vascular compromise of the distal loops with bowel necrosis.

- *Strangulation.* Vascular compromise can be identified by circumferential **thickening** of the wall of the bowel frequently accompanied by reduction or **absence** of normal bowel wall enhancement following intravenous contrast administration. There may be associated edema of the mesentery and ascites (Fig. 14.13).

## MECHANICAL OBSTRUCTION: LARGE BOWEL

- **Pathophysiology**
  - A lesion, either inside or outside the colon, causes obstruction to the lumen.
  - Over time, from the point of obstruction *backward*, the **large bowel dilates** and the **cecum frequently attains the greatest diameter** even if the obstruction is as far away as the sigmoid colon.
  - The large bowel normally functions to reabsorb water, so there are **usually few or no air-fluid levels** in the obstructed colon.
  - As time passes, continuing peristaltic waves from the point of obstruction *forward* empty the colon distal to **the obstruction.**
  - **Usually little or no air is seen in the rectum in a mechanical large bowel obstruction.**
- **Causes of a mechanical large bowel obstruction** are summarized in Table 14.5

- **Key imaging features of a mechanical large bowel obstruction**
  - **The colon is dilated to the point of obstruction.**
    - Because there are a limited number of large bowel loops, they tend not to overlap (as do the loops of small bowel) so **it is sometimes possible to identify the site of obstruction** as the **last air-containing** segment of the colon (Fig. 14.14).
    - Regardless of the point of obstruction, the **cecum** is **often the most dilated** part of the colon. When the

| **TABLE 14.5** | **Causes of a Mechanical Large Bowel Obstruction** |
|---|---|
| **Cause** | **Remarks** |
| **Tumor (carcinoma)** | Most common cause of LBO; more frequently obstructs when it involves the left colon |
| **Hernia** | May be visible on conventional radiographs if air is seen over the obturator foramen |
| **Volvulus** | Either the sigmoid (more commonly) or cecum may twist on its axis and obstruct the colon and/or small bowel (Box 14.2) |
| **Diverticulitis** | Uncommon cause of colonic obstruction |
| **Intussusception** | Colo-colic intussusception usually occurs because of a tumor acting as a lead point |

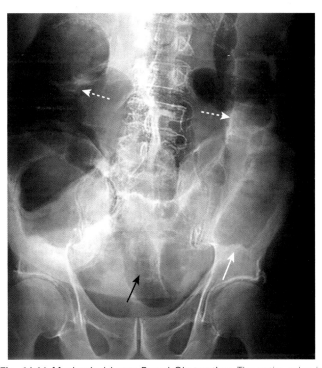

**Fig. 14.14** Mechanical Large Bowel Obstruction. The entire colon is dilated *(dashed white arrows)* to a cut-off point in the distal descending colon *(solid white arrow)*, the site of this patient's obstructing carcinoma of the colon. Some gas has passed backward through an incompetent ileocecal valve and outlines a dilated ileum *(solid black arrow)*. Notice that the large bowel is disproportionately dilated compared to the small bowel, consistent with a large bowel obstruction.

cecum reaches a diameter **above 12 to 15 cm,** there is **danger** of cecal rupture.

- The **small bowel is not dilated** (unless the ileocecal valve becomes *incompetent;* see later discussion).
- **The rectum usually contains little or no air** since it is distal to the point of obstruction.
- Because the large bowel functions to reabsorb water, there are **usually no (or very few) air-fluid levels in the large bowel.**

---

### ❗ DIAGNOSTIC PITFALLS

- **A large bowel obstruction can mimic the appearance of a small bowel obstruction** if the intracolonic pressure rises high enough that the **ileocecal valve opens** (such a valve is called *incompetent*) and **gas from the dilated large bowel decompresses backward into the small bowel,** much like the air escaping from a balloon (Fig. 14.15).

---

- **Oral contrast containing barium is usually not administered to a patient with a suspected large bowel obstruction** in part because water will be absorbed from the barium when it reaches the obstructed colon, increasing the viscosity of the barium.
- **Recognizing a large bowel obstruction on CT**
  - CT is obtained to identify the cause of the obstruction, assess for free intraperitoneal air, and identify associated lesions, such as metastases to the liver or lymph nodes if the obstruction is produced by a malignancy.
  - The large bowel is **dilated** to the **point of obstruction** (the **transition point**), then **normal** in caliber **distal** to the obstructing lesion.
  - The point of obstruction, frequently a carcinoma, can usually be located on CT as a **soft-tissue mass.** Hernias containing large bowel are also easy to identify on CT (Fig. 14.16).

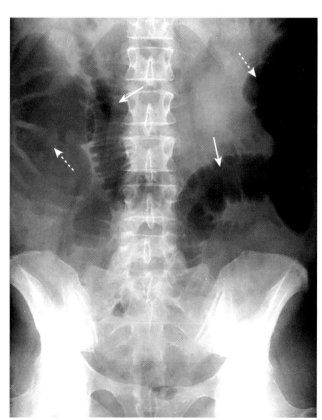

**Fig. 14.15 Large Bowel Obstruction Masquerading as a Small Bowel Obstruction.** There are air-filled and dilated loops of small bowel *(solid arrows)* in this patient who actually had a mechanical large bowel obstruction from a carcinoma of the mid-descending colon. The pressure in the colon was sufficient to open the ileocecal valve, which then allowed much of the gas in the colon to decompress backward into the small bowel. The ascending and descending colon are dilated and still contain air *(dashed arrows),* a clue that this is really a distal large bowel obstruction. Abdominal CT can resolve the question of whether the large or small bowel is obstructed.

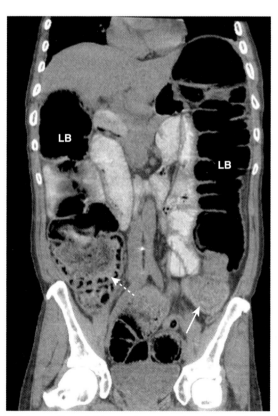

**Fig. 14.16 Large Bowel Obstruction from Carcinoma of the Colon.** This coronal-reformatted CT scan of the abdomen and pelvis shows a dilated cecum containing stool *(dashed arrow)* and dilated large bowel (LB) to the level of the distal descending colon where a large soft-tissue mass is identified *(solid arrow).* This mass was surgically removed and was an adenocarcinoma of the colon.

# VOLVULUS OF THE COLON

- Volvulus of the colon is a particular kind of large bowel obstruction that produces a striking and characteristic picture that is summarized in Box 14.2 (Fig. 14.17).

# COLONIC PSEUDOOBSTRUCTION (OGILVIE SYNDROME)

- *Ogilvie syndrome (acute colonic pseudoobstruction)* is an uncommon disease that usually occurs in elderly individuals, frequently those who are already hospitalized or at chronic bed rest.
  - Its etiology is not known. Drugs like anticholinergics, antidiarrheals, opioids, calcium channel blockers, and anti-parkinsonian agents may cause or exacerbate the condition.
- The syndrome is characterized by acute and sometimes **massive dilatation of the right colon or the entire colon resembling a large bowel obstruction** (Fig. 14.18).
  - Unlike a mechanical obstruction, **no obstructing lesion can be demonstrated** on CT. Unlike a generalized adynamic ileus, **patients have more marked abdominal distension** and bowel sounds may be **normal or hyperactive** in almost half of patients with Ogilvie syndrome.
- The supine abdominal radiograph shows **marked bowel dilatation, almost always confined to the colon.**
- Management can be **pharmacologic stimulation of colonic contractions**, with drugs such as neostigmine, or decompressive sigmoidoscopy/colonoscopy.

---

## BOX 14.2  Volvulus: A Cause of Mechanical Large Bowel Obstruction

- Either the cecum or the sigmoid colon can twist upon its mesentery producing a mechanical obstruction known as a volvulus.
- **Sigmoid volvulus** is **more common** and tends to occur in older men.
- The volvulated sigmoid can assume a massive size unmatched by any other bowel obstruction, rising up from the pelvis with the wall between the twisted loops of sigmoid forming a line that points from the left lower to the right upper quadrant.

- The appearance of the dilated sigmoid has been likened to a **coffee bean** (Fig. 14.17).
- When the **cecum** volvulates, it usually moves across the midline into the left upper quadrant producing loops of bowel separated by a line that characteristically points from the right lower to the left upper quadrant.
- Endoscopic decompression is the usual treatment for a sigmoid volvulus. Sigmoid colectomy may be used to reduce or prevent recurrent volvulus.

---

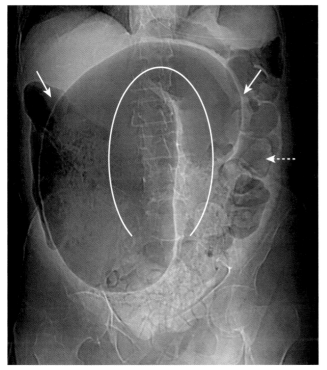

**Fig. 14.17 Sigmoid Volvulus, Supine Abdomen.** There is a massively dilated sigmoid colon *(solid arrows)* that is twisted upon itself at some point in the pelvis. The dilated sigmoid has a **coffee-bean** shape *(oval)*. Because the point of obstruction is in the distal colon, there is air and stool in the more proximal portion of the colon *(dashed arrow)*. Volvulus can produce massively dilated loops of sigmoid colon.

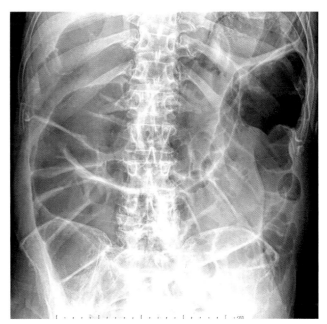

**Fig. 14.18 Ogilvie Syndrome.** This syndrome most often occurs in elderly and bedridden patients who are already severely ill and results in acute, massive dilatation of the colon, particularly the right colon and cecum, without mechanical obstruction. It can result in perforation and peritonitis and has a high overall mortality. Treatment may include a nasogastric tube, colonoscopic decompression, or pharmacologic stimulation of the bowel.

## CASE QUIZ 14 ANSWER

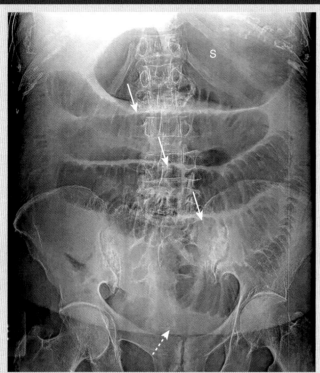

There are multiple dilated loops of small bowel *(solid arrows)* and the stomach (S) is also dilated. There is no bowel gas in the rectum *(dashed arrow)*. The combination of findings suggests a mechanical obstruction in the mid- to distal small bowel. The obstruction was secondary to adhesions from prior surgery.

## 🏠 TAKE HOME POINTS

- Abnormal bowel gas patterns can be divided into two main groups: **functional ileus** and **mechanical obstruction.**
- There are two varieties of functional ileus: **localized** ileus (sentinel loops) and **generalized** adynamic ileus. There are two varieties of mechanical obstruction: **small bowel obstruction (SBO)** and **large bowel obstruction (LBO).**
- In **mechanical obstructions,** the gut reacts in predictable ways: loops proximal to the obstruction become dilated, peristalsis attempts to propel intestinal contents through the bowel, and loops distal to the obstruction eventually are evacuated. The loop(s) that become the most dilated will either be the loop of bowel with the largest resting diameter or the loop(s) of bowel just proximal to the obstruction.
- The key findings of a **localized ileus** are two to three dilated loops of small bowel (**sentinel loops**) with air in the rectosigmoid and an underlying irritative process that frequently is adjacent to the dilated loops.
- Some causes of **sentinel loops** include pancreatitis (LUQ), cholecystitis (RUQ), diverticulitis (LLQ), and appendicitis (RLQ). They can be readily identified using ultrasound or CT.
- The key findings in a **generalized adynamic ileus** are dilated loops of large and small bowel; gas in the rectosigmoid; and long, air-fluid levels. Postoperative patients develop generalized adynamic ileus.

- The key imaging findings in a **mechanical small bowel obstruction** are disproportionately dilated and fluid-filled loops of small bowel with little or no gas in the rectosigmoid. CT is best at identifying the cause and site of obstruction, or its complications.
- The most common cause of an SBO is **adhesions;** other causes include hernias, intussusception, gallstone ileus, malignancy, and inflammatory bowel disease, such as Crohn disease.
- A **closed-loop obstruction** is one in which two points of the bowel are obstructed in the same location producing the closed loop. In the small bowel, a closed-loop obstruction carries a higher risk of strangulation of the bowel. In the large bowel, a closed-loop obstruction is called a volvulus.
- The key imaging findings in **mechanical LBO** include dilatation of the colon to the point of the obstruction and absence of gas in the rectum with no dilatation of the small bowel as long as the ileocecal valve remains competent. CT will often demonstrate the cause of the obstruction.
- Causes of mechanical LBO include malignancy, hernia, diverticulitis, and intussusception.
- **Ogilvie syndrome** is characterized by acute and frequently massive dilatation of the entire colon resembling a large bowel obstruction, but without a demonstrable point of obstruction; it can sometimes be radiographically confused for a generalized adynamic ileus.

 Additional content is available online including chapters on Nuclear Medicine, Artificial Intelligence, Radiation Dose and Safety, an Early History of Radiology, and a compendium of 200 Diagnostic Radiology Signs.

# 15

# Recognizing Extraluminal Air in the Abdomen

*William Herring, MD, FACR*

Recognition of extraluminal air is an important finding that can have an immediate effect on the course of treatment. Air is normally not present in the peritoneal or extraperitoneal spaces, bowel wall, or biliary system. **Air outside of the bowel lumen** is called *extraluminal air.*

- **The four most common locations of extraluminal air are:**
  - Intraperitoneal *(pneumoperitoneum)* (frequently called *free air*)
  - Retroperitoneal air
  - Air in the bowel wall *(pneumatosis intestinalis)*
  - Air in the biliary system *(pneumobilia)*

## FREE INTRAPERITONEAL AIR

> ### ⏵⏵ IMPORTANT POINTS
>
> - The **three major radiographic signs of free intraperitoneal air** are arranged below in the order in which they are most commonly seen:
>   - **Air beneath the diaphragm**
>   - **Visualization of both sides of the bowel wall**
>   - **Visualization of the falciform ligament**

### Air Beneath the Diaphragm

- Free air will generally rise to the highest part of the abdomen. In the upright position, **free air** will usually reveal itself **under the diaphragm** as a **crescentic lucency**

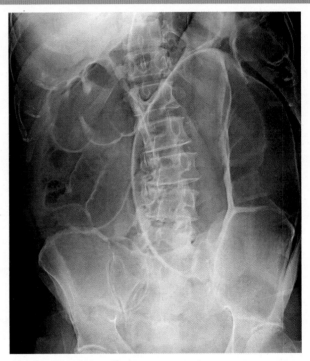

A 48-year-old male presented to the emergency department with severe abdominal pain and a tympanitic abdomen. A supine radiograph of the abdomen was obtained and is shown. Some time later, the patient was discharged after undergoing which one of these most likely events? (a) neostigmine administration, (b) insertion of a rectal tube, (c) abdominal surgery, or (d) polypectomy. See the answer at the end of the chapter.

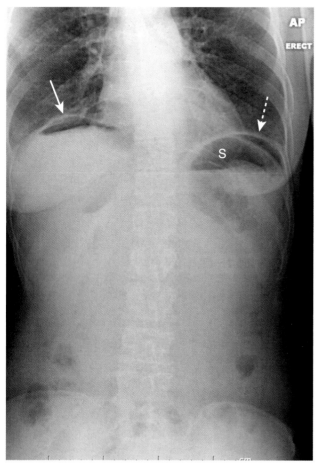

**Fig. 15.1 Free Air Beneath the Diaphragm.** There are thin crescents of air beneath both the right *(solid arrow)* and left *(dashed arrow)* hemidiaphragms representing free intraperitoneal air. There is normally an air-fluid level in the stomach (S) beneath the left hemidiaphragm. The patient had undergone abdominal surgery 2 days earlier.

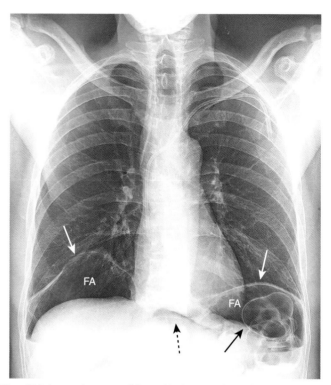

**Fig. 15.2 Large Amount of Free Air.** Upright view of the chest demonstrates a large amount of free air (FA) beneath each hemidiaphragm *(white arrows)*. Both sides of the splenic flexure's bowel wall are also seen *(solid black arrow)* as is the **cupola sign** of free air *(dashed black arrow)*, described in the online Radiology Signs section. The patient had a perforated gastric ulcer.

that parallels the undersurface of the diaphragm (Fig. 15.1).

- The **size of the crescent** will be **roughly proportional to the amount of free air.** The smaller the amount of free air, the thinner the crescent; the larger the amount of free air, the larger the crescent (Fig. 15.2).
- **Although free air is best demonstrated on CT scans of the abdomen** because of its greater sensitivity in detecting very small amounts of free air (Fig. 15.3), most surveys of the abdomen begin with conventional radiographs. Conventional radiographs **serve as an important screening tool** on which many previously unsuspected cases of free air are discovered.

### ▶▶ IMPORTANT POINTS

- On conventional radiographs, **free air is best demonstrated with the x-ray beam directed parallel to the floor** (i.e., a horizontal beam) (see Fig. 12.14). **Small amounts of free air will not be visible on** radiographs in which the x-ray beam is directed vertically downward, such as supine or prone views.

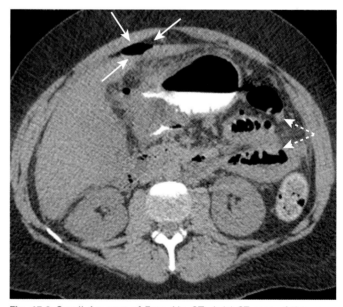

**Fig. 15.3 Small Amount of Free Air, CT.** Axial CT scan of the upper abdomen performed with the patient supine shows a very small collection of free air beneath the anterior abdominal wall *(solid arrows)*. Characteristically, free air has no surrounding bowel wall, as does air within bowel loops *(dashed arrows)*. This amount of free air was not visible on conventional radiographs.

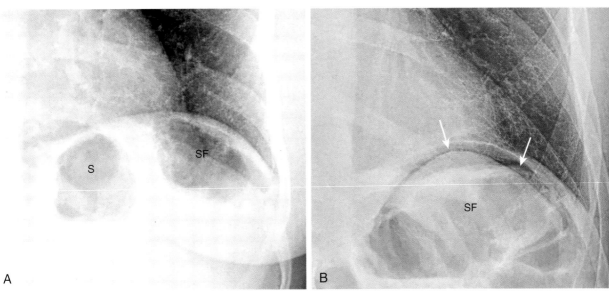

**Fig. 15.4** Normal Left Hemidiaphragm (A) and Free Air Under Hemidiaphragm (B). (A) It is more difficult to detect free air in the left upper quadrant than the right because of the presence of normal air-containing structures like the stomach (S) and splenic flexure (SF). (B) In another patient, there is a crescent of free air *(arrows)* below the left hemidiaphragm and above the SF.

- Free air is **easier to recognize under the right hemidiaphragm** because that is normally the location of the liver, which has soft-tissue density. Free air is **more difficult to recognize under the left hemidiaphragm** because air-containing structures, such as the fundus of the **stomach** and the splenic flexure of the **colon,** already reside in that location, and they may mimic or hide free air (Fig. 15.4).
- If the patient is unable to stand or sit upright, then a view of the abdomen with the patient lying on their left side (meaning the right side is pointing up) taken with a horizontal x-ray beam may show free air rising above the right edge of the liver (see Fig. 12.15). This is called a **left lateral decubitus view** of the abdomen (Fig. 15.5).

> **!  DIAGNOSTIC PITFALLS**
>
> - *Chilaiditi sign*
>   - Occasionally, **normal colon** may be interposed between the dome of the liver and the right hemidiaphragm and, unless a **careful search** is made **for the presence of haustral folds** characteristic of the colon, it may be mistaken for free air (Fig. 15.6). This normal interposition of the colon between the liver and right hemidiaphragm is called the ***Chilaiditi sign*** (pronounced kyla-ditty). If in doubt, obtain a left lateral decubitus view of the abdomen or, if necessary, a CT scan of the abdomen.

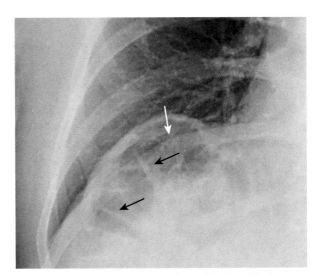

**Fig. 15.6** Chilaiditi Sign. Close-up of the right hemidiaphragm on a conventional chest radiograph demonstrates air beneath the diaphragm that could be confused for free air *(white arrow)*. Careful evaluation of this air shows that it contains several haustral folds *(black arrows)* that indicate this is a loop of colon interposed between the liver and the diaphragm rather than free air.

Foot                    Head

**Fig. 15.5** Left Lateral Decubitus View, Free Air. Close-up of the right upper quadrant in a patient lying on their left side in the left lateral decubitus position shows a crescent of air *(dashed white arrows)* above the outer edge of the liver *(black arrow)*, beneath the right hemidiaphragm *(solid white arrow)*. The head/foot orientation of the patient is indicated.

## Visualization of Both Sides of the Bowel Wall

- On the **normal** abdominal radiograph, we visualize only the air **inside** the lumen of the bowel, **not the wall of the bowel itself.** This is because the wall is soft-tissue density and is normally surrounded by intraperitoneal tissues of the same density.
- Introduction of **air into the peritoneal cavity enables us to visualize the wall of the bowel itself** because the wall is now surrounded on both inside and outside by air.
- The **ability to see both sides of the bowel wall is a sign of free intraperitoneal air** called the *Rigler sign* (Fig. 15.7).
- The Rigler sign can be seen on supine, upright, or prone films of the abdomen so long as there is a relatively large amount of free air present.

> **! DIAGNOSTIC PITFALLS**
>
> - When **dilated loops** of small bowel **overlap**, they may occasionally produce the mistaken impression that you are seeing both sides of the bowel wall (Fig. 15.8). If in doubt, confirm the presence of free air with an upright or left lateral decubitus view of the abdomen, or a CT scan of the abdomen.

## Visualization of the Falciform Ligament

- The **falciform ligament** courses over the **free edge of the liver anteriorly** just to the **right of the upper lumbar spine.** It contains a remnant of the obliterated umbilical vein. **It is normally invisible,** composed of soft tissue, and surrounded by tissue of similar density.
- When a (usually) large amount of free air is present and the **patient is in the supine position, free air** may rise over the anterior surface of the liver **on both sides of the falciform ligament** and **render it visible.** Visualization of the falciform

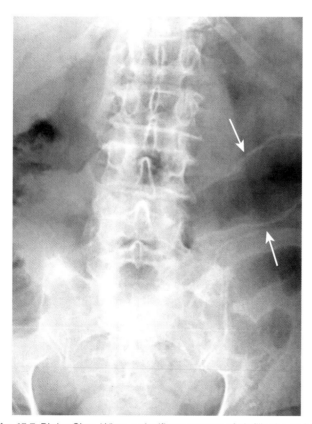

**Fig. 15.7 Rigler Sign.** When a significant amount of air fills the peritoneal cavity, both sides of the bowel wall will be outlined by air, making the bowel walls visible as discrete lines *(arrows)*. This is known as the ***Rigler sign*** and indicates the presence of a pneumoperitoneum. This patient had a perforated ulcer.

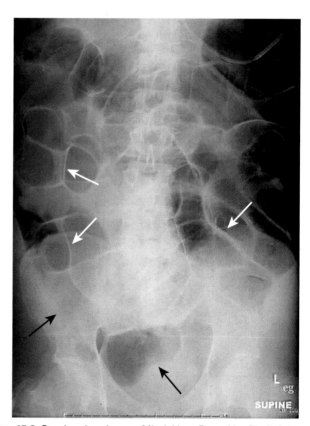

**Fig. 15.8 Overlapping Loops Mimicking Free Air.** Don't let overlapping loops of dilated small bowel *(white arrows)* fool you into thinking you are seeing both sides of the bowel wall due to free air. Notice that where the loops do not overlap, both sides of the bowel wall are not seen *(black arrows)*. This has been called a ***pseudo-Rigler sign.***

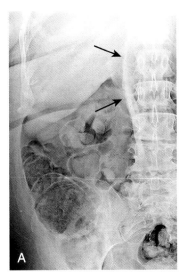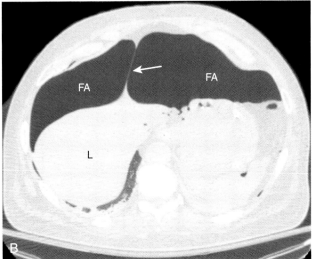

**Fig. 15.9** Falciform Ligament Sign. (A) Free intraperitoneal air surrounds the normally invisible falciform ligament on the anterior edge of the liver causing that soft-tissue structure to become visible *(arrows)* just to the right of the upper lumbar spine. This patient had a large pneumoperitoneum from a perforated gastric ulcer. (B) On CT in another patient, the falciform ligament *(arrow)* is outlined by free air (FA) on either side of it, anterior to the liver (L).

ligament is aptly called the *falciform ligament sign* (Fig. 15.9).

- The linear appearance of the falciform ligament combined with a large, oval-shaped amount of free air that distends the abdomen has been likened to the appearance of a football with its laces and is called the *football sign* (Fig. 15.10).
- Table 15.1 summarizes the **three major signs of free air** on conventional radiographs.

## Causes of Free Air

- The **most common cause of free intraperitoneal air is rupture of an air-containing loop of bowel**, either stomach or small or large bowel.
  - **Perforated peptic ulcer** is the most common cause of a perforated stomach or duodenum and is still the most common noniatrogenic cause of free air.
- **Trauma**, whether accidental or iatrogenic, can also produce free air. **Free air following penetrating trauma** usually **implies a perforation of the bowel**, not free air generated simply by penetration of the abdominal wall itself.

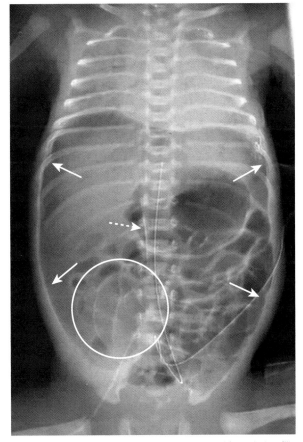

**Fig. 15.10** Football Sign. There is a large amount of free air that fills and distends the entire abdominal cavity *(solid arrows)* with visibility of the falciform ligament *(dashed arrow)* and both sides of bowel wall *(circle)* in this infant with pneumoperitoneum from necrotizing enterocolitis. The combination of the oval-shaped abdomen and the line of "laces" made by the falciform ligament led to this being named the *football sign.* This infant also has hyaline membrane disease of the lungs and two umbilical catheters in place.

| TABLE 15.1 | **Three Signs of Free Air** |
| --- | --- |
| **Sign** | **Remarks** |
| **Air beneath diaphragm** | Requires patient to be in the upright or left lateral decubitus position and a horizontal x-ray beam, unless free air is massive in amount |
| **Visualization of both sides of the bowel wall** | Usually requires large amount of free air; will be visible in any position |
| **Visualization of the falciform ligament** | Usually requires large amount of free air; best seen when patient is supine |

- For several days following abdominal surgery ($\approx 5$ to 7 days), whether the surgery had been performed on the bowel or not, **it is normal to see free air** on postoperative studies. The **amount** of free air following surgery **should diminish with each successive study.** A complication of the surgery or of the original disease should be considered **if free air persists for longer than a week** or if the amount **increases** on successive studies.
- **Perforated diverticulitis** and **perforated appendicitis** usually produce walled-off abscess collections around the site of the perforation and **rarely lead to significant amounts of free air.**
- **Perforation of a carcinoma**, most often of the colon, is unusual but can also lead to free air.

# EXTRAPERITONEAL AIR (RETROPERITONEAL AIR)

- Unlike the collections of free intraperitoneal air that outline loops of bowel and usually move freely in the abdomen, **extraperitoneal air** can be recognized by:
  - **Streaky, linear appearance outlining extraperitoneal structures**
  - **Mottled, blotchy appearance** (anterior pararenal space, especially)
  - **Relatively fixed position, moving little** if at all **with changes in patient positioning**
- Extraperitoneal air may outline extraperitoneal structures such as:
  - **Psoas muscles**
  - **Kidneys, ureters, or urinary bladder**
  - **Aorta or inferior vena cava** (Fig. 15.11)
  - Inferior border of the diaphragm by collecting in the **subphrenic tissues**
- **Extraperitoneal air may extend through a diaphragmatic hiatus into the mediastinum** (and produce *pneumomediastinum*) or **may extend to the peritoneal cavity** through openings in the peritoneum (and produce *pneumoperitoneum*).
- Box 15.1 summarizes the signs of extraperitoneal air.

## Causes of Extraperitoneal Air

- Extraperitoneal air is **most frequently** the result of **bowel perforation** secondary to either:
  - **Inflammatory disease (e.g., ruptured appendix)**, or
  - **Ulcerative disease (e.g., Crohn disease** of the ileum or colon)

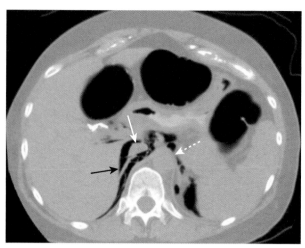

**Fig. 15.11 Extraperitoneal Air Seen on CT.** Air is seen in the retroperitoneum *(black arrow)* on this axial CT scan of the upper abdomen. Air outlines the inferior vena cava *(solid white arrow)* and the aorta *(dashed white arrow)*. Unlike free air, extraperitoneal air is streaky, relatively fixed in position, and outlines extraperitoneal structures.

---

## BOX 15.1  Signs of Extraperitoneal Air

- Streaky, linear collections of air that outline extraperitoneal structures
- Mottled, blotchy collections of air that remain in a fixed position

---

- **Other causes of extraperitoneal air** include:
  - **Blunt or penetrating trauma**
  - **Iatrogenic manipulation** (e.g., perforation of the bowel during **sigmoidoscopy**)
  - **Foreign body** (e.g., perforation of extraperitoneal ascending colon by an ingested foreign body)
  - **Gas-producing infection** originating in extraperitoneal organs (e.g., **perforated diverticulitis**)

# AIR IN THE BOWEL WALL

- Air in the bowel wall is called *pneumatosis intestinalis.*
- Pneumatosis intestinalis is **most easily recognized** on abdominal radiographs **when it is seen in profile** producing a **linear radiolucency (black line) whose contour exactly parallels the bowel lumen** (Fig. 15.12).

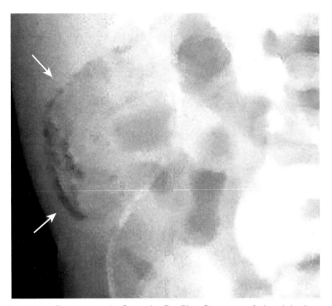

**Fig. 15.12 Pneumatosis Seen in Profile.** Close-up of the right lower quadrant in an infant demonstrates a thin curvilinear lucency that parallels the lumen of the adjacent bowel *(arrows),* an appearance characteristic of gas in the bowel wall seen in profile. In infants, the most common cause for this finding is **necrotizing enterocolitis**, a disease found mostly in premature infants in which the terminal ileum is most affected (see Chapter 27). Pneumatosis intestinalis is pathognomonic for necrotizing enterocolitis in infants.

- **Air in the bowel wall seen *en face* is more difficult to recognize** but frequently has a **mottled appearance** that resembles air mixed with fecal material (Fig. 15.13).
  - Clues to help differentiate pneumatosis from fecal material include:
    - Presence of such mottled air in an area of the abdomen unlikely to contain colon
    - **Lack of change** in the appearance of the mottled air pattern over several images in **different positions**
- Table 15.2 summarizes the signs of air in the bowel wall.

## Causes and Significance of Air in the Bowel Wall

- Pneumatosis intestinalis can be divided into two major categories.
  - A rare, **primary form called *pneumatosis cystoides intestinalis*** that usually **affects the left colon,** producing

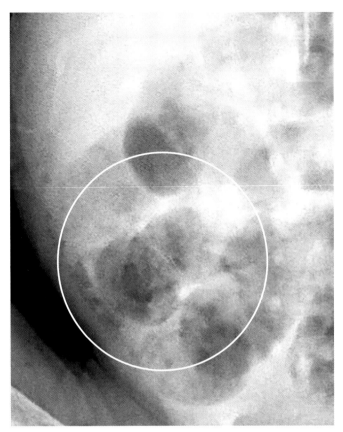

**Fig. 15.13 Pneumatosis Seen En Face.** Close-up of the right lower quadrant in another infant shows multiple faint, mottled lucencies in the right lower quadrant *(circle)* that are the appearance of pneumatosis intestinalis when seen *en face.* The density has the same appearance as air mixed with stool. This infant also had necrotizing enterocolitis.

| TABLE 15.2 Signs of Air in the Bowel Wall | |
|---|---|
| **Sign** | **Remarks** |
| **Linear radiolucency paralleling the contour of air in the adjacent bowel lumen** | Appearance when seen in profile |
| **Mottled appearance that resembles air mixed with fecal material** | Appearance when seen *en face;* may occur in an area of the abdomen not expected for colon; does not change over time |
| **Globular, cyst-like collections of air that parallel the contour of the bowel** | Unusual, benign condition affecting the colon, most often left colon |

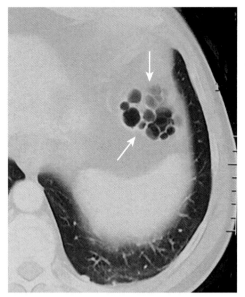

**Fig. 15.14** Pneumatosis Cystoides Intestinalis. Axial CT scan of the upper abdomen windowed for lung technique shows a cluster of air-containing cysts *(arrows)* associated with the left colon, characteristic of *pneumatosis cystoides intestinalis,* a rare condition of unknown etiology. The cysts are usually subserosal or submucosal in location and the patient is often asymptomatic.

cyst-like collections of air in the submucosa or serosa (Fig. 15.14).
- A **more common, secondary form** that can occur in:
  - **Chronic obstructive pulmonary disease,** presumably secondary to air from ruptured blebs dissecting through the mediastinum to the abdomen
  - Diseases in which there is **necrosis of the bowel** wall such as:
    - **Necrotizing enterocolitis** in infants (see Figs. 15.12 and 15.13)
    - **Ischemic bowel disease** in adults (Fig. 15.15)

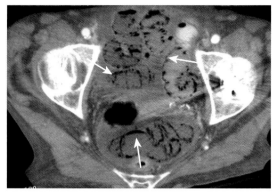

**Fig. 15.15** Necrosis of Bowel from Mesenteric Ischemia. Axial CT image of the pelvis demonstrates multiple loops of bowel with curvilinear collections of air throughout their walls consistent with pneumatosis *(arrows).* The patient had widespread ischemia of bowel from mesenteric vascular disease. Pneumatosis that results from bowel necrosis is an ominous sign.

- **Obstructing lesions of the bowel,** which raise intraluminal pressure such as:
  - *Hirschsprung disease* or *pyloric stenosis* in children
  - **Obstructing carcinomas** in adults

**▶▶ IMPORTANT POINTS**

- **Pneumatosis intestinalis associated with** diseases that produce **necrosis of bowel** is usually **a more ominous prognostic sign** than pneumatosis associated with **obstructing lesions of the bowel** or chronic obstructive pulmonary disease.

- **Complications of pneumatosis intestinalis** can include:
  - **Rupture into the peritoneal cavity** leading to intraperitoneal free air (pneumoperitoneum)
  - Dissection of air into the portal venous system (Fig. 15.16)

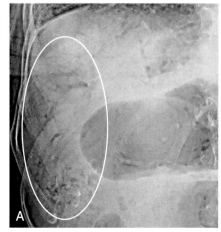
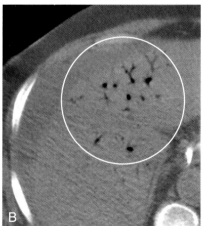

**Fig. 15.16** Portal Venous Gas. (A) Numerous small black branching structures are visible over the periphery of the liver *(oval).* This is air in the portal venous system, a finding most often associated with necrotizing enterocolitis in infants but can also be seen in adults, usually with bowel necrosis. Unlike air in the biliary system, this air is peripheral rather than central and has numerous branches rather than the few tubular structures seen with pneumobilia. (B) Close-up of axial CT scan through the liver shows air in the portal venous system *(circle)* in a patient with mesenteric vascular disease.

# AIR IN THE BILIARY SYSTEM

- Air in the biliary system *(pneumobilia)* presents as **one or two tube-like, branching lucencies in the right upper quadrant overlying the central portion of the liver that conform to the location and appearance of the major bile ducts** (i.e., the common duct, cystic duct, and/or the major hepatic ducts) (Fig. 15.17).
- Box 15.2 summarizes the signs of **air in the biliary system.**

## Causes of Air in the Biliary System

- Air in the biliary system **may be a "normal" finding** if the sphincter of Oddi, which guards the entrance of the common bile duct as it enters the duodenum, is open (said to be *incompetent*).
- Prior **sphincterotomy,** such as might be done to allow gallstones to exit from the ductal system into the bowel.
- **Prior surgery** that results in the **reimplantation of the common bile duct** into another part of the bowel (i.e., choledochoenterostomy) is frequently accompanied by the persistent presence of air in the biliary ductal system.
- **Pathologic conditions** that can produce pneumobilia include **uncommon causes,** such as:
  - *Gallstone ileus,* in which a **gallstone erodes through the wall of the gallbladder** into the **duodenum** (usually) producing a **fistula between the bowel and the biliary system.** The **gallstone impacts in the small bowel,** most often in the narrower terminal ileum, and produces a mechanical small bowel obstruction (which has historically been called an "ileus" even though it is a mechanical obstruction) (Fig. 15.18).
- **Gas-forming pyogenic cholangitis,** particularly from *Escherichia coli*

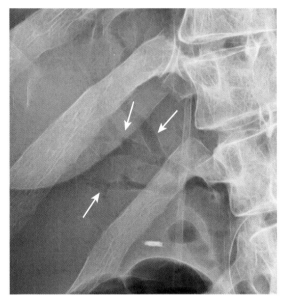

**Fig. 15.17 Air in the Biliary Tree (Pneumobilia).** Close-up view of the right upper quadrant shows several air-containing tubular structures over the central portion of the liver consistent with air in the biliary system *(arrows)*. This patient had a history of a prior sphincterotomy for gallstones so that reflux of air into the biliary system would be expected.

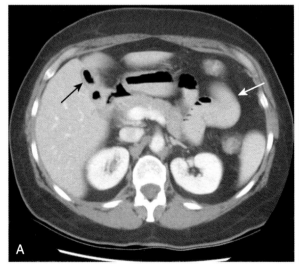
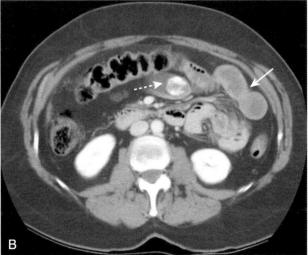

**Fig. 15.18 Gallstone Ileus.** The three key findings of gallstone ileus are present on this study. (A) Axial CT scan of the upper abdomen shows **air in the lumen of the gallbladder** *(black arrow)* and dilated small bowel *(white arrow)* consistent with a mechanical **small bowel obstruction.** (B) At a lower level, another axial CT scan of the abdomen shows a **large calcified gallstone** inside the small bowel *(dashed arrow)* and additional proximal, dilated loops of small bowel *(solid arrow)*.

## CASE QUIZ 15 ANSWER

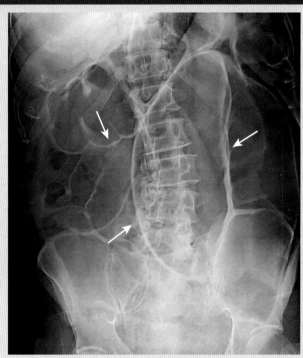

There is a massive amount of free air in the abdomen evidenced by visualization of both sides of the bowel wall (Rigler sign) *(arrows)*. The patient underwent emergent **abdominal surgery** to repair a perforated gastric ulcer. The correct answer is (C).

## TAKE HOME POINTS

- Gas in the abdomen outside of the normal confines of the bowel is called **extraluminal air.**
- The four most common locations for extraluminal air are intraperitoneal (**pneumoperitoneum,** frequently called **free air**), extraperitoneal air, air in the bowel wall (pneumatosis), and air in the biliary system (pneumobilia).
- The three key signs of free air are air beneath the diaphragm, visualization of both sides of the bowel wall (**Rigler sign**), and visualization of the falciform ligament.
- The most common causes of free air are perforated peptic ulcer, trauma whether accidental or iatrogenic, perforated diverticulitis, and perforation of a carcinoma, usually of the colon.
- The key signs of **extraperitoneal (retroperitoneal) air** are a streaky, linear appearance or a mottled, blotchy appearance outlining extraperitoneal structures and its relatively fixed position, moving little or at all with changes in patient positioning.
- Extraperitoneal air outlines extraperitoneal structures such as the psoas muscles, kidneys, aorta, and inferior vena cava.
- Causes of extraperitoneal air include bowel perforation secondary to either inflammatory or ulcerative disease, blunt or penetrating trauma, iatrogenic manipulation, and foreign body ingestion.
- The key signs of **air in the bowel wall** include linear radiolucencies paralleling the contour of air in the adjacent bowel lumen, a mottled appearance

that resembles air mixed with fecal material or, uncommonly, globular, cyst-like collections of air that parallel the contour of the bowel.
- Causes of air in the bowel wall **(pneumatosis intestinalis)** include a rare primary form called **pneumatosis cystoides intestinalis.** A more common secondary form includes diseases in which there is **necrosis of the bowel** wall, such as necrotizing enterocolitis in infants, ischemic bowel disease in adults, and obstructing lesions of the bowel that raise intraluminal pressure, such as Hirschsprung disease in children and obstructing carcinomas in adults.
- Pneumatosis intestinalis associated with diseases that produce **necrosis** of bowel is usually a **more ominous** prognostic sign than pneumatosis associated with obstructing lesions of the bowel or chronic obstructive pulmonary disease.
- Signs of **air in the biliary system** (pneumobilia) include tube-like, branching lucencies in the right upper quadrant overlying the liver that are central in location and few in number as well as gas in the lumen of the gallbladder.
- Causes of pneumobilia include incompetence of the sphincter of Oddi, prior sphincterotomy, prior surgery that resulted in the reimplantation of the common bile duct into another part of the bowel, and gallstone ileus.
- The triad of findings in **gallstone ileus** are air in the biliary system, small bowel obstruction, and visualization of the gallstone itself.

 Additional content is available online including chapters on Nuclear Medicine, Artificial Intelligence, Radiation Dose and Safety, an Early History of Radiology, and a compendium of 200 Diagnostic Radiology Signs.

# 16

# Recognizing Abnormal Calcifications and Their Causes

*William Herring, MD, FACR*

Soft-tissue calcifications lend themselves to a systematic approach that connects a diverse group of diseases. Although this chapter focuses primarily on abdominal calcifications, the same principles and approach apply to dystrophic calcification found anywhere in the body.

## CASE QUIZ 16 QUESTION

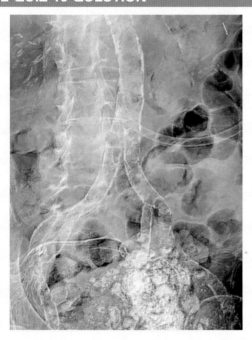

This is a supine abdominal radiograph of a 56-year-old female with chronic renal disease. The image demonstrates two of the four classic patterns of calcification described in this chapter. What are they and in what structures are they located? The answers are at the end of the chapter.

- Most soft-tissue calcification occurs in tissue that is already abnormal. Such calcification is called *dystrophic calcification.*
- The **nature of most calcifications can be determined by examining two of their characteristics:**
  - Their **pattern of calcification**
  - Their **anatomic location**
    - CT can easily identify the location of such calcifications.

## PATTERNS OF CALCIFICATION

- Calcifications **tend to occur in one of four distinct patterns,** depending on the type of structure that has calcified.
- The patterns are:
  - **Rim-like**
  - **Linear or track-like**
  - **Lamellar (or laminar)**
  - **Cloudlike, amorphous, or popcorn**

### Rim-Like Calcification

- Rim-like calcification implies calcification that has occurred **in the wall of a hollow viscus.** A "hollow viscus" in this context means a structure containing fluid, fat, or air and is enclosed by an outer wall.
- Examples of structures that manifest rim-like calcifications include:
  - **Cysts:** calcification in any one of the following is relatively uncommon.
    - **Renal cysts**
    - **Splenic cysts**
      - And **extraabdominal** sites, such as:
        - Mediastinal cysts, such as pericardial and bronchial cysts (Fig. 16.1)
        - Popliteal cysts

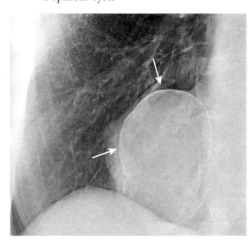

**Fig. 16.1** Calcified Pericardial Cyst. There is a **rim-like calcification** *(arrows)* that identifies the structure containing the calcification as cystic or saccular. The calcification's location is ideal for a pericardial cyst. Pericardial cysts almost always occur on the right side and are usually asymptomatic, discovered when a chest radiograph is obtained for another reason.

- **Aneurysms**
  - **Aortic aneurysms**
    - These can sometimes be recognized on radiographs of the lumbar spine, especially in the lateral projection.
    - The abdominal aorta should **normally** measure less than **3 cm in diameter**, a measurement that usually requires both opposing walls be visible (Fig. 16.2).
  - **Splenic artery** or **renal artery** aneurysms
  - And **extraabdominal sites** like:
    - Femoral artery aneurysms
    - Cerebral aneurysms
- **Saccular organs,** such as the gallbladder or urinary bladder
  - **Porcelain gallbladder**
    - This uncommon entity (named after the porcelain-like gross appearance of the gallbladder) that occurs with **chronic inflammation** and **stasis** of the gallbladder is associated with **gallstones** in over 90% of cases. It may possibly be associated with an increased incidence of carcinoma of the gallbladder (Fig. 16.3).

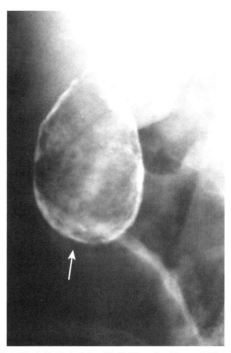

**Fig. 16.3** Calcified Gallbladder Wall. The **rim-like** calcification *(arrow)* identifies this as one that occurs in the wall of a cyst or saccular organ. The calcification is in the right upper quadrant, the location of the gallbladder. This is a **porcelain gallbladder,** so named because of its bluish color and brittle nature at the time of surgery.

- **Urinary bladder**
  - Calcification of the bladder wall is an uncommon occurrence in diseases such as **schistosomiasis, bladder cancer,** and **tuberculosis.**
- Table 16.1 highlights key facts about rim-like calcifications.

## Linear or Track-Like Calcification

- Linear or track-like calcification implies calcification that has occurred in the **walls of tubular structures.**

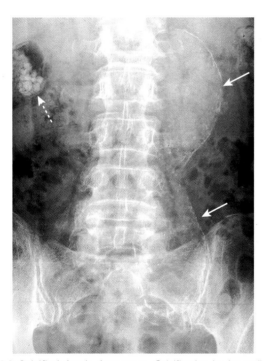

**Fig. 16.2** Calcified Aortic Aneurysm. Calcification in the wall of the abdominal aorta is a common finding in atherosclerosis, especially in those with diabetes mellitus. In this patient, the aorta demonstrates a **rim-like** calcification *(solid arrows)* in a large, bi-lobed abdominal aortic aneurysm. There are also multiple calcifications in the right upper quadrant *(dashed arrow)* consistent with gallstones. When the diameter of the abdominal aorta exceeds its normal diameter by more than 50%, an aneurysm is present.

| TABLE 16.1 | Rim-Like Calcifications |
|---|---|
| **Organ of Origin** | **Remarks** |
| **Renal cyst** | Thick and irregular calcifications, although uncommon, may indicate the presence of renal cell carcinoma |
| **Splenic cysts** | May be a manifestation of hydatid cyst, old trauma, or prior infection |
| **Aortic aneurysms** | Occurs more often in diabetics with advanced atherosclerosis |
| **Gallbladder** | Associated with chronic stasis; called **porcelain gallbladder** for its gross appearance; possible slightly higher incidence of carcinoma of the gallbladder |

- Examples include calcifications in the walls of:
  - **Arteries** (Fig. 16.4)
    - **Common in atherosclerosis** and can be seen anywhere in the body
  - Walls of veins do not calcify.
    - In veins, **long, linear thrombi or small, focal thrombi** (the latter called *phleboliths*) may calcify (see Fig. 12.18).
  - **Other tubular structures**
    - **Fallopian tubes and vas deferens**
      - Seen more often in diabetics (Fig. 16.5)
    - **Ureter**
      - Uncommon finding seen in schistosomiasis and even more rarely in tuberculosis (TB)
- Table 16.2 highlights key facts about linear or track-like calcifications.

## Lamellar or Laminar Calcification

- Lamellar (or laminar) calcification implies calcification that **forms around a nidus inside a hollow lumen.** A "hollow lumen" refers to a walled structure such as the gallbladder or urinary bladder, which both contain a fluid.

> **IMPORTANT POINTS**
>
> - **Calcification in concentric layers** begins with a central nidus around which alternating layers of calcified and noncalcified material form because of the prolonged movement of the stone within the hollow viscus (Fig. 16.6).

- Lamellar or laminated calcifications are usually called *stones* or *calculi* (singular: calculus) and include:

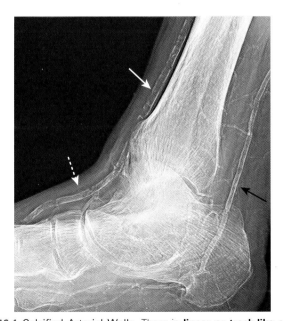

**Fig.16.4 Calcified Arterial Walls.** There is **linear or track-like** calcification present in the arteries around the ankle and foot which implies calcification that has occurred in the walls of tubular structures. There is calcification of the anterior tibial *(solid white arrow)*, posterior tibial *(black arrow)*, and dorsalis pedis arteries *(dashed white arrow)*. Many smaller arteries are also calcified. Such wall calcification occurs in arteries, not veins, and is usually secondary to atherosclerosis, frequently associated with diabetes, or in patients with chronic renal disease.

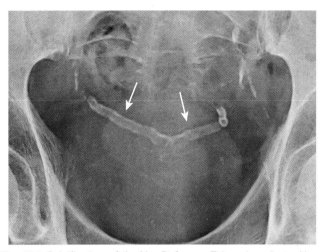

**Fig. 16.5 Calcification of the Vas Deferens.** This male patient with an enlarged prostate manifests two symmetric **track-like** calcifications *(arrows)*. The type of calcification identifies it as occurring in the wall of a tubular structure. Calcification in the walls of the vas deferens occurs more commonly and earlier in diabetics than as a natural, degenerative process.

| TABLE 16.2 | **Linear or Track-Like Calcifications** |
|---|---|
| **Organ of Origin** | **Remarks** |
| **Walls of smaller arteries** | Mostly seen in atherosclerosis accelerated by diabetes and renal disease |
| **Fallopian tubes or vas deferens** | Usually accelerated by diabetes |
| **Ureters** | Uncommon occurrence described with schistosomiasis and, rarely, tuberculosis |

- **Renal calculi**
  - CT is the study of choice for the detection of renal and ureteral calculi.

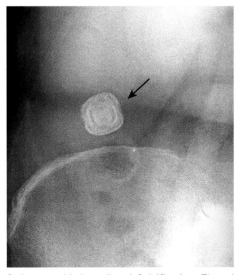

**Fig. 16.6 Gallstone with Lamellated Calcification.** There is a **lamellated** calcification in the right upper quadrant *(arrow)*. The alternating bands of calcium and less dense material identify it as a calculus that has formed in a viscus in this region. The anatomic location places it in the region of the gall bladder. Ultrasound is the most accurate imaging modality to detect gallstones.

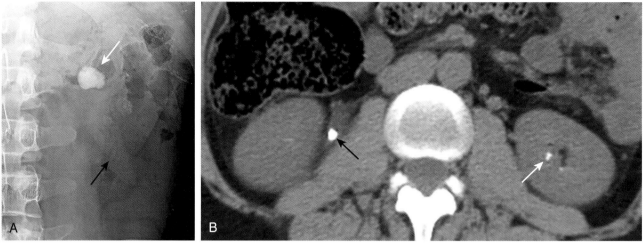

**Fig. 16.7** Renal Calculus, Conventional Radiograph and Axial CT Scan. (A) There is a calcification *(white arrow)* that overlies the shadow of the left kidney *(black arrow)*. Although it is too small to recognize lamination (lamellation), its location suggests a renal calculus. (B) In a different patient, an image from an unenhanced axial CT called a ***stone search*** reveals a large calcification in the proximal right ureter *(black arrow)* and smaller calcifications in the left intrarenal collecting system *(white arrow)*. Because of its greater sensitivity, a CT stone search done without intravenous contrast has mostly replaced conventional radiography for the identification of renal and ureteral calculi.

- Conventional radiographs are only about 50% to 60% sensitive for displaying renal calculi despite the fact that about 90% of renal calculi contain calcium (Fig. 16.7).
- **Gallstones**
  - **Ultrasound** is the study of choice for the detection of gallstones.

- Only about 10% to 15% of gallstones contain enough calcification to be visible on conventional radiographs (Fig. 16.8).
- **Bladder stones**
  - Bladder stones usually develop secondary to **chronic bladder outlet obstruction**; they are very susceptible to developing lamination (Fig. 16.9).

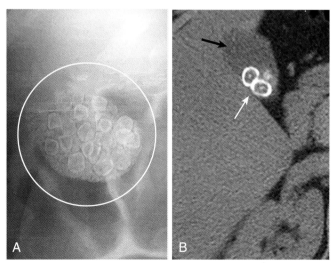

**Fig. 16.8** Gallstones, Conventional Radiographs and Axial CT Scan. (A) There are multiple **lamellar** calcifications *(circle)* which have interlocking edges, suggesting that they all formed in a viscus in proximity to each other producing ***facets*** on some of the stones. (B) In a different patient, a close-up view of an unenhanced axial CT scan of the right upper quadrant shows several gallstones *(white arrow)*, two of which clearly have a central nidus surrounded by laminated, concentric rings of noncalcified and calcified material. The gallbladder *(black arrow)* contains bile fats and is less dense than the adjacent liver.

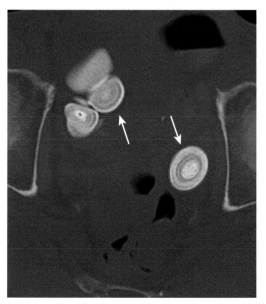

**Fig. 16.9** Urinary Bladder Stones. There are **lamellar** calcifications *(arrows)* seen on this axial CT scan through the level of the pelvis and windowed to show the laminations better. The laminations imply that these calcifications have formed inside of a viscus. The anatomic location of these calculi places them in the urinary bladder.

- Table 16.3 highlights key facts about laminated/lamellar calcifications.

## Cloudlike, Amorphous, or "Popcorn" Calcification

- Cloud-like, amorphous, or popcorn calcification is a calcification that has **formed inside of a solid organ or tumor** and examples include:
  - **Body of the pancreas**
    - Pathognomonic for chronic pancreatitis (Fig. 16.10)
  - **Leiomyomas of uterus**
    - Uterine fibroids or leiomyomas very commonly degenerate and calcify over time (Fig. 16.11).

### TABLE 16.3 Laminar or Lamellated Calcifications

| Organ of Origin | Remarks |
| --- | --- |
| **Kidney** | Most calcified renal stones are composed of calcium oxalate crystals; mostly form because of stasis, infection |
| **Gallbladder** | Most calcified gallstones are calcium bilirubinate; form because of chronic infection and stasis |
| **Urinary bladder** | Most bladder calculi contain urate crystals; most often from chronic outlet obstruction |

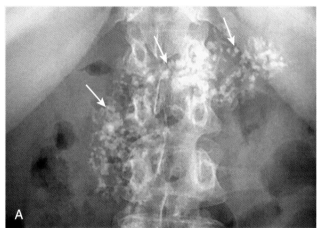 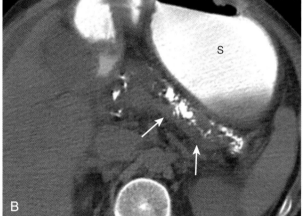

**Fig. 16.10** Chronic Calcific Pancreatitis, Conventional Radiograph and Axial CT Scan. (A) A close-up view of the upper abdomen on a conventional radiograph shows **amorphous** calcifications *(arrows)* implying calcification in a solid organ or tumor. The anatomic distribution of the calcification corresponds to the location of the pancreas. (B) In another patient, a nonenhanced CT image of the upper abdomen displays amorphous calcifications distributed along the course of the body and tail of the pancreas *(arrows)*. There is oral contrast in the stomach (S). These calcifications are pathognomonic of chronic pancreatitis, an irreversible disease occurring mostly secondary to alcoholism that leads to atrophy of the gland and diabetes.

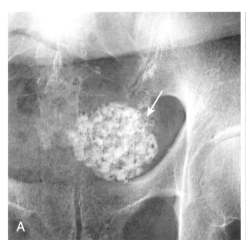 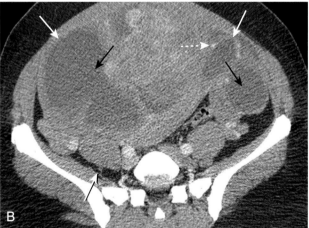

**Fig. 16.11** Calcified Uterine Leiomyoma (Fibroid) on Conventional Radiograph and CT. (A) There is an **amorphous** or **popcorn** calcification *(arrow)* in the pelvis of this 48-year-old female. The type of calcification suggests formation in a solid organ or tumor. This is the anatomic location and the classical appearance of calcified uterine leiomyomas (fibroids). (B) CT on another patient shows large uterine fibroids *(solid white arrows)*, portions of which have necrosed *(solid black arrows)* and calcified *(dashed white arrow)*. Ultrasound is the study of choice in diagnosing uterine fibroids.

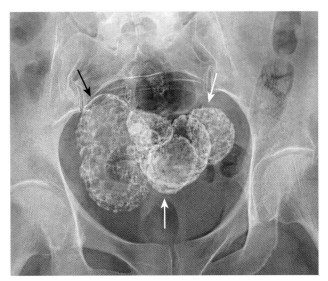

**Fig. 16.12** Calcified Rims in Uterine Leiomyomas. This is a **rim-like** calcification *(arrows)* in the pelvis of a female patient so that it would be appropriate to consider that this calcification formed in the wall of a saccular structure, like a cyst. In fact, this is a characteristic pattern of calcification in the outer walls of degenerated uterine leiomyomas (fibroids). They are rim-like calcifications, but the structure in which it originally formed was solid.

> **! DIAGNOSTIC PITFALLS**
>
> • Sometimes a **solid tumor will outgrow its blood supply and the center of the tumor will undergo necrosis** leaving only a viable outer shell. The subsequent calcification will be **more rim-like than amorphous.** Uterine fibroids are especially likely to develop this appearance (Fig. 16.12).

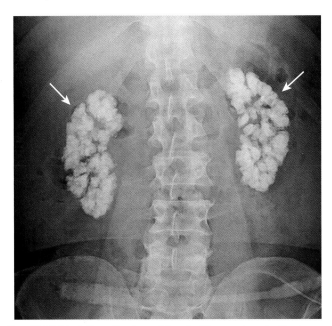

**Fig. 16.13** Medullary Nephrocalcinosis (Hypercalcemic Nephropathy). There are **cloudlike** calcifications seen bilaterally *(arrows)* suggesting these calcifications have formed within a solid organ or tumor. The calcifications conform to the anatomic locations of the renal collecting systems. This is *medullary nephrocalcinosis,* a condition associated with hypercalcemia. This patient had primary hyperparathyroidism, the most common cause of nephrocalcinosis in adults.

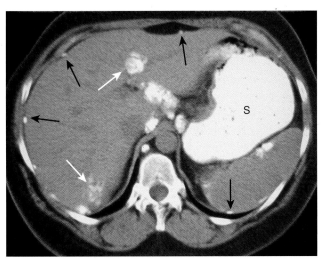

**Fig. 16.14** Calcified Ovarian Metastases. An unenhanced axial CT scan of the upper abdomen shows multiple **amorphous** calcifications, some within the liver *(white arrows)* and others which stud the peritoneal surface of the abdomen *(black arrows)*. This patient had a mucin-producing adenocarcinoma of the ovary which metastasized to the peritoneum and liver. Mucin-producing tumors of the stomach and colon can also produce calcified metastases, but ovarian malignancy would be the most common to metastasize to the peritoneum. There is oral contrast in the stomach (S).

- **Lymph nodes**
  - Can calcify anywhere in the body, mostly from prior granulomatous infection, such as old TB.
- **Kidneys**
  - *Medullary nephrocalcinosis* is macroscopic calcification deposited in the pyramids of the renal medulla, usually secondary to a metabolic derangement such as hyperparathyroidism (Fig. 16.13).
- **Mucin-producing adenocarcinomas** of the stomach, ovary, and colon may produce calcifications in both their primary tumors and in metastatic deposits (Fig. 16.14).
- And, outside of the abdomen, in structures like:
  - **Meningiomas**
- Table 16.4 highlights key facts about amorphous, cloud-like, or popcorn calcifications.

### TABLE 16.4 Amorphous, Cloud-Like, or Popcorn Calcifications

| Organ of Origin | Remarks |
|---|---|
| **Pancreas** | Chronic pancreatitis, frequently secondary to alcoholism |
| **Uterine fibroids (leiomyomas)** | Degenerating fibroids calcify |
| **Mucin-producing tumors** | Mucin-producing tumors of the ovary, stomach, or colon may calcify as can their metastases |
| **Meningioma** | Benign, extraaxial brain tumor of older individuals that calcifies about 20% of the time |

## TABLE 16.5  Identifying the Four Types of Abnormal Calcification

| Type of Calcification | Implies | Examples |
| --- | --- | --- |
| Rim-like | Formed in wall of hollow viscus | Cysts, aneurysms, gallbladder wall |
| Linear or track-like | Formed in walls of tubular structures | Ureters, arteries, ducts |
| Lamellar or laminar | Formed in stones | Renal, gallbladder, and bladder calculi |
| Amorphous, cloud-like, popcorn | Formed in a solid organ or tumor | Uterine fibroids; some mucin-producing tumors |

- Table 16.5 summarizes the key findings of the four patterns of abnormal calcification.

### ▶▶ IMPORTANT POINTS

- **No matter what its cause, the presence of calcification implies a process that is subacute or chronic.**

## LOCATION OF CALCIFICATION

- Identifying the **pattern** of calcification helps in identifying its **type.**
- Identifying the anatomic **location** of the calcification helps to identify its **organ or tissue of origin.**
  - Combining the **type** of calcification with its **anatomic location** should provide the key to the **cause** of most pathologic calcifications.
- Table 16.6 summarizes some of the possible locations of calcifications in the abdomen.

## TABLE 16.6  Location, Location, Location

| Anatomic Quadrant in the Abdomen | Pattern of Calcification | Possible Organ of Origin | Cause |
| --- | --- | --- | --- |
| RUQ | Rim-like | Gallbladder wall | Chronic infection |
| | Track-like | Hepatic artery | Atherosclerosis |
| | Laminated | Gallbladder | Gallstones |
| | Amorphous | Head of pancreas | Chronic pancreatitis |
| LUQ | Rim-like | Splenic cyst | Amoebic infection |
| | Track-like | Splenic artery | Atherosclerosis |
| | Laminated | Kidney | Renal stone |
| | Amorphous | Tail of pancreas | Chronic pancreatitis |
| RLQ | Rim-like | Iliac artery | Iliac artery aneurysm |
| | Track-like | Iliac artery | Atherosclerosis |
| | Laminated | Appendix | Appendicolith |
| | Amorphous | Uterus | Fibroids |
| LLQ | Rim-like | Iliac artery | Iliac artery aneurysm |
| | Track-like | Iliac artery | Atherosclerosis |
| | Laminated | Unlikely location for such a calcification | |
| | Amorphous | Uterus or ovaries | Fibroids; ovarian tumors |

*LLQ*, Left lower quadrant; *LUQ*, left upper quadrant; *RLQ*, right lower quadrant; *RUQ*, right upper quadrant.

## CASE QUIZ 16 ANSWER

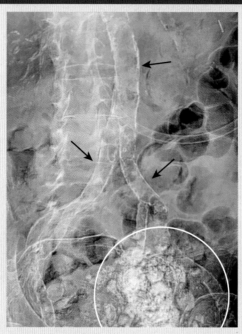

There are **linear** or **track-like** calcifications implying calcification in the wall of a tubular structure and conforming to the anatomic location of the abdominal aorta and iliac arteries *(arrows)*. Such calcifications can occur with atherosclerosis but are more likely in patients with diabetes and renal disease. As a bonus, there are also **amorphous** or **popcorn** calcifications in the pelvis *(circle)* consistent with calcified uterine leiomyomas.

## 🏠 TAKE HOME POINTS

- Soft-tissue calcifications can be characterized by the pattern of their calcification and their anatomic location.
- There are four distinct patterns: (1) rim-like, (2) linear or track-like, (3) lamellar (or laminar), and (4) cloud-like, amorphous, or popcorn.
- **Rim-like calcifications** imply calcification that has occurred in the wall of a hollow viscus (i.e., a saccular structure containing fluid).
- Examples of rim-like calcifications include the walls of cysts, aneurysms, or saccular organs, such as the gallbladder.
- **Linear or track-like calcifications** imply calcification that has occurred in the walls of tubular structures.
- Examples of track-like calcifications include the walls of arteries and tubular structures, such as the ureters, fallopian tubes, and vas deferens.

- **Lamellar (or laminar) calcifications** imply calcification that forms around a nidus inside a hollow (usually fluid-containing) lumen.
- Examples of lamellar calcifications include renal calculi, gallstones, and bladder stones.
- **Cloud-like, amorphous, or popcorn calcification** is calcification that has formed inside a solid organ or tumor.
- Examples of amorphous or popcorn calcifications include chronic pancreatitis, leiomyomas of the uterus, old inflammatory disease in lymph nodes, and mucin-producing adenocarcinomas.
- Combining the type of calcification with its anatomic location should provide the key to the causes of most pathologic calcifications. CT scans will demonstrate the anatomic location easily.

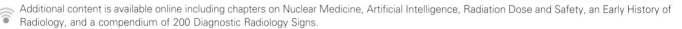

📶 Additional content is available online including chapters on Nuclear Medicine, Artificial Intelligence, Radiation Dose and Safety, an Early History of Radiology, and a compendium of 200 Diagnostic Radiology Signs.

# 17

# Recognizing Gastrointestinal, Hepatobiliary, and Urinary Tract Abnormalities

*Susan L. Summerton, MD, FACR*

In this chapter, you will learn how to recognize some of the most common abnormalities in the abdomen. We will also discuss selected hepatic abnormalities. Chapter 18, on ultrasound, describes some of the more common biliary and pelvic abnormalities.

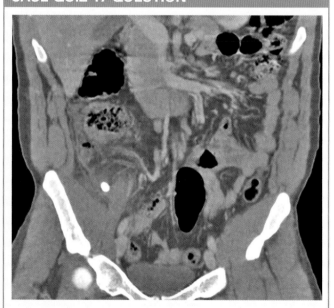

**CASE QUIZ 17 QUESTION**

This is a coronal view of the lower abdomen from an abdominal CT scan performed **without** oral contrast on a 20-year-old male with right lower quadrant pain for 5 hours. What is the diagnosis? The answer is at the end of this chapter.

## BARIUM STUDIES OF THE GASTROINTESTINAL TRACT

- CT, ultrasound, and MRI have essentially replaced conventional radiography and, in many instances, barium studies for the evaluation of the gastrointestinal (GI) tract and the visceral abdominal organs.
- To review some of the terminology used for fluoroscopic studies of the GI tract, see **e-Appendix D. Key Terminology and Glossaries.**

## ESOPHAGUS

- Single- and/or double-contrast examinations of the esophagus are performed with the patient drinking liquid barium, either by itself *(single contrast)* or accompanied by a gas-producing agent that provides the "air" in a ***double-contrast examination.*** Because both the single- and double-contrast techniques have their own strengths, many esophagrams are routinely performed with **both** techniques, called a *biphasic examination.*
- *Video esophagography* (**video swallowing function**) is a study of the **swallowing mechanism,** usually performed with fluoroscopy and frequently captured dynamically either digitally, on videotape, or on film. This is the study of choice for diagnosing and documenting **aspiration,** in which ingested substances pass into the trachea below the level of the vocal cords (see Case Quiz in Chapter 8; Video 17.1).
- **Fluoroscopic observation** of the esophagus can also **reveal abnormalities in esophageal motility.** For example, *tertiary waves* are a common but nonspecific abnormality of esophageal motility, representing disordered and nonpropulsive contractions of the esophagus. They can be observed fluoroscopically and captured on spot films (Video 17.2).

### Esophageal Carcinoma

- Esophageal carcinoma continues to have a very **poor prognosis** as more than **50% of patients will have metastases on initial presentation.** The **lack of an esophageal serosa** and a **rich supply of lymphatics** aid in the extension and dissemination of esophageal carcinoma. Long-term alcohol and tobacco use are associated with a higher risk of esophageal carcinoma.

- Esophageal malignancies are either **squamous cell carcinomas** or **adenocarcinomas,** the latter of which is **increasing in prevalence. Adenocarcinomas** arise in esophageal epithelium that has undergone metaplasia from **squamous** to **columnar epithelium** *(Barrett esophagus),* a process in which **gastroesophageal reflux** *(GERD)* plays a major role.
- Barium esophagrams are **frequently the initial study** in patients with symptoms that suggest this diagnosis, such as dysphagia (Fig. 17.1).

## Hiatal Hernia and Gastroesophageal Reflux (GERD)

- Hiatal hernias are divided into the *sliding type* (almost all) in which the **esophagogastric junction lies above the diaphragm** or the *paraesophageal type* (1%) in which a **portion of the stomach herniates through the esophageal hiatus, but the esophagogastric junction remains below the diaphragm.** In general, hiatal hernia increases in incidence with age.
- **Most hiatal hernias are asymptomatic,** but there is an association between the presence of some hiatal hernias and clinically significant **gastroesophageal reflux.**
  - Gastroesophageal reflux also occurs in patients without any visible hiatal hernia, usually because of some dysfunction of the lower esophageal sphincter that

normally acts to prevent gastric acid from repeatedly refluxing into the esophagus.

> ⯈ **IMPORTANT POINTS**

- **The radiologic findings of hiatal hernia include:**
  - **A bulbous area** of the distal esophagus containing oral contrast at the level of the diaphragm with **failure of the esophagus to narrow** on multiple images **as it passes through the esophageal hiatus** of the diaphragm
  - **Extension of multiple gastric folds above the diaphragm**
  - Sometimes, visualization of a thin, circumferential filling defect in the distal esophagus called a ***Schatzki ring*** (Fig. 17.2)

- **Gastroesophageal reflux may be evident during fluoroscopy** when barium is seen to move from the stomach retrograde into the esophagus, but reflux is intermittent so this event may not occur during the course of the examination. The absence of reflux during the study **does not exclude reflux,** and demonstration of reflux **does not necessarily indicate the patient has the complications of GERD (i.e., esophagitis, stricture, and Barrett esophagus).**

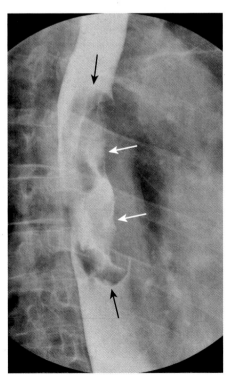

**Fig. 17.1 Esophageal Carcinoma.** Liquid barium fills the esophageal lumen except where it coats a space-occupying **polypoid mass** that arises from the left lateral wall of the esophagus *(white arrows)*. The tumor produces classical ***overhanging edges*** at its proximal and distal margins *(black arrows)*. Note that throughout this chapter, barium may be depicted as either white or black.

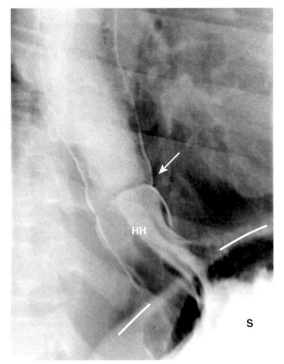

**Fig. 17.2 Hiatal Hernia.** The stomach (S) extends above the level of the diaphragm *(lines)* as a hiatal hernia (HH). Gastric folds are seen radiating from the stomach into the hernia. Notice that the esophagus does not narrow (as it normally does) when passing through the esophageal hiatus. A ***Schatzki ring*** *(arrow)* marks the position of the esophagogastric junction and its appearance above the diaphragm automatically indicates the presence of a sliding hiatal hernia.

# STOMACH AND DUODENUM

- Today, the lumen of the stomach is most often studied by upper endoscopy and the wall thickness and structures outside of the stomach are studied by CT examination of the abdomen with oral contrast. Nevertheless, biphasic upper gastrointestinal (UGI) examinations, which include a study of the esophagus, stomach, and duodenum, remain a sensitive, cost-effective, readily available, and noninvasive examination.

## Gastric Ulcers

- In the United States, the incidence of **gastric ulcer disease has been declining.** In adults, infection with *Helicobacter pylori* accounts for almost three out of four cases of gastric ulcer disease. **Nonsteroidal antiinflammatory agents** account for most of the rest.

### ⟫ IMPORTANT POINTS

- Most gastric ulcers occur on the **lesser curvature** or **posterior wall** in the region of the **body or antrum.** About **95% of all gastric ulcers are benign.** The other **5% will represent ulcerations in gastric malignancies** (Fig. 17.3).

## Gastric Carcinoma

- There has been a dramatic **decline in the incidence of gastric carcinoma in the United States.** The **mortality, however, remains quite high** as gastric carcinomas are frequently not diagnosed until after they have spread. Most gastric carcinomas (actually, they are adenocarcinomas) **occur in the distal third of the stomach** along the **lesser curvature** (Fig. 17.4).
- Double-contrast UGI images and CT scans of the abdomen can demonstrate gastric carcinomas. CT is used for staging the extent of the tumor and degree of spread.
- Other mass lesions may resemble gastric carcinoma, including **leiomyomas,** a benign, wall lesion that characteristically ulcerates, and **lymphoma,** which may produce diffusely thickened folds or multiple masses in the stomach.

## Duodenal Ulcers

### ⟫ IMPORTANT POINTS

- **Duodenal ulcers are two to three times more common than gastric ulcers.** Almost all duodenal ulcers occur in the **duodenal bulb,** the majority on the **anterior wall** of the bulb. They are **overwhelmingly caused by** *H. pylori* infection (85% to 95%).

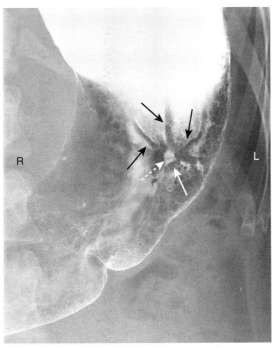

**Fig. 17.3 Benign Gastric Ulcer.** A central collection of barium (the ulcer) *(dashed white arrow)* is surrounded by a mound of edema *(solid white arrow).* There are numerous gastric folds *(black arrows)* that radiate to the ulcer margin. This was a benign gastric ulcer. *L,* Patient's left; *R,* patient's right.

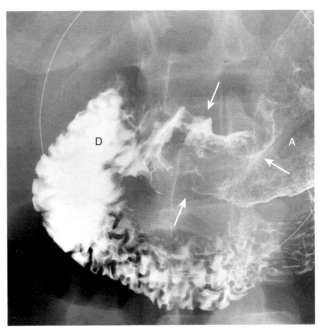

**Fig. 17.4 Carcinoma of the Stomach.** There is a large, lobulated mass in the antrum (A) of the stomach that displaces the barium around it and disrupts the normal smooth contour of the stomach *(arrows).* This was an adenocarcinoma of the stomach. *D,* Duodenum.

- A double-contrast UGI series has a sensitivity that exceeds 90% in detecting duodenal ulcers (Fig. 17.5).

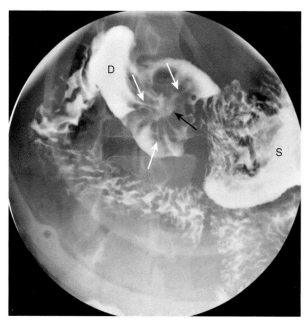

**Fig. 17.5** Acute Duodenal Ulcer. Contained within the duodenal bulb (D) is an irregularly shaped collection of barium *(black arrow),* shown to be **persistent** on a number of other images, representing a duodenal ulcer. It is surrounded by a **zone of edema** and **radiating folds** *(white arrows)* that displace the barium from around the base of the ulcer. When duodenal ulcers heal, they are likely to do so with scarring that deforms the normal triangular contour of the bulb. *S,* Stomach.

- **Complications** of duodenal ulcers, best demonstrated by CT, include **obstruction, perforation** (into the peritoneal cavity) (Fig. 17.6), **penetration** (e.g., into the pancreas), or **hemorrhage.**

## SMALL AND LARGE BOWEL

### General Considerations

- **Opacification** and **distension** of the bowel lumen is necessary for proper evaluation of the bowel no matter what modality is used.

> **! DIAGNOSTIC PITFALLS**
>
> - **Collapsed or unopacified loops of bowel can introduce errors of diagnosis** related to an inability to **visualize** and **differentiate** real from artifactual findings or to accurately characterize the abnormality even if recognized. On CT scans of the abdomen and pelvis, unopacified loops of bowel may mimic masses or adenopathy and wall thickness is difficult to assess if the bowel is not distended.

- Therefore, **orally administered contrast,** frequently given in doses divided over time to allow earlier contrast to reach the colon while later contrast opacifies the stomach, is **routinely utilized for most abdominal CT scans.** Exceptions might include those studies performed for **trauma,** the **stone search study** for ureteral calculi, and studies specifically directed toward evaluating vascular structures, such as the **aorta.** Oral contrast used for CT examinations is either a dilute solution containing barium or iodinated contrast.

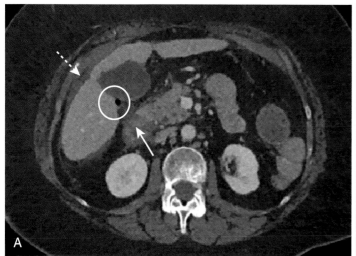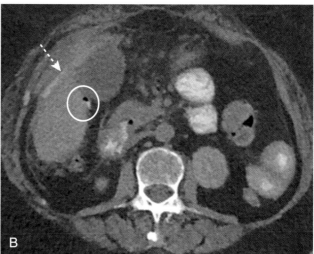

**Fig. 17.6** Perforated Duodenal Ulcer. (A) There is discontinuity of the duodenal wall *(solid arrow)* with intraperitoneal air *(circle)* posterior to the gallbladder as well as fluid around the liver *(dashed arrow).* (B) is the same patient with views obtained after oral contrast was administered; the air behind the gallbladder now also contains contrast *(circle)* and there is contrast around the liver *(dashed arrow)* that could only have occurred via a perforation in the bowel (i.e., the duodenum).

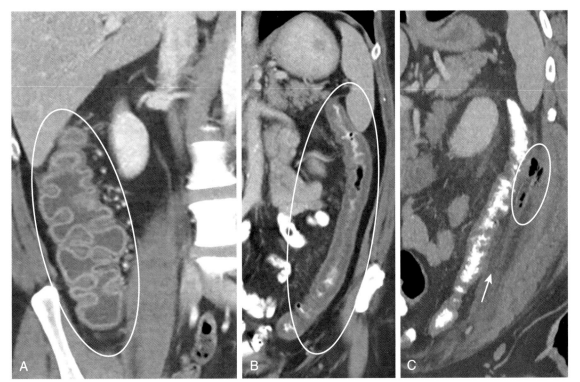

**Fig. 17.7 Key Findings on CT of the GI Tract.** These are findings applicable to any part of the bowel and are keys to the diagnosis of bowel abnormalities on CT. (A) There is **thickening and enhancement** of the wall of the colon *(oval)*. Normally the colonic wall is thin and becomes even thinner with distension of the colon. (B) **Submucosal infiltration** is seen producing thickening and irregularity of the wall and narrowing of the lumen *(oval)*. In this case of ischemic colitis, it most likely represents edema with some hemorrhage. (C) There is **infiltration of the surrounding fat** of the descending colon *(arrow)*, a sentinel finding that usually heralds adjacent inflammation as in this case of diverticulitis. A small amount of extraluminal air is also present *(oval)*.

---

## ⯈ IMPORTANT POINTS

- **Several key findings** are common to any part of the bowel and they are important to the diagnosis of bowel abnormalities by CT. All are demonstrated in Fig. 17.7. They include:
  - **Thickening of the bowel wall** (Fig. 17.7A).
  - **Submucosal edema or hemorrhage.** Submucosal infiltration produces varying degrees of ***thumbprinting,*** nodular indentations into the bowel lumen representing focal areas of submucosal infiltration by edema, hemorrhage, inflammatory cells, tumor (lymphoma), or amyloid (Fig. 17.7B).
  - **Hazy or strand-like infiltration of the surrounding fat.** Extension of inflammatory reaction outside of the bowel into the adjacent fat is a sentinel finding that points to associated disease (Fig. 17.7C).
  - **Extraluminal contrast or extraluminal air** indicates the presence of a bowel perforation (see Fig. 17.6B).

## Crohn Disease

- Crohn disease is a **chronic, relapsing granulomatous inflammation of the small bowel and colon** resulting in ulceration, obstruction, and fistula formation. Crohn disease typically **involves the ileum and right colon,** presents with ***skip areas*** (abnormal bowel interposed between normal bowel), is prone to **fistula formation,** and has a propensity for **recurring** following surgical resection and reanastomosis in whatever loop of bowel serves as the new terminal ileum.
- Crohn disease may be imaged either with a barium **small bowel follow-through** (series) or **CT of the abdomen and pelvis.**

## ⯈ IMPORTANT POINTS

- Imaging findings in Crohn disease include:
  - **Narrowing, irregularity, and ulceration of the terminal ileum,** frequently with proximal small bowel dilatation
  - **Separation of the loops of bowel** due to fatty infiltration of the mesentery surrounding the ileum making the affected loop(s) stand apart from the surrounding loops of small bowel (called a ***proud loop***)
  - The ***string sign,*** narrowing of the terminal ileum into a near slit-like structure by spasm and fibrosis
  - **Fistulae,** especially between the ileum and colon but also to the skin, vagina, and urinary bladder (Fig. 17.8)

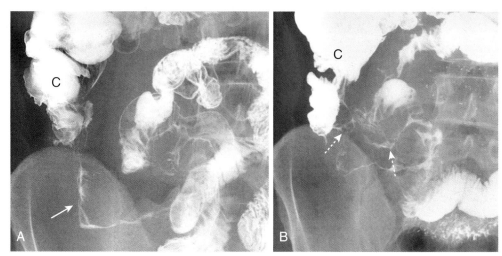

**Fig. 17.8 Crohn Disease.** (A) A close-up image of the right lower quadrant from a small bowel follow-through study displays a markedly narrowed terminal ileum *(arrow)* **(string sign)** that stands apart from other loops of small bowel **(proud loop).** (B) A similar study in another patient shows streaks of barium representing multiple enteric **fistulae** connecting adjacent abnormal loops of small bowel *(arrows).* Fistula formation is a common complication of this disease. *C,* Cecum.

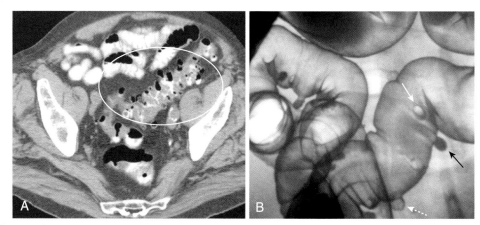

**Fig. 17.9 Diverticulosis.** (A) In this CT scan of the pelvis, diverticula contain air and contrast and appear as small, usually round out-pouchings, especially in the region of the sigmoid colon *(white oval).* (B) There are numerous diverticula seen in the sigmoid colon of this air-contrast barium enema examination. Some diverticula are filled with barium *(black arrow)* while others contain air outlined by barium *(dashed white arrow).* Where an air-containing diverticulum is seen *en face,* it produces a circular density *(solid white arrow)* that can mimic the appearance of a polyp.

## LARGE BOWEL

- The intraluminal surface of the colon is most often studied with optical colonoscopy or CT colonography and/or double-contrast barium enema examination. Structures outside of the colon are usually studied by CT examination of the abdomen and pelvis with oral or rectal contrast.

### Diverticulosis
- **Colonic diverticula,** like most diverticula of the GI tract, represent herniation of the mucosa and submucosa through a defect in the muscular layer *(false diverticula).*

>> **IMPORTANT POINTS**

- Colonic diverticula occur more frequently with increasing age and may be caused, at least in part, by an increase in intraluminal pressure and weakening of the colonic wall. They are **usually multiple (diverticulosis),** are almost always **asymptomatic** ($\approx 90\%$ of the time), but **can become inflamed** or **bleed. Diverticulosis is the most common cause of massive lower GI bleeding.** When they bleed, the **right-sided** diverticula tend to bleed more than those on the left.

- They occur most often in the sigmoid colon and are readily **identified on either barium enema or CT examination as small spikes or smoothly contoured pouches attached to the colon containing either air and/or contrast** (Fig. 17.9).

## Diverticulitis

- Diverticula can become **inflamed** and then **perforate** (*diverticulitis*), most often secondary to mechanical irritation and/or obstruction. **CT is the modality of choice** for the **diagnosis of diverticulitis** because the pericolonic soft tissues can be visualized with CT, which is impossible with either a barium enema or optical endoscopy.

### ▶▶ IMPORTANT POINTS

- CT findings of diverticulitis require the **presence** of at least one **diverticula** and include:
  - **Thickening** of the adjacent colonic wall (>4 mm)
  - **Pericolonic inflammation**: hazy areas of increased attenuation and/or streaky and disorganized linear and amorphous densities in the pericolonic fat
  - **Abscess formation**: multiple small bubbles of air or pockets of fluid contained within a pericolonic soft-tissue, mass-like density
  - **Perforation of the colon**: extraluminal air or contrast, either around the site of the perforation (Fig. 17.10) or, less likely, free in the peritoneal cavity

## Colonic Polyps

- The **incidence of polyps increases with age** and the **incidence of malignancy increases with the size** of the polyp. Patients with **polyposis syndromes**, in which multiple adenomatous polyps are present, have a much higher risk of developing a colonic malignancy.

### ▶▶ IMPORTANT POINTS

- Most colonic polyps are **hyperplastic polyps** that have **no malignant potential**. **Adenomatous polyps** carry a **low potential** for malignancy that **increases with the size of the polyp** so that those greater than **1.5 cm in size** have about a **10% chance of being malignant**. Therefore, the early detection and removal of adenomatous polyps will decrease the chances of malignant transformation.

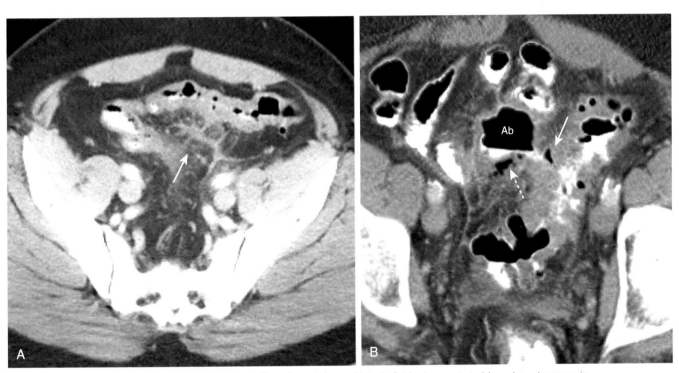

**Fig. 17.10** Diverticulitis, CT. (A) **Infiltration** of the pericolonic fat is demonstrated by a hazy increase in attenuation (*arrow*) of the normal fat. Focal infiltration of fat is a common characteristic of inflammatory disease. (B) There is an **abscess cavity** (Ab) seen in this close-up of a CT scan of the lower abdomen. Air is seen in a diverticulum (*solid arrow*) and there are adjacent small bubbles of **extraluminal gas** (*dashed arrow*) present. These findings are secondary to a confined perforation with abscess formation from diverticulitis.

- Colonic polyps can be visualized using barium enema examination, CT colonography, or optical colonoscopy.
- *CT colonography* is a technique made possible by newer, faster CT scanners and complex computer algorithms that allow for the three-dimensional reconstruction of the appearance of the **inside** of the bowel lumen, including time-of-flight (motion) displays without the use of an endoscope. CT colonography also allows for visualization of the other abdominal structures outside of the colon (Fig. 17.11A, Video 17.3).

- Polyps may be *sessile* (attached directly to the wall) or *pedunculated* (attached to the wall by a **stalk**) (Fig. 17.11B).
- Occasionally, a polyp may serve as a **lead point** for an *intussusception*, in which the polyp drags and prolapses one part of the bowel into the lumen of the bowel immediately ahead of it. The bowel proximal to the intussusception may become obstructed and therefore dilates. Intussusception may produce a characteristic *coiled-spring* appearance on imaging studies (Fig. 17.12).

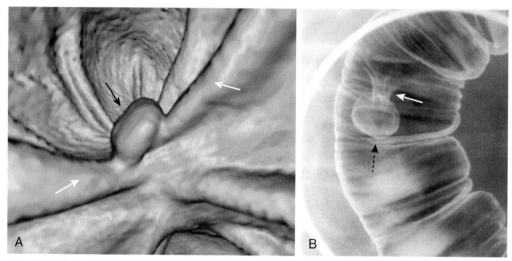

**Fig. 17.11** Colonic Polyps. (A) **CT colonography** utilizes CT scanning of the abdomen to allow for the three-dimensional reconstruction of the appearance of the **inside** of the bowel lumen without the use of an endoscope. A polyp in the descending colon *(black arrow)* is seen as a distinct mass while the normal haustral folds *(white arrows)* are ridge-like structures present throughout the large bowel. (B) Example of an **air-contrast barium enema** on another patient with a polypoid mass in the sigmoid colon outlined by barium *(black arrow)*. In this patient, the polyp is attached to the wall of the colon by a **stalk** *(white arrow)*. Polyps on a stalk are called *pedunculated polyps.*

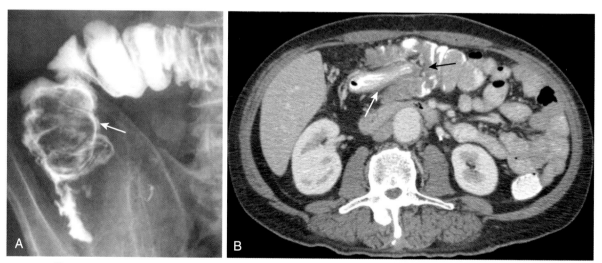

**Fig. 17.12** Intussusception, Barium Enema and CT Scan. (A) When one loop of bowel prolapses inside the loop immediately distal to it, the resultant obstruction produces a *coiled-spring* appearance on barium enema examination as two loops of bowel are superimposed on one another *(arrow)*. (B) CT on another patient with an intussusception shows a loop of large bowel *(white arrow)* prolapsing into the loop distal to it *(black arrow)* producing a filling defect and obstructing the lumen.

## Colonic Carcinoma

- The **imaging findings** of carcinoma of the colon include:
  - The presence of a **persistent, large polypoid filling defect**
  - **Annular constriction** of the colonic lumen producing an *apple-core* lesion (Fig. 17.13)
  - **Frank perforation or microperforation** manifest by infiltration of the pericolonic fat with streaky or hazy densities of increased attenuation with or without the presence of extraluminal air
- **Other findings** of carcinoma of the colon can include **large bowel obstruction** (see Fig. 14.14) and **metastases,** especially to the liver and the lungs.

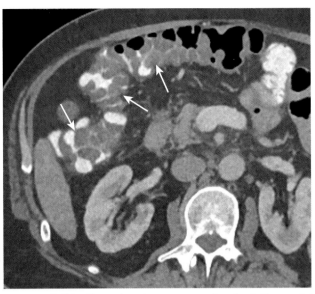

**Fig. 17.14 Colitis.** The colon demonstrates ***thumbprinting,*** nodular indentations on the lumen *(arrows),* and an overall pattern that is called the ***accordion sign.*** This patient had *C. difficile* colitis, formerly called ***pseudomembranous colitis*** and now known to be caused almost exclusively by toxins produced by *Clostridium difficile.* It frequently follows antibiotic therapy. The diagnosis is usually made clinically by visualization of the pseudomembrane on endoscopy. The accordion sign represents contrast that is trapped between enlarged folds and indicates the presence of marked edema or inflammation, but it is not specific for *C difficile* colitis.

## Colitis

- Colitis is **inflammation of the large bowel.** There are **numerous causes** of colitis, including infectious, ulcerative and granulomatous, ischemic, radiation-induced, and antibiotic-associated etiologies. Because many forms of colitis appear similar radiologically, **clinical history is of paramount importance.**

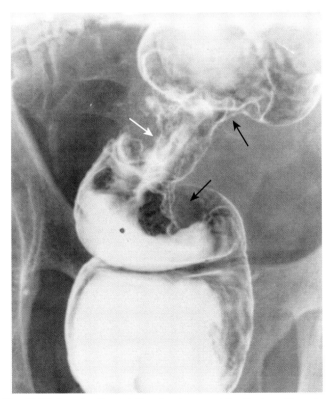

**Fig. 17.13 Annular Constricting Carcinoma of the Rectum.** There is a characteristic ***apple-core*** lesion of the rectum caused by circumferential growth of a colonic carcinoma. The margins of the lesion *(black arrows)* demonstrate what is called an **overhanging edge** where tumor tissue projects into and overhangs the normal lumen, typical of this type of lesion. The "core" of the "apple" *(white arrow)* is composed of tumor tissue rather than normal colonic mucosa. Identification of such a lesion is pathognomonic for carcinoma.

## Appendicitis

- Pathophysiologically, the development of appendicitis is invariably preceded by **obstruction** of the **appendiceal lumen.** CT or ultrasound are now the modalities of choice in diagnosing appendicitis. Appendicitis may also be visualized with MRI.
- An *appendicolith* **is a calcified concretion found in the appendix** of about 15% of all people. It will be visible, especially on CT, as a calcification in the appendiceal lumen. The combination of **abdominal pain** and the **presence of**

an appendicolith is associated with **appendicitis about 90% of the time** and indicates a higher probability for perforation.

> ### ▶▶ **IMPORTANT POINTS**
>
> * **The key CT findings of acute appendicitis** are:
>   * Identification of a **dilated appendix** (>6 mm) that does **not fill** with oral contrast
>   * **Periappendiceal inflammation,** which is evidenced by streaky, disorganized, linear high-attenuation densities in the surrounding fat (Fig. 17.15A)
>   * **Increased contrast enhancement of the wall of the appendix** due to inflammation.
>   * **Perforation** occurs in up to 30% of cases and is **recognized by small quantities of periappendiceal, extraluminal air,** or a **periappendiceal abscess.** Because obstruction of the appendiceal lumen is a prerequisite for appendicitis, the presence of a **large amount** of free intraperitoneal air should point to **another diagnosis** (Fig. 17.15B).

* The use of ultrasound in appendicitis will be discussed in Chapter 18.
* Included online, **e-Appendix D. Key Terminology and Glossaries** of this book (not to be surgically removed) lists

the **studies of first choice** for **different clinical scenarios,** some relating to **abdominal pain.**

## Lower Gastrointestinal Bleeding

* **Diverticulosis** is one of the main causes of lower gastrointestinal bleeding *(LGIB).* LGIB is defined as bleeding that originates between the ileocecal valve and the rectum. Other causes of LGIB include angiodysplasias, inflammatory bowel disease, and neoplasms.
* In acute (overt) lower GI bleeding, there are several diagnostic approaches. **Colonoscopy, catheter angiography, and CT angiogram (CTA)** are the diagnostic studies most often employed for evaluation of acute LGIB. Radionuclide bleeding scans may also be used.
* Both **colonoscopy** and **catheter angiography** have the added benefit of allowing **treatment** of the cause of bleeding after identification of its site. Colonoscopy is frequently utilized as the initial modality in **hemodynamically stable** patients (with adequate bowel preparation). Angiography is especially helpful in those who are **hemodynamically unstable** and have massive lower GI bleeding.
* **CT angiography** requires a certain rate of active arterial bleeding (at least 0.5 mL/min) to effectively show **extravasation of contrast into the bowel lumen** so as to identify a bleeding site. It is less invasive than colonoscopy or catheter

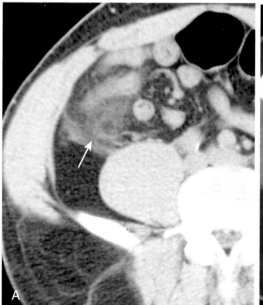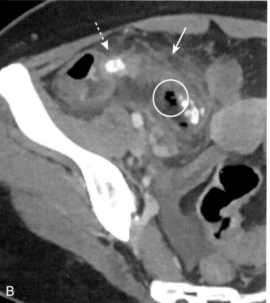

**Fig. 17.15 Appendicitis, CT.** (A) There is infiltration of the periappendiceal fat in the right lower quadrant manifest by the increased attenuation in the mesenteric fat *(arrow).* Focal infiltration of fat is a common characteristic of inflammatory diseases and helps in their localization. (B) Contained within the lumen of the appendix is a small calcification *(dashed arrow)* or **appendicolith,** in a different patient. There is inflammatory infiltration of the surrounding fat producing high attenuation *(solid arrow).* A very small amount of air is present outside of the appendiceal lumen from a confined perforation *(circle).*

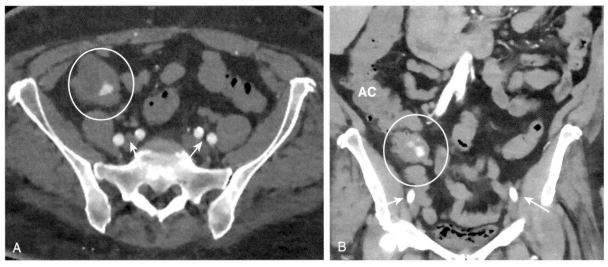

**Fig. 17.16 CT Angiogram (CTA) of Lower GI Bleed.** Active GI bleeding is diagnosed by demonstrating extravasation of intravenously injected contrast into the bowel lumen. (A) Axial image of the pelvis after IV, but no oral, contrast shows an amorphous collection of contrast **in the lumen** of the cecum *(circle)*, representing extravasated blood. (B) Coronal reconstruction on the same patient demonstrates several collections of intraluminal contrast in the cecum *(circle)*. The arrows on both images identify opacified iliac vessels. The patient was bleeding from a vascular malformation of the cecum. *AC,* Ascending colon.

angiography, is **readily available,** and may demonstrate lesions in the **small bowel,** which colonoscopy cannot (Fig. 17.16).

- **Nuclear scintigraphy bleeding scans** are a sensitive diagnostic tool for GI hemorrhage but suffer from a relatively low specificity because of their limited resolution compared with endoscopy or angiography.

poorer prognostic significance. They usually develop **early** in the course of the disease and require intravenous contrast administration for visualization.

- **Pseudocyst formation.** Fibrous tissue can encapsulate a walled-off collection of pancreatic juices released from the inflamed pancreas. The **wall of a pseudocyst is**

# PANCREAS

## Pancreatitis

- The two **most common causes of pancreatitis** are **alcoholism** and **gallstones.** In children, abdominal trauma may play a role. Inflammation of pancreatic tissue leading to disruption of the ducts and spillage of pancreatic juices occurs readily, in part because of the lack of a capsule surrounding the pancreas.

> ### ▶▶ IMPORTANT POINTS
>
> - Pancreatitis is a **clinical diagnosis** with CT serving to document either a **cause** (e.g., gallstones) or a **complication** (e.g., pseudocyst formation).

- Recognizing acute pancreatitis on CT:
  - **Enlargement** of all or part of the pancreas (normal measurements for the pancreas are **3 cm for the head, 2.5 cm for the body,** and **2 cm for the tail**).
  - **Peripancreatic stranding** or **fluid collections** (Fig. 17.17)
  - **Low-attenuation** lesions in the pancreas from **necrosis** may represent areas of nonviable pancreas and have a

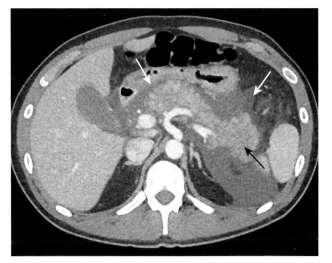

**Fig. 17.17 Acute Pancreatitis.** The pancreas is markedly enlarged and irregular in appearance *(black arrow).* There is extensive infiltration of the peripancreatic fat *(white arrows).* Severe abdominal pain, often radiating to the back, is an almost universal symptom of acute pancreatitis. This patient had a markedly elevated amylase and lipase.

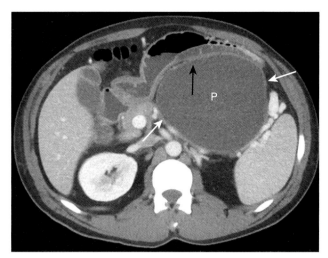

**Fig. 17.18** Pancreatic Pseudocyst. A pseudocyst (P) of the pancreas is a collection of fluid, usually high in pancreatic enzymes, outside of the pancreas and enclosed by a wall of fibrous and granulation tissue. The wall may contrast enhance *(white arrows)*. The cyst is indenting a loop of adjacent bowel *(black arrow)*. This type of indentation on a loop of bowel by an extrinsic mass, whatever its origin, is called a **pad sign**.

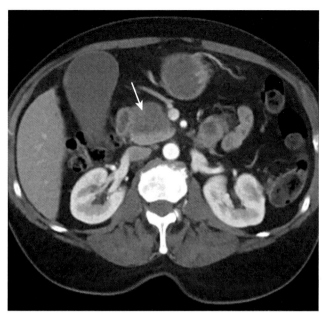

**Fig. 17.19** Pancreatic Adenocarcinoma. The head of the pancreas is enlarged by a mass *(arrow)*. The symptoms of pancreatic adenocarcinomas are frequently vague, laboratory findings are nonspecific, and the lesions are difficult to image, especially in patients with concomitant changes of chronic pancreatitis.

usually visible by CT and **may contrast enhance** (Fig. 17.18).

## Chronic Pancreatitis

- Chronic pancreatitis is a continuous and irreversible disease of the pancreas, most often secondary to **alcohol abuse**, leading to **fibrosis, atrophy of the gland, ductal dilatation**, and, frequently, **diabetes**.

> **IMPORTANT POINTS**
> - The **hallmarks** of the disease are **multiple, amorphous calcifications** that form within the **dilated ducts** of the **atrophied gland** (see Fig. 16.10).

## Pancreatic Adenocarcinoma

- Risk factors for pancreatic adenocarcinoma include **alcoholism, cigarette smoking, chronic pancreatitis**, and **diabetes**. Pancreatic adenocarcinoma has an **exceedingly poor prognosis**: most tumors are unresectable and incurable at the time of diagnosis. **Most of the time** (75%), the tumor is located in the **head** of the pancreas; about 10% occur in the body and 5% in the tail. About half of the patients

present with **jaundice** and, most of the time, **there is associated pain**.
- **Ultrasound is the study of choice in the initial work-up of the jaundiced patient** (see Chapter 18).

> **IMPORTANT POINTS**
> - **Recognizing pancreatic adenocarcinoma on CT:**
>   - **Focal pancreatic mass,** usually **hypodense** to the remainder the gland (Fig. 17.19)
>   - **Ductal dilatation,** usually involving **both the pancreatic and biliary ducts.** The normal **pancreatic duct** measures **less than 4 mm** in the head and tapers to the tail; the **common duct** should be **less than 7 mm** in diameter.
>   - Other findings of pancreatic carcinoma include spread to contiguous organs, enlarged lymph nodes, and/or ascites.

## HEPATOBILIARY ABNORMALITIES

### Liver: General Considerations

- CT evaluation of **liver masses** is usually done with a **sequence of scans obtained before** and then **twice after intravenous contrast** injection, which is called a *triple-phase scan*. The

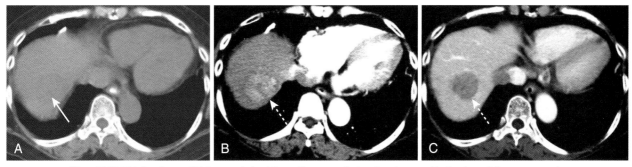

**Fig. 17.20** Triple-phase CT Scan of the Liver, Hepatocellular Carcinoma. Evaluation of liver masses is usually done with a combination of scans including an **unenhanced** scan (A) and then two postcontrast scans: one obtained quickly (B), called the **hepatic-arterial phase,** and a second about a minute later (C), called the **portal-venous phase.** This case shows the typical findings of a focal hepatocellular carcinoma. Most are low density (hypodense) or the same density as normal liver (isodense) **without contrast** (arrow in A), **enhance** on the arterial phase with IV contrast (hyperdense) (arrow in B), and then return to **hypodense or isodense** on the venous phase (arrow in C).

combination of images helps to best define and characterize liver masses (Fig. 17.20).

- **MRI** is increasingly utilized as the modality of choice in the evaluation of both focal and diffuse liver disease. MRI can often definitively characterize hepatic lesions described as indeterminate on CT, such as cysts, benign hepatic neoplasms such as hemangioma and focal nodular hyperplasia, hepatocellular carcinoma, and metastatic disease. It is **particularly useful in the evaluation of small (≤1 cm) lesions** compared with CT.

- For routine MRI imaging of the liver, an intravenous contrast agent called *gadolinium* is typically administered, and multiple postgadolinium-enhanced images are obtained. Gadolinium will be discussed in Chapter 20.

## Fatty Infiltration

- The term **nonalcoholic fatty liver disease** refers to a spectrum of diseases of the liver ranging from *hepatic steatosis* (fatty infiltration of the liver) to *nonalcoholic steatohepatitis (NASH)* to *cirrhosis.*

### ▶▶ IMPORTANT POINTS

- **Fatty infiltration of the liver** (hepatic steatosis) is a **very common** abnormality in which there is fat accumulation in the hepatocytes in such diseases as obesity, diabetes, hepatitis, or cirrhosis. Most patients with a fatty liver are **asymptomatic.** The **fatty infiltration** may be **diffuse** or **focal,** and focal lesions may be **solitary** or **multiple.**

- Normally on **noncontrast** CT scans, the **liver** is always **denser** than or **equal** to the density of the **spleen.** With **fatty infiltration of the liver, the spleen appears denser than the liver** without intravenous contrast (Fig. 17.21).

- When the fatty infiltration is diffuse, the **liver is usually slightly enlarged.** The **blood vessels stand out prominently** but are usually **neither obstructed nor displaced.**

### ❗ DIAGNOSTIC PITFALLS

- **Focal** fatty infiltration can produce an appearance that **mimics a tumor.** Unlike a tumor, fatty infiltration usually produces **no mass effect** and has the ability to **appear and disappear** in a matter of weeks, quite unlike tumor masses.

- **MRI is the most accurate modality in the evaluation of a fatty liver,** using a phenomenon called *chemical shift imaging* to detect the presence of microscopic, intracellular lipid

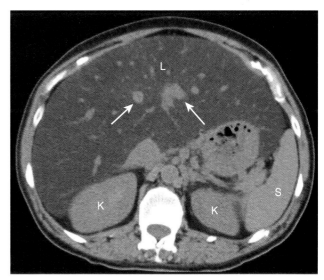

**Fig. 17.21** Diffuse Fatty Liver, Unenhanced CT. In this patient with diffuse fatty infiltration of an enlarged liver (L), the spleen (S) is denser than the liver, the reverse of normal on a nonenhanced scan. In this case, the degree of fatty infiltration is such that the vessels stand out in the fatty liver (arrows). K, Kidneys.

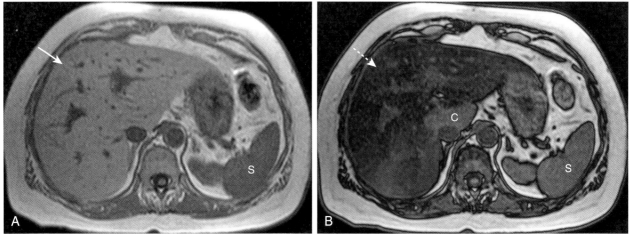

**Fig. 17.22** Fatty Liver, MRI. Using a phenomenon called **chemical shift imaging** to detect the presence of intracellular lipid present in a fatty liver, MRI provides the most accurate identification of a fatty liver. (A) The liver *(arrow)* appears normal, brighter than the spleen (S). (B) This is called an **opposed-phase image** and it demonstrates marked signal loss (signal dropout) throughout the liver *(arrow)*, indicating a fatty liver. Most of the liver is now darker than the spleen (S), except for the caudate lobe (C), which is normal.

present in such a liver. Chemical shift relates to the way that lipid and water protons behave in the magnetic field (Fig. 17.22).

## Cirrhosis

- Cirrhosis is a chronic, irreversible disease of the liver that features destruction of normal liver cells and diffuse fibrosis that appears to be the final common pathway of many abnormalities, including **hepatitis B** and **C**, **alcoholism**, **nonalcoholic fatty infiltration of the liver,** and miscellaneous diseases such as **hemochromatosis** and **Wilson disease.** Complications of cirrhosis include **portal**

**hypertension, ascites, renal dysfunction, hepatocellular carcinoma, hepatic failure,** and **death.**

### ▶▶ IMPORTANT POINTS

- **Recognizing cirrhosis of the liver on CT:**
  - **Early** in the disease, the liver may demonstrate **diffuse fatty infiltration.** As the disease progresses, the liver **contour becomes lobulated.** The **liver shrinks in volume** with the **right lobe** characteristically becoming **smaller** whereas the **caudate lobe** and **left lobe become disproportionately larger**, especially in alcoholic cirrhosis (Fig. 17.23).

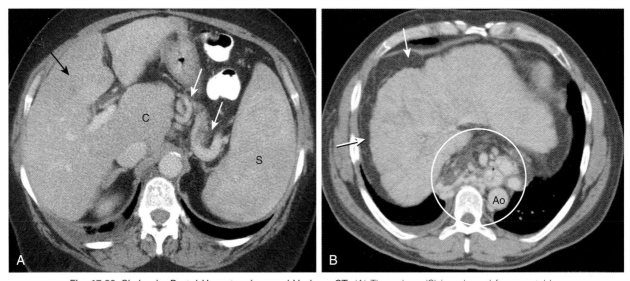

**Fig. 17.23** Cirrhosis, Portal Hypertension, and Varices, CT. (A) The spleen (S) is enlarged from portal hypertension secondary to cirrhosis. There is characteristic enlargement of the caudate lobe (C) relative to the right lobe of the liver *(black arrow)*. There are several contrast-enhanced dilated veins (varices) around the stomach and splenic hilum *(white arrows)*. (B) Another patient shows the typical nodular and shrunken appearance of the cirrhotic liver *(arrows)* along with numerous contrast-enhanced, peri-esophageal varices *(circle)*. *Ao,* Descending aorta.

---

### BOX 17.1  Differentiating Ascites from Pleural Effusion

- Patients may have a combination of ascites and pleural effusion for a number of reasons, including cirrhosis, ovarian tumors, metastatic disease, hypoproteinemia, and congestive heart failure.
- Differentiation between ascitic fluid and pleural fluid at the lung base on axial CT examinations may be difficult because **both may appear posterior to the liver.**

- **Ascitic fluid** will appear **anterior to the hemidiaphragm** in the axial plane. **Pleural effusion** will be located **posterior to the hemidiaphragm** (Fig. 17.24A).
- Ascitic fluid **will not spread to the *bare* area of the liver posteriorly** where there is no peritoneal lining (see Fig. 13.3).
  - Therefore, **fluid that appears posterior to the bare area of the liver is pleural in location** (Fig. 17.24B).

---

### ▶▶ IMPORTANT POINTS—cont'd

- There is a **mottled**, **inhomogeneous** appearance to the liver parenchyma following intravenous contrast enhancement due to a mixture of regenerating nodules, focal fatty infiltration, and fibrosis.
- **Portal hypertension** may develop, which can lead to **dilated vessels** around the stomach, splenic hilum, and esophagus, representing ***varices.***
- **Splenomegaly** may result (see Fig. 17.23A).
- **Ascites** may be present. Sometimes it can be difficult to differentiate between ascites and pleural effusion on CT examinations (Box 17.1, Fig. 17.24).

- CT studies are best at demonstrating liver masses when performed **both with and without contrast** as either study alone may fail to reveal an ***isodense*** mass (i.e., one that has identical attenuation to the surrounding normal tissue), therefore hiding its presence.
- **MRI is useful in characterizing liver masses,** particularly small lesions 10 mm or less.

## Metastases

### ▶▶ IMPORTANT POINTS

- Metastases are the **most common malignant hepatic masses.** Although **most are multiple**, metastases also represent the **most common cause** of a **solitary** malignant mass in the liver.

## Space-Occupying Lesions of the Liver

- One of the primary aims of imaging studies, no matter the body part, is to accurately differentiate between benign and malignant processes with techniques that do not place patients in danger or subject them to unnecessary pain. This is the central goal in evaluating liver masses as well.

- **Most liver metastases originate in the GI tract**, in particular the **colon,** and almost all reach the liver via the bloodstream. Other primary sites of metastatic spread to the liver

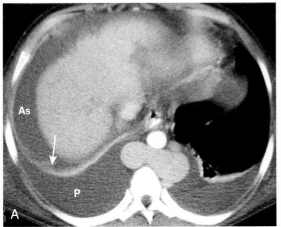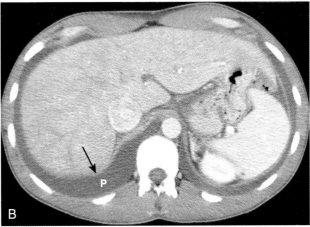

**Fig. 17.24 Differentiating Pleural Effusion from Ascites.** (A) Patients with cirrhosis may have a combination of ascites and pleural effusions. Ascitic fluid (As) will appear anterior to the hemidiaphragm *(arrow)* in the axial plane. Pleural effusion (P) will be located posterior to the hemidiaphragm. (B) Ascites will never completely encircle the dome of the liver because of the ***bare area*** *(arrow)*, not covered by peritoneum (see Fig. 13.3). Fluid posterior to the bare area must be in the pleural space (P).

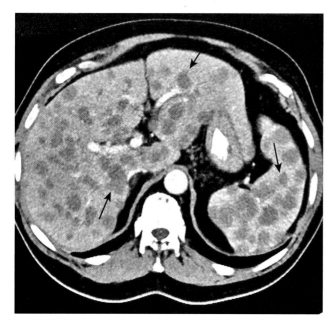

**Fig. 17.25 Metastases to the Liver and Spleen.** Numerous, low-attenuation metastatic masses fill the liver and spleen *(arrows* point to only a few) on this contrast-enhanced CT scan. The patient had a primary adenocarcinoma of the colon.

include the stomach, pancreas, esophagus, lung, breast, and malignant melanoma.

- **Recognizing liver metastases on CT and MRI:**
  - Metastases are usually **multiple, low-attenuation masses** (Fig. 17.25). **Larger metastases** may demonstrate areas of necrosis that can be recognized as mottled areas of low attenuation within the mass. **Mucin-producing carcinomas**, such as those originating in the stomach, colon, or ovary, can **calcify** at the site of both the primary tumor and the metastases (see Fig. 16.14).
  - MRI is **as sensitive** as CT in detecting liver metastases, but it is usually used in a **problem-solving role.** In

general, MRI is more expensive than CT scanning and may suffer from more motion artifact than CT.

## Hepatocellular Carcinoma (Hepatoma)

- Hepatocellular carcinoma is the **most common primary malignancy** of the liver. Virtually all arise in livers with pre-existing abnormalities such as **cirrhosis** and/or **hepatitis. Most are solitary**, but up to one out of five can be multiple, mimicking metastases. **Vascular invasion is common**, particularly of the portal system.

>> **IMPORTANT POINTS**

- **Recognizing hepatocellular carcinoma on CT and MRI:**
  - Hepatocellular carcinomas (HCC) can be a **solitary mass** (see Fig. 17.20), **multiple masses,** or **diffusely infiltrating.**
  - On CT, most HCCs are **low density *(hypodense)*** or the same density as normal liver *(isodense)* **without contrast**, **enhance** on the **arterial phase** with intravenous contrast *(hyperdense)*, and then return to **hypodense** or **isodense** on the **venous phase** (Fig. 17.26).
  - Low-attenuation areas due to tumor **necrosis** are common. **Calcification** occurs relatively frequently.
  - **MRI** can demonstrate certain features that are fairly specific for **hepatocellular carcinoma,** as well as detect intrahepatic metastases and venous invasion. Unlike benign lesions, such as hemangiomas of the liver that tend to retain intravenously administered gadolinium contrast, hepatocellular carcinomas **show washout** of the contrast material.

## Cavernous Hemangiomas

- Cavernous hemangiomas are the **most common** *primary liver tumor* and **second in frequency to metastases for localized liver masses.** More common in **women,** they are usually **solitary** and are almost always **asymptomatic.** They are complex structures composed of multiple large vascular channels lined by a single layer of endothelial cells.

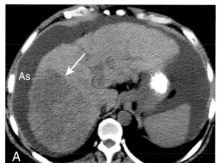
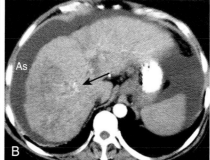

**Fig. 17.26 Diffuse Hepatocellular Carcinoma of the Liver, CT.** There are three major patterns of appearance for hepatocellular carcinoma: **solitary mass** (see Fig. 17.20), **multiple nodules,** or **diffuse infiltration** throughout a segment or lobe (as in this case) or the entire liver. The overall volume of this liver is decreased and the contour is lobulated from underlying cirrhosis. (A) A typical low-attenuation lesion is seen in the right lobe of the liver on the nonenhanced scan *(arrow).* (B) The arterial phase demonstrates patchy enhancement *(arrow)* indicating the probability of tumor necrosis in the low-attenuation areas. There is ascites present (As).

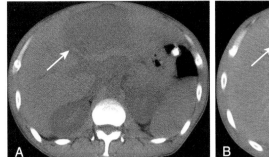
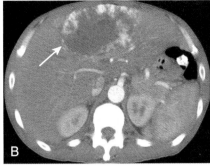
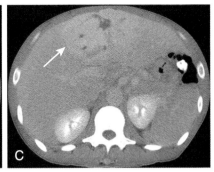

**Fig. 17.27** Cavernous Hemangioma of the Liver, Triple-phase CT Study. (A) Cavernous hemangiomas *(arrows on all images)* are usually **hypodense** lesions on unenhanced scans. (B) They characteristically **enhance from the periphery** inward following injection of intravenous contrast during the **arterial phase** and eventually become isodense. (C) Contrast then tends to be retained within the numerous vascular spaces of the lesion so that they characteristically appear **denser** than the rest of the liver on **delayed scans**.

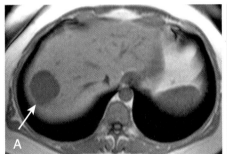
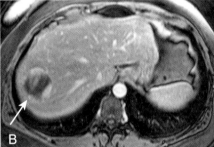
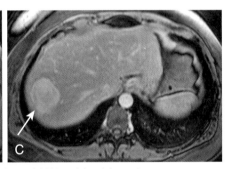

**Fig. 17.28** Cavernous Hemangioma of the Liver, MRI. (A) This image (an axial T1-weighted image) demonstrates a well-circumscribed, slightly lobular dark mass in the right hepatic lobe *(arrow on all images)*. (B) Subsequent images following the administration of intravenous contrast (gadolinium) show peripheral-to-central enhancement until the entire mass homogeneously enhances on a delayed 10-minute image (C). The combination of this enhancement pattern and the signal characteristics of the lesion allows an unequivocal diagnosis of hemangioma.

## ≫ IMPORTANT POINTS

- **Recognizing cavernous hemangiomas of the liver on CT and MRI:**
  - **Cavernous hemangiomas** have a characteristic appearance on triple-phase, unenhanced, and enhanced CT scans of the liver (Fig. 17.27).
  - **MRI is frequently the preferred modality** in the evaluation of hemangiomas; it is **more sensitive** than nuclear medicine tagged-red blood cell scans and more specific than a multiphase CT scan.
  - Similar to CT, **hemangiomas on MRI** usually have a characteristic nodular **enhancement starting from the periphery inward** following injection of intravenous contrast. Contrast tends to be retained within the numerous vascular spaces of hemangiomas so that they typically appear brighter than the rest of the liver on delayed (10-minute) scans (Fig. 17.28, Video 17.4).

## Hepatic Cysts

- The characteristics of hepatic cysts are shown in Fig. 17.29.

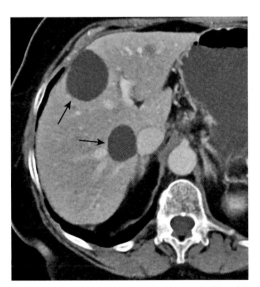

**Fig. 17.29** Hepatic Cysts, CT. Believed to be **congenital** in origin, they are easily identified as **sharply marginated** lesions of **low attenuation (fluid density)** compared to the remainder of the liver, on both unenhanced and enhanced CT scans. MRI is much better than CT at characterizing cysts. They are often **multiple** and are **homogeneous** in density *(arrows)*.

# BILIARY SYSTEM

## Magnetic Resonance Cholangiopancreatography

- Magnetic resonance cholangiopancreatography (MRCP) is a **noninvasive** way to image the biliary tree **without requiring injection of contrast material.** MRCP uses MRI imaging sequences that make fluid-filled structures such as the bile ducts, pancreatic ducts, and gallbladder extremely bright, and everything else dark. Patients are imaged during a single-breath hold (Fig. 17.30).

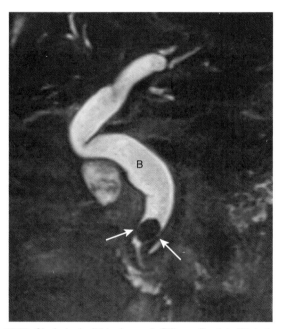

Fig. 17.30 Choledocholithiasis and Biliary Ductal Dilatation on Magnetic Resonance Cholangiopancreatography (MRCP). This is a coronal close-up of the right upper quadrant utilizing MR imaging. There is a large obstructing oval-shaped gallstone that appears dark *(arrows)* in the distal common bile duct (B), which appears white. Because of the signal characteristics of bile, an MRCP can be done **without** the need for the injection of contrast.

- MRCP is excellent at depicting **biliary or ductal strictures, ductal dilatation, stones in the bile ducts (choledocholithiasis), gallstones, adenomyomatosis of the gallbladder, choledochal cysts, and pancreas divisum.**
- If there is a concern for malignancy (e.g., pancreatic adenocarcinoma or cholangiocarcinoma) as the cause of pancreaticobiliary ductal dilatation, then additional pulse sequences following the administration of gadolinium contrast can be obtained. Contrast administration allows better detection of malignancy.

# URINARY TRACT

## Kidneys: General Considerations

- The kidneys are retroperitoneal organs, encircled by varying amounts of fat and enclosed within a fibrous capsule. So long as they are functioning properly, the **kidneys are the route** through which intravenously injected, **iodinated contrast (and gadolinium-based MRI contrast) agents are excreted from the body.** Following initial injection of iodinated contrast agents, the kidneys will therefore normally **enhance.**

## Space-Occupying Lesions
### Renal Cysts

- Simple renal cysts are a **very common** finding on CT and US scans of the abdomen; they occur in more than half of the population over 55 years of age.

> ▶▶ **IMPORTANT POINTS**
>
> - Simple cysts are **benign, fluid-filled** structures that are frequently **multiple** and **bilateral.** On CT scans, they tend to have a **sharp margin** where they meet the normal renal parenchyma. They have density measurements (Hounsfield numbers) of **water density** ($-10$ to $+20$). They **do not contrast enhance** (Fig. 17.31A).

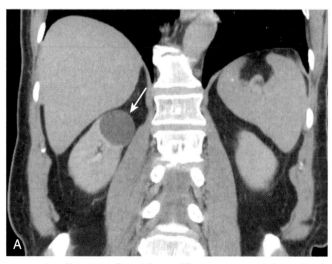
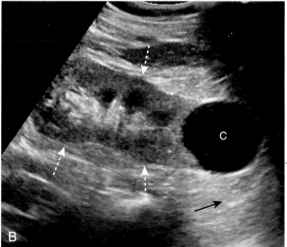

Fig. 17.31 Renal Cysts, CT Urogram and US. (A) This is a coronal image from a CT urogram that demonstrates a low-attenuation mass *(arrow)* in the upper pole of the right kidney that is homogeneous in density and sharply marginated from the rest of the kidney. These findings are characteristic of a simple cyst. (B) A sagittal ultrasound of the kidney *(white arrows)* in another patient demonstrates an anechoic mass *(C = cyst)* with strong through-transmission *(black arrow)*, features consistent with a simple cyst of the lower pole.

- On **ultrasound examinations,** simple cysts are **echo-free** (anechoic) masses with **strong through-transmission** of the ultrasound signal; they have **sharp borders** where they meet the renal parenchyma and **round or oval shapes.** Thickening of the wall or dense internal echoes raise suspicion for a malignant lesion (Fig. 17.31B).

## Renal Cell Carcinoma (Hypernephroma)

- Renal cell carcinoma is the **most common primary renal malignancy** in **adults.** Solid masses in the kidneys of adults are usually renal cell carcinomas. They have a propensity for **extending into the renal veins,** into the **inferior vena cava,** and metastasizing via the bloodstream to produce **nodules in the lung.** When they metastasize to bone, their metastases are **purely lytic** and **often expansile.**

> ### ⟩⟩ IMPORTANT POINTS
>
> - **Recognizing renal cell carcinoma on CT:**
>   - A dedicated CT scan for renal cell carcinoma usually consists of images obtained before and after intravenous contrast administration.
>   - Ranging from **completely solid** to **completely cystic**, renal cell carcinomas are **usually solid lesions that may contain low-attenuation areas of necrosis.** Even though renal cell carcinomas **enhance with intravenous contrast,** they still tend to remain **lower in density than the surrounding normal kidney.**
>   - **Renal vein invasion** occurs in up to one in three cases and may produce filling defects in the lumen of the renal veins (see Fig. 17.32A).

- Ultrasound is used in the characterization of renal masses, particularly in assessing their cystic or solid nature and involvement of the collecting system or surrounding vessels.
- On **ultrasound,** smaller renal cell carcinomas are **usually hyperechoic;** as the lesion increases in size and undergoes necrosis it may be hypoechoic. The wall of a renal cell carcinoma should be thicker and more irregular than a simple cyst (Fig. 17.32B).
- The primary role of **MRI of the kidneys** is in the evaluation of **small masses** less than 1.5 cm or in any renal mass characterized as **indeterminate** for malignancy by either CT or US.

## PELVIS

### General Considerations

- **Ultrasound is the study of first choice in evaluation of suspected abnormalities of the female pelvis** (see Chapter 18).
- **MRI** has assumed an increasingly important role in defining the anatomy of the uterus and ovaries and in clarifying questions in patients in whom US findings are confusing. MRI is also used in staging and surgical planning.
- MRI can be particularly useful in evaluating ovarian dermoid cysts, endometriosis, and hydrosalpinges (fluid-filled fallopian tubes), and in determining whether an ovarian cystic lesion is simple (benign) or contains a solid component (possibly malignant) (see Fig. 20.4).

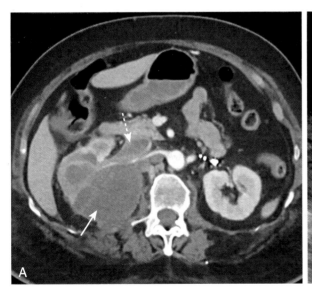
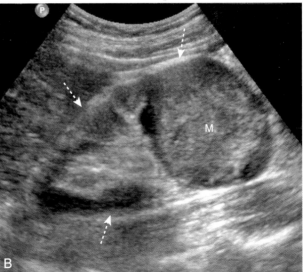

**Fig. 17.32 Renal Cell Carcinomas, CT and US.** (A) There is a large, low-density mass involving the right kidney *(solid white arrow).* The tumor extends directly into the right renal vein *(dashed white arrow),* a feature of renal cell carcinomas. (B) Sagittal ultrasound on another patient with renal cell carcinoma shows an echogenic mass (M) occupying the midportion of the kidney *(arrows).* Compare the absence of internal echoes for the renal cyst (see Fig. 17.31B) and the increased echogenicity of this renal cell carcinoma.

# URINARY BLADDER

## Bladder Tumors

- Most malignant bladder tumors are **urothelial tumors** (transitional cell tumors). Urothelial tumors may occur simultaneously from the lining uroepithelium anywhere in the bladder, ureter, and kidney. The **primary tumor** appears as **focal thickening of the bladder wall** and/or produces a **filling defect in the contrast-filled bladder** (Fig. 17.33).

# ADENOPATHY

## Lymphoma

- Lymphoma can involve any part of the GI or genitourinary tract. Thoracic lymphoma is almost always caused by Hodgkin disease, whereas **the stomach is the most common extranodal site of gastrointestinal non-Hodgkin lymphoma.**

- **Extranodal involvement** and **noncontiguous spread** to other organs or nodes are features of non-Hodgkin lymphoma.

>> **IMPORTANT POINTS**

- **Recognizing the CT findings of abdominal lymphoma:**
  - **Multiple enlarged lymph nodes.** Pelvic lymph nodes are considered pathologically enlarged if they exceed 1 cm in their shortest dimension.
  - **Conglomerate masses of coalesced nodes.** Bulky tumor masses that can encase and obstruct vessels
  - Lymphadenopathy will classically **displace the aorta and/or vena cava anteriorly** (Fig. 17.34).

- Other malignancies can produce abdominal and/or pelvic adenopathy besides lymphoma and even benign disease like sarcoid can produce abdominal adenopathy.

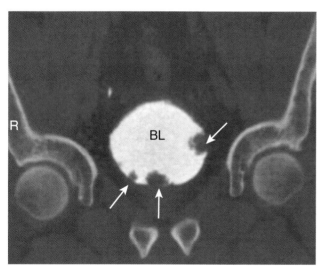

**Fig. 17.33** Urothelial Carcinomas of the Bladder, CT Urogram. There are multiple filling defects in the contrast-filled bladder *(arrows)* representing multiple bladder tumors. Urothelial tumors can occur in the kidneys, ureters, and bladder. Bladder cancer tends to have a high recurrence rate. *R,* Patient's right. *BL,* bladder.

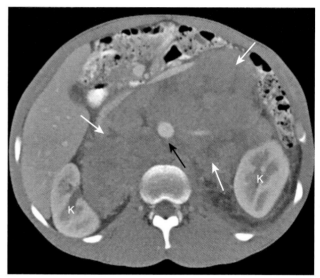

**Fig. 17.34** Massive Lymphadenopathy, Lymphoma. There is massive abdominal lymphadenopathy occupying most of the abdomen *(white arrows)* and displacing the kidneys (K) laterally and the aorta *(black arrow)* anteriorly far from its normal location next to the spine. The patient had non-Hodgkin lymphoma.

## CASE QUIZ 17 ANSWER

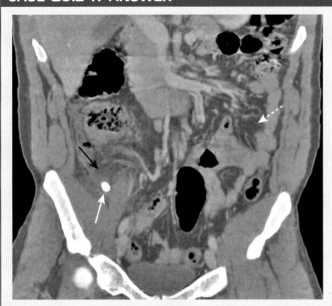

There is a calcification in the right lower quadrant *(solid white arrow)* that represents an **appendicolith**. Adjacent to the calcification, there is infiltration of the surrounding fat *(black arrow)* indicating inflammation in this area. Compare the fat infiltration in the right lower quadrant with normal-appearing fat *(dashed white arrow)*. The findings are those of **acute appendicitis**.

## 🏠 TAKE HOME POINTS

- CT, US, and MRI have essentially replaced conventional radiography and, in many instances, barium studies for the imaging evaluation of the GI tract.
- **Esophageal carcinoma** has a poor prognosis, with an increasing incidence of adenocarcinomas forming in Barrett esophagus, a condition in which gastroesophageal reflux plays a major role in stimulating metaplasia of the squamous to columnar epithelium.
- **Hiatal hernias** are a common abnormality that may be associated with GERD, although GERD can occur even in the absence of a demonstrable hernia. They are usually of the **sliding** variety in which the esophagogastric junction lies above the diaphragm.
- The radiologic findings of **gastric ulcer** include a persistent collection of barium, usually along the lesser curvature or posterior wall in the region of the body or antrum. The ulcer may have radiating folds that extend to the ulcer margin and a surrounding margin of edema.
- The key finding in **gastric carcinoma** is a mass that protrudes into the lumen and produces a filling defect, displacing barium. Gastric carcinomas may be associated with rigidity of the wall and nondistensibility of the lumen as well as irregular ulceration or thickening of the gastric folds (>1 cm), especially localized to one area of the stomach.
- The radiologic findings of **duodenal ulcers** include a persistent collection of contrast in the duodenal bulb, with surrounding spasm and edema. Healing of duodenal ulcers frequently occurs with scarring and deformity of the duodenal bulb.
- Any imaging evaluation of the bowel should ideally be carried out with the bowel distended with air or contrast because collapsed and unopacified loops of bowel can introduce artifactual errors of diagnosis.
- Key abnormal findings of bowel disease on CT are **thickening** of the bowel wall, **submucosal edema or hemorrhage**, **hazy infiltration** of fat, and **extraluminal air** or contrast.
- **Crohn disease** is a chronic, relapsing, granulomatous inflammation of the small bowel and colon, usually involving the terminal ileum, resulting in ulceration, obstruction, and fistula formation. It may have skip areas and has a propensity for recurring following surgical removal of an involved segment.

- Colonic **diverticulosis** increases in incidence with increasing age. It most often involves the sigmoid colon and is almost always asymptomatic, although it can lead to diverticulitis or massive GI bleeding, especially from right-sided diverticula.
- CT is the study of choice for imaging **diverticulitis** and the findings include pericolonic inflammation, thickening of the adjacent colonic wall (>4 mm), abscess formation, and/or confined perforation of the colon.
- Most **colonic polyps** are hyperplastic and have no malignant potential. Adenomatous polyps carry a malignant potential that is related, in part, to their size. Colonic polyps can be visualized with barium enema examination, CT colonography, or optical colonoscopy.
- Imaging signs of colonic polyps include a persistent filling defect in the colon, with or without a stalk.
- The imaging findings of **colonic carcinoma** are a persistent, polypoid, or annular constricting filling defect of the colon that occasionally perforates or causes large bowel obstruction. It may metastasize, especially to the liver and the lungs.
- **Colitis** of any etiology can cause thickening of the bowel wall, narrowing of the lumen, and infiltration of the surrounding fat.
- CT or ultrasound are the studies of choice in diagnosing **appendicitis**. Findings include a dilated appendix (>6 mm) that does not fill with oral contrast, periappendiceal inflammation, increased enhancement of the wall of the appendix with intravenous contrast, and sometimes identification of an appendicolith (fecalith).
- **Lower gastrointestinal bleeding** is frequently caused by diverticulosis. CT angiography, tagged-red blood cell bleeding scans, catheter angiography, and optical colonoscopy can be used to visualize the site of bleeding with the latter two also capable of treating the cause.
- The two most common causes of **pancreatitis** are gallstones and alcoholism. Pancreatitis is a clinical diagnosis with CT serving to document a cause or a complication of the disease. CT findings include enlargement of the pancreas, peripancreatic stranding, pancreatic necrosis, and pseudocyst formation.

- **Pancreatic adenocarcinoma** has a very unfavorable prognosis. It occurs most often in the pancreatic head and usually manifests as a focal hypodense mass on CT that may be associated with dilatation of the pancreatic and/or biliary ducts.
- **Fatty infiltration** of the liver is very common and can produce focal or diffuse areas of decreased attenuation that characteristically do not displace or obstruct the hepatic vessels. With it, the liver appears less dense than the spleen on unenhanced CT scans.
- In its later stages, **cirrhosis** produces a small liver (especially the right lobe) with a lobulated contour, inhomogeneous appearance of the parenchyma, prominent left and caudate lobes, splenomegaly, varices, and ascites.
- Evaluation of liver masses is frequently done with a **triple-phase CT scan** that includes a precontrast scan and two postcontrast scans, one in the hepatic-arterial phase and then another in the portal-venous phase.
- **Metastases** are the most common malignant hepatic masses and they mostly originate in the GI tract. They appear as multiple, low-density masses that may necrose as they become larger.
- **Hepatocellular carcinoma** is the most common primary hepatic malignancy. They are usually solitary and typically enhance with intravenous contrast on CT.

- **Cavernous hemangiomas** are usually solitary, more common in females, and typically produce no symptoms. They have a characteristic "outside-in" pattern of enhancement and frequently retain contrast longer than the remainder of the liver.
- **MRCP** is a noninvasive way to image the biliary tree without requiring injection of contrast material. It can be used to demonstrate biliary strictures, gallstones, and congenital anomalies.
- **Renal cysts** are a very common finding. They are frequently multiple and bilateral, do not enhance, and typically have sharp margins where they meet the normal renal parenchyma. On US, simple cysts are well-defined anechoic masses.
- **Renal cell carcinoma**, the most common primary renal malignancy, shows a propensity for extension into the renal vein and for metastasizing to lung and bone. On CT, renal cell carcinoma is usually a solid mass that enhances with intravenous contrast but remains less dense than the normal kidney. On US, they frequently produce echogenic masses.
- **Ultrasound** is the imaging study of first choice in evaluating the **female pelvis.**
- **Abdominal and/or pelvic adenopathy** may be caused by lymphoma, other malignancies, or benign diseases such as sarcoid. Multiple enlarged nodes or conglomerate masses of nodes may be seen on CT.

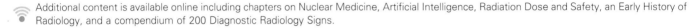

Additional content is available online including chapters on Nuclear Medicine, Artificial Intelligence, Radiation Dose and Safety, an Early History of Radiology, and a compendium of 200 Diagnostic Radiology Signs.

# 18

# Ultrasonography: Understanding the Principles and Its Uses in Abdominal and Pelvic Imaging

*Peter S. Wang, MD*

**Ultrasound** is a diagnostic imaging tool that makes use of *probes (transducers)* that can produce an acoustical frequency that is hundreds of times greater than humans can hear and that utilizes acoustical energy to localize and characterize human tissues.

## CASE QUIZ 18 QUESTION

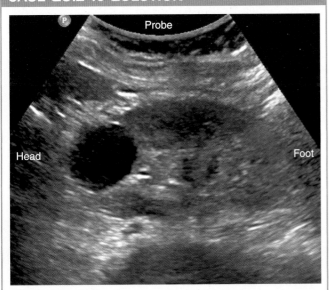

An abnormality in the upper pole of the kidney was discovered incidentally during an ultrasound examination for another reason. A sagittal view of the kidney is shown. What is the abnormality and what does it most likely represent? See the answer at the end of this chapter.

## HOW IT WORKS

- Ultrasonography is performed by placing the transducer on a body surface while sweeping back and forth as real-time images are displayed on a monitor. Adequate contact between the transducer and the body surface is essential to obtain a good sonographic image. Therefore, a **coupling gel** is applied to produce the best contact between the transducer and the body surface by eliminating air gaps (Video 18.1).

- The body surface that is scanned may be **external,** such as the skin surface in *transabdominal* sonography, or **internal,** such as in *transvaginal, transrectal, transesophageal,* and *endovascular* sonography.

### ▶▶ IMPORTANT POINTS

- The creation of a sonographic image *(sonogram)* depends on three major components:
  - Production of **high-frequency sound waves**
  - Reception of a **reflected wave** or **echo**
  - Conversion of that echo into the actual **image**

- The sound wave is produced by the **probe** or **transducer** that sends out extremely short bursts of acoustical energy at a given frequency.

- As with all sound waves, the pulses produced by the transducer travel at different speeds depending on the **density** of the medium through which they are traveling.

- Where the wave strikes an *interface* between tissues of **differing densities,** some of the sound wave will be **transmitted forward** while some will be **reflected back** to the transducer (Fig. 18.1).

- How much sound is transmitted versus how much is reflected depends on the property of the tissues that make up the interface and is called *acoustical impedance.* **Small differences** in acoustical impedance will result in **greater sound transmission; large differences** in acoustical impedance will result in **greater sound reflection.**

- For example, if the pulse encounters a gallstone, the acoustical impedance is **high** and most of the acoustical energy is

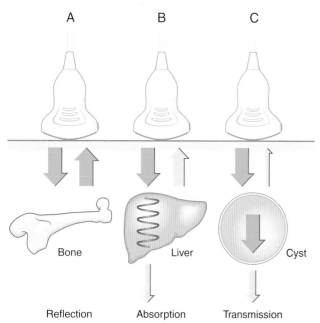

**Fig. 18.1** Diagram of Three Probes on Skin Surface. The amount of sound that is transmitted or reflected depends on the acoustic impedance of the tissues. (A) Large differences in acoustic impedance are encountered with bone and result in predominant **reflection** of the sound with little or no transmission. (B) As the sound passes through tissues, such as the liver, its intensity decreases as some of it is **absorbed** and transformed to heat while some may be transmitted. (C) Small differences in acoustic impedance such as encountered in a fluid-filled cyst result in predominant **transmission** of the sound.

reflected back. If the tissue that is encountered is extremely dense, such as bone, so much of the energy is reflected that there are not enough transmitted sound waves to define tissues deeper to the bone (see Fig. 18.1A).

- If a pulse traveling through soft tissue encounters fluid, the acoustical impedance (difference in densities) is relatively **low** and most of the acoustical energy is **transmitted** (see Fig. 18.1C).
- As the sound waves pass through tissue, their intensity decreases as they are absorbed by the tissue and converted into heat energy.
- When the reflected echo arrives back at the transducer (a matter of microseconds), it is converted from **sound** into **electrical pulses** that are then sent to the scanner itself.
- Using an on-board computer, the scanner determines the **length of time** it took for the echo to be received, the **frequency** of the reflected echo, and the **magnitude (amplitude)** of the signal.
- With this information, a sonographic image of the scanned body part can be generated by the computer and displayed on the screen. The images may then be captured as **single, static images** or recorded as a **cine loop** that is composed of a set of images that can be played as a video. Both this chapter and the next feature cine loops of US studies that can be viewed online (Videos 18.1–18.8 and Videos 19.1–19.7).

## Echogenicity

>> **IMPORTANT POINTS**

- The **echogenicity** (brightness or darkness) of a tissue on US is determined by the amount of sound waves the tissue transmits or reflects.

- A tissue that **reflects more** echoes is depicted **brighter or whiter** on the sonogram and is called **echogenic (hyperechoic).**
- A tissue that **transmits more** echoes (resulting in less echoes reflected back to the transducer) is depicted **darker** on the image and is called **sonolucent (hypoechoic).**
- A tissue that essentially transmits **all** the echoes is depicted as **black** on the sonogram and is called **anechoic.**
- When a very dense structure such as a gallstone or bone reflects so many echoes that virtually no sound waves are transmitted, the tissue deeper to this structure is displayed as hypoechoic and this phenomenon is called **posterior acoustic shadowing.**
- When a structure transmits more echoes than the surrounding tissues, such as a cyst in the liver might, the sound waves deeper to this structure compared to surrounding structures are depicted as hyperechoic and this phenomenon is called **posterior acoustic enhancement.**
- The typical appearances of different types of commonly encountered tissues and structures are described in Table 18.1.

## Imaging Planes

- Images can be produced in any plane of the body by adjusting the direction of the probe (see Fig. 1.6). By convention, two common imaging planes are utilized.

| TABLE 18.1 **Appearance of Commonly Encountered Tissues on Ultrasound** | | |
| --- | --- | --- |
| **Tissue** | **Appearance** | **Examples** |
| **Fluid** | Hypoechoic or anechoic, depending whether the fluid is **simple** or **complex** (containing debris, pus, or blood); may have **posterior acoustic enhancement** | Cysts, abscesses, gallbladder, urinary bladder, spinal fluid, blood in vessels |
| **Calcium** | Hyperechoic; may have **posterior acoustic shadowing** | Gallstones, renal stones, bones, calcifications in soft tissue |
| **Air** | Hyperechoic foci; may cause posterior acoustic shadowing | Gas-forming infections (abscesses, Fournier's gangrene, endometritis), intraperitoneal air, necrotizing enterocolitis, portal venous gas, pneumobilia |

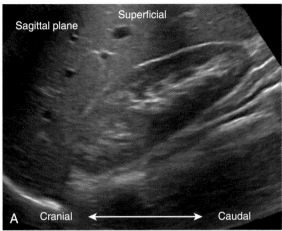

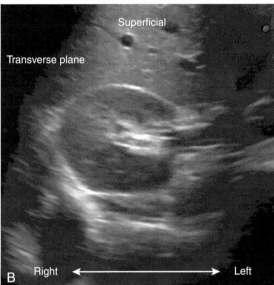

Fig. 18.2 Sagittal and Transverse Ultrasound Images of the Right Kidney. (A) The sagittal plane is along the long axis of the body or long axis of the body part being scanned and is viewed with the patient's head toward the left and feet toward the right. (B) The transverse plane is perpendicular to the sagittal plane and is typically viewed with the patient's right side on the left of the image and the patient's left side on the right of the image, just as most radiologic images are. In both planes, the **upper** part of the image is more **superficial** and closer to the transducer probe and the **lower** part of the image is **deeper** and farther from the probe.

- The *sagittal (or longitudinal) plane* is obtained along the **long axis** of the body or body part being scanned and is viewed with the **patient's head toward the left** and **feet toward the right.** The **upper part** of the image is more **superficial or closer to the transducer** and the **lower part** of the image is **deeper and farther from the probe** (Fig. 18.2A).
- The *transverse plane* is obtained **perpendicular to the long axis** of the body or body part being scanned and is conventionally viewed with the patient's right on your left side and the patient's left on your right side (Fig. 18.2B).

## FREQUENCY AND RESOLUTION

- The **frequency of the soundwaves** utilized in any given US study plays an integral role in the **resolution** of the US images.
- **Higher frequencies** result in **higher resolution** images and **more detail.** However, the higher the frequency, the **shorter the penetration** distance. Therefore, while higher frequencies will provide more detail, they cannot display deeper tissues because of their shorter penetration.
- US transducers produce inherently different frequencies of sound waves, usually labeled on the probe. Choosing the proper transducer for the type of study is important in order to provide as much **detail** as possible while also providing enough **penetration** to reach the desired tissue.
- In general, **higher frequency** transducers are appropriate for **superficial structures** or those that require fine detail, and **lower frequency** transducers are appropriate for **deep structures.**

## TYPES OF ULTRASOUND

- Several types of US are used in medical imaging. They are described in Table 18.2.

### Doppler Ultrasonography

- You are probably familiar with the common examples of the *Doppler effect* illustrated by a passing train whistle or police siren. The effect generally states that sound **changes in frequency** as the object producing the sound either **approaches** or **recedes** from your ear (Video 18.2).

| TABLE 18.2 | Types of Ultrasound |
|---|---|
| **A-Mode** | Simplest; spikes along a line represent the signal amplitude at a certain depth; used mainly in ophthalmology. |
| **B-Mode** | Mode most often used in diagnostic imaging; each echo is depicted as a dot and the **sonogram** is made up of thousands of these dots; can depict real-time motion. |
| **M-Mode** | Used to show moving structures, such as blood flow or motion of the heart valves. |
| **Doppler** | Uses the **Doppler effect** to assess blood flow; used for vascular US. ***Pulsed Doppler*** devices emit short bursts of energy that allow for an accurate localization of the echo source. |
| **Duplex ultrasonography** | Used in vascular studies; refers to the simultaneous use of grayscale (or color Doppler) to visualize the **structure** of, and flow within, a vessel and spectral (waveform) Doppler to **quantitate** flow (see Video 18.1). |

- Sonography makes use of the Doppler effect to determine whether an object, usually blood, is **moving toward** or **away** from the transducer and at what velocity it is moving. Here is how it works:
  - The transducer sends out a signal of **known frequency;** the frequency of the echo returned is **compared** to the frequency of the original signal.
  - If the returning echo has a **lower frequency** than the original, then the object is **moving away** from the transducer. If the returning echo has a **higher frequency** than the original, then the object is **moving toward** the transducer.

> ## ▶▶ IMPORTANT POINTS
>
> - The **direction of flow** is represented by the colors red and blue. By convention, **red** indicates **flow toward** and **blue** indicates **flow away** from the transducer.

## ADVERSE EFFECTS OR SAFETY ISSUES

- US procedures are **well-tolerated.** Scans can be obtained relatively quickly, done at the bedside if necessary, and, for the most part, require no patient preparation other than abstinence from food before abdominal studies (Table 18.3).
- US has the short-term potential of causing **minor elevation of heat** in the area being scanned, though **not** at levels used in diagnostic imaging.
- **No known long-term side effects** have been scientifically demonstrated from the use of medical US in humans. Nevertheless, like all medical procedures, it should be utilized only when medically necessary. The United States Food and Drug Administration warns against the use of US during pregnancy to produce "keepsake photos or videos."
- The **advantages of US** over CT and conventional angiography include the **absence of the use of ionizing radiation, lack of the need for intravenous iodinated contrast,** and the **portability** of US.

## MEDICAL USES OF ULTRASONOGRAPHY

- We will look at several common abnormalities in which US plays a primary imaging role.

### TABLE 18.3 Advantages and Disadvantages of Ultrasonography

| Advantages | Disadvantages |
| --- | --- |
| **No ionizing radiation** | Difficulty penetrating through bone |
| **No known long-term side effects** | Gas-filled structures reduce its utility |
| **"Real-time" images** | Obese patients may be difficult to penetrate |
| **Produces little or no patient discomfort** | Dependent on the skills of the operator scanning |

## Biliary System

- Ultrasound is the **study of first choice** for abnormalities of the biliary system. Patients who present with the relatively common complaint of right upper quadrant abdominal pain usually undergo an US examination as their first imaging study. CT may be helpful in cases with difficult or unusual anatomy, for detecting masses, or in determining the extent of disease already diagnosed, but **CT is less sensitive than US in detecting gallstones.**

### Normal Gallbladder Anatomy: Ultrasound

- The **gallbladder** is an elliptical sac that lies between the right and left lobes of the liver in the interlobar fissure. Although different layers of its wall have different echogenic properties, the gallbladder overall consists of a **fluid-filled sonolucent lumen** surrounded by an **echogenic wall.** In the fasting patient, the gallbladder is about **4 x 10 cm in size** and the **wall** is normally **no thicker than 3 mm** (Fig. 18.3).

### Gallstones and Acute Cholecystitis

- **Cholelithiasis** is estimated to affect more than 20 million in the United States. In almost all cases, acute cholecystitis starts with a **gallstone impacted in the neck of the gallbladder or cystic duct.** The presence of gallstones does not, by itself, mean that the source of a patient's pain is the gallbladder since asymptomatic gallstones are common. Cholecystitis can also occur, though less commonly, in the **absence** of stones *(acalculous cholecystitis).*
- Because of gravity, **gallstones usually fall to the most dependent part of the gallbladder,** which will be influenced by the patient's position at the time of the scan. This helps to differentiate gallstones from polyps or tumors that may be

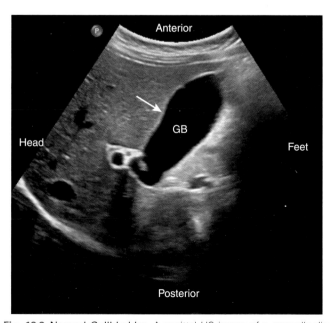

**Fig. 18.3 Normal Gallbladder.** A sagittal US image of a normally distended gallbladder (GB) filled with anechoic fluid, i.e., bile. The normal wall thickness is less than 3 mm *(arrow).*

attached to a nondependent surface. Gallstones are characteristically **echogenic** and produce **posterior acoustic shadowing** (Fig. 18.4).

- *Biliary sludge* can be found in the lumen of the gallbladder and is an aggregation that may contain cholesterol crystals, bilirubin, and glycoproteins. It is often associated with **biliary stasis.** Although it may be echogenic, **sludge does not produce acoustic shadowing** as gallstones do (Fig. 18.5). Sludge layers along the dependent gallbladder wall or may appear as a rounded, mobile "mass" that is called *tumefactive sludge.*

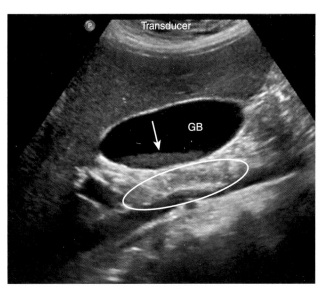

**Fig. 18.5** Sludge in the Gallbladder. *Sludge (arrow)* in the gallbladder (GB) is associated with biliary stasis. The sludge is more echogenic than the normal anechoic bile, but it transmits enough sound waves *(oval)* that it does not result in posterior acoustic shadowing associated with gallstones.

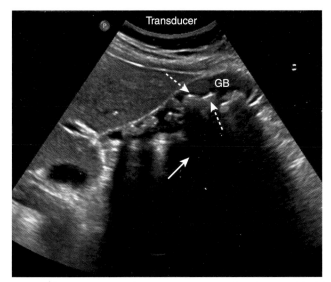

**Fig. 18.4** Gallstones with Posterior Acoustical Shadowing. Multiple echogenic gallstones *(dashed arrows)* are in this gallbladder (GB). When most of the sound waves are reflected back toward the transducer by the stones, the result is a paucity of sound waves deep (posterior) to the stones creating a hypoechoic area or **posterior acoustic shadowing** *(solid arrow).*

> ▷▷ **IMPORTANT POINTS**
>
> - **Recognizing acute cholecystitis on US:**
>   - **Thickening of the gallbladder wall** (>3 mm) (Fig. 18.6A)
>   - *Pericholecystic fluid* (fluid around the gallbladder) (Fig. 18.6B)
>   - A *positive sonographic Murphy sign* (i.e., pain that is elicited by compression of the gallbladder with the US probe).

- If gallstones are present (see Fig. 18.4) in addition to these other US features, the diagnosis of *acute calculous cholecystitis* can be made. In the presence of gallstones and

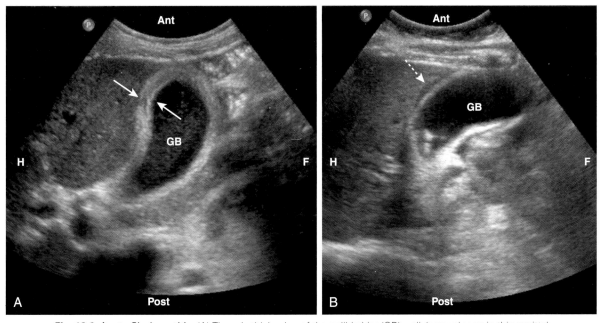

**Fig. 18.6** Acute Cholecystitis. (A) There is thickening of the gallbladder (GB) wall *(arrows)* seen in this sagittal view. The wall is normally 3 mm or less. This wall is markedly thickened at 6 mm. (B) There is an echo-free crescent *(arrow)* surrounding a thickened gallbladder (GB) wall representing *pericholecystic fluid.* The patient had a **positive sonographic Murphy's sign.**

gallbladder wall thickening, US has a positive predictive value for acute cholecystitis as high as 94%.

- If these features exist in the absence of gallstones, the patient may have **acalculous cholecystitis**, which typically tends to occur in critically ill patients.
- Radionuclide scans (**hepatoiminodiacetic acid [HIDA] scans**) are also used in the diagnosis of acute cholecystitis.
  - Hepatoiminodiacetic acid (HIDA), which is physiologically absorbed by the liver and excreted into the biliary system, is tagged with a radioactive tracer (**technetium-99m**) and injected intravenously. The tagged HIDA can then be imaged with a special camera to demonstrate its normal physiologic uptake by the liver and subsequent excretion into the bile ducts, gallbladder, and small intestine.
  - In patients with **obstruction of the cystic duct,** the tracer will **not appear** in the **gallbladder;** in patients with **obstruction of the common bile duct,** the tracer will **not appear** in the **small intestine.** Either finding is typically caused by an obstructing stone (Fig. 18.7).

### Normal Bile Duct Anatomy: Ultrasound

- **Ultrasound plays a key role in evaluation of the intrahepatic and extrahepatic bile ducts and the pancreatic duct.** The intrahepatic biliary radicals drain into the left and right hepatic ducts, which join to form the common hepatic duct (CHD). The common bile duct (CBD) begins where the cystic duct from the gallbladder joins with the CHD. It drains into the second portion of the duodenum either within or adjacent to the head of the pancreas via the ampulla of Vater.
- The **CBD** lies **anterior** to the **portal vein** and **lateral** to the **hepatic artery** in the **porta hepatis** (Fig. 18.8A).

- The CHD and proximal CBD can be visualized on virtually all US studies of the right upper quadrant. The **CHD** measures **no more than 4 mm** (inner wall to inner wall) in diameter, and the **CBD** measures **no more than 6 mm** in diameter (Fig. 18.8B). The **pancreatic duct** measures **less than 2 mm.**

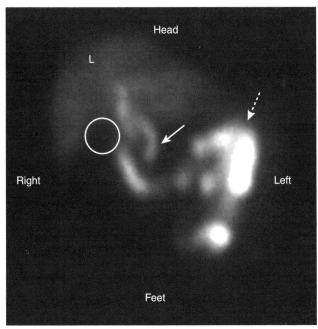

**Fig. 18.7 HIDA Scan in Cystic Duct Obstruction.** Normally, HIDA tagged with a radioisotope will concentrate in the liver (L) after which the HIDA will collect in the gallbladder via a patent cystic duct and be excreted through the common bile duct *(solid arrow)* into the small intestine *(dashed arrow).* When the cystic duct is obstructed by a gallstone, as in this case, the gallbladder does not fill with the radioisotope tagged HIDA and will appear ***photopenic* (dark)** *(circle).*

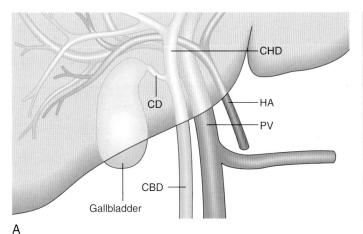

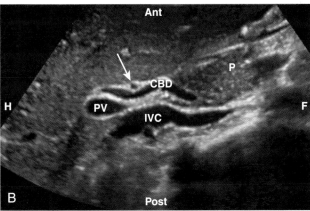

**Fig. 18.8 Normal Common Bile Duct, Portal Vein, and Hepatic Artery—Illustration and Sagittal View.** (A) The illustration demonstrates the normal relationships of some of the structures in the porta hepatis. (B) A sagittal view of the right upper quadrant shows the common bile duct (CBD), which measures 3 mm (normal <6 mm). The arrow points to the hepatic artery, seen on end. The portal vein (PV) is posterior to the common duct and the inferior vena cava (IVC) is seen posterior to the portal vein. The pancreas (P) is anterior to the CBD. *CD,* Common bile duct; *CHD,* common hepatic duct; *HA,* hepatic artery.

- Normally, the **intrahepatic bile ducts** are **not visible** on US. However, they may become dilated over time when there is prolonged CBD obstruction. Dilated intrahepatic ducts appear as additional, tubular sonolucent structures adjacent to the portal veins, which results in a ***tram-track*** appearance (Fig. 18.9).

- **Causes of bile duct obstruction** include gallstones, pancreatic carcinoma, strictures, sclerosing cholangitis, cholangiocarcinoma, and metastatic disease.

## Urinary Tract

### Normal Renal Anatomy: Ultrasound

- The kidneys normally measure **9 to 12 cm in length, 4 to 5 cm in width, and 3 to 4 cm thick.** The **renal sinus** is home to the **renal pelvis** and the major branches of the renal artery and vein. Because the renal sinus contains fat, it normally appears **brightly echogenic.** The **calyces** are **normally not visible.** The **pyramids** are hypoechoic. The **renal parenchyma** has **uniformly low echogenicity,** which is usually **less** than that of the **adjacent liver and spleen** (Fig. 18.10).
- Renal masses are discussed in Chapter 17.

### Hydronephrosis

- *Hydronephrosis* is defined as **dilatation of the renal pelvis and calyces.** Renal pelvis dilatation by itself is called ***pelviectasis*** and calyceal dilatation alone is called ***caliectasis.***
- In patients experiencing **renal colic,** US is used primarily to evaluate for the **presence of hydronephrosis.** Because the ureters may be difficult to visualize on US, **stone searches** are usually carried out by CT scanning (see Fig. 16.7).
- However, in the hands of an experienced sonographer, even stones in the ureter can often be found, eliminating the additional expense and radiation associated with a CT scan.

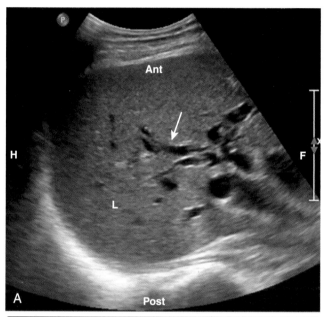

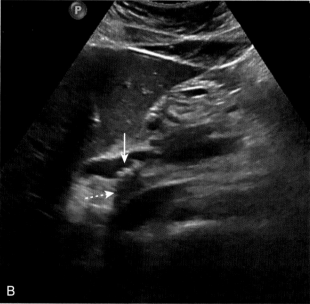

**Fig. 18.9 Dilated Intrahepatic and Extrahepatic Ducts in Two Different Patients, Sagittal Images.** (A) The intrahepatic biliary ducts are normally not visible with US. In this case, they are dilated *(arrow)* from obstruction by a pancreatic carcinoma (not visible). (B) The common bile duct is dilated to 1 cm due to multiple echogenic gallstones *(solid arrow)* producing posterior acoustical shadowing *(dashed arrow). L,* liver.

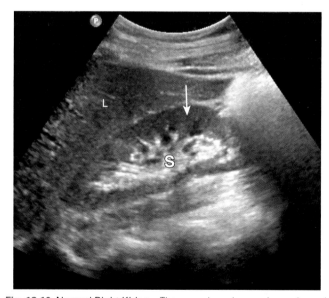

**Fig. 18.10 Normal Right Kidney.** The normal renal parenchyma *(arrow),* seen here sagittally, is homogenous in echogenicity and either similar or slightly less echogenic than the adjacent liver (L) or spleen. The **renal sinus** (S) is mainly composed of fat that is more echogenic than the parenchyma. Branches of the renal artery and vein and the renal collecting system are also located in the renal sinus.

- The typical appearance of obstructive uropathy is a **dilated calyceal system.**
- The echogenic renal sinus contains a dilated, fluid-filled, and therefore **anechoic renal pelvis.**
- The **ureter** may be **dilated** to the level of the obstructing stone.
- Severe **hydronephrosis** may distort the appearance of the kidney (Fig. 18.11).

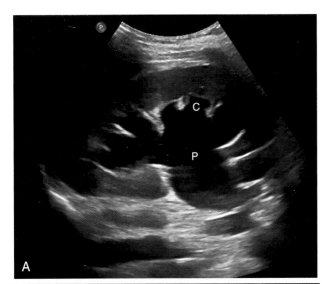

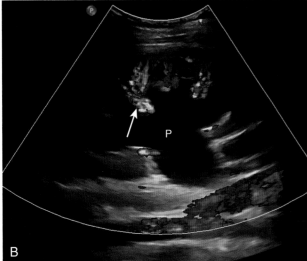

**Fig. 18.11 Hydronephrosis, Sagittal Grayscale and Color Doppler Views, Right Kidney.** (A) In this sagittal grayscale image of the right kidney, the renal pelvis (P) and calyces (C) are markedly dilated and filled with anechoic fluid (urine) representing hydronephrosis. (B) The lack of color Doppler flow helps to differentiate the dilated renal collecting system (P) from blood vessels *(arrow)* that would fill with color.

## Medical Renal Disease

- *Medical renal disease* refers to a host of diseases that primarily affect the **renal parenchyma.** They include such diseases as glomerulonephritis, diseases that cause the nephrotic syndrome, and renal involvement in collagen vascular diseases.
- In the early stages of medical renal disease, the kidneys may appear normal on US. As the disease advances, the **renal parenchyma becomes more echogenic (brighter) than the liver and spleen,** the reverse of the normal echo pattern (Fig. 18.12). However, these changes usually cannot differentiate between the numerous causes of medical renal disease. A biopsy using US guidance may be performed to determine the etiology of the disease.
- **Renal size** may be a helpful indicator of disease chronicity. When associated with abnormal renal parenchymal echotexture, **renal sizes smaller than normal indicate more chronic disease.**

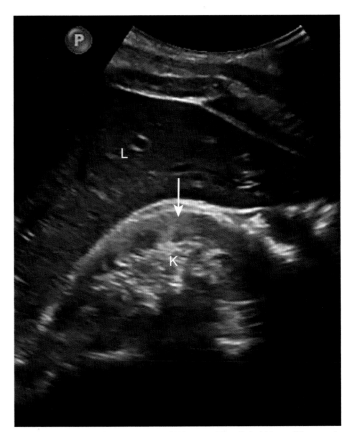

**Fig. 18.12 Chronic Medical Renal Disease.** The right kidney (K), seen in sagittal view, is small and has a thin cortex *(arrow)* which is more echogenic than the adjacent liver (L), the reverse of the normal echogenic pattern.

## Urinary Bladder

- As a fluid-filled structure, the urinary bladder lends itself well to US evaluation. Ultrasound of a fluid-distended bladder can be used to assess bladder wall thickness and the presence of bladder **tumors, stones, and diverticula** (Fig. 18.13). The **postvoid residual bladder volume** can also be estimated, which is helpful in the assessment of **urinary incontinence, bladder outlet obstruction,** and in patients with a **neurogenic bladder.**
- A full, fluid-filled bladder is also used as an *acoustic window,* a portal to avoid image-degrading, air-filled bowel and allowing easier assessment of the prostate in men and pelvic structures in women.

## Scrotal Ultrasound

- Differential diagnosis of **acute scrotal pain** includes epididymitis, orchitis, testicular torsion, testicular trauma, and herniation of abdominal contents into the scrotum. Prompt intervention is required in cases of testicular torsion and trauma to salvage the affected testis.
- *Testicular torsion,* which usually occurs in adolescents, is an especially important diagnosis because **timely detorsion is curative,** while a missed torsion can result in loss of the testicle. **Color Doppler US** (which can reveal scrotal blood flow) is used in the assessment of suspected torsion; there

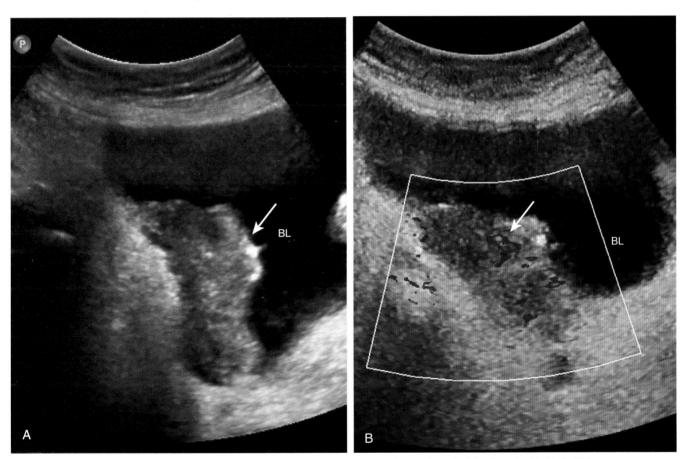

**Fig. 18.13 Bladder Tumor, Sagittal Views.** (A) There is a polypoid mass *(arrow)* arising from the bladder's (BL) posterior wall seen in this grayscale image. (B) Color Doppler demonstrates vascular flow *(arrow)* in the mass, which helps to differentiate a tumor from debris or blood clot, neither of which would have vascular flow.

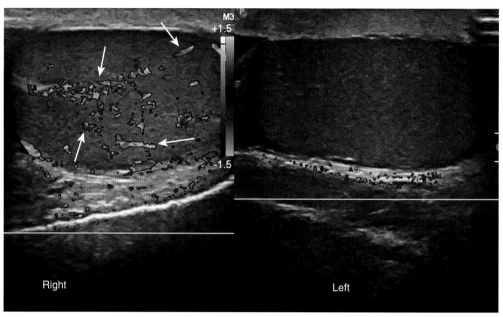

**Fig. 18.14 Scrotal Ultrasound, Left Testicular Torsion.** A dual screen image of the right and left testicles was obtained using the same Doppler sensitivity settings demonstrating normal color Doppler blood flow *(arrows)* in the right testicle and lack of color Doppler blood flow in the left testicle, which is the result of torsion of the spermatic cord structures with subsequent loss of the blood supply to the ipsilateral testicle.

is usually **no flow in the torsed testis** (Fig. 18.14). Adjacent to the testicle, identification of a twisted vascular pedicle (which has a swirling appearance) *(whirlpool sign)* confirms the diagnosis (Video 18.3).

## Abdominal Aortic Aneurysms

- An *aneurysm* is defined as a localized dilation of an artery by **50% or more above its normal size.** Most aortic aneurysms occur in the abdominal aorta **inferior to the origin of the renal arteries and frequently extend into one or both common iliac arteries.**
- Most aortic aneurysms are either **fusiform** in shape or produce **uniform dilatation** of the entire vessel.

> ⟫ **IMPORTANT POINTS**
>
> - The **abdominal aorta normally measures no more than 3 cm in diameter** (outer wall to outer wall).

- The **size** of an aneurysm is directly related to its **risk of rupture.** For aneurysms **less than 4 cm** in diameter, there is a **less than 10% chance** of rupture; aneurysms **4 to 5 cm** in diameter have almost a **25% risk of rupture.**
- **Recognizing an abdominal aortic aneurysm:**
  - US is the screening study of choice when there is an asymptomatic, pulsatile abdominal mass.
  - **Flowing blood** within the lumen of the aorta will appear **anechoic; thrombus** in the wall of the aneurysm will appear **echogenic** (Fig. 18.15).
  - Unenhanced CT has the advantage of depicting the absolute size of the aneurysm, but to define the extent of

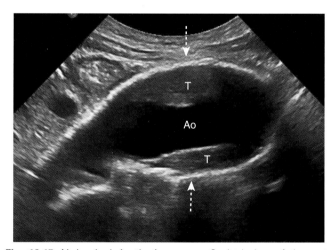

**Fig. 18.15 Abdominal Aortic Aneurysm.** Sagittal view of the aorta displays a fusiform dilation of the abdominal aorta of 4.3 cm *(between dashed arrows).* The aneurysm contains echogenic mural thrombus (T), and the remaining patent aortic lumen (Ao) with flowing blood is anechoic. For aneurysms 4 to 5 cm in diameter, the risk of rupture increases to almost 25%.

mural thrombus and the presence of dissection, intravenous contrast must be used.

## FEMALE PELVIC ORGANS

- **Ultrasound is the imaging study of choice in evaluating a pelvic mass or pelvic pain in the female.** *Leiomyomas (fibroids)* confined to the myometrium are the most common tumors of the uterus. **Endometrial carcinomas** are usually

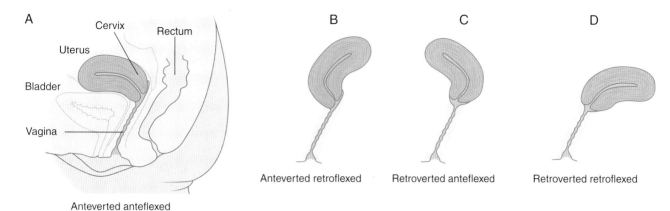

**Fig. 18.16 Normal Variations in Uterine Position.** The position of the uterus in the body is described by its **version** (i.e., the angle of the **cervix** relative to the **vagina**) and **flexion** (i.e., the angle of the **uterine body** relative to the **cervix**). **Anteversion** (A and B) occurs when the cervix is angled anteriorly relative to the vagina. **Anteflexion** (A and C) occurs when the uterine body is angled anteriorly relative to the cervix. In **retroversion** (C and D) and **retroflexion** (B and D), the cervix and body are angled posteriorly relative to the vagina and cervix, respectively. **Usually, the uterus is anteverted and anteflexed** as in (A).

confined to the uterus at the time of discovery. The most common premenopausal ovarian mass is a *functional cyst.* Generally, **uterine masses** are **solid** and **ovarian masses** are **cystic.**

## Normal Uterine Anatomy: Ultrasound

- The uterus is made up of a thick muscular layer *(myometrium)* and a mucous surface *(endometrium).* It is divided into a *body* (with *cornu* to receive the *fallopian tubes)* and the *cervix.* Anterior to the uterus is the peritoneal space called the *anterior cul-de-sac.* The *posterior cul-de-sac* is also called the *rectouterine recess.*
- The position of the uterus in the body is described by its *version* (i.e., the angle of the cervix relative to the vagina) and *flexion* (i.e., the angle of the uterine body relative to the cervix). These relationships are shown in Fig. 18.16. **Usually, the uterus is anteverted and anteflexed.**
- In the adult, the uterus has a **pear shape** with maximum dimensions of approximately **8 cm in length, 5 cm in width, and 4 cm in the anteroposterior dimension.** The size of the normal uterus increases with multiparity; with aging, the uterus decreases in size (Fig. 18.17).
- The normal *endometrial cavity* is in a collapsed state, forming a **thin, echogenic stripe or line** between the apposing surfaces of the endometrium. By convention, the endometrial thickness is measured by including both walls on a sagittal view of the mid-uterus. The appearance of both the endometrium and the ovaries varies, depending on the phase of the menstrual cycle.
- Normal **fallopian tubes** are collapsed and not usually visualized on US.
- The standard *transabdominal* **(through the abdominal wall)** study of the uterus is done with a **full urinary bladder.** The full bladder provides an **acoustic window** to the uterus by pushing bowel loops upward out of the pelvis and helps to delineate the bladder itself.

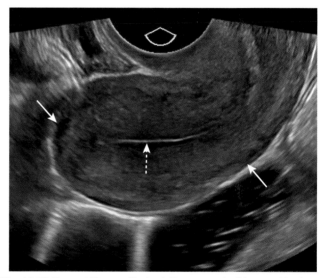

**Fig. 18.17 Normal Uterus, Sagittal.** The uterus *(solid arrows)* is shown in the sagittal plane. In a premenopausal woman, the endometrium changes in appearance depending on the stage of menstrual cycle. During the early proliferative phase, the endometrium appears as a thin, linear, echogenic structure *(dashed arrow)* in the uterus.

- *Transvaginal* studies are done with higher frequency probes and thus provide better resolution images. They are done with the **bladder empty.** Transabdominal and transvaginal studies are considered complementary techniques.
- *Sonohysterography* is a procedure in which saline is instilled in the endometrial cavity while transvaginal US images are obtained. The saline distends the normally collapsed endometrial cavity and separates the endometrial walls to allow for the delineation of **endometrial polyps, submucosal myomas, and adhesions** (Video 18.4).

## Uterine Leiomyomas (Fibroids)

- **Leiomyomas** are **benign smooth muscle tumors** of the uterus that occur in up to 50% of women over the age of 30. Most women with fibroids are asymptomatic. When symptoms occur, it is usually due to the size of the fibroid and can include pain, infertility, menorrhagia, and urinary and bowel symptoms.
- **Pelvic US is the imaging study of choice in evaluating uterine fibroids.** Magnetic resonance imaging may be used to evaluate complicated cases or in surgical planning.

>> **IMPORTANT POINTS**

- **Recognizing uterine leiomyomas on US:**
  - They are **heterogeneously hypoechoic, solid masses,** meaning they may display areas of varying echogenicity (brightness or darkness).
  - Fibroids may be intramural, submucosal, or subserosal. **Intramural** fibroids are surrounded by myometrium, **submucosal** fibroids project into the uterine cavity, and **subserosal** fibroids project outward from the uterine surface (Fig. 18.18A).
  - **Intramural** fibroids are the most common. When submucosal fibroids lie completely in the uterine cavity, they are characterized as **intracavitary.** Fibroids that are attached to the uterus by a stalk are **pedunculated** (Fig. 18.18).
  - Fibroids may undergo **degeneration** and **calcify.** These calcifications may reflect enough sound to produce **acoustic shadowing.** Fibroid degeneration may also manifest as cystic or fatty components.

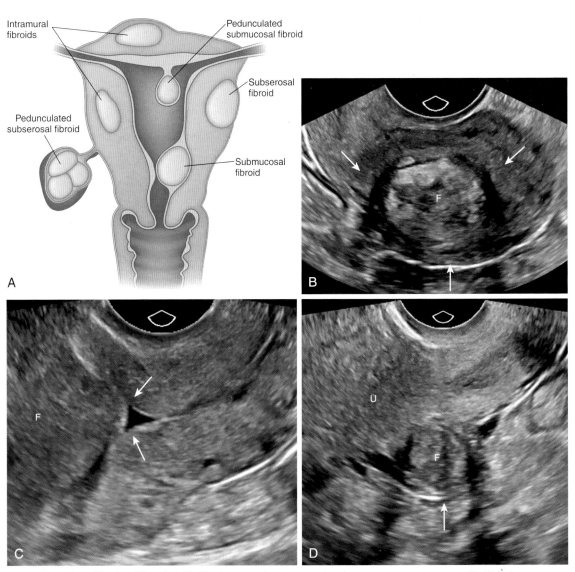

**Fig. 18.18 Uterine Fibroids.** (A) Fibroids may be intramural, submucosal, or subserosal. (B) This is an **intramural fibroid** (F) in the uterine body surrounded by myometrium *(arrows).* (C) A **submucosal fibroid** (F) is seen projecting into the uterine cavity and splaying the endometrium *(arrows).* A small amount of anechoic fluid is in the uterine cavity. (D) This is a **subserosal fibroid** (F) that protrudes from the uterus (U) and is not completely surrounded by myometrium (lack of myometrium indicated by an *arrow).*

- **Recognizing uterine leiomyomas on CT scans:**
  - Fibroids typically appear as **rounded, lobulated soft tissue uterine masses.** They may contain **amorphous** or *popcorn calcifications* indicating degeneration or they may undergo central necrosis, which manifests as low-attenuation areas (see Fig. 16.11).
  - Although fibroids are frequently visualized on CT scans, their extent may be more difficult to assess on CT than on US or MRI because they have a similar density to normal uterine myometrium and endometrium.
- The **location** of fibroids is important to aid in treatment planning (either surgical or interventional).

## Adenomyosis

- **Adenomyosis** refers to **ectopic endometrial tissue within the myometrium** (Fig. 18.19). It usually occurs in women 35 to 50 years old and may be the cause of **dysmenorrhea** and **menorrhagia.** It can be associated with ectopic endometrial tissue **outside** of the uterus (i.e., *endometriosis*). Symptoms will usually abate after menopause.

## Normal Ovarian Anatomy/Physiology: Ultrasound

- Ultrasound is the **imaging study of choice** for evaluating the **ovaries.**
- In **premenopausal women,** the ovaries are approximately **2 x 3 x 4 cm in size** ($\approx$ 5–15 mL in volume), frequently containing **cystic follicles** (Fig. 18.20). The ovaries atrophy after menopause.
- The normal ovary changes in appearance not only with age but also with the phases of each menstrual cycle. Under normal hormonal stimulation, one egg-containing *follicle* becomes **dominant** and attains a size of about 2.5 cm at the time of ovulation (Fig. 18.21).

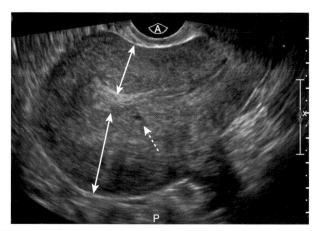

**Fig. 18.19 Adenomyosis of the Uterus.** This sagittal, transvaginal image of the uterus demonstrates several sonographic findings of adenomyosis, including a markedly thickened myometrium *(double arrows)* and a myometrial cyst *(dashed arrow).* Other findings of adenomyosis include a globular uterine shape, a heterogeneous myometrial echo-texture, and asymmetric uterine wall thickening (more often posterior wall). *A,* anterior; *P,* posterior.

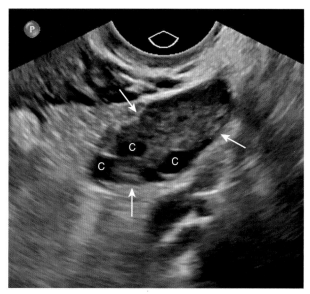

**Fig. 18.20 Normal Left Ovary.** The normal ovary *(arrows),* seen here in the sagittal plane, in premenopausal women is approximately 2 x 3 x 4 cm in size and contains small anechoic follicles (C).

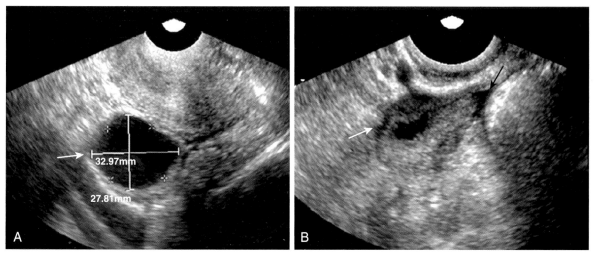

**Fig. 18.21 Dominant Follicle Ruptures During Scan.** Under normal hormonal stimulation, one egg-containing follicle becomes dominant and attains a size of about 2.5 cm at the time of ovulation. (A) The dominant follicle is 3.3 x 2.8 cm at the start of the study *(arrow).* (B) A few minutes later, during the study, the follicle ruptures (ovulation occurs) and the follicle shrinks dramatically in size *(white arrow).* A small, physiologic amount of free fluid appears in the peritoneal cavity *(black arrow).*

## Ovarian Cysts

- The **majority** of ovarian cysts in **premenopausal women** are *functional cysts* that include *follicular cysts* and *corpus luteal cysts.* These cysts occur as a result of the hormonal stimuli associated with ovulation and usually involute within one or two menstrual cycles.
    - A **follicular cyst** forms when a **nondominant** follicle fills with fluid and does not rupture.
    - A *corpus luteum* forms after an egg is expunged from a **dominant** ovarian follicle. If the corpus luteum fills with fluid, it then becomes a *corpus luteal cyst.*

> ### ▶ IMPORTANT POINTS
>
> - **Functional cysts** are characteristically **well-defined, thin-walled, anechoic** structures with **homogenous internal fluid echogenicity** (Fig. 18.22). These cysts are **physiologic** and **do not require follow-up** or other imaging in the asymptomatic patient. Occasionally, a functional cyst may contain blood that will appear as lacy reticular echoes (Fig. 18.23).

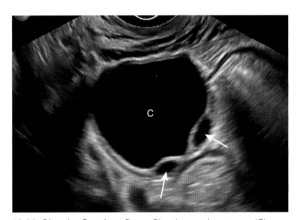

**Fig. 18.22 Simple Ovarian Cyst.** Simple ovarian cysts (C) are well-defined, thin-walled, and anechoic fluid-filled structures. There are also two separate follicles adjacent to the simple cyst in this sagittal view of the ovary *(arrows).*

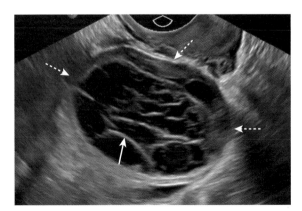

**Fig. 18.23 Hemorrhagic Ovarian Cyst.** Sagittal US image of the right ovary *(dashed arrows)* demonstrates a cystic mass that contains lacy reticular echoes *(solid arrow)* consistent with a hemorrhagic cyst. Hemorrhagic cysts may also contain a retracting clot, not shown here, which typically appears as avascular echogenic material in the cyst with angular, straight, or concave margins.

- *Polycystic ovarian disease* is an endocrine abnormality that allows for numerous ovarian follicles (>25/ovary) to develop in various stages of hormonal growth and atresia. When associated with **oligomenorrhea, hirsutism, and obesity,** the constellation is called the *Stein-Leventhal syndrome* (Fig. 18.24).
- **Nonfunctional cystic lesions** of the ovary include *dermoid cysts* and *endometriomas.* A specific diagnosis can usually be made with US.
    - **Dermoid cysts** are **mature teratomas** composed of cells from all three germ layers that can produce hair, bone, teeth, and fat in the cyst (Fig. 18.25). They are most commonly found in **women of reproductive age,** are **bilateral** in up to 25% of cases, and may serve as a lead point for **ovarian torsion.**

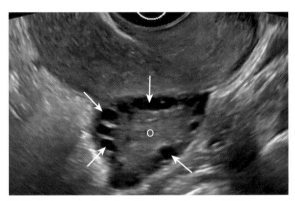

**Fig. 18.24 Polycystic Ovarian Disease.** A sagittal US image shows an enlarged left ovary (O) containing multiple small peripherally located follicles *(arrows)* consistent with a polycystic ovary. **Polycystic ovarian syndrome** (also called Stein-Leventhal syndrome) is diagnosed when two of the following three criteria are met: (1) ovulatory dysfunction (oligo- or anovulation), (2) clinical or biochemical signs of hyperandrogenism, and (3) polycystic ovarian morphology on US.

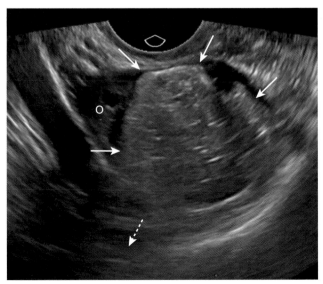

**Fig. 18.25 Ovarian Dermoid Cyst.** A US image demonstrates a solid echogenic mass *(solid arrows)* in the right ovary (O) with mild posterior acoustical shadowing *(dashed arrow)* consistent with a dermoid cyst or teratoma. Dermoid cysts may also contain calcification, teeth, and hair.

- *Endometriomas,* part of the disease **endometriosis,** are cystic ovarian lesions, sometimes called *chocolate cysts* because they are filled with brownish-red blood. They are frequently bilateral. Endometriomas can become large and multilocular (Fig. 18.26).

## Ovarian Tumors

- **Most ovarian tumors are cystic** and arise from the **surface epithelium** that covers the ovary and include **serous or mucinous tumors.** The **majority** of serous tumors *(serous cystadenomas)* and the overwhelming number of mucinous tumors *(mucinous cystadenomas)* are **benign.** Malignant tumors are designated *serous or mucinous adenocarcinomas.* **Staging** of ovarian cancer is best done with **CT or MRI.**

> ## IMPORTANT POINTS

- In contrast to benign ovarian cysts, features of **malignant ovarian cysts** include thick and irregular walls, **thick and irregular septations, internal vascular flow,** and **solid papillary projections** in the tumors (Fig. 18.27).

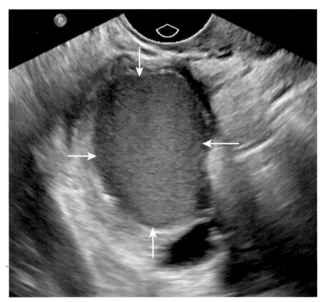

**Fig. 18.26** Endometrioma. A transverse US image demonstrates a right ovary containing a cystic mass *(arrows)* that contains diffuse, fine low-level echoes creating a *snow-storm* appearance that is consistent with an endometrioma.

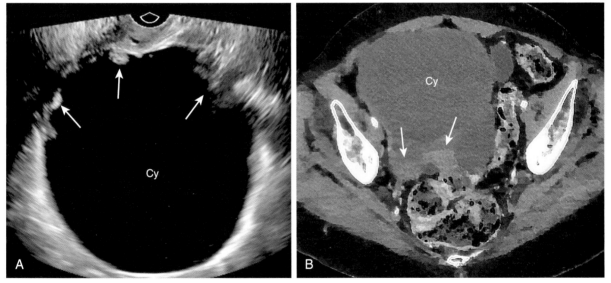

**Fig. 18.27** Ovarian Tumor, US and CT. (A) This transverse grayscale US image displays a large right ovarian cyst (Cy) that has multiple peripheral nodular papillary projections *(arrows).* (B) An axial, contrast-enhanced CT image through the pelvis of the same patient shows the large cystic mass (Cy) with enhancing solid components corresponding to nodular projections similar to those seen on US *(arrows).*

## Ovarian Torsion

- Like testicular torsion, **ovarian torsion is a surgical emergency,** and its timely diagnosis and treatment is essential to prevent loss of the ovary. The typical presentation is the **acute onset of excruciating adnexal pain.**

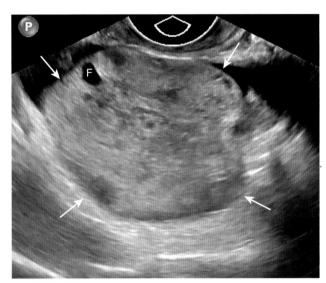

**Fig. 18.28 Ovarian Torsion.** A transverse US image in a patient with severe, acute right adnexal pain shows a markedly enlarged right ovary *(arrows)* that is of heterogeneous echogenicity. A follicle (F) is located peripherally in the ovary. In the setting of acute adnexal pain and an asymmetrically enlarged ovary, ovarian torsion is the most likely diagnosis and should be considered even if color and spectral Doppler blood flow can still be demonstrated in the ovary.

- Unlike testicular torsion, the **diagnosis of ovarian torsion** largely depends on the **morphologic appearance of the ovary.** The torsed ovary will appear **asymmetrically enlarged** and may have **increased stromal echogenicity** (Fig. 18.28).

## Pelvic Inflammatory Disease

- *Pelvic inflammatory disease* (PID) is a term used to describe a group of **infections affecting the uterus, fallopian tubes, and ovaries.** Most cases of PID begin as a **transient endometritis** and ascend to infection of the tubes and ovaries. Patients can have pain, vaginal discharge, adnexal tenderness, fever, and elevated white blood cell counts. Complications include infertility, chronic pain, or ectopic pregnancy.

> **IMPORTANT POINTS**
>
> - **Recognizing PID on US:**
>   - The **ovaries are enlarged** with **multiple cysts** and periovarian inflammation.
>   - The fallopian tubes may be **fluid-filled** and **dilated** *(pyosalpinx)* (Fig. 18.29A).
>   - There may be **fusion of the dilated fallopian tube and ovary** *(tubo-ovarian complex)* (Fig. 18.29B).
>   - A **multiloculated mass** with septations *(tubo-ovarian abscess)* may be present.
> - CT can be used for cases of complicated PID or for patients whose history may not suggest the diagnosis.

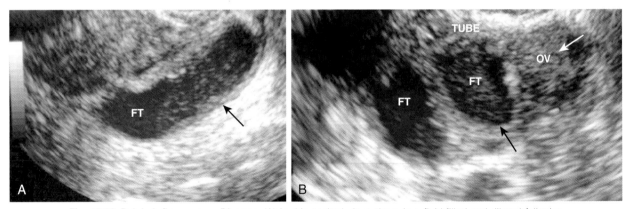

**Fig. 18.29 Pelvic Inflammatory Disease.** (A) In this sagittal view, there is a fluid-filled and dilated fallopian tube (FT) containing pus and debris *(arrow)* representing a pyosalpinx. (B) Because of progressive inflammation, this transverse view shows fusion of a dilated and tortuous fallopian tube *(black arrow-FT)* and the adjacent ovary *(white arrow)* producing a **tubo-ovarian complex.**

# PREGNANCY

- Ultrasound has provided a **safe and reliable** means of visualizing the fetus *in utero* and the ability to do so repeatedly during the course of a pregnancy, if necessary. The overwhelming majority of pregnant women in North America and Western Europe undergo at least one US evaluation sometime during pregnancy.
- Even before pregnancy, US can be used to determine ovulation time to aid in the process of successful fertilization.
- The uses of US during pregnancy are outlined in Box 18.1.
- The goals of sonography during pregnancy may differ depending on the timing of the scan.
    - During the **first trimester**, the goals are to exclude an ectopic pregnancy, estimate the age of the pregnancy, determine viability, and determine the number of embryos.
    - During the **second and third trimesters**, goals may include estimates of amniotic fluid volume, detection of fetal anomalies, determination of placental and fetal positioning, or guidance for invasive studies to determine the likelihood of fetal viability in the event of a premature birth (Video 18.5).
- We will look at three important uses of US during pregnancy.

## Ectopic Pregnancy

- Most ectopic pregnancies are **tubal in location** and occur near the **fimbriated (ovarian) end.** The classical clinical findings of **pain, abnormal vaginal bleeding, and a palpable adnexal mass** occur in only about half of cases. The incidence of ectopic pregnancies is increasing, most likely because of increasing risk factors, but the mortality

rate has declined, in part because of their early diagnosis by US.
- Using transvaginal scanning, **US is best at identifying the presence** of an **intrauterine pregnancy** and is less effective at visualizing the actual ectopic pregnancy itself.

> ### ▶▶ IMPORTANT POINTS
>
> - If a ***gestational sac*** (the earliest sonographic findings in pregnancy, appearing at about 4–5 weeks gestational age) or a ***yolk sac*** (the first structure to be seen normally in the gestational sac) or **embryo** is identified **in the uterine cavity**, an ectopic pregnancy is effectively **excluded.** Endovaginal US examinations are usually performed to find the gestational sac (Fig. 18.30).

- Simultaneous intrauterine and extrauterine pregnancies, also called ***heterotopic pregnancies,*** are **extremely rare** except in those undergoing fertility treatment. Therefore, identification of an ***intrauterine pregnancy*** effectively **excludes** the likelihood of an ***ectopic pregnancy.***

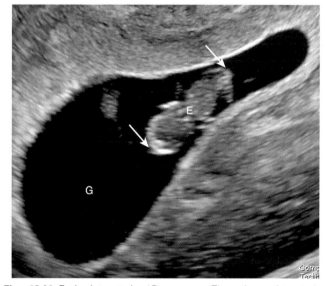

**Fig. 18.30 Early Intrauterine Pregnancy.** There is an intrauterine gestational sac (G) (which is a fluid-filled anechoic structure) containing a single, live embryo (E) seen in this sagittal view. The gestational age can be estimated by the ***crown-rump length*** *(between arrows),* which is this case was 1.8 cm and corresponded to a gestational age of 8 weeks, 2 days. Sonographic gestational age is estimated from the first day of the last menstrual cycle.

---

### BOX 18.1 Uses of Ultrasound During Pregnancy

- Fetal presence and gestational age
- Fetal abnormalities and viability
- Presence of multiple pregnancies
- Placental localization
- Amniotic fluid volume
- Intrauterine growth retardation
- Helping guide invasive studies like amniocentesis, chorionic villus sampling, and intrauterine transfusions

- Conversely, the demonstration of a **live embryo outside of the uterus is diagnostic of an ectopic pregnancy.** However, this is not a common occurrence with most ectopic pregnancies (Fig. 18.31).

> ## ▶▶ IMPORTANT POINTS
>
> - Most often, the ectopic location is diagnosed by a combination of findings that includes **absence** of an identifiable **intrauterine pregnancy,** often accompanied by an **extrauterine, extraovarian** solid or cystic **mass.**

- **Serum human chorionic gonadotropin hormone (β-HCG)** is produced by placental tissue shortly after the implantation of a fertilized ovum in the uterus. Combined with US, the β-HCG level may be helpful in distinguishing between intrauterine pregnancy, ectopic pregnancy, and early abortion (Fig. 18.32).
- An ectopic pregnancy is presumed present when there are **large amounts of free fluid (blood) inside the abdominal cavity. Small amounts** of free fluid can occur from other causes, such as spontaneous abortion, ruptured ovarian cysts, and normal ovulation.
- Ectopic pregnancies are **managed** either **surgically** (usually laparoscopic surgery) or **medically** with an abortifacient such as methotrexate. Some spontaneously resolve.

## Fetal Abnormalities

- Ultrasound is used extensively to monitor normal **fetal growth** and **development.**
- Certain fetal anomalies can be recognized by US *in utero* that are known to be universally fatal after birth, such as **anencephaly** (Fig. 18.33) or complete **ectopia cordis.** The accurate interpretation of sonograms by someone trained and experienced in obstetric US is important in detecting such anomalies.

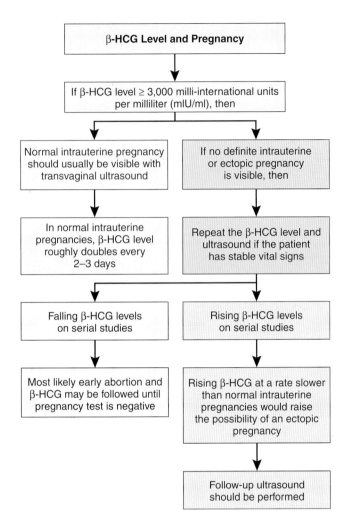

Fig. 18.32 Serum Human Chorionic Gonadotrophin and Pregnancy.

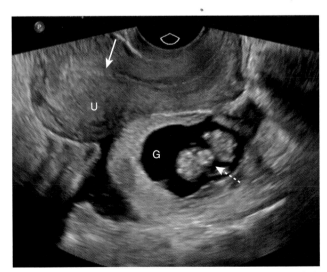

**Fig. 18.31 Ectopic Pregnancy.** A sagittal US image of the pelvis during early pregnancy demonstrates a uterus (U) with a normal endometrium *(arrow)* and no intrauterine gestational sac. Posterior to the uterus, in the right adnexa, is an extrauterine gestational sac (G) containing a single, live embryo *(dashed arrow)* consistent with a tubal ectopic pregnancy.

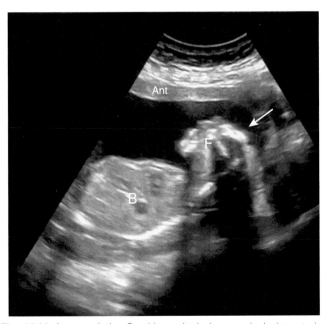

**Fig. 18.33 Anencephaly.** On this sagittal view, a single intrauterine pregnancy is seen. The body (B) and face (F) are present, but the cranium and all of the cerebrum and cerebellum are absent *(arrow).* Anencephaly involves a failure of closure of the neural tube during the 3rd to 4th weeks of development. It virtually always leads to fetal demise, stillbirth, or neonatal death.

## TABLE 18.4   In Utero Abnormalities Diagnosable by Ultrasound

| Organ System | Abnormalities |
|---|---|
| **Central nervous system** | Hydrocephalus, abnormalities of the prosencephalon, agenesis of the corpus callosum, intrauterine infections, cysts, meningomyelocele, anencephaly (Fig. 18.33) |
| **Skeletal anomalies** | Dwarfism, skeletal dysplasias, achondroplasia, osteogenesis imperfecta, asphyxiating thoracic dysplasia, limb anomalies |
| **Gastrointestinal abnormalities** | Esophageal atresia and tracheoesophageal fistula, duodenal atresia, small and large bowel obstruction, abdominal wall defects, congenital diaphragmatic hernias, choledochal cyst |
| **Genitourinary tract abnormalities** | Renal agenesis, congenital ureteropelvic junction and ureterovesical junction obstruction, bladder outlet obstruction, multicystic dysplastic kidney, polycystic kidney disease |
| **Cardiac anomalies** | Hypoplastic left heart syndrome, tricuspid atresia, endocardial cushion defects, Ebstein's anomaly, tetralogy of Fallot, transposition of the great vessels, coarctation of the aorta, cardiac arrhythmias |

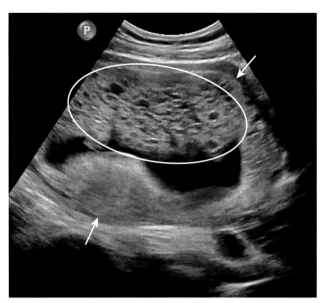

**Fig. 18.34 Molar Pregnancy.** A sagittal, transabdominal US image of the uterus *(arrows)* in a pregnant woman demonstrates a mass containing multiple small cystic spaces *(white oval)*. There is no normal-appearing fetus. These findings combined with a markedly elevated beta-HCG are consistent with a molar pregnancy.

- Some of the many fetal anomalies that can be diagnosed by US *in utero* are shown in Table 18.4.
- In detecting fetal anomalies, US has played a major role in obstetric management of pregnancy. As more reliable markers for chromosome abnormalities that can be quickly assessed without prolonged waiting periods become available, its role may increase.

## Molar Pregnancy

- *Molar pregnancy* is the most common group of disorders of the **placenta** that also includes *invasive mole* and *choriocarcinoma.* Pathologically, molar pregnancies feature **cystic (grape-like or hydatidiform) degeneration of chorionic villi** and proliferation of the placental trophoblast.

### ▶ IMPORTANT POINTS

- A molar pregnancy (Fig. 18.34) is suggested by uterine size that is **disproportionately large** for the gestational age, β-HCG levels in **excess of 100,000 mIU/mL** (normal pregnancies are less than 60,000 mIU/mL), **vomiting, vaginal bleeding,** and **toxemia.**

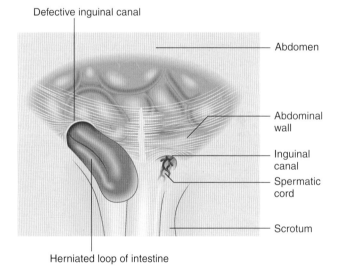

**Fig. 18.35 Graphic Representation of a Right Inguinal Hernia.** The most common location of an abdominal wall hernia is in the inguinal region. The herniated tissue may contain a combination of fat, bowel (as shown here), and/or visceral organs. The defect in the abdominal wall may pinch the herniated bowel, causing bowel obstruction, or compress blood vessels supplying the bowel, causing bowel ischemia (strangulation).

- Treatment of a molar pregnancy is **uterine evacuation.** About 20% of those with complete molar pregnancies may harbor persistent trophoblastic tissue, so follow-up is carried out with serial HCG determinations.

## ABDOMINAL HERNIAS

- An abdominal hernia is a protuberance of tissue, usually bowel, through a defect or hole in the abdominal wall (Fig. 18.35).
- Ultrasound evaluation for inguinal hernias is initially performed with the patient supine. Under real-time US, the patient performs the ***Valsalva maneuver,*** which increases the intraabdominal pressure and may elicit a hernia that is not normally present at rest (Video 18.6).
  - If a hernia is not detected in the supine position, having the patient **stand** while performing the Valsalva maneuver further increases the intraabdominal pressure and improves elicitation of a hernia. The ability of US to evaluate the inguinal region under real-time imaging either in the supine or standing position affords it an advantage over other imaging modalities.

## APPENDICITIS

- The appendix is a blind-ending tube that arises from the cecum. The **normal diameter** of the appendix is **less than 6 mm.** When visible, the normal appendix **will compress** when pressure is applied with the transducer.
- The **pathophysiology** of acute appendicitis begins with obstruction of the appendiceal lumen, followed by progressive distension of the obstructed appendix until perforation occurs and a periappendiceal abscess forms.

> ## ► IMPORTANT POINTS
>
> - In **acute appendicitis,** the abnormal appendix may be recognized on US as a blind-ending, aperistaltic tube with a diameter of **6 mm or more.** The inflamed appendix is **noncompressible** (using a technique called **graded compression).** It may also be tender when palpated with the probe. In about one-third of appendicitis cases, a **fecalith** will be present (Fig. 18.36, Video 18.7).

- The CT findings of appendicitis are discussed in Chapter 17.
- In addition to appendicitis and abdominal wall hernias, US can be used for other gastrointestinal abnormalities such as bowel wall thickening, masses, and intussusception. Endoscopic US allows for further characterization of the bowel wall and helps in guidance for biopsies.

## ASCITES

- Normally, the peritoneal cavity contains only a few milliliters of fluid. Excessive accumulation of fluid in the cavity is called

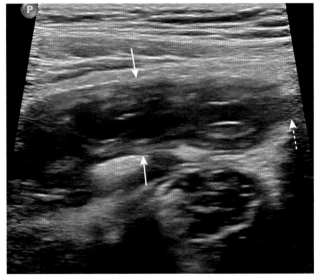

**Fig. 18.36 Acute Appendicitis.** A US image of the right lower abdomen shows a sagittal view of a thickened tubular structure *(solid arrows)* with a blind end *(dashed arrow)* consistent with acute appendicitis. An appendicolith obstructing this appendix and demonstrating posterior acoustical shadowing can be seen in an accompanying online video (Video 18.7).

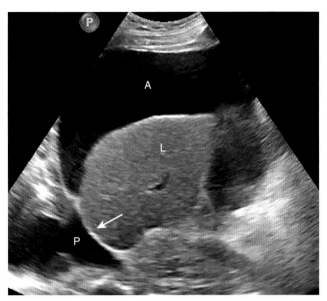

**Fig. 18.37 Ascites.** A sagittal US image of the right upper abdomen demonstrates ascites (A) around the liver (L). The ascitic fluid is anechoic consistent with transudate. Exudative ascitic fluid may contain internal echoes. The diaphragm *(arrow)* is a thin, linear echogenic structure between the liver and right lung. In this patient, a pleural effusion (P) is interposed between the diaphragm and the base of the lung.

*ascites.* When a large amount of ascites is present, it is easily identified in all four quadrants of the abdomen on US.
- However, smaller amounts may only be detectable in certain areas such fluid typically accumulates. The **right upper quadrant** between the liver and diaphragm is one of the first locations in which ascites collects, because the fluid flows up the right paracolic gutter to the right subphrenic space in the recumbent position.
- Other common locations for the detection of ascitic fluid are the *pouch of Douglas* in women and *rectovesical pouch* in men, which are the most dependent locations of the peritoneal cavity.
  - Ascitic fluid that is a **transudate** is primarily **sonolucent or anechoic.** Fluid collections that are **exudates** or contain hemorrhage or pus **may contain echoes** (Fig. 18.37).
- Ultrasound is frequently used to identify the largest accessible pocket of fluid that, in turn, provides image-guidance for the safe removal of the fluid via *paracentesis.*

## MUSCULOSKELETAL SYSTEM

- Although the musculoskeletal system is typically assessed with MRI, US is increasingly used for the evaluation of the musculoskeletal system.
- Ultrasound has the advantages of **real-time imaging, lower cost,** and **lack of contraindications** associated with a strong magnetic field used in MRI.

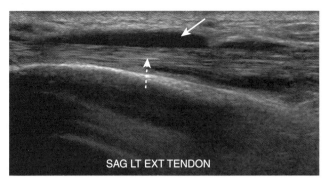

**Fig. 18.38 Extensor Pollicis Longus Tendon.** The normal tendon appears as a band of echogenic striations *(dashed arrow)*. There is anechoic fluid *(solid arrow)* surrounding this tendon which is consistent with tenosynovitis.

- **Real-time US imaging** allows a structure to be evaluated in **different positions,** including the position that elicits the patient's pain. For example, tendon subluxation may only occur in certain positions and subtle tendon or ligament tears may only be seen when they are stretched in certain positions.

> ⟩⟩ **IMPORTANT POINTS**
>
> - **Tendinopathy** can be diagnosed by US when the tendon appears thickened or when there is fluid around the tendon (Fig. 18.38). A tendon **tear** appears as **fluid in** the tendon or **discontinuity** of the tendon fibers.

- Ultrasound is also useful at the **point of care** to identify **foreign bodies** in the superficial soft tissues. Wood splinters, which may not be visible on conventional radiographs, can be **echogenic** on US and readily visible. Other materials such as metal, glass, and plastic can also appear as echogenic structures and may be visible on US (Fig. 18.39).
- Musculoskeletal US can also be used to evaluate joint effusions, superficial ligaments, musculature, and small joints in the hands and feet. It can also be used to guide therapeutic and diagnostic injections.

## CONTRAST-ENHANCED ULTRASOUND

- Contrast-enhanced US is increasingly used in the United States to aid in the diagnosis of a wide variety of pathologies. It involves the use of a *microbubble* contrast agent with specialized US imaging software to demonstrate **vascular flow and soft tissue perfusion.**
- The enhancement pattern of masses in abdominal organs such as the liver and kidneys can be assessed on contrast-enhanced

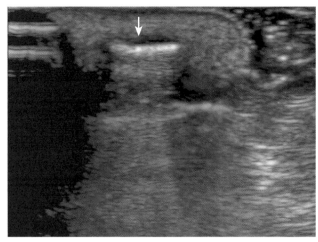

**Fig. 18.39 Foreign Body in the Ear Lobe.** The patient complained of swelling and redness in the left earlobe. An US image of the earlobe demonstrates a linear echogenic structure *(arrow)* corresponding to the plastic backing of an earring accidentally pulled into the earring tract of the earlobe. *(Courtesy Ryan K. Cunningham, MD.)*

US (Fig. 18.40, Video 18.8). The presence or lack of enhancement as well as the enhancement pattern itself aids in the diagnosis, especially of soft tissue tumors.
- The microbubble contrast agent is safe with no nephrotoxicity or risk of nephrogenic systemic fibrosis as can accompany the contrast agents used for CT and MRI, respectively.

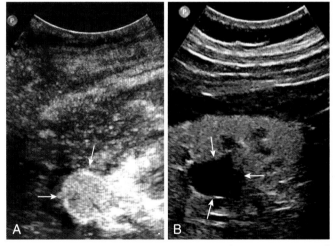

**Fig. 18.40 Contrast-Enhanced Ultrasound.** (A) Contrast-enhanced US of the right kidney demonstrates a mass *(arrows)* with internal enhancement that is consistent with a renal cell carcinoma. (B) Contrast-enhanced US of a different patient with a left renal mass shows no internal enhancement, consistent with a simple cyst *(arrows)*. Another example of an enhancing renal mass consistent with renal cell carcinoma is shown in Video 18.8.

## CASE QUIZ 18 ANSWER

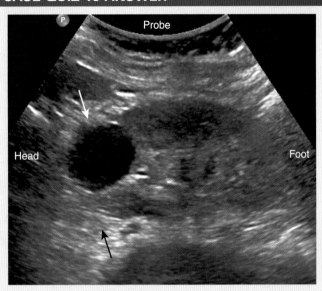

There is a sonolucent mass in the upper pole of the kidney *(white arrow)* with strong through transmission *(black arrow)* consistent with a simple cyst of the kidney. Simple cysts are relatively common, are almost always clinically silent, and rarely may hemorrhage and cause acute pain.

## 🏠 TAKE HOME POINTS

- Creation of a sonographic image **(sonogram)** depends on three major components: the production of a high-frequency sound wave, the reception of a reflected wave or echo, and the conversion of that echo into an image.
- **Echogenic (hyperechoic)** is a sonographic term used to describe tissue that reflects many echoes and appears bright or white on the sonogram. **Hypoechoic or anechoic** are sonographic terms used to describe tissue that reflects few or no echoes and appears dark or black on the sonogram.
- The **Doppler effect** is used in US to determine and display the direction and velocity of a moving object, usually blood.
- There are no known long-term side effects that have been scientifically demonstrated to be caused by the medical use of US in humans.
- **Gallstones** are characteristically echogenic and produce an **acoustical shadow** because they reflect most of the sound waves.
- **Biliary sludge** can also be seen in the gallbladder. Although sludge may also appear echogenic, it does not produce acoustic shadowing as gallstones do.
- **Obstructive uropathy** typically appears as a dilated calyceal system and is depicted as a fluid-filled, dilated, hypoechoic collecting system on US.
- In **medical renal disease,** the renal parenchyma becomes more echogenic than the liver and spleen, which is the reverse of the normal echo pattern.
- **Scrotal torsion** is a medical emergency and appears as an absence of blood flow on color Doppler imaging in the torsed testicle.
- Ultrasound is the study of choice to screen for **abdominal aortic aneurysms** when an asymptomatic, pulsatile abdominal mass is palpated.
- **Leiomyomas (fibroids),** the most common tumor of the uterus, appear as heterogeneously hypoechoic, solid masses. **Adenomyosis** refers to ectopic endometrial tissue in the myometrium and presents as small, cystic spaces in the myometrium of an enlarged, globular uterus.
- The most common ovarian mass is a **functional cyst,** which appears as a thin-walled anechoic structure on US. The cyst may be echogenic if it contains hemorrhage.
- **Nonfunctional ovarian cysts** include dermoid cysts and endometriomas.
- **Ovarian tumors** most often arise from the surface epithelium and are either serous or mucinous.
- **Pelvic inflammatory disease (PID)** is a term used to describe a group of infectious diseases affecting the uterus, fallopian tubes, and ovaries, with most beginning as transient endometritis.
- Ultrasound is a safe and reliable means of visualizing the fetus *in utero* and provides the ability to do so repeatedly during the course of a pregnancy, if necessary.
- Most **ectopic pregnancies** are tubal in location and can be effectively **excluded** if an intrauterine pregnancy is present and **included** if the extrauterine pregnancy is demonstrated.
- A **molar pregnancy** is suggested by uterine size that is disproportionately large for the dates of gestation and markedly elevated β-HCG levels of greater than 100,000 mIU/mL.
- An **abdominal hernia** is a protuberance of tissue through a defect in the abdominal wall. It can be diagnosed on US by visualizing the intraabdominal contents (usually fat and/or bowel) herniated through abdominal wall, with detection improved if intraabdominal pressure is increased by having the patient stand and perform the Valsalva maneuver.
- The appendix is a blind-ending, aperistaltic tube that can become inflamed in **acute appendicitis.** On US, the appendix appears thickened (diameter >6 mm) and noncompressible in acute appendicitis. The patient may be tender when palpated with the US probe.
- Ultrasound may be used to evaluate superficial tendons, ligaments, musculature, and for the presence of joint effusions. Superficial foreign bodies may also be detected by US as echogenic structures, even when they cannot be visualized on radiographs.
- **Contrast-enhanced US** is increasingly used in the United States and involves the injection of a microbubble contrast agent to determine vascular flow and tissue perfusion.

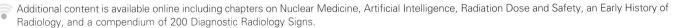

Additional content is available online including chapters on Nuclear Medicine, Artificial Intelligence, Radiation Dose and Safety, an Early History of Radiology, and a compendium of 200 Diagnostic Radiology Signs.

# 19

# Vascular, Pediatric, and Point-of-Care Ultrasound

*Peter S. Wang, MD*

In this chapter, we will discuss some additional applications of ultrasound (US), including vascular ultrasound, pediatric applications of ultrasound, and point-of-care ultrasound.

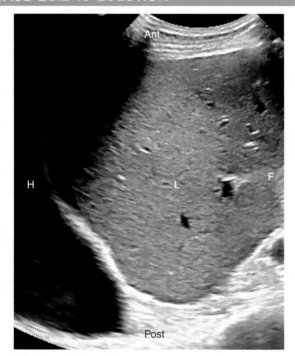

This is a sagittal US image of the chest/right upper quadrant in a 75-year-old who had increasing shortness of breath from congestive heart failure. What complication of that disease is depicted on the image? The answer is at the end of this chapter. *Ant,* Anterior; *F,* foot; *H,* head; *L,* liver; *Post,* posterior.

## VASCULAR ULTRASOUND

- **Vascular US** uses both *B-mode* **(gray-scale) US** and *Doppler ultrasonography*—a combination called *duplex sonography*—to display the morphologic appearance of vessels while recording the **flow direction** and **velocity of moving blood** in those vessels.

- Duplex sonography ensures that the direction and flow measurements are made in the exact anatomic location of interest (Video 19.1).
- The two most common types of Doppler US are *color Doppler* and *spectral Doppler.*
  - Color Doppler can provide specific, but limited, information over a relatively large region, whereas spectral Doppler provides more precise information about a smaller region. The two modes are complementary.

> ### ▶▶ IMPORTANT POINTS
>
> - **Color Doppler US** superimposes color on the gray-scale image to indicate the presence and direction of moving blood. By convention, **red** indicates **movement toward the transducer** and **blue** indicates **movement away from transducer** (Fig. 19.1).

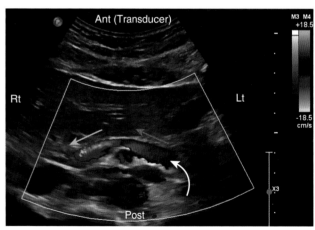

**Fig. 19.1** Color Doppler Image. By convention, color Doppler depicts flow **toward** the transducer as **red** and flow **away** from the transducer as **blue**. This is an image of the **splenic vein** *(curved arrow)*. When imaged anteriorly at the midline, the splenic vein to the left of midline has blood flowing anteriorly toward the transducer *(red arrow)* and to the right of midline has blood flowing posteriorly away from the transducer *(blue arrow)*. Therefore, color Doppler depicts flow both as red and blue in same vessel. Throughout this chapter, many figures will have one or more of the following abbreviations to aid in orientation: *Ant,* Anterior; *F,* foot of the patient; *H,* head of the patient; *Lt or L,* left; *Post,* posterior; *Rt or R,* Right.

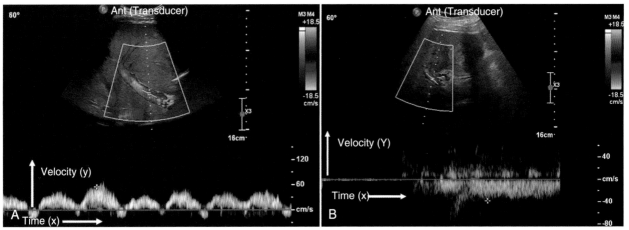

**Fig. 19.2** Normal Color and Spectral Doppler Images. (A) This image of the main portal vein demonstrates normal flow direction depicted as red (toward the transducer) and the periphery of the liver. (B) In a different patient who has cirrhosis and portal hypertension, the flow direction in the main portal vein is reversed and flows toward the liver hilum. Thus the flow direction is depicted as blue (away from the transducer). The spectral Doppler waveforms are located below the color portions of the ultrasound images and are drawn on a time-velocity scale with the **x-axis** depicting **time** and the **y-axis** depicting **velocities**. The portal vein waveform in (A) is above the baseline (the baseline is the thin, horizontal line) indicating blood flow toward the transducer. The waveform in the main portal vein in (B) is below the baseline indicating blood flow away from the transducer.

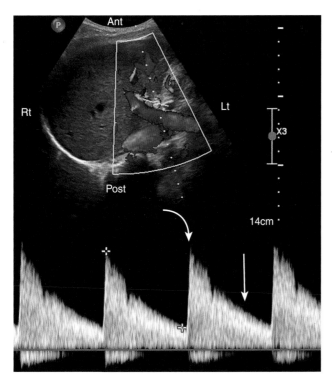

**Fig. 19.3** Normal Color and Spectral Doppler Images of the Hepatic Artery: Low Resistance. End organs like the liver have a vascular bed with low resistance to blood flow from their supplying arteries because they require a continuous blood supply. Therefore, flow in the hepatic artery is normally toward the liver throughout the cardiac cycle during both systole *(curved arrow)* and diastole *(straight arrow)*.

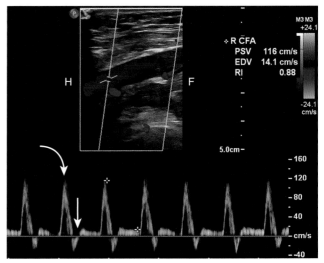

**Fig. 19.4** Normal Color and Spectral Doppler Images of Common Femoral Artery: High Resistance. Extremities at rest normally have a constricted vascular bed and therefore a high resistance to flow from their supplying arteries. Consequently, flow in the common femoral artery (which supplies the lower extremity) typically has a high-resistance waveform. The flow is toward the foot (above the baseline) during the high pressures of systole *(curved arrow)* and may stop or reverse (below the baseline) during the low pressures of diastole *(straight arrow)*.

- **Spectral Doppler ultrasound** is displayed as a **waveform,** which is a graphic representation of the **velocity of flow** measured **over time** within a **focused area.** It is depicted

along an **X** (**time**) and **Y** (**velocity**) axis. By convention, **flow toward** the transducer is displayed **above the baseline** and **flow away** is **below the baseline** (Fig. 19.2).
- There are distinctive arterial spectral Doppler waveforms, depending on the **resistance** to blood flow in the vascular bed that the artery supplies (Figs. 19.3 and 19.4). Venous waveforms can also vary depending on their proximity to the heart, the cardiac function, and phase of respiration.

- If a US signal is reflected from a **stationary object**, the returning signal should theoretically retain the **same frequency** with which it was transmitted. But based on the principles of Doppler US, the frequency of a signal reflected from **moving objects**, such as blood cells, will **change** in proportion to the **velocity** of the target.
- With this information, we can **interrogate** (i.e., systematically examine) **vessels** to determine whether they are **narrowed** or **occluded** because an **arterial stenosis** leads to an **increase in blood velocity** through the area of narrowing. If we gradually advance the Doppler probe along the path of a blood vessel, we can identify a stenotic lesion and its location.
- This is analogous to the velocity of water flowing through the open end of a garden hose. When the opening of the garden hose is narrowed, the velocity of the flowing water must increase for the same volume of water to flow through the smaller lumen (Fig. 19.5).
- Because of changes in blood flow, abnormalities in the spectral waveforms can also suggest narrowing or occlusion that occurs in a part of the vessel that is more **proximal** or **distal** to the area being studied.

## ARTERIAL STENOSIS
### Carotid Arteries
- **Carotid ultrasonography** has become the study of choice for the noninvasive assessment of **extracranial atherosclerotic disease.** Carotid US is also used to evaluate bruits, as preoperative screening prior to other major vascular surgery, and to assess the patency of the vessel after endarterectomy.

- When there is **greater than 50% stenosis** of the carotid artery lumen, the **velocity** of flow becomes **elevated.** Significant stenosis alters the Doppler waveform at points **proximal**, **at**, and **distal** to the stenosis.
- Ultrasound is also used to assess the **thickness of the vessel wall** (it gets thicker with atherosclerosis) and the presence and nature of **plaque.**

### Peripheral Arteries
- **Peripheral artery disease** occurs when **atherosclerotic plaques** are deposited in the arteries feeding the extremities. Significant narrowing or occlusion of the peripheral arteries usually occurs in the **lower extremities** and can result in *claudication* (i.e., leg pain during exertion) or pain at rest.
  - **Risk factors** include smoking, diabetes, hypertension, hyperlipidemia, male gender, and Black ethnicity.
- The peripheral arteries in the extremities **normally** have what is called a *high-resistance waveform* because **at rest**, the vascular bed in the muscles they supply is constricted (see Fig. 19.4).
- **Significant narrowing of a peripheral artery** will cause an **elevation in the velocities** of the flowing blood.

> ## ▶ IMPORTANT POINTS
> - **Screening** for peripheral arterial disease typically involves obtaining the *ankle-brachial index (ABI)*, which is the **ratio** of the systolic blood pressure in the **ankle** divided by the systolic blood pressure in the **arm** (i.e., brachial artery).
>
> $$ABI = \frac{\text{systolic blood pressure in a ankle}}{\text{Systolic blood pressure in arm}}$$

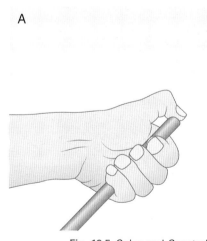

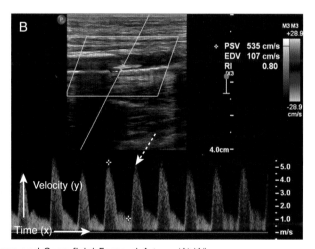

**Fig. 19.5** Color and Spectral Doppler Image of a Narrowed Superficial Femoral Artery. (A) When you position your thumb to narrow the opening of a garden hose, the water flows significantly faster because the same volume of water must travel through a smaller opening. (B) Similarly, when an artery is significantly narrowed by atherosclerotic disease, the velocity of blood flow through the stenosis must increase *(dashed arrow)* for the same volume of blood to travel through the smaller lumen (in this case the velocities are over 500 cm/sec). In addition, the arterial waveform may change to monophasic (which has flow remaining on one side of the spectral Doppler baseline) because there is relatively less resistance after the stenosis when the artery opens to a normal caliber lumen (see Fig. 19.3).

- Blood pressures are measured by **detecting arterial flow** with a **Doppler probe** on the artery instead of with a stethoscope. Pressures are usually taken in **both arms** and the posterior tibial and dorsalis pedis arteries in **each leg** by inflating blood pressure cuffs past the point where flow and Doppler sounds **cease,** then slowly deflating the cuffs until flow and Doppler sounds **return.**
- Normally, the systolic blood pressures in the ankle should be equal to that in the arm resulting in an **ABI of 1.** As the blood pressure in the ankle falls due to peripheral vascular disease in the legs and because ankle pressures are the numerator for the ABI, there will be a **decrease** in the value of the ABI, and an **ABI of 0.5 or less** usually indicates **severe arterial disease.**

## PSEUDOANEURYSM

- One of the complications following an invasive vascular procedure, such as cardiac catheterization, is the development of a *pseudoaneurysm,* most often at the **catheter entrance site.** This is usually in the **groin** at the common femoral artery or in the **arm** at the brachial artery.
- A pseudoaneurysm forms when there is a **rupture or injury to the arterial wall,** but the blood leaking through the defect **remains confined** either by an intact, thin outer layer of the arterial wall itself or by the surrounding perivascular tissues. Because the wall or perivascular tissue containing the pseudoaneurysm is very thin, it is at **high risk for further rupture and extravasation.** In contradistinction, a **true aneurysm's** arterial walls are intact but the **caliber** of the artery is abnormally **dilated.**

> ### ▶▶ IMPORTANT POINTS
>
> - On US, a pseudoaneurysm appears as a **hypoechoic outpouching** arising from an artery (Video 19.2). Occasionally, the pseudoaneurysm may be connected to the artery by a thin neck or stalk. **Blood flowing into and out of a pseudoaneurysm** results in a **distinctive appearance** on color and spectral Doppler images (Fig. 19.6).

- Ultrasound is also used for the **treatment** of pseudoaneurysms by applying direct **compression with the US probe** to occlude the aneurysm sac, especially if the sac is small. Ultrasound can also be used to guide thrombin injection resulting in thrombosis or occlusion of the pseudoaneurysm.

## DEEP VEIN THROMBOSIS (DVT)

- Ultrasound is the **study of choice** when **deep vein thrombosis** is suspected in the upper or lower extremities. **Local symptoms** can include pain, tenderness, and warmth in the affected area, although most patients with DVT are asymptomatic. The most serious complication of DVT is **pulmonary embolism.**
- The highest-yield sonographic examination for DVT in the leg occurs in the **symptomatic patient** who manifests local symptoms **above the knee.** Ultrasound has a much lower sensitivity in asymptomatic patients.
- Sonographic evaluation of deep venous thrombosis is usually performed in the legs but can also evaluate the arms. In the leg, it involves the use of the transducer to systematically **compress** the deep veins while scanning along **certain anatomic landmarks,** including the common femoral vein,

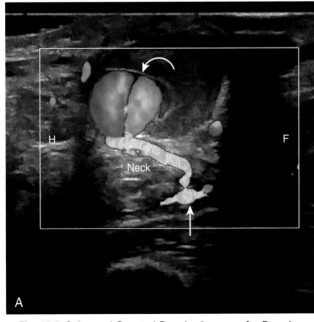
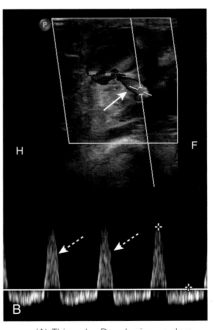

**Fig. 19.6** Color and Spectral Doppler Images of a Pseudoaneurysm. (A) This color Doppler image demonstrates a **pseudoaneurysm** *(curved arrow)* arising from the common femoral artery *(straight arrow)* via a thin neck. Because of flow into and out of the pseudoaneurysm, a typical pattern of red and blue color Doppler flow similar to a **yin-yang** symbol is displayed. (B) Spectral Doppler interrogation of the pseudoaneurysm neck *(solid arrow)* demonstrates flow into and out of the pseudoaneurysm as flow above *(dashed arrows)* and below the baseline. The pseudoaneurysm developed from the common femoral artery after cardiac catheterization.

proximal deep femoral vein, greater saphenous vein, femoral vein, popliteal vein, and the posterior tibial and peroneal veins. Similarly, DVT evaluation of the arms includes the internal jugular, subclavian, axillary, and brachial veins.

> ## ▶ IMPORTANT POINTS
>
> • **Normal venous structures** have elastic walls and will **easily compress** and **completely collapse** when pressure is applied by the transducer. Veins containing **thrombus *will not* completely collapse**. The echogenic thrombus itself may be visualized on gray-scale imaging. Duplex sonography can also be used to determine the presence or absence of flow in the vein (Fig. 19.7).

## PEDIATRICS

• Ultrasound's **lack of ionizing radiation** is especially useful in pediatric patients because younger and developing patients are more susceptible to the effects of radiation and have a relatively longer lifespan to develop potential complications. In addition, the smaller body habitus of a child allows better penetration of the US signal and permits the use of higher frequency transducers to provide higher resolution images.

• Many uses of US are specific to the pediatric age group, several of which are discussed in the following sections.

### Germinal Matrix Hemorrhage

• A *sonographic window* describes an anatomic **pathway** for the US signal to travel that is relatively free of bone or gas, both of which would degrade the US image. The intracranial contents of the neonate are particularly accessible by US because of the sonographic windows provided by the **open fontanelles.**

• Many of the structures in the supratentorial and infratentorial spaces, including the brain parenchyma and extraaxial spaces, can be evaluated. In the neonate, one such use is for the evaluation of **intracranial hemorrhage.**

• **Neonatal intracranial hemorrhage** can cause significant morbidity and mortality, particularly in **premature infants.**

Normal

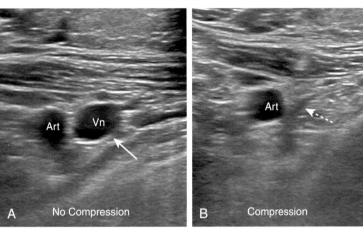

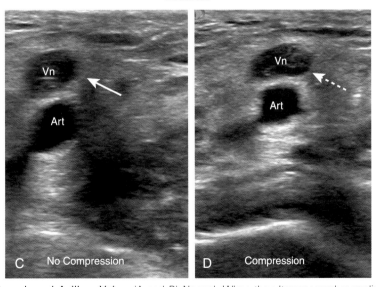

Abnormal

**Fig. 19.7 Normal and Thrombosed Axillary Veins.** (A and B) Normal. When the ultrasonographer applies compression using the transducer, the normal axillary vein (Vn) will completely collapse between its precompression *(solid arrow)* and postcompression *(dashed arrow)* states because of its elastic walls. (C and D) Abnormal. In a patient with a slightly different orientation of the artery and vein, acute deep venous thrombus in the axillary vein (Vn) prevents its normal collapse between precompression *(solid arrow)* and postcompression *(dashed arrow)* states.

These hemorrhages **most commonly occur in the *germinal matrix,*** which is only transiently present before 34 weeks of gestation. The germinal matrix is the source in the developing fetal brain that gives rise to the neuronal cells that will later migrate out to constitute the gray matter of the brain. It occurs in the vessel-rich ***caudothalamic groove,*** which is in the subependymal region between the caudate nucleus and thalamus (Fig. 19.8A).

> ### ▶ IMPORTANT POINTS
>
> • **Germinal matrix hemorrhage** appears as an area of **echogenic material** in the caudothalamic groove that can expand into the ventricle and brain parenchyma (Fig. 19.8B).

• Germinal matrix hemorrhages are divided into four grades, usually by US imaging, with increasing predicted mortality as the grade increases. Injury to the germinal matrix has substantial mortality and morbidity consequences.

## Developmental Dysplasia of the Hip (DDH)

• Developmental dysplasia of the hip is a relatively common disorder of newborns that can result in **dislocation or subluxation of the hip.** It is more common in females, firstborn children, breech presentation, and children whose parents had DDH. The left hip is also more commonly affected.

• Physical examination findings that suggest DDH include positive **Ortolani** and **Barlow tests.**
   • In the ***Ortolani test,*** the hip is **externally rotated** and **abducted.** A positive test occurs when a "click" or "clunk" is felt or heard during this test due to **reduction** of the dislocated or subluxed hip.

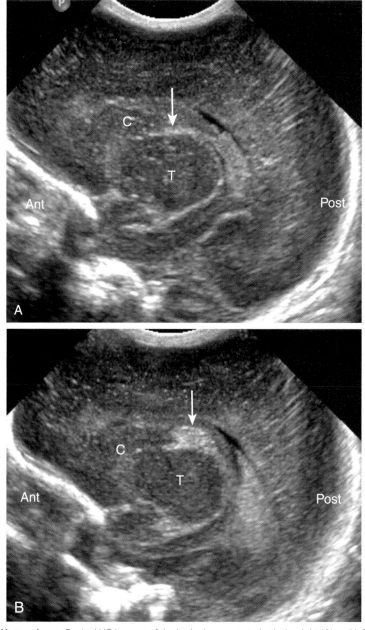

**Fig. 19.8 Germinal Matrix Hemorrhage.** Sagittal US images of the brain demonstrate both the right (A) and left (B) caudothalamic grooves. (A) The normal right caudothalamic groove is depicted as a thin, echogenic line *(arrow)* between the thalamus (T) and caudate (C). (B) On the left side of the brain, globular, echogenic material *(arrow)* located in the caudothalamic groove represents a germinal matrix hemorrhage.

- In the *Barlow test,* the hip is **flexed, internally rotated, and adducted** with posterior pressure on the femoral head. A positive test occurs when a "click" or "clunk" is felt from the **hip dislocating.**
- In infants with a high risk of DDH or abnormal physical examination findings, the morphology of the acetabulum may be assessed by US at 4 to 6 weeks of age while the femoral head epiphysis is still cartilaginous. An **abnormal morphology of the acetabulum** or **frank dislocation** of the femoral head indicates DDH (Fig. 19.9). The Barlow maneuver can also be performed under real-time US to depict any subluxation or dislocation of the hip.

- **Once the epiphysis ossifies**, which occurs at approximately 3 to 4 months of age, **radiographs are needed** for assessment because US cannot penetrate the ossified bone to evaluate the acetabulum.

## Necrotizing Enterocolitis (NEC)

- **Necrotizing enterocolitis** most commonly affects **premature infants** within the first weeks of life. It can be a life-threatening gastrointestinal condition in neonates. The pathophysiology has been postulated to involve the breakdown of the intestinal mucosa, translocation of intestinal bacteria, and an inflammatory response that can lead to **dissection of gas**

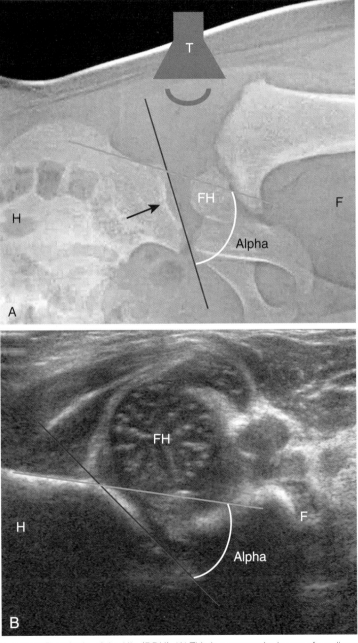

**Fig. 19.9** Evaluating Developmental Dysplasia of the Hip (DDH). (A) This is a composite image of a radiograph on an older infant in order to show the transducer's (T) position relative to the infant as the infant lays on its side during scanning. The femoral head (FH) normally resides in the acetabulum, composed in part by the acetabular roof *(arrow, red line)*. The acetabular roof is contiguous with the lateral border of the ilium *(green line)*. The angle formed by the intersection of the two lines is called the **alpha angle**. The alpha angle is normally **greater** than 55° in a newborn and **greater** than 60° at 4 to 6 weeks of age. (B) A similarly oriented ultrasound image of a younger infant's hip with DDH demonstrates the cartilaginous FH, acetabular roof *(red line)*, and ilium *(green line)*. In DDH, the slope of the acetabular roof *(red line)* is abnormally shallow and steep, which causes the alpha angle to **decrease** and increases the risk of the FH subluxing or dislocating.

into the bowel wall and **portal venous system.** Severe cases of NEC may result in bowel perforation and free intraperitoneal air (see Chapter 27).

- Although **conventional abdominal radiographs** are the **study of choice** for the diagnosis of NEC, US may be complementary.

---

**▶▶ IMPORTANT POINTS**

- Ultrasound can depict **air dissecting into the bowel wall** (intramural gas or ***pneumatosis intestinalis***) (Fig. 19.10), free **intraperitoneal gas**, **bowel wall thickening**, and **portal venous gas** (Fig. 19.11). Small amounts of gas difficult to detect on radiographs may be readily seen on US.

---

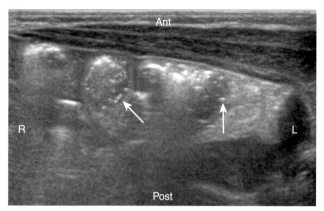

**Fig. 19.10 Pneumatosis Intestinalis.** Ultrasound image of the left upper quadrant in a neonate demonstrates multiple, nondependent echogenic foci *(arrows)* representing gas in the bowel wall consistent with pneumatosis intestinalis from necrotizing enterocolitis.

## Intussusception

- Intussusception occurs when a segment of bowel **telescopes forward** into the lumen of an adjacent bowel loop, causing **bowel obstruction** (Fig. 19.12). In children, intussusception typically occurs between **6 months and 2 years** of age, is most frequently **ileocolic** (i.e., the ileum telescopes into the colon), and is most often **idiopathic** in origin.

- Clinically, it is characterized by vomiting, intermittent and colicky abdominal pain, and passage of blood per rectum, although this classical triad occurs in only about a third of patients.

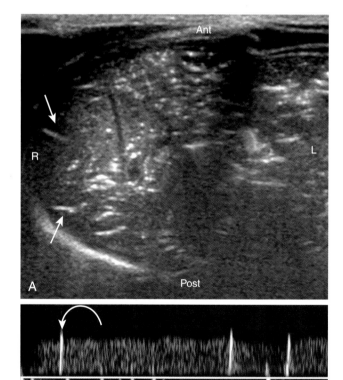

**Fig. 19.11 Portal Venous Gas.** (A) Transverse US of the liver demonstrates multiple linear and branching echogenic foci *(straight arrows)* that extend to the periphery of the liver consistent with portal venous gas. (B) Spectral Doppler interrogation of the main portal vein in the same patient demonstrates characteristic spikes *(curved arrow)* along the spectral waveform due to small air bubbles passing intermittently in the blood flowing through the portal vein.

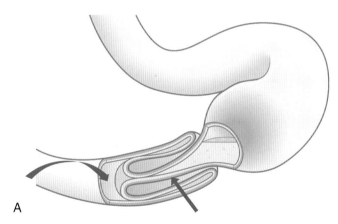

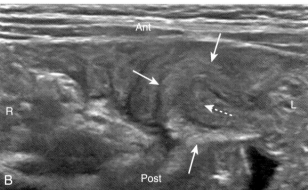

**Fig. 19.12 Intussusception.** (A) The bowel loop that telescopes into another is called the ***intussusceptum (straight blue arrow).*** The bowel loop that receives the telescoping segment is called the ***intussuscipiens (curved blue arrow).*** (B) US image of the left abdomen demonstrating an intussusception of the small bowel including the intussusceptum *(dashed arrow)* and intussuscipiens (solid arrows). The intussusception occurred in the direction of the dotted white arrow.

### ▶ IMPORTANT POINTS

- On a transverse US image, intussusception may display a **target or donut** appearance as a result of the multiple alternating hypoechoic and hyperechoic layers of the bowel walls imaged tightly adjacent to each other. In the sagittal plane, the intussusception might have a **bowel-within-bowel appearance** and may sometimes display the **pseudokidney sign** (Fig. 19.13).

## Hypertrophic Pyloric Stenosis (HPS)

- Hypertrophic pyloric stenosis occurs when there is hypertrophy (thickening) of the gastric pyloric musculature that results in **gastric outlet obstruction.** It typically presents at

**4 to 6 weeks of age** with **nonbilious vomiting** that becomes more **frequent** and **projectile** over time. The enlarged pylorus, called an *olive,* may be palpable in the right upper quadrant or epigastrium in about 60% to 80% of infants.

### ▶ IMPORTANT POINTS

- Ultrasound is the imaging study of choice. On US, **pyloric musculature that is thickened to more than 3 mm** or a **pyloric channel longer than 15 mm** is considered abnormal and indicative of hypertrophic pyloric stenosis (Fig. 19.14).

## POINT-OF-CARE ULTRASOUND

- Ultrasound is increasingly being used at the **point-of-care** or **bedside** to help facilitate diagnoses and direct **management and therapy.** Point-of-care US (sometimes abbreviated *POCUS*) is a highly focused interrogation that quickly determines the presence or absence of a specific pathologic condition. Although extremely useful, **it does not replace detailed, routine sonographic evaluation.** Incidental findings that may be detected during point-of-care US often require follow-up detailed sonography to determine their etiology.

### Focused Assessment with Sonography in Trauma (FAST)

- The **FAST examination** is part of the Advanced Trauma Life Support protocol and is performed simultaneously with other resuscitative measures in the trauma patient.
- The primary goal of the FAST examination is to identify **intraperitoneal bleeding** because the presence of

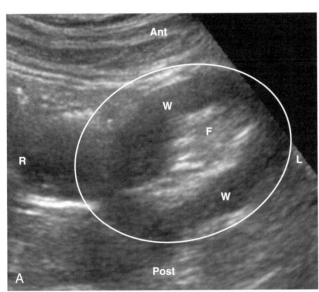

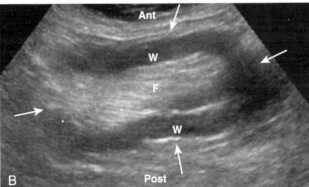

**Fig. 19.13 Intussusception, Transverse and Sagittal Images.** (A) On the transverse image, the intussusception has a **target** or **donut** appearance *(oval)* with the echogenic, mesenteric fat (F) of the intussusceptum in the center surrounded by the hypoechoic, bowel wall (W) of the intussuscipiens. (B) On the sagittal image, the ring of hypoechoic, bowel wall (W) is seen partially encasing the hyperechoic, mesenteric fat (F), creating what is called the **pseudokidney sign** *(arrows)* because of its similar appearance to the sagittal image a normal kidney (see Fig. 18.10).

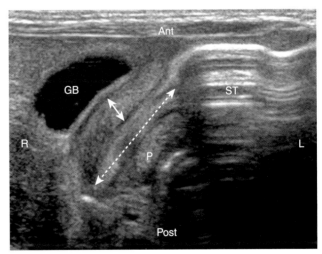

**Fig. 19.14 Hypertrophic Pyloric Stenosis.** Sagittal US of the pylorus (P) in a 2-month-old with projectile vomiting. The stomach (ST) and gallbladder (GB) are also included in the image. The pylorus has a thickened wall *(solid double arrow)* and elongated channel *(dashed double arrow)* consistent with hypertrophic pyloric stenosis.

**hemoperitoneum** in a hemodynamically **unstable patient** will generally lead to **emergent laparotomy.**

- The FAST examination has largely replaced diagnostic peritoneal lavage, but CT still remains much more sensitive for detecting abdominal and thoracic injuries.

> ▶▶ **IMPORTANT POINTS**
>
> - A typical FAST examination involves the **search for blood or fluid in the pericardium and peritoneum.** The peritoneal search focuses on the area between the liver and right kidney and posterior pelvis (between the rectum and bladder in men and between the rectum and uterus in women) as they are the **most dependent portions of the abdominopelvic cavity** when the patient is supine (Fig. 19.15).

## Pleural Effusion

- A pleural effusion is fluid that **accumulates between the visceral and parietal pleura** (see Chapter 7). Although radiographs and CTs are generally used to evaluate the presence of pleural effusions, US can detect **small amounts of pleural fluid** and is increasingly used at the point-of-care.
- Ultrasound can also help to determine whether a radiographic opacity is due to **pleural fluid** and/or **parenchymal lung disease.** In addition, US may be used for **image-guided**

thoracentesis, especially if the amount of fluid is small or the fluid is loculated.

> ▶▶ **IMPORTANT POINTS**
>
> - A simple effusion will be **anechoic** on US and is depicted as a fluid collection just above the diaphragm. The diaphragm appears as a highly echogenic, curvilinear structure that abuts the liver (Fig. 19.16). The presence of **echoes within an effusion** suggests an **exudative effusion**, which may contain pus or blood.

## Pneumothorax

- Ultrasound has become a useful and reliable modality in the diagnosis of pneumothorax. In the trauma patient, US has been shown to be **more sensitive than radiographs** for the diagnosis of **small pneumothoraces.** In the critical care patient, US is especially helpful because small pneumothoraces may be difficult or impossible to visualize radiographically in the supine patient (see Chapter 24).
- In a **supine patient,** air from a pneumothorax will **rise to the most superior** part of the chest that is located **anteriorly** between the **second and fourth intercostal spaces** near the **midclavicular line.**

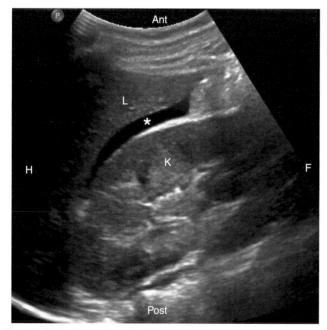

**Fig. 19.15** Ascites. A sagittal image of the right upper quadrant, including the liver (L) and right kidney (K), is shown. A small amount of anechoic fluid *(asterisk)* is present between the liver and kidney, representing ascites in **Morrison's pouch.** Morrison's pouch is the most dependent portion of the peritoneum in the right upper quadrant in the supine position and therefore is one of the most sensitive areas for evaluation of peritoneal fluid.

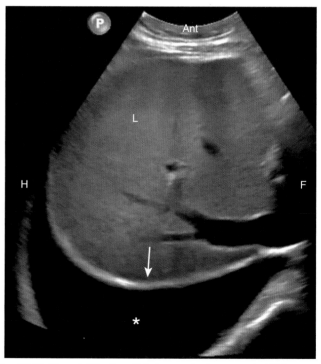

**Fig. 19.16** Pleural Effusion. This is a sagittal, gray-scale US image of the right upper quadrant including the liver (L). Pleural fluid *(asterisk)* is demonstrated as anechoic fluid above the diaphragm, which is depicted as a highly echogenic curvilinear structure *(arrow).*

- Normally the **pleura appears as an echogenic line** deep to and between the ribs (Fig. 19.17). During real-time US, the parietal and visceral pleurae can normally be seen **sliding** across each other as the patient breathes (Video 19.3).

> ### ▶▶ IMPORTANT POINTS
>
> - When a patient has a **pneumothorax**, air in the pleural cavity separates the parietal and visceral pleurae, which **prevents the sliding motion** and results in a **stationary echogenic pleural line** on US (Videos 19.4 and 19.5).

## Pericardial Effusion

- Ultrasound is a useful tool for the bedside diagnosis of pericardial effusions and cardiac tamponade.

> ### ▶▶ IMPORTANT POINTS
>
> - **Pericardial effusions** will appear as **anechoic fluid** collections surrounding the heart (Fig. 19.18 and Video 19.6). Echoes within the fluid would suggest a **hemopericardium.**

- *Cardiac tamponade* occurs when a pericardial effusion prevents blood from filling the **right atrium** and **right ventricle**

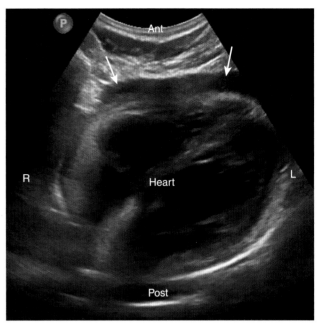

**Fig. 19.18 Pericardial Effusion.** Gray-scale US image demonstrates hypoechoic fluid *(arrows)* around the heart from a pericardial effusion. If a diagnosis of cardiac tamponade is made, emergency drainage of the pericardial fluid by either pericardiocentesis or surgery is the usual course of treatment.

during **diastole.** It can be caused by as little as 50 mL of fluid. Real-time sonography is useful in detecting tamponade by demonstrating complete **collapse of the right atrium or ventricle** or a **flattening or concavity of the right atrial or ventricular wall** during diastole.

## Cardiac Function

- Certain aspects of cardiac function can be quickly assessed at the point-of-care and may be valuable in trauma and critical care patients.
- Bedside US can identify patients with poor cardiac output by allowing estimation of the **left ventricular ejection fraction,** which is the percentage of blood pumped out of the left ventricle during systole. Normally, the **ejection fraction is above 50%.**
- The ejection fraction may be estimated subjectively by **visual evaluation** during real-time US based on a **change in the size** of the left ventricle between end-diastole and end-systole. Severely decreased left ventricular function is present when there is **less than 30% difference** between the size of the left ventricle during end-diastole and end-systole.
  - Other methods of determining ejection fraction involve the use of additional software packages on the US machine that can calculate the left ventricular size during end-diastole and end-systole.
- **Right heart (right ventricular) strain** can also be assessed at the point-of-care. It refers to the presence of right ventricular dysfunction **without** an underlying cardiomyopathy as its cause. It might occur with pulmonary embolism, pulmonary hypertension, or chronic obstructive pulmonary disease.

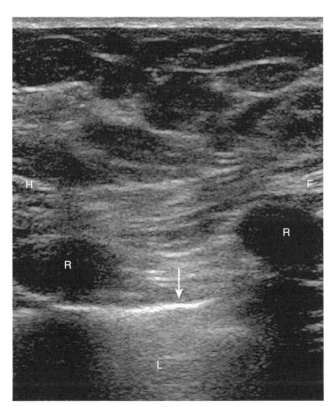

**Fig. 19.17 Normal Pleural Line.** This is a sagittal, gray-scale US image of the chest. The pleura is displayed as a highly echogenic line *(arrow)* between the ribs (R) and lung (L). **Video 19.3** displays the **normal, sliding motion** of the pleural line during respiration. **Video 19.4** demonstrates the **absence** of the sliding motion of the pleural line when a pneumothorax is present.

- Normally the **right ventricle** is **smaller** than the **left ventricle**. Enlargement of the right ventricle to the **same size or larger** than the left ventricle is **abnormal** and indicates right heart strain.

## Central Venous Pressure

- Central venous pressure refers to the **blood pressure in the intrathoracic vena cava** and may be assessed via bedside US.
- Multiple etiologies can cause **elevated** central venous pressure, including heart failure, hypervolemia, massive pulmonary embolism, cardiac tamponade, tension pneumothorax, large pleural effusions, and mechanical ventilation itself. **Decreased** central venous pressure can occur with hypovolemia and shock.
- Because the vena cava is a thin-walled vessel, it normally **expands and contracts with respiration.**
  - During **inspiration**, the vena cava **decreases** in size because the **negative intrathoracic pressure** allows more blood to drain from the vena cava into the right atrium. Conversely, the vena cava **increases** in size during **expiration** as the blood flow out of the vena cava decreases with the **positive intrathoracic pressure.**
  - The inferior vena cava (IVC) typically averages about 2 cm in diameter during the respiratory cycle (in a nonventilated patient). An IVC diameter that is greater than 2 cm throughout the respiratory cycle and collapses **less than 50%** at end-inspiration suggests **elevated** central venous pressure (Fig. 19.19, Video 19.7). An IVC diameter that is less than 2 cm throughout the respiratory cycle and that collapses **more than 50%** at end-expiration suggests **decreased** central venous pressure.

## Ocular Ultrasound

- Ophthalmologic emergencies account for approximately 3% of visits to the emergency department. Because the eye is a superficial, fluid-filled structure, US can be used to assess the internal structures of the eye at the point-of-care, especially if the **eyelid is swollen shut,** preventing direct visualization with an ophthalmoscope.
- Common indications for the performance of ocular US include **eye trauma, sudden decrease or loss of vision, ocular pain,** and **suspected foreign body.**
- The closed eye can be scanned gently with a high-frequency, linear transducer providing high-resolution sonographic images.
- Normal structures that can be visualized during ocular US include the **cornea, anterior chamber, iris and ciliary body, lens, vitreous chamber, retina,** and **optic nerve** (Fig. 19.20).
- Pathologic conditions in the orbit that can be diagnosed with point-of-care ocular US include globe perforation, retinal detachment, lens dislocation, vitreous hemorrhage, intraocular foreign body, and retrobulbar hematoma.

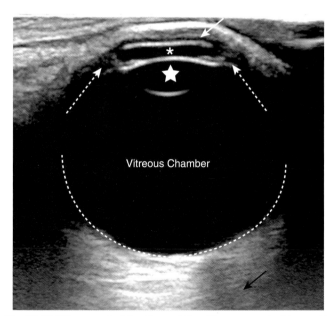

**Fig. 19.20** Ultrasound of the Normal Eye. The **cornea** *(solid arrow)* is depicted as a thin echogenic line just beneath the eyelid. The **anterior chamber** *(asterisk)* is an anechoic, fluid-filled space posterior to the cornea. The **lens** *(star)* is an ovoid, anechoic structure between the echogenic iris and ciliary body *(dashed arrows)*. The **vitreous chamber** is the large fluid-filled anechoic space posterior to the lens. The **retina** *(curved dashed line)* is located along the periphery of the vitreous chamber and cannot be differentiated from the choroidal layers on US. The **optic nerve** *(black arrow)* is located posterior to the globe.

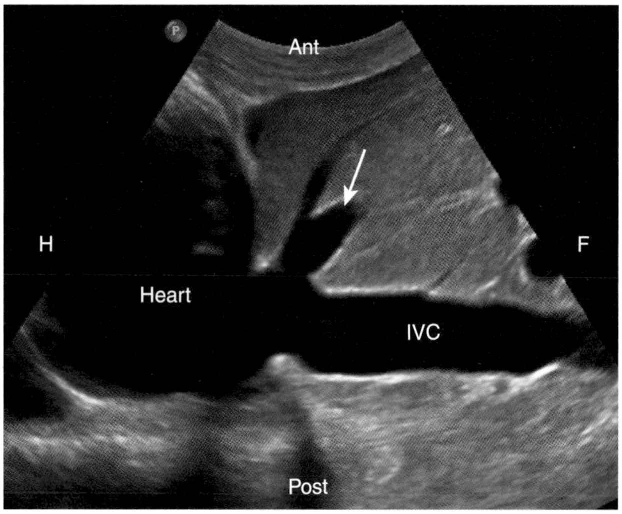

**Fig. 19.19** Central Venous Pressure Elevation. This is a sagittal, grayscale US image of the inferior vena cava (IVC), heart, and hepatic veins *(arrow)* obtained at end-inspiration in a patient with congestive heart failure. The IVC measured 2.5 cm at end-inspiration in this patient, which is consistent with an elevated central venous pressure.

## CASE QUIZ 19 ANSWER

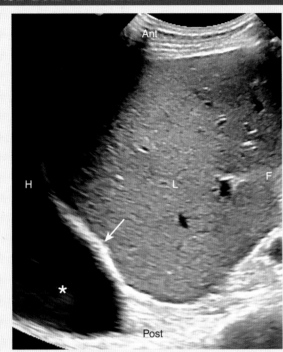

The right hemidiaphragm is depicted by the highly echogenic white line *(arrow).* The liver (L) lies below it and there is anechoic fluid *(asterisk)* **above** the hemidiaphragm in the posterior costophrenic recess of the pleural space. This is the expected location for a **pleural effusion** in a supine patient. *Ant,* Anterior; *F,* foot; *H,* head; *L,* liver; *Post,* posterior.

## 🏠 TAKE HOME POINTS

- **Vascular ultrasound** uses gray-scale and Doppler ultrasonography to display the morphologic appearance of vessels and the direction and velocity of blood flow simultaneously.
- Significant **arterial narrowing** typically causes an elevation in blood flow velocities. Ultrasound is used to evaluate for carotid artery stenosis and for peripheral vascular disease, especially in the lower extremities.
- A **pseudoaneurysm** is formed when there is a rupture or injury to the arterial wall, but the blood leaking through the rupture is confined by an intact, thin outer layer of the arterial wall or the surrounding perivascular tissues. Pseudoaneurysms are at high risk of further rupture and bleeding.
- Sonographic evaluation of **deep venous thrombosis** is based on the principle that veins have thin, elastic walls that are easily compressible by the US probe. Thrombus in a vein will prevent it from being easily compressed. The echogenic thrombus itself may also be seen on gray-scale US imaging.
- The **germinal matrix** has a rich network of microscopic vessels that are at risk of bleeding in the premature infant. Germinal matrix hemorrhages appear as echogenic material in the caudothalamic groove and can extend into the ventricle and brain parenchyma with increasing morbidity and mortality.
- **Developmental dysplasia of the hip** can be evaluated on US at 4 to 6 weeks of age during which time the femoral head epiphysis is cartilaginous. Once the epiphysis ossifies, radiographs are needed to assess the acetabular morphology and femoral head location.
- **Necrotizing enterocolitis** is a life-threatening gastrointestinal condition in neonates that can result in bowel perforation. Ultrasound may be complementary to radiographs in the diagnosis of necrotizing enterocolitis and has the ability to visualize pneumatosis intestinalis, free intraperitoneal air, portal venous gas, and bowel wall thickening.
- **Intussusception** typically occurs between 6 months and 2 years of age and is most frequently ileocolic and idiopathic. Ultrasound may demonstrate a bowel-within-bowel (pseudokidney) appearance or a target or donut appearance.

- **Hypertrophic pyloric stenosis** results in gastric outlet obstruction, leading to nonbilious projectile vomiting. The abnormally thickened pyloric musculature and elongated pyloric channel may be depicted on US.
- **Point-of-care ultrasound** is a highly focused interrogation that can quickly determine the presence or absence of a specific pathologic condition, facilitating treatment or often suggesting further, more extensive studies for evaluation.
- The **focused assessment with sonography in trauma (FAST) examination** is used in the trauma patient to detect intraperitoneal bleeding, especially in those hemodynamically unstable and unable to undergo more sensitive CT or US imaging.
- Ultrasound can detect a small amount of **pleural fluid** and can be used to guide thoracentesis.
- In the supine patient, **pneumothoraces** rise to the most superior part of the chest. Normally, the parietal and visceral pleurae can be seen sliding across each other on real-time US, but a pneumothorax prevents that sliding motion from occurring.
- **Pericardial effusions** are readily visible on US as hypoechoic or anechoic fluid around the heart. **Cardiac tamponade** occurs when the pericardial fluid prevents adequate filling of the right atrium and right ventricle.
- Cardiac function, including an estimate of the **left ventricular ejection fraction,** can be assessed at the bedside using US. Normally, the ejection fraction is above 50%.
- An elevated or decreased **central venous pressure** is depicted on US by the caliber of the inferior vena cava during inspiration and expiration. The normal inferior vena cava is usually around 2 cm throughout the respiratory cycle.
- As a superficial, fluid-filled structure, the **eye** is readily assessed by US, especially if the eyelid is swollen closed preventing direct visualization. Point-of-care ocular US can be used to diagnose globe perforation, retinal detachment, lens dislocation, vitreous hemorrhage, foreign bodies, and retrobulbar hematoma.

🛜 Additional content is available online including chapters on Nuclear Medicine, Artificial Intelligence, Radiation Dose and Safety, an Early History of Radiology, and a compendium of 200 Diagnostic Radiology Signs.

# 20

# Magnetic Resonance Imaging: Understanding the Principles and Recognizing the Basics

*Daniel J. Kowal, MD*

- **Magnetic resonance imaging (MRI)** is a diagnostic modality capable of producing both anatomic and physiologic data that utilizes the molecular composition of tissues, especially water, to generate images with **extraordinary contrast** between soft tissues, surpassing the sensitivity of other imaging modalities.
- To achieve this **sensitivity**, MRI studies are designed using specific **scanning protocols** based on the clinical question that allows the signal from certain tissues to be maximized while minimizing competing signal from other tissues.
- Some understanding of these protocols is necessary to comprehend how these contrast differences are generated and then to recognize what imaging protocol was used in order to correctly interpret the images.

## HOW MRI WORKS

- MRI uses a **very strong magnetic field** to manipulate the electromagnetic activity of atomic nuclei in a way that releases energy in the form of **radiofrequency signals**, which are recorded by the scanner's **receiving coils** and then computer-processed to form an image.
  - **Clinical MRI scanners** utilize the properties of **hydrogen nuclei** (which contain one proton) due to their abundance in the human body.
- Each proton has a **positive electrical charge**, and because protons also have a *spin*, this charge is **constantly moving.** You might remember that a **moving electrical charge** is also an **electrical current**, and because an electrical current

### CASE QUIZ 20 QUESTION

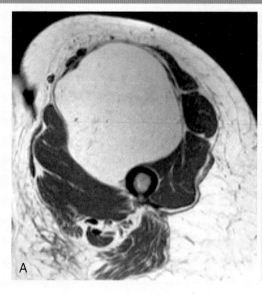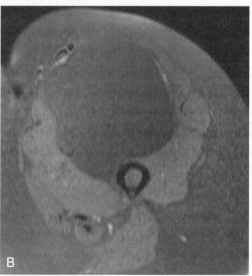

This patient is a 61-year-old female who presented with a large mass in her anterior left thigh that could not be fully characterized by ultrasound. These are both axial T1-weighted images, but what additional technique was added to the sequence in (B), and how does that help us make the diagnosis? The answer is at the end of this chapter.

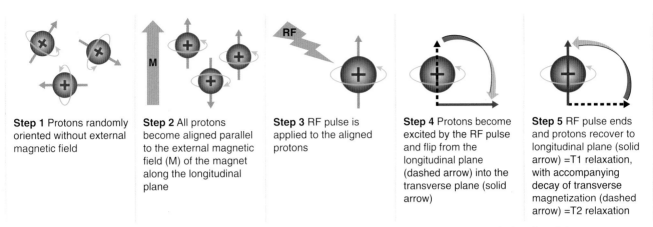

**Step 1** Protons randomly oriented without external magnetic field

**Step 2** All protons become aligned parallel to the external magnetic field (M) of the magnet along the longitudinal plane

**Step 3** RF pulse is applied to the aligned protons

**Step 4** Protons become excited by the RF pulse and flip from the longitudinal plane (dashed arrow) into the transverse plane (solid arrow)

**Step 5** RF pulse ends and protons recover to longitudinal plane (solid arrow) =T1 relaxation, with accompanying decay of transverse magnetization (dashed arrow) =T2 relaxation

**Fig. 20.1 Relaxing on the Job.** This graphic explains the various steps in the excitation and relaxation of the hydrogen protons in producing the T1 and T2 relaxation times.

induces a **magnetic field,** each proton has its own small magnetic field (called a *magnetic moment*).

- When a patient enters an MRI scanner, the mini-magnet protons all align with the more powerful external magnetic field of the MRI magnet. Most of these protons will point **parallel to the field** and others point **antiparallel** to the field, but they will all align with the external magnetic field of the MRI.
- Protons do not like to be couch potatoes, so they *precess* (i.e., **wobble** like a spinning top) along the magnetic field lines of the MRI (Fig. 20.1).
- We will return to our little wobbling protons in a (magnetic) moment.

# HARDWARE THAT MAKES UP AN MRI SCANNER

## Main Magnet

- The main magnet in an MR scanner is usually a *superconducting magnet.*
- Superconducting magnets contain a conducting coil that is cooled down to **superconducting temperatures** (4° K or −269° C) in order to carry the current. At temperatures that low (close to absolute zero), **resistance to the flow of electricity in the conductor practically disappears.**

### ▶ IMPORTANT POINTS

- An electric current sent once through this ultra-cold conducting material will **flow continuously** and create a **permanent** magnetic field. The **main magnet** in an MRI scanner is **always "on"** whether there is a patient present or not.

- Most scanners today have a **magnetic *field strength*** between **0.5 and 3 Tesla (T).** *Open MRI scanners,* those that do not completely encircle the patient in the scanning circle, have **lower field strengths of 0.2−1.0 T, which results in** decreased image quality compared to closed-bore MRI. By comparison, the earth's magnetic field is only about **50 microTesla.**

## Coils

- The *coils* placed within the magnet are an important part of the MRI scanner. These coils are responsible for either **transmitting** the *radiofrequency (RF) pulses* (**transmitter coils**) that excite the protons, or **receiving** the signal (or *echo*) given off by these excited protons (**receiver coils**) (Fig. 20.2).

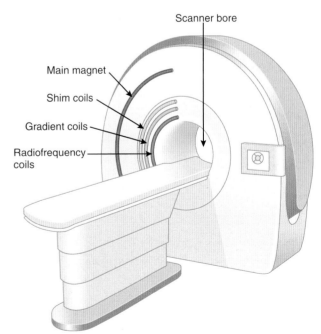

Scanner bore

Main magnet

Shim coils

Gradient coils

Radiofrequency coils

**Fig. 20.2 Scanner Schematic.** The **main magnet** produces the intense and stable magnetic field around the patient. **Shim coils** help make the magnetic field more homogeneous. The **gradient coils** are lower strength than the main magnetic field and produce a variable field adjusted to different body parts. **Radiofrequency coils** direct a pulse toward the area to be examined and are also adjusted for different body parts. The **scanner bore** is the horizontal tube in which the patient rests. The actual magnets reside inside the gantry housing.

- These coils are subjected to strong electrical currents and exist within a strong magnetic field that produces the repetitive "knocking" sound during an MRI scan.

## Computer

- A computer dedicated to the MRI scanner processes the radiofrequency signals obtained by the receiver coils and converts them into an image.

## WHAT HAPPENS ONCE SCANNING BEGINS

- When the patient is placed in the scanner magnet, recall that the spinning protons in the patient will have already **aligned** parallel or antiparallel to the magnetic field of the main magnet.
- Then, the **transmitter coils** send a short (measured in milliseconds) electromagnetic pulse—the **radiofrequency (RF) pulse.**
- This radiofrequency pulse is sent at a particular frequency that **changes the orientation** of the protons.
- When the **RF pulse is turned off,** the displaced protons *relax and realign* with the main magnetic field, and **energy** subsequently **released in** the **form of radiofrequency signals** (the *echo*) is **detected** by the **receiver coils.**

> ▶ **IMPORTANT POINTS**
>
> - The **times** it takes for this *recovery* and *decay* to occur and the **echo** to be generated are called **T1** and **T2.**

- **T1 relaxation** (or *recovery*) is the time it takes for the tissue to recover to its **longitudinal state** (parallel to the magnetic field), i.e., the time before the RF pulse was administered (see Fig. 20.1).
- **T2 relaxation** (or *decay*) is the time it takes for the tissue to regain its **transverse orientation** (perpendicular to the magnetic field) before the RF pulse was administered.
- **In summary,** as soon as the RF pulse stops, relaxation begins, and the spinning nuclei release energy that is subsequently detected by the receiver coil and ultimately used to produce an image.

## Pulse Sequences

- *Pulse sequences* consist of a set of **imaging parameters** determined in advance by protocols for **specific diseases** and **body parts** and then preselected by the MRI technologist at the computer control console. They are based on the patient's clinical issue. A particular **imaging protocol** (e.g., a routine MRI brain protocol) **consists of a series of multiple pulse sequences,** which determine the way different tissues will subsequently appear. A pulse sequence can last between 20 seconds to 15 minutes.

> ▶ **IMPORTANT POINTS**
>
> - There are **two main pulse sequences: *spin echo (SE)* and *gradient-recalled echo (GRE)*.** Spin echo sequences have a higher signal-to-noise ratio, which is desirable, but gradient-recalled echo sequences are faster sequences preferred for rapid imaging techniques. **All of the pulse sequences used in MRI scanning are based on these two pulse sequences.**

- TR and TE
  - These parameters are set by the MRI operator at the console prior to scanning and determine how the image is *weighted.*
  - TR is the *repetition time* **between two RF pulses,** and it influences the amount of **T1 weighting.**
    - Pulse sequences that feature a **short TR** (meaning a short amount of time between the RF pulses) will create what is called a *T1-weighted image.*
  - TE is the *echo time* **between a pulse and its resultant echo,** and it influences the amount of **T2 weighting.**
    - Pulse sequences that feature a **long TE** (meaning a long amount of time between the RF pulse and the echo) will create what is called a *T2-weighted image.*

## HOW TO IDENTIFY A T1-WEIGHTED OR T2-WEIGHTED IMAGE

- **Different tissues** have different T1 (recovery) and T2 (decay) values, which is why fat, muscle, and bone, for example, will appear differently from each other. But it is also important to remember that the **same tissue** may have **different appearances** on different pulse sequences, and it is fundamental to understand **how** the image was obtained in order to interpret it correctly.
- **Tissues** that have a **short T1** will be **bright.**
- **Tissues** with a **long T2** will be **bright.**
- **Bright** translates into **whiter** or having *increased signal intensity* on MRI scans. **Dark** translates into **blacker** or having *decreased signal intensity* on MRI.

> ▶ **IMPORTANT POINTS**
>
> - A key point is that **water** will be **dark** on **T1-weighted images** and **bright** on **T2-weighted images. Water is T1-dark and T2-bright.**
> - A "bright" way to remember this fact is that the number 2 is both in **$H_2O$ (water)** and **T2-weighted image.**
>   - Therefore, when looking at any MR image, **first try to find something you know is fluid (water),** such as the **CSF in the ventricles** and **spinal canal** or **urine** in the bladder, for example.
>   - If the fluid is **dark,** then you are probably looking at a **T1-weighted sequence** (Fig. 20.3A).
>   - If the fluid is **bright,** then chances are you are looking at a **T2-weighted sequence** (Fig. 20.3B).

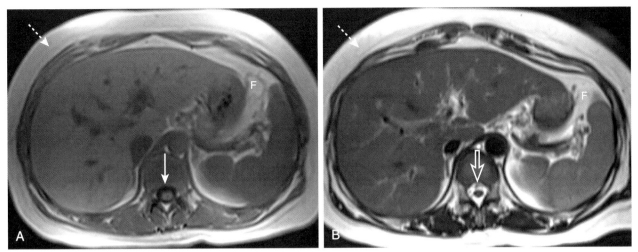

**Fig. 20.3** Normal T1-Weighted and T2-Weighted Axial Images of the Abdomen. Because cerebrospinal fluid surrounding the cord is similar to water, it appears **dark** on the **T1-weighted image** (A) *(solid arrow)* and **bright** on the **T2-weighted image** (B) *(open arrow)*. Subcutaneous fat *(dashed arrows)* and intraabdominal fat (F) are bright on both T1- and T2-weighted images.

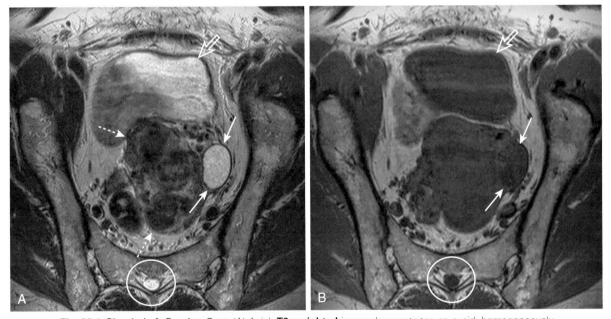

**Fig. 20.4** Simple Left Ovarian Cyst. (A) Axial, **T2-weighted** image demonstrates an ovoid, homogeneously bright lesion in the left ovary *(solid arrows)* adjacent to a fibroid uterus *(dashed arrows)*. Note that urine in the bladder *(open arrow)* and CSF in the spinal canal *(white circle)* are both bright, which helps us identify this image as a T2-weighted image. (B) Axial, **T1-weighted** image shows that this left ovarian lesion is dark *(solid arrows)* and therefore consistent with simple fluid. Urine in the bladder *(open arrow)* and CSF in the spinal canal *(circle)* are also dark. MRI is an excellent tool for evaluating the tissue characteristics of both abdominal and pelvic masses.

- Understanding the appearance of **water** and **fat** on MRI
  - Just like water elsewhere in the body, **simple cysts** containing water that originate in the kidneys, liver, ovaries, and other organs will be **dark** on T1-weighted images and **bright** on T2-weighted images (Fig. 20.4), as will the water component in **cystic tumors** or solid tumors with **cystic degeneration** (Fig. 20.5).
- **Edema** will also behave like water, and when present can help identify trauma (Fig. 20.6), tumoral edema (see Fig. 20.5), infarction, infection, and inflammation.

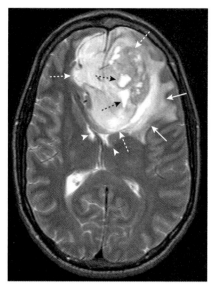

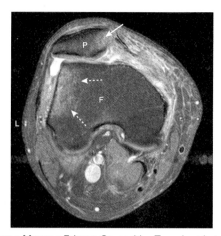

**Fig. 20.6** Bone Marrow Edema Caused by Transient Lateral Patellar Dislocation. Axial, proton-density, fat-saturated image (a T2-like sequence) demonstrates bright bone marrow edema involving the lateral (L) femoral (F) condyle *(dashed arrows)* and medial aspect of the patella (P) *(solid arrow)*. This edema pattern helps us make the diagnosis of bony contusion from recent lateral patellar dislocation causing the patella to strike the femur. MRI is the most sensitive and specific imaging modality for the detection of bone marrow edema.

**Fig. 20.5** Glioblastoma Multiforme with Surrounding Edema. Axial, T2-weighted image demonstrates bright vasogenic-type edema *(solid white arrows)* surrounding a large, lobulated frontal lobe mass *(dashed white arrows)* representing glioblastoma multiforme, an aggressive malignant brain tumor. There are a few bright areas of cystic degeneration *(dashed black arrows)* within this mass. Mass effect compresses the frontal horns of the lateral ventricles *(arrowheads)*. Because of its superior tissue contrast resolution, MRI is generally preferred to CT to determine the extent of tumor and to assist in neurosurgical planning. Also, detection of edema can aid clinicians in understanding and treating the patient's symptoms.

- **Unlike** water, **fat** will be **bright** on **both T1-weighted and T2-weighted images.**
- This bright fat signal can be seen normally in subcutaneous and intraabdominal fat (see Fig. 20.3), fat within yellow bone marrow, and abnormally in fat-containing tumors.

- **Suppression**
  - A useful feature of MRI is the ability to **cancel out** or *suppress* the signal from certain tissues selectively, thus making that tissue look **dark** on the image, and making other structures and pathology more conspicuous.
  - The body tissue that is most **often suppressed** is **fat.**
  - Although **fat** is normally bright on T1-weighted and T2-weighted images, **it can be made to appear dark on fat-suppressed images** (Fig. 20.7).

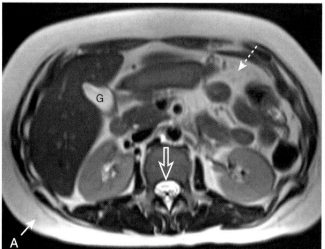

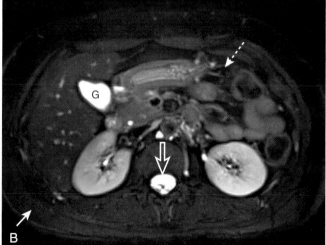

**Fig. 20.7** Normal T2-weighted Axial Images of the Abdomen without and with Fat Suppression. (A) We can tell that this is a **T2-weighted** image because the CSF in the spinal canal is bright *(open arrow)*. When there is **no fat suppression**, subcutaneous fat *(solid arrow)* and intraabdominal fat *(dashed arrow)* are normally bright. (B) With the addition of **fat suppression**, the fat-containing areas become dark. Note also that fluid-containing structures like the gallbladder (G) and CSF *(open arrow)* become even brighter and more conspicuous when the surrounding fat is suppressed, a helpful feature that also improves detection of pathologic fluid or edema.

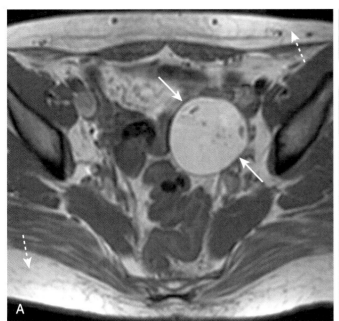

**Fig. 20.8 Fat in an Ovarian Dermoid Cyst.** (A) Axial **T1-weighted** image of the pelvis shows a bright, rounded left ovarian mass *(solid arrows)* in a female patient. (B) Axial **T1-weighted, fat-suppressed** image demonstrates that this bright signal is now dark indicating a fat-containing mass *(solid arrows)*. This appearance is highly specific for and diagnostic of a ***dermoid cyst,*** also known as a mature cystic teratoma, the most common ovarian neoplasm. Note that the fat signal in the dermoid cyst behaves similarly to the subcutaneous fat *(dashed arrows)*.

- This feature is useful when attempting to identify or characterize fat-containing lesions such as **lipomas, ovarian dermoid cysts, adrenal myelolipomas,** and **liposarcomas,** as they will appear to change from **bright** on the **non-fat-suppressed** images to **dark** on the **fat-suppressed images** (Fig. 20.8).
- Fat suppression is **also essential** for evaluation of tissues **after the administration of gadolinium contrast.**
- In addition to fat, certain tissues and structures are also typically **bright on T1-weighted images,** but **unlike fat** will **remain bright** on fat-suppressed images. Examples include:
  - **Protein-rich fluid:** proteinaceous, nonsimple cysts, and proteinaceous cystic tumors
  - **Melanin,** e.g., melanoma (Fig. 20.9)
  - **Gadolinium and other paramagnetic substances (manganese, copper)**
- **Hemorrhage** is unique in that its degree of brightness on MRI depends on its **age.**
  - On T1-weighted images, hemorrhage will be bright when it is **subacute** (Fig. 20.10A).
  - On T2-weighted images, hemorrhage will be bright when it is **hyperacute** or **subacute** (Fig. 20.10B).

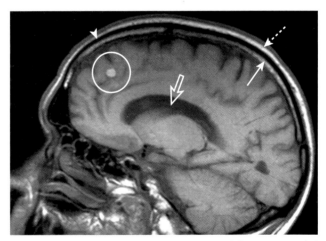

**Fig. 20.9 Metastatic Melanoma.** Sagittal, **T1-weighted** image of the brain demonstrates a bright mass *(circle)* in the frontal lobe representing metastatic melanoma. This appearance is not specific for melanoma, as a hemorrhagic brain metastasis could also be T1-bright. The outer cortical bone of the skull creates a signal void and appears dark *(arrowhead)*, but notice that both the fatty yellow bone marrow of the inner skull *(solid arrow)* and the overlying subcutaneous fat of the scalp *(dashed arrow)* are bright. We can tell that this is a T1-weighted image because the CSF in the lateral ventricles is dark *(open arrow)*.

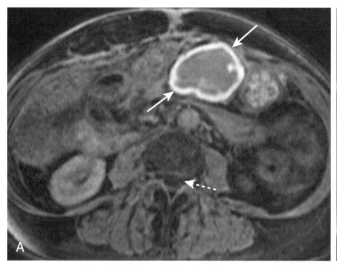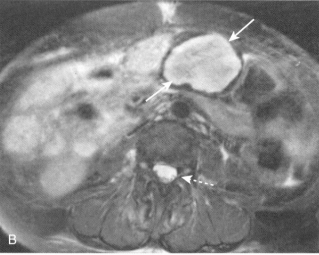

**Fig. 20.10** Intraabdominal hematoma. (A) Axial, **T1-weighted, fat-suppressed** image demonstrates an anterior abdominal mass with a bright rim *(solid arrows)*. We can tell that this is a T1-weighted image because the CSF in the spinal canal is dark *(dashed arrow)*. (B) Axial, **T2-weighted, fat-suppressed** image demonstrates that the mass has a corresponding bright rim *(solid arrows)*. Note that the bright CSF signal allows us to recognize this image as a T2-weighted image *(dashed arrow)*. On CT scan, it was unclear if this mass represented a hematoma or recurrent malignancy, but on MRI this combination of T1 and T2 rim brightness helps us make the diagnosis of subacute hematoma. The central part of the hematoma has different signal due to the presence of fluid mixing with various states of hemoglobin.

- Notice that **both fat and subacute hemorrhage will be T1-bright and T2-bright.**
- A summary of T1 and T2 brightness is shown in Table 20.1.
- There are many other pulse sequences besides T1-weighted and T2-weighted images that typically comprise a particular MRI scan protocol, such as *diffusion-weighted images (DWI), proton density–weighted images,* and an entire alphabet soup of catchy acronyms like **ADC, STIR, FLAIR, TOF, etc.**
- *Functional MRI (fMRI)* correlates the brain's changing **blood flow** requirements with changes in **neural activity** and translates them into differences in the MRI signal. It is being increasingly used to map neural activity in the brain, although it remains most commonly utilized in research as opposed to the clinical setting.

## TABLE 20.1  What Is Bright on MRI?

| Bright on T1-weighted Image | Bright on T2-weighted Image |
| --- | --- |
| • Fat | • Fat |
| • Hemorrhage (subacute) | • Hemorrhage (hyperacute and subacute) |
| • Protein-rich fluid (proteinaceous cysts, proteinaceous cystic tumors) | • Water (simple cysts, cystic tumors) |
| • Melanin | • Edema (trauma, tumoral edema, infarction, infection, and inflammation) |
| • Paramagnetic substances (gadolinium, manganese, copper) | |

## MRI CONTRAST

- *Gadolinium* is the most common intravenous contrast agent used in clinical MRI imaging.
  - Gadolinium is a **rare-earth, heavy-metal ion** that is chelated to different compounds to form MRI contrast agents. When chelated to an acid known as DOTA, it forms *gadoterate meglumine,* also known as the commonly used macrocyclic-structured contrast agent *Dotarem.*
- Gadolinium is **used in the same way that iodinated contrast media is used in CT.** It can be injected either by an intravascular or intraarticular route.
- After intravenous injection, gadolinium enters the blood pool, enhances organ parenchyma, and then is **excreted by the kidneys** via glomerular filtration.
  - Other special types of gadolinium-based contrast agents have a component of biliary excretion.
- **Gadolinium's effect is to shorten the T1 relaxation times** of hydrogen nuclei (and to a lesser extent also shorten T2).
- **T1 shortening will cause a brighter signal on T1-weighted images** than the same images without gadolinium, and it is for this reason that **images obtained after gadolinium administration are usually T1-weighted** to take advantage of this effect.
- Remember that fat is bright on T1 even before the administration of gadolinium. To increase detection of contrast enhancement in areas surrounded by fat, the precontrast and postcontrast images are typically fat suppressed

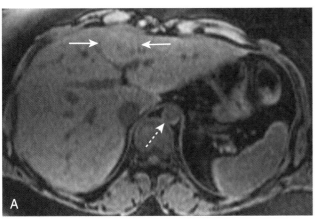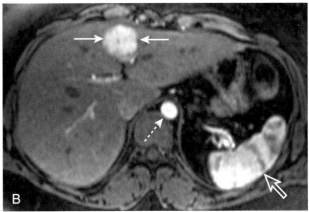

Fig. 20.11 Enhancing Hepatic Mass Following the Administration of Intravenous Gadolinium. (A) **T1-weighted**, fat-suppressed, **noncontrast** image shows a subtle mass in the left hepatic lobe *(solid arrows)*, isointense to the surrounding liver. The aorta *(dashed arrow)* is relatively dark, a clue that intravenous contrast has not been administered. (B) **T1-weighted**, fat-suppressed, **postgadolinium** image shows a now robustly enhancing mass. This example highlights how intravenous contrast can make masses much more visible on MRI, and in this case allows us to make the diagnosis of ***focal nodular hyperplasia,*** the second most common benign liver tumor after cavernous hemangioma. Note also how the aorta *(dashed arrow)* brightly enhances with gadolinium, and the spleen *(open arrow)* demonstrates characteristic heterogeneous enhancement on this early contrast-enhanced image.

(meaning darkened) to enhance the effect of the gadolinium (Fig. 20.11).

> ## ⓘ IMPORTANT POINTS
>
> - Structures that become **bright on postgadolinium images are typically vascular** (such as tumors) (see Fig. 20.11) or **inflammatory** and are described as ***enhancing.***

# MRI SAFETY ISSUES

## Claustrophobia

- Compared with CT scans, the MRI bore is a narrower, more confined space than the CT gantry, and MRI examinations have a longer scan time. Patients can therefore occasionally suffer such extreme claustrophobia in the small confines of the MR scanner that **they will be unable to begin or complete** the study. Pretreatment with sedatives may help in the appropriate clinical situation.
- Many manufacturers now produce MRI units with a larger, 70 cm opening (compared to the traditional 60 cm) known as *wide-bore MRI,* providing more room and comfort for patients while maintaining image quality.
- Alternatively, the patient can be scanned in an *open magnet* **(i.e., open on three to four sides),** which is even less confining. The trade-off, however, is that open magnets, in general, have lower magnetic field strengths and poorer spatial resolution.

## Ferromagnetic Objects

- Any ferromagnetic object inside the patient **can be moved** by the magnetic field of the MR scanner and potentially damage adjacent tissues. Such internal ferromagnetic objects also hold the potential to be **heated and cause burns** to surrounding tissues.

> ## ⓘ IMPORTANT POINTS
>
> - **Ferromagnetic objects inserted in a location where motion of the object may be harmful to the patient represent an absolute contraindication to MR imaging.** These objects can include medically inserted items such as cerebral aneurysm repair clips, vascular clips, and surgical staples. Many vascular clips and staples are now manufactured to be MRI compatible.

- Some **foreign bodies, such as bullets, shrapnel,** and **metal in the eyes** (as can sometimes be found in metal workers) can also be ferromagnetic.
  - Patients who have a history of possible metallic foreign bodies in the eyes must have conventional orbital radiographs before undergoing an MRI and, if metal is present, an alternative means of imaging should be utilized.
- Ferromagnetic objects **outside** of the patient, such as **oxygen tanks, scissors, scalpels,** and **metallic tools,** also pose a risk to the patient as **they could become airborne** once they enter the magnetic field and for this reason are strictly forbidden in the MRI scanning room.

| TABLE 20.2 | Is That Device MRI Compatible? |
|---|---|
| **Device Label** | **Meaning** |
| **MRI safe** | An item poses no known hazards in any MRI environment (e.g., plastic tubing) |
| **MRI conditional** | The item is safe under predetermined conditions in some MRI environments (e.g., up to a certain field strength such as 3 Tesla) |
| **MRI unsafe** | An item that is known to pose hazards in all MRI environments (e.g., a pair of ferromagnetic scissors) |

**Source:** American Society for Testing and Materials (ASTM) International, Designation: F2503-05. *Standard Practice for Marking Medical Devices and Other Items for Safety in the Magnetic Resonance Environment.* West Conshohocken, PA: ASTM International; 2005.

- The current terminology applied to identifying the safety of devices and whether they can enter an MRI environment is shown in Table 20.2.

## Mechanical or Electrical Devices

- MRI cannot usually be performed in patients who have **pacemakers, pain stimulator implants, insulin pumps,** other **implantable drug infusion pumps,** and **cochlear implants.** Exceptions include devices specifically engineered as MRI conditional, such as newer FDA-approved types of pacemakers designed to safely undergo MRI.

## Pregnant Patients

- Unlike CT and plain radiography, MRI uses no ionizing radiation making it more suitable for use on younger or pregnant patients. Although there are no known biologic risks associated with MR imaging in adults, the effects of MRI on the fetus are not definitely known.
- Current data yields no evidence of definite harmful effects on the developing fetus using MRI with a field strength of 1.5 T or 3 T. Therefore, the American College of Radiology states that pregnant patients **can** undergo MRI scans at any stage of pregnancy if it is decided that the risk-benefit ratio to the patient weighs in favor of performing the study (Fig. 20.12).
- **Gadolinium is not recommended in pregnant patients,** as gadolinium crosses the placenta, is subsequently excreted by the fetal kidneys, and its effects on the fetus are not known.

## Nephrogenic Systemic Fibrosis

- In patients with renal insufficiency, gadolinium has been associated with a rare, painful, debilitating, and sometimes fatal disease called *nephrogenic systemic fibrosis (NSF).*
- NSF produces fibrosis of skin, eyes, joints, and internal organs resembling scleroderma.

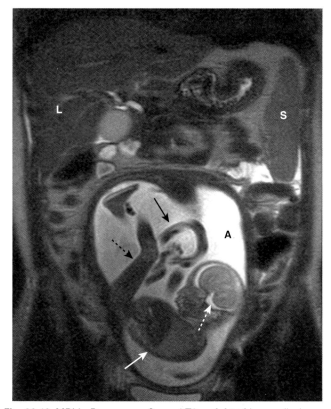

**Fig. 20.12 MRI in Pregnancy.** Coronal **T2-weighted** image displays an intrauterine pregnancy. The maternal liver (L) and spleen (S) are partially imaged. The bright amniotic fluid (A) and fetal CSF *(dashed white arrow)* help us to recognize this image as a T2-weighted image. The fetal body *(solid white arrow)* and leg *(dashed black arrow)* can be seen clearly. The umbilical cord *(solid black arrow)* is partially visualized.

- Patients with **end-stage or severe chronic kidney disease,** especially those on dialysis, were thought to be at the **greatest risk.**
  - However, the latest guidelines indicate that the now more-commonly used gadolinium-based contrast agents (known as group II agents) have negligible if any risk of NSF and can even be administered to patients with end-stage renal disease on dialysis.
- It has been discovered that gadolinium can deposit in brain tissue, particularly in patients that have received multiple doses of gadolinium-based contrast agents. The significance of this deposition is being actively investigated, but there is currently no known health risk or neurotoxicity associated with this phenomenon.

## DIAGNOSTIC APPLICATIONS OF MRI

- Some of the many clinical uses of MRI are outlined in Table 20.3. The chapters in which some of the diseases are discussed in greater detail are indicated.

## TABLE 20.3   Diagnostic Applications of MRI

| System | Organ | Diseases |
|---|---|---|
| **Musculoskeletal** | Evaluate bone marrow, menisci, tendons, muscles | Meniscal tears; ligamentous and tendon injuries; contusions |
| | Bones | Occult or stress fractures |
| | Osteomyelitis | High negative predictive value if normal |
| | Spine **(see Chapter 22)** | Disk disease and marrow infiltration; differentiating scarring from prior surgery from new disease; evaluating spinal cord |
| **Neurologic** | Brain **(see Chapter 26)** | Ideal for studying brain, especially posterior fossa; tumor, infarction, hemorrhage; multiple sclerosis |
| | Peripheral nerves | Impingement; injury |
| **GI** | Liver **(see Chapter 17)** | Characterize liver lesions; detect small lesions; cysts, hemangiomas; hepatocellular carcinoma; focal nodular hyperplasia; fatty infiltration; hemochromatosis |
| | Biliary system **(see Chapter 17)** | Magnetic resonance cholangiopancreatography for ductal dilatation, choledocholithiasis, strictures |
| | Small and large bowel | MR enterography; appendicitis in pregnant females |
| **Endocrine/ reproductive** | Adrenal glands | Adenomas; adrenal hemorrhage |
| | Female pelvis | Anatomy of uterus and ovaries; leiomyomas; adenomyosis; ovarian dermoid cysts; endometriosis; hydrosalpinx; staging of cervical and endometrial carcinoma |
| | Male pelvis | Staging of rectal, bladder, and prostate carcinoma |
| **GU** | Kidneys | Renal masses; cysts versus tumors |

## CASE QUIZ 20 ANSWER

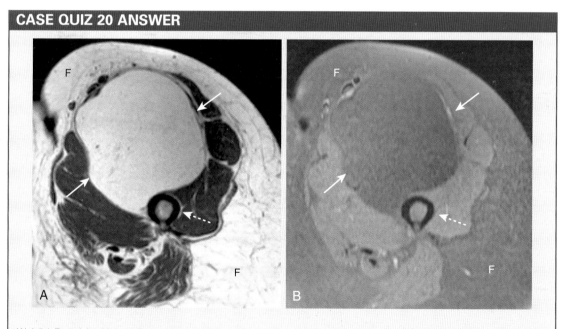

(A) Axial, T1-weighted image shows a large intramuscular mass *(solid arrows)* in the left thigh anterior to the femur *(dashed arrows in A and B)*. The mass is T1-bright, which makes us think of either fat or subacute hemorrhage. Note that the mass is isointense to the surrounding subcutaneous fat of the thigh (F). (B) Fat suppression has been applied to this axial, T1-weighted image, and we can see that the bright signal from the mass now appears dark *(solid arrows)*, along with the signal of subcutaneous fat (F), thus excluding hematoma. The homogeneous signal of this fat-containing mass is diagnostic for a **simple lipoma**. MRI is superior to ultrasound in the characterization of large lipomas given that the ultrasound beam can have difficulty penetrating deep tissues.

## TAKE HOME POINTS

- MRI uses a very strong magnetic field to influence the electromagnetic activity of hydrogen nuclei, also called protons.
- **Protons** each have a charge and possess a spin. The constant movement of protons generates a small magnetic field causing the proton to behave like a mini-magnet. When the protons are placed in the much more powerful magnetic field of the MRI scanner, they all align with this external magnetic field.
- A **radiofrequency (RF) pulse**, transmitted by a transmitter coil, displaces the protons from their original alignment with the external magnetic field of the scanner.
- When the RF pulse is turned off, the displaced protons **relax and realign** with the main magnetic field, producing a radiofrequency signal (the echo) as they do so. Receiver coils receive this signal (or echo) given off by the excited protons. A computer reconstructs the information from the echo to generate an image.
- The main magnet in an MRI scanner is usually a **superconducting magnet** that is cooled to extremely low temperatures in order to carry the electrical current.
- **Pulse sequences** consist of a set of imaging parameters that determine the way a particular tissue will appear. The two main pulse sequences upon which all MRI pulse sequences are based are called **SE** and **GRE**.
- **T1 and T2** are both time constants. T1 is called the **longitudinal** relaxation time, and T2 is called the **transverse** relaxation time.
- **TR** is the repetition time between two RF pulses. A short TR creates a T1-weighted image.
- **TE** is the echo time between a pulse and its resultant echo. A long TE creates a T2-weighted image.

- On T1-weighted images, fat, subacute hemorrhage, proteinaceous fluid, melanin, and gadolinium are typically **bright (white)**.
- On T2-weighted images, fat, water, edema, inflammation, infection, cysts, and hyperacute/subacute hemorrhage are typically **bright.**
- In summary, **fat is T1-bright and T2-bright. Water is T1-dark and T2-bright.**
- **Suppression** is a feature of MRI that will cancel out or eliminate signal from certain tissues and is most often used for fat. Although normally T1-bright, fat will be dark on T1-weighted, **fat suppressed** images. Fat suppression is particularly useful for tissue characterization after administration of gadolinium.
- **Gadolinium** is the most common intravenous contrast agent used in clinical MR imaging, and its effect is to **shorten the T1 relaxation time** of hydrogen nuclei yielding a **brighter signal.** Vascular structures such as tumors and areas of inflammation enhance after gadolinium administration and become more conspicuous.
- **Ferromagnetic objects** must be kept outside of the MRI scanning room as they could become airborne when exposed to the magnetic field. Patients who may have metallic foreign bodies in their eyes must first have conventional orbital radiographs to determine whether metal is present.
- In **pregnancy**, MRI can be performed at any stage if the risk-to-benefit ratio is deemed appropriate, but gadolinium is contraindicated.
- **Nephrogenic systemic fibrosis** is a debilitating fibrotic disease that can occur in patients with renal insufficiency who receive intravenous gadolinium. However, there is negligible risk with newer group II gadolinium agents that are typically safe for patients with chronic renal disease.

 Additional content is available online including chapters on Nuclear Medicine, Artificial Intelligence, Radiation Dose and Safety, an Early History of Radiology, and a compendium of 200 Diagnostic Radiology Signs.

# Recognizing Nontraumatic Abnormalities of the Appendicular Skeleton and Arthritis

*William Herring, MD, FACR*

## CONVENTIONAL RADIOGRAPHY, CT, AND MRI IN BONE IMAGING

- Most examinations of bone start with **conventional radiographs** obtained with at least **two views** exposed at a **90-degree angle** to **each other** (called *orthogonal views*) so as to localize abnormalities better and to visualize as much of the bone as possible (Fig. 21.1).
- Still, conventional radiographs cannot visualize the entire circumference of a tubular bone and they are not particularly sensitive for demonstrating musculoskeletal soft-tissue abnormalities other than significant soft-tissue swelling.
  - It is important to remember that, although the cortex completely surrounds the entire bone, on conventional radiographs it is best seen where it is viewed in profile (i.e., where the x-ray beam passes **tangentially** to the bone).
- CT and MRI are able to demonstrate the entire circumference and internal matrix of bone including, especially with MRI, the **surrounding soft tissues** not visible on conventional radiographs. This is accomplished by computer-

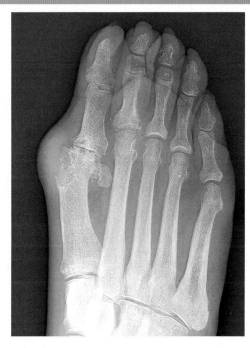

The patient is a 63-year-old male with chronic pain in his right great toe. What clinical diagnosis does this conventional radiograph of the foot confirm? The answer is at the end of the chapter.

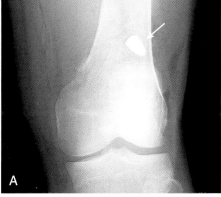 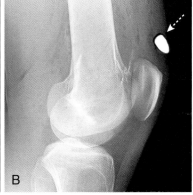

**Fig. 21.1** Importance of Orthogonal Views. (A) On this frontal view of the knee, a bullet *(solid arrow)* appears to lie within the distal femur. (B) The lateral view demonstrates that the bullet, in fact, is in the suprapatellar soft tissue *(dashed arrow)*, not the femur. Conventional views of bone require two images at roughly 90 degrees to each other to help localize a finding.

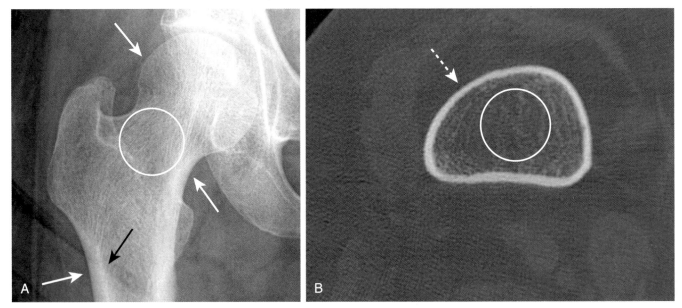

**Fig. 21.2 Normal Appearance of Bone.** (A) This is an anteroposterior radiograph of the hip. When viewed in tangent, the cortex is seen as a smooth, white line, varying in thickness in different parts of the bone *(white arrows)*. The **medullary cavity** lies within the **cortical shell** and contains an interlacing network of trabeculae *(circle)*. The **corticomedullary junction** is the interface between the inner margin of the cortex and the medullary cavity *(black arrow)*. (B) An axial CT scan through the femoral shaft depicts the entire 360° circumference of the cortex *(dashed arrow)* surrounding the less-dense medullary cavity containing both bony trabeculae and fat *(circle)*. This image is optimized to display bone, which is why the muscles and subcutaneous fat are less well seen.

aided reformatting and a superior ability to display more subtle differences in tissue densities (Fig. 21.2).

- **MRI** is an excellent means of studying the components of marrow, a fact that makes it so useful in the study of **marrow pathology.** Whereas the cortex is the part of the bone most easily visualized on conventional radiographs, **cortical bone has a very low signal intensity on conventional MRI** sequences (Fig. 21.3).

## NORMAL BONE AND JOINT ANATOMY

- On conventional radiographs, visualized long bones exhibit a dense **cortex** of **compact bone** that completely envelopes a less-dense **medullary cavity** containing **cancellous bone** arranged as **trabeculae,** separated primarily by blood vessels, hematopoietic cells, and fat. The shaft of the bone is the *diaphysis,* capped on each end by the *epiphyses.* Where the diaphysis and epiphysis join (i.e., the *metaphysis*) is the site of the *epiphysial growth plate* in children.
- The proportions of cortical versus trabecular bone vary in different skeletal sites and even at different locations in the same bone (i.e., the **cortex is naturally thicker in some places than in others**) (see Fig. 21.2A).

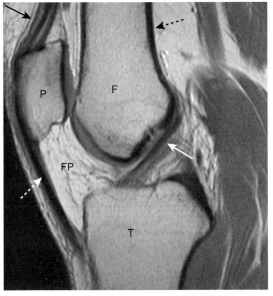

**Fig. 21.3 Normal MRI, Knee.** The outstanding display on MRI of the internal matrix of bone and the surrounding soft tissues is seen in this sagittal view of the knee. There is fatty marrow in the distal femur (F), proximal tibia (T), and patella (P). The quadriceps *(solid black arrow)* and patellar *(dashed white arrow)* tendons are shown. The anterior cruciate ligament *(solid white arrow)* is visible. There is high signal fat in the infrapatellar fat pad (FP). Notice how the bone's cortex has a very weak signal, appearing dark *(dashed black arrow)*.

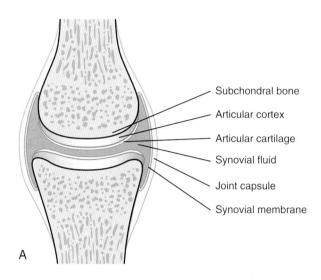

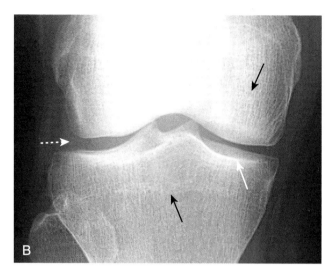

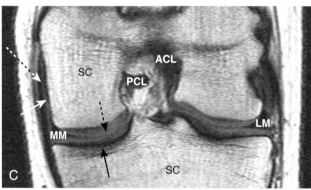

**Fig. 21.4 Diagram, Radiograph and MRI Image of a True Joint.** (A) Drawing of synovial joint shows the *articular cortex,* which corresponds to the thin, white line within the *joint capsule* that is usually capped by hyaline, *articular cartilage*. The bone immediately beneath the articular cortex is called **subchondral bone.** Within the joint capsule is the **synovial membrane** and **synovial fluid.** (B) On conventional radiographs, the articular cortex *(solid white arrow)* and subchondral bone *(solid black arrows)* are visible, but the cartilage and synovial fluid are not *(dashed white arrow)*. (C) A T1-weighted, coronal MRI of the knee shows the medial (MM) and lateral (LM) menisci, anterior (ACL) and posterior (PCL) cruciate ligaments, articular cartilage *(dashed black arrow)*, joint capsule *(dashed white arrow)*, synovial fluid *(solid white arrow)*, and marrow in the subchondral bone (SC). The cortex of the bone *(solid black arrow)* produces little signal and is dark.

- Fig. 21.4 contains a diagram of a typical synovial joint and compares the structures visualized on conventional radiographs and MRI.

# DISEASES THAT AFFECT BONE DENSITY

## The Effect of Bone Physiology on Bone Anatomy

- Bones reflect the general metabolic status of the individual. Their composition requires a **protein-containing, collagenous matrix** *(osteoid)* upon which **bone mineral**, principally **calcium phosphate**, is transformed into cartilage and bone.
- Bones are continuously undergoing remodeling processes that include **resorption of old or diseased bone by**

**osteoclasts** and **formation of new bone by** *osteoblasts.* Osteoblasts are responsible for bone matrix production, whereas osteoclasts resorb both the matrix and mineral.
- Both osteoclastic and osteoblastic activity depend on the presence of a **viable blood supply** to bring those cells to the bone.
- Bones also **respond to mechanical forces,** for example, the contractions of muscles and tendons, the process of bearing weight, constant use, or prolonged disuse, which help to form and/or maintain the shape as well as the content of each bone.
- In this section, we arbitrarily divide abnormalities of **bone density** into two major categories based primarily on their appearance on conventional radiographs: those that produce

**TABLE 21.1 Changes in Bone Density**

| Density | Extent | Examples Used in This Chapter |
|---|---|---|
| **Increased density** | Diffuse | Diffuse osteoblastic metastases |
| | Focal | Localized osteoblastic metastases |
| | | Avascular necrosis of bone |
| | | Paget disease |
| **Decreased density** | Diffuse | Osteoporosis |
| | | Hyperparathyroidism |
| | Focal | Localized osteolytic metastases |
| | | Multiple myeloma |
| | | Osteomyelitis |

a pattern of either **increased** or **decreased** bone density (Table 21.1).

# DISEASES THAT INCREASE BONE DENSITY

## Recognizing an Increase in Bone Density

- On conventional radiographs and CT, an increase in bone density produces *sclerosis* (increased whiteness) to the affected part. If the entire bone is sclerotic, there is a loss of the demarcation of the **normal cortico-medullary junction** because of the abnormally increased density of the medullary cavity relative to the cortex (Fig. 21.5).
- Examples of diseases that cause increased bone density include osteoblastic metastatic disease, avascular necrosis of bone, and Paget disease.

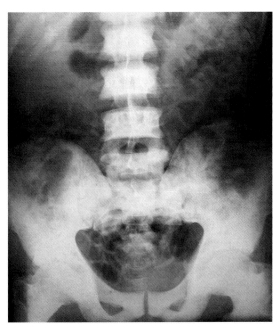

**Fig. 21.6 Diffuse Osteoblastic Metastatic Disease.** The bones are diffusely sclerotic from abnormal osteoblastic activity. You can no longer see the normal trabeculae or the junction between the medullary cavity and the cortex. This patient had widespread metastases from prostate carcinoma.

## Osteoblastic Metastatic Disease

- Diffuse, blood-borne, metastatic disease from **carcinoma of the prostate** is the **prototype** for a **generalized increase in bone density.** Osteoblastic metastatic disease, like that from the prostate, can also produce **focal areas** of increased bone density as well. These osteoblastic lesions are **most often** seen in the **vertebrae, ribs, pelvis, humeri,** and **femora** (Fig. 21.6). Osteoblastic activity occurs beyond the control of normal physiologic constraints.

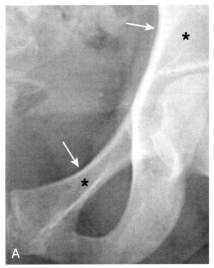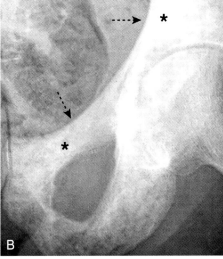

**Fig. 21.5 Corticomedullary Junction, Normal and Abnormal.** (A) The cortex normally projects as a smooth, white line of varying thickness at the periphery of bone on conventional radiographs *(arrows)*, distinguishable from the less-dense medullary cavity *(asterisks)*. (B) Diseases that cause a generalized increase in bone density cause the medullary cavity *(asterisks)* and the cortex to appear equally dense *(arrows)*. This obliterates the cortico-medullary interface seen in normal bones. This patient had diffuse, osteoblastic metastatic prostate carcinoma.

- **Focal sclerotic lesions** can affect either the cortex, the medullary cavity, or both. Those that affect the **cortex** will usually produce **periosteal new bone formation *(periosteal reaction)*,** which leads to an appearance of **thickening of the cortex.** Those that affect the **medullary cavity** will result in **punctate, amorphous, sclerotic lesions** surrounded by the normal medullary cavity (Fig. 21.7).
- Metastatic disease to bone is found in a **significant percentage of autopsied patients with carcinoma of the prostate. Multiple** bone **metastases** from carcinoma of the prostate occur much **more frequently** than do **solitary bone lesions,** which are discussed later in this chapter (Box 21.1).

## ►► IMPORTANT POINTS

- The **radionuclide bone scan is currently the study of choice for detecting skeletal metastases**, regardless of the suspected primary (Box 21.2). With diffuse bone metastases, a so-called *superscan* may be seen on radionuclide bone scan. The superscan demonstrates high radiotracer uptake throughout the skeleton, with poor or absent renal excretion of the radiotracer (Fig. 21.8).

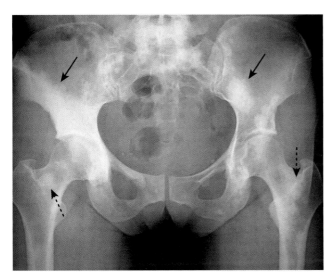

**Fig. 21.7** Focal Sclerotic Metastases from Carcinoma of the Breast. There are focal sclerotic lesions seen in the right and left ilium *(solid arrows)* and both proximal femurs *(dashed arrows)*. Additional sclerotic lesions are also present. Metastatic breast carcinoma can be both osteoblastic and osteolytic.

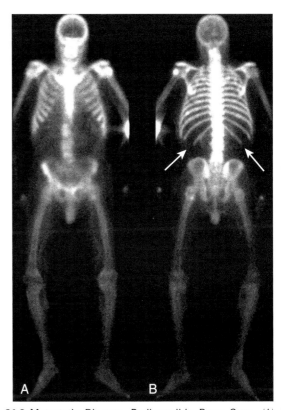

**Fig. 21.8** Metastatic Disease, Radionuclide Bone Scan. (A) Anteroposterior and (B) posteroanterior views of the axial and appendicular skeleton show the distribution of bone radiotracer uptake throughout the skeleton. This is the picture of the so-called *superscan* produced by osteoblastic metastatic disease involving every bone, leading to very high uptake throughout the skeleton and very little renal excretion of the radiotracer *(arrows* point to the absence of excretion by the kidneys, a characteristic of a superscan).

## Avascular Necrosis of Bone

- *Avascular necrosis (AVN)* of bone (also called **ischemic necrosis, aseptic necrosis, osteonecrosis**) results from cellular death and eventually leads to the collapse of the affected bone. It usually involves those bones that have a relatively **poor collateral blood supply** (e.g., scaphoid in the wrist, femoral head) and tends to affect the hematopoietic elements of marrow earliest so that **MRI is the most sensitive modality for detecting AVN.**
- There are numerous causes of avascular necrosis. Some of the more common are shown in Table 21.2.
- On conventional radiographs, the devascularized bone becomes **denser** and therefore appears more sclerotic

than the remainder of the bone. This especially occurs in the **femoral head** (Fig. 21.9) and **humeral head** (Fig. 21.10).
- On **MRI,** there is usually a **decrease from the normal high signal** produced by fatty marrow (Fig. 21.11).
- On conventional radiographs, **old medullary bone infarcts** are recognized as dense, amorphous deposits of bone within

### TABLE 21.2  Some Causes of Avascular Necrosis of Bone

| Location | Example of Disease |
| --- | --- |
| Intravascular | Sickle cell disease<br>Polycythemia vera |
| Vascular | Vasculitis (Lupus and radiation-induced) |
| Extravascular | Trauma (fractures) |
| Idiopathic | Exogenous steroids and Cushing disease<br>Legg-Calvé-Perthes disease |

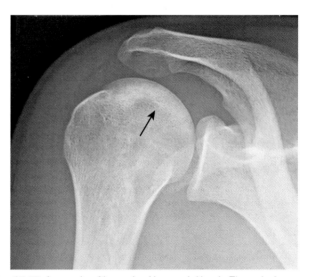

Fig. 21.10 Avascular Necrosis, Humeral Head. There is increased density seen at the very top of the humeral head *(arrow)* in this patient with sickle cell disease. Because the white cap on the bone was thought to resemble snow on a mountain-top, this sign of avascular necrosis has been called ***snow-capping***. Avascular necrosis in sickle cell disease does not usually manifest until young adulthood and, with the sensitivity of MRI, is more prevalent than had been originally thought using conventional films alone.

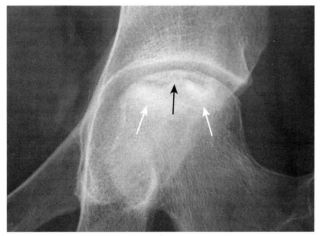

Fig. 21.9 Avascular Necrosis, Femoral Head. A close-up view of the left femoral head shows a zone of increased sclerosis in the superior aspect of the femoral head *(white arrows)*, a characteristic finding of avascular necrosis of the head. The linear, subcortical lucency *(black arrow)* represents subchondral fractures seen with this disease, called the ***crescent sign***. Notice that the disease is isolated to the femoral head and involves neither the joint space nor the acetabulum, i.e., it is not an arthritis. The patient was on long-term steroids for lupus erythematosus.

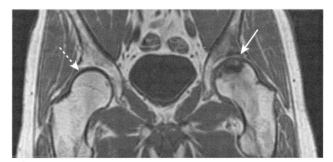

Fig. 21.11 Avascular Necrosis, MRI. A T1-weighted coronal view of both hips demonstrates normal, high signal from the fatty marrow in the right femur *(dashed arrow)* but decreased signal in the left femoral head extending to the subchondral bone of the left hip joint *(solid arrow)*. The joint space is preserved. MRI is the most sensitive method of detecting avascular necrosis of the hip.

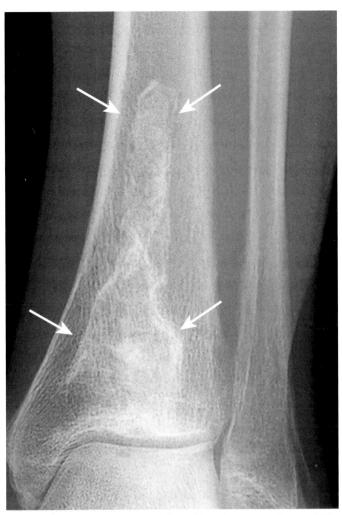

**Fig. 21.12** Old Medullary Bone Infarct. There is an amorphous calcification in the medullary cavity of the distal tibia *(arrows)*. In general, the differential diagnosis for such an intramedullary calcification includes bone infarct or enchondroma. The characteristic sclerotic membrane surrounding this lesion suggests it is more likely an old bone infarct. This patient had been on long-term steroids for asthma.

the medullary cavities of long bones, frequently marginated by a thin, sclerotic membrane (Fig. 21.12).

## Paget Disease

- Paget disease is a **chronic disease of bone**, most often occurring in older men, now believed to be caused by chronic paramyxoviral infection. It is **characterized by varying degrees of increased bone resorption and increased bone formation** with bone formation predominating in those cases seen in more progressive forms of the disease.
- The end result is almost always a **denser bone** that, despite its density, is **mechanically inferior** to normal bone and thus susceptible to *pathologic fractures* or bone-softening deformities such as *bowing*. The **pelvis** is **most frequently**

involved, followed by the **lumbar spine, thoracic spine, proximal femur,** and **calvarium.**

---

> ### ⟩⟩ IMPORTANT POINTS
>
> - Paget disease is usually diagnosed with conventional radiography. **The imaging hallmarks of Paget disease are:**
>   - **Thickening of the cortex.**
>   - **Coarsening and thickening of the trabecular pattern** (Fig. 21.13).
>   - **Increase in the size of the bone involved.** The "classic" history for Paget disease, rendered less useful since fashions have changed, was a gradual increase in a person's hat size as the calvarium increased in size from this disease.

---

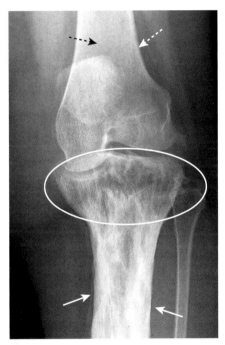

**Fig. 21.13** Paget Disease of the Tibia. The proximal tibia demonstrates three of the major signs of Paget disease: (1) An overall **increase in bone density**, (2) **accentuation** and **coarsening** of the trabeculae *(oval)*, and (3) **thickening** of the cortex *(solid white arrows)*. Compare the appearance of the tibia with the normal cortex *(dashed white arrow)* and medullary cavity *(dashed black arrow)* of the femur.

## DISEASES THAT DECREASE BONE DENSITY

### Recognizing a Decrease in Bone Density

- As bones decrease in radiographic density, there may be a **diffuse loss of the normal network of bony trabeculae in the medullary cavity** because of the decreased number and thinning of many of the smaller trabecular structures.
- **Accentuation of the cortex** may be present, in which the cortex, although thinner than normal, **stands out more**

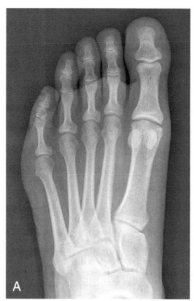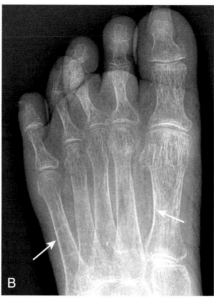

**Fig. 21.14 Normal and Osteoporotic Foot.** (A) Normal frontal view of the foot to contrast with (B) in the same patient some weeks later after prolonged immobilization. (B) There is overall decreased density of the bone and thinning of the cortices *(arrows)* secondary to disuse osteoporosis. Conventional radiographs are subject to technical variations that can mimic osteoporosis even in a healthy individual.

**strikingly** because of the **lower density** of the **medullary cavity** (Fig. 21.14).

- **Compression of vertebral bodies** may occur (see Chapter 22).
- There may be **pathologic fractures** in the hip, pelvis, or vertebral bodies (see Chapter 23).
- Examples of diseases that cause a **diffuse decrease** in bone density include osteoporosis and hyperparathyroidism.

## Osteoporosis

- **Osteoporosis** is defined as a systemic skeletal disorder in which there is **low bone mineral density** (BMD) and is generally divided into **postmenopausal** and **age-related bone loss.**
  - *Postmenopausal osteoporosis* is characterized by **increased bone resorption** due to increased osteoclastic activity relative to that of osteoblasts.
  - *Age-related bone loss* begins around age 45 to 55 and is characterized by a **loss of total bone mass.**
- Additional factors that **increase the risk of osteoporosis** include exogenous steroid administration, Cushing disease, estrogen deficiency, inadequate physical activity, and alcoholism.
- Osteoporosis **predisposes to pathologic fractures** in the femoral neck, compression fractures of the vertebral bodies, and fractures of the distal radius *(Colles fractures).*
- **Conventional radiographs** are relatively **insensitive for detecting osteoporosis.** Almost **50% of the bone mass must be lost** before it is **recognizable** on conventional radiographs. Findings on conventional radiographs include **overall decreased density of bone, thinning of the cortex, and decrease in the visible number of trabeculae in the medullary cavity** (see Fig. 21.14B).

- Currently, **DEXA (d**ual-**e**nergy **x**-ray **a**bsorptiometry**) scans are the most accurate** and widely recommended method for bone mineral density measurements.
  - DEXA scans are obtained by using a filtered x-ray source that produces two distinct energies that are differentially absorbed by bone and soft tissue, respectively. This allows for the more accurate calculation of bone density by digitally subtracting the error introduced by varying amounts of overlying soft tissue. The x-ray dose is very low and the spine or hip are generally used for density measurements.

## Hyperparathyroidism

- *Hyperparathyroidism* is a condition caused by excessive secretion of **parathormone (PTH)** by the parathyroid glands. Parathormone exerts its effects on bones, the kidneys, and the gastrointestinal tract. Its **effect on bones is to increase resorption** by stimulating osteoclastic activity. Calcium is removed from the bone and deposited in the bloodstream.
- There are **three forms** of hyperparathyroidism, which are listed in Table 21.3.

### TABLE 21.3  Forms of Hyperparathyroidism

| Type | Remarks |
| --- | --- |
| **Primary** | Usually caused by a single adenoma in most patients (80%–90%) and almost always results in hypercalcemia |
| **Secondary** | Results from hyperplasia of the glands secondary to imbalances in calcium and phosphorous levels, seen mostly with chronic renal disease |
| **Tertiary** | Occurs in patients with long-standing secondary hyperparathyroidism in whom autonomous hypersecretion of parathyroid hormone develops, leading to hypercalcemia |

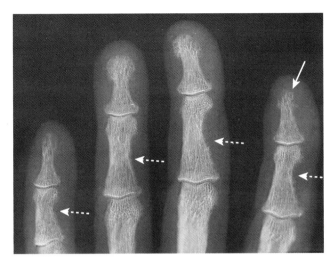

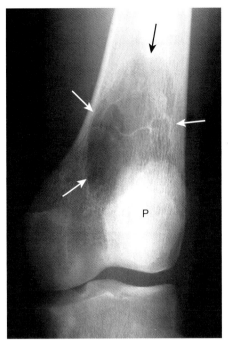

**Fig. 21.15** Subperiosteal Resorption in Hyperparathyroidism. There is characteristic subperiosteal bone resorption, seen especially well on the radial aspect of all the middle phalanges *(dashed arrows)*. The cortex appears shaggy and irregular, compared to the cortices on the opposite sides of the same bones, which are well-defined. This patient also displays partial resorption of the terminal phalanx of the index finger *(solid arrow)* called **acro-osteolysis**.

- The **diagnosis of hyperparathyroidism is based on clinical and laboratory findings,** but there are numerous findings of the disease on conventional radiographs and there are other imaging studies utilized to aid if surgery on the parathyroid glands is indicated. Imaging studies of the parathyroid glands themselves may include ultrasound, nuclear medicine parathyroid scans, and MRI scans.

**Fig. 21.17** Brown Tumor. There is a geographic, lytic lesion in the distal femur *(arrows)*. Brown tumors (also called **osteoclastomas**) are benign lesions that represent the osteoclastic resorption of a localized area of (usually) cortical bone and its replacement with fibrous tissue and blood. Their high hemosiderin content gives them a characteristic brown color; they were not named after a "Dr. Brown." These bone lesions can mimic osteolytic metastases or multiple myeloma, so the clinical history of hyperparathyroidism is key. They can be seen with both primary and secondary hyperparathyroidism. *P,* Patella.

---

>> **IMPORTANT POINTS**

- Some of the **findings of hyperparathyroidism on conventional radiographs** include:
  - Overall **decrease in bony density.**
  - **Subperiosteal bone resorption,** especially on the **radial** side of the **middle phalanges** of the **index and middle fingers** (Fig. 21.15).
- **Erosion** of the distal clavicles (Fig. 21.16).
- **Well-circumscribed lytic lesions** in the long bones called **brown tumors** (Fig. 21.17)

---

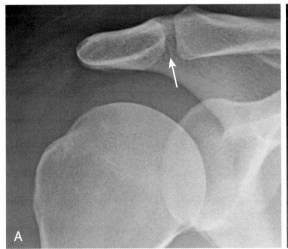

**Fig. 21.16** Erosion of Distal Clavicle in Hyperparathyroidism. Another relatively common site of bone resorption in hyperparathyroidism is the distal end of the clavicle. (A) The normal width of the acromioclavicular joint is no more than 7 to 8 mm and the cortical margins are distinct *(arrow)*. (B) The distal clavicle has been resorbed and is irregular in appearance *(dashed arrow)* and there is increased distance between it and the acromion *(solid arrow)*. Other sites of bone resorption in hyperparathyroidism might include the lamina dura of the teeth and portions of the medial aspects of the tibia, humerus, and femur.

## Focal Decreases in Bone Density

- Examples of diseases that cause a **focal decrease** in bone density include osteolytic metastatic disease, multiple myeloma, and osteomyelitis.

### Osteolytic Metastatic Disease

- **Osteolytic metastatic disease** can produce focal destruction of bone (see Box 21.1). These lesions are most often produced by **focal infiltration of bone by cells other than osteocytes.**
- The **medullary cavity is almost always involved**, from which the disease may erode into and destroy the cortex as well. When the medullary cavity alone is involved, there must be almost a 50% reduction in mass in order for the lesion to be recognizable on **conventional radiographs** when viewed *en face.*
- MRI, on the other hand, is **excellent** at demonstrating the status of the medullary cavity and so is much more sensitive to the presence of metastatic disease than conventional radiography (Fig. 21.18).
- In **some cases, only the cortex is involved.** Cortical metastases may be easier to visualize on conventional radiographs because relatively less cortical destruction is needed for them to become apparent, especially if the lesions happen to be viewed in tangent.

---

### ▶▶ IMPORTANT POINTS

- On conventional radiographs, the **classical findings of osteolytic metastases** include:
  - **Irregularly shaped, lucent bone lesions,** which can be single or multiple.
    - These lytic lesions are frequently characterized as belonging to one (or sometimes more) of three patterns: **geographic, mottled, or permeative**, in order of decreasing size of the most discrete lesion visible (Fig. 21.19).

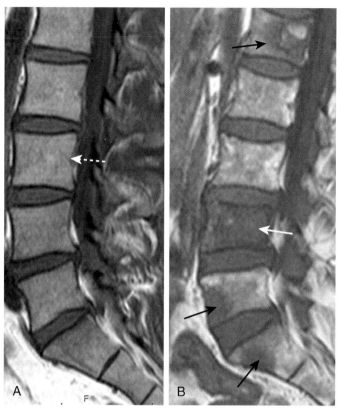

**Fig. 21.18 Metastases to Lumbar Spine: MRI.** (A) There is normal signal in the lumbar vertebral bodies *(dashed arrow)* on this T1-weighted sagittal view of the lumbar spine. (B) In another patient, this one with a primary breast carcinoma, there are multiple metastatic deposits replacing the normal marrow in the lumbar spine and sacrum *(black arrows)*. The body of L4 is completely replaced by tumor *(white arrow)*.

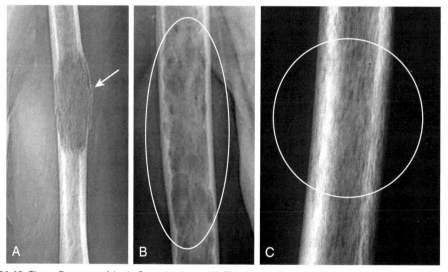

**Fig. 21.19 Three Patterns of Lytic Bone Lesions.** (A) This is a solitary, slightly expansile **geographic** bone lesion *(arrow)* with a relatively narrow zone of transition between it and surrounding normal bone in a patient with a primary lung carcinoma. (B) A close-up of the humerus in another patient with lung cancer demonstrates multiple, ill-defined lytic lesions *(oval)* with indistinct margins implying a more aggressive malignancy. This appearance is called a **moth-eaten pattern.** (C) This is a close-up of the femur in a patient with multiple myeloma that shows innumerable, small, irregular lucencies throughout the bone *(circle)* called a **permeative pattern.** Permeative lesions are called **round cell lesions** for the shape of the cells that produce them. Such diseases include Ewing's sarcoma, myeloma, and leukemia.

- Osteolytic metastases typically **incite little or no reactive bone formation** around them. They can be **expansile** and **soap-bubbly** (i.e., contain bony septations), especially in renal and thyroid carcinoma (Fig. 21.20).
- In the spine, they may preferentially **destroy the pedicles,** because of their blood supply (the **pedicle sign**), which can help to differentiate metastases from multiple myeloma (see next section) that tends to spare the pedicle early in the disease (Fig. 21.21).

| TABLE 21.4 **Causes of Osteoblastic and Osteolytic Bone Metastases** | |
|---|---|
| **Osteoblastic** | **Osteolytic** |
| Prostate carcinoma (most common in older men) | Lung cancer (most common osteolytic lesion in male patients) |
| Breast carcinoma is usually osteolytic, but can be osteoblastic, especially if treated | Breast cancer (most common osteolytic lesion in female patients) |
| Lymphoma | Renal cell carcinoma |
| Carcinoid tumors (rare) | Thyroid carcinoma |

- The most common causes of osteoblastic and osteolytic bone metastases are listed in Table 21.4.

### Myeloma

- **Myeloma,** the most common primary malignancy of bone in adults, can occur in a **solitary form,** often seen as a soap-bubbly, expansile lesion in the spine or pelvis (called a *solitary plasmacytoma*) or a **disseminated form** with multiple, **punched-out** lytic lesions throughout the axial and proximal appendicular skeleton.

- **Findings of multiple myeloma on conventional radiographs:**
  - The most common early manifestation is **diffuse and usually severe osteoporosis.**
  - **Plasmacytomas** appear as **expansile, septated lesions, frequently with associated soft-tissue masses** (Fig. 21.22).
  - Later, in its disseminated form, **multiple, small, sharply circumscribed** (described as *punched-out*) **lytic lesions of approximately the same size** are present, usually without any accompanying sclerotic reaction around them (Fig. 21.23).

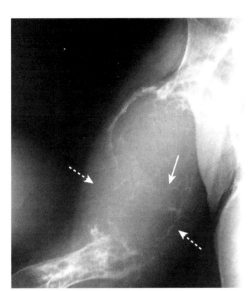

**Fig. 21.20 Expansile Renal Cell Carcinoma Metastasis.** This is a very **aggressive** and **expansile** osteolytic metastasis in the humerus from a primary renal cell carcinoma. Notice that the cortex has been destroyed in several areas *(dashed arrows)* and the lesion has a characteristic **soap-bubbly** appearance produced by fine septae *(solid arrow).* Thyroid carcinoma and a solitary plasmacytoma could also produce these findings.

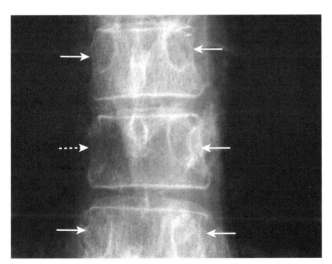

**Fig. 21.21 Pedicle Sign.** Each vertebral body should normally have two oval-shaped pedicles, one on each side, visible on the frontal radiograph of the spine *(solid arrows).* The right pedicle of T10 *(dashed arrow)* is missing because it has been destroyed by metastatic tumor. This is called the **pedicle sign.** Most metastatic lesions to the spine will also involve the vertebral body.

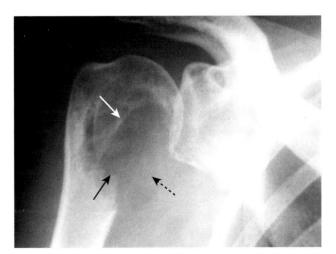

**Fig. 21.22 Solitary Plasmacytoma.** There is a large, lytic lesion in the proximal humerus *(solid black arrow)* that destroys the cortex *(dashed black arrow)* and contains multiple septations *(white arrow).* Solitary plasmacytomas can be a precursor to the more disseminated form of multiple myeloma. Renal cell and thyroid carcinoma can also produce such a picture (see Fig. 21.20).

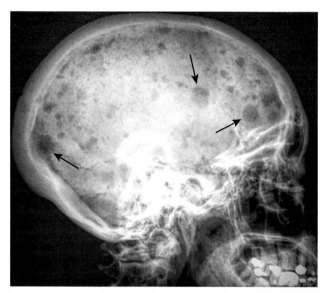

**Fig. 21.23 Multiple Myeloma.** Innumerable lytic lesions *(arrows)* are seen in this lateral view of the skull. They are small and have well-marginated edges, the so-called **punched-out** lytic defects characteristic of multiple myeloma. Metastases to the skull can produce a similar picture but tend to be fewer in number and less well-defined.

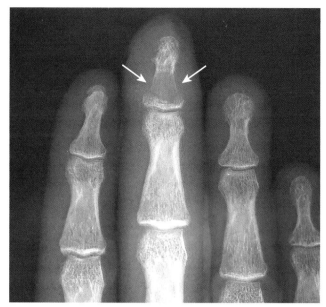

**Fig. 21.24 Osteomyelitis, Middle Finger.** Close-up view of the hand shows a lytic lesion in the terminal phalanx of the middle finger with destruction of a part of the cortex *(arrows)*. The soft tissue of the finger was edematous and the patient had history of a penetrating injury to the finger weeks earlier.

- Classically, **conventional radiographs are more sensitive in detecting the lesions of multiple myeloma than radionuclide bone scans** that tend to underestimate the number and extent of lesions because of the absence of reactive bone formation.

### Osteomyelitis

- **Osteomyelitis** refers to the **focal destruction of bone**, most often by a blood-borne **infectious agent,** the most common of which is *Staphylococcus aureus.*
- **In children,** the osteolytic lesion **tends to occur at the metaphysis** because of its rich blood supply.

> **IMPORTANT POINTS**
>
> - **Findings of acute osteomyelitis on conventional radiographs:**
>   - **Focal cortical bone destruction** (Fig. 21.24)
>   - **Periosteal new bone formation**
>   - Inflammatory changes accompanying the infection may produce **soft-tissue swelling** and **focal osteoporosis** from hyperemia

- In **adults,** the **infection** tends to **involve the joint space more** often than it does in **children,** producing not only osteomyelitis but also **septic arthritis.**
- **Conventional radiographs can take up to 10 days to display the first findings of osteomyelitis** so that other imaging modalities, such as MRI and nuclear medicine studies, are frequently used for earlier diagnosis.
- A variety of radionuclide bone scans can demonstrate osteomyelitis, the most specific of which is currently a **tagged, white-cell scan** in which a sample of the patient's white

blood cells is removed, tagged with a radioactive isotope (frequently indium), and injected back into the patient who is then imaged with a camera specific for nuclear studies to detect a site of abnormally increased radioactive tracer uptake.

## DISEASES OF THE JOINTS: AN APPROACH TO ARTHRITIS

- Imaging studies play a key role in the diagnosis and management of arthritis and are the method by which many arthritides are first diagnosed. Other arthritides are initially diagnosed on clinical and laboratory grounds and imaging is used to document the severity, extent, and course of the disease (Table 21.5).

| TABLE 21.5  **Arthritis: Who Makes the Diagnosis?** | |
| --- | --- |
| **Usually Diagnosed Clinically** | **Frequently Diagnosed Radiologically** |
| Septic (pyogenic) arthritis | Osteoarthritis |
| Psoriatic arthritis | Early rheumatoid arthritis |
| Gout, hemophilia | Calcium pyrophosphate deposition disease |
| | Ankylosing spondylitis |
| | Septic (TB) |
| | Charcot (neuropathic) joint—late |

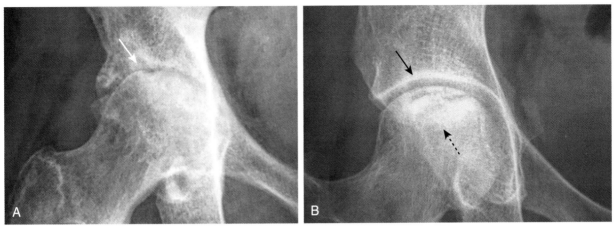

**Fig. 21.25** Arthritis or Not? (A) There is narrowing of the hip joint and both the femoral head and the acetabulum are abnormal *(arrow)*. This meets the criteria for an arthritis and represents osteoarthritis of the hip. (B) There is sclerosis of the femoral head *(dashed arrow)* but the joint space remains normal as is the acetabulum *(solid arrow)*. This is avascular necrosis of the femoral head, not an arthritis.

- **Conventional radiographs remain the study of first choice** in evaluating for the presence of arthritis. Conventional radiographs will demonstrate abnormalities of the **articular cortex** and the **subchondral bone** and will provide late, indirect evidence of the integrity of the articular cartilage. MRI is more sensitive in directly visualizing the soft tissues in and around a joint.

## Classification of Arthritis

- An **arthritis is a disease that affects a joint and usually the bones on either side of the joint,** almost always accompanied by **joint space narrowing** (Fig. 21.25).
- We divide arthritides into **three main categories** (Table 21.6):
  - *Hypertrophic arthritis* is characterized, in general, by **bone formation** at the site of the involved joint(s). The bone formation may occur within the confines of

## TABLE 21.6  Classification of Arthritis

| Category | Hallmarks | Types | Remarks |
|---|---|---|---|
| **Hypertrophic arthritis** | Bone formation Osteophytes | Primary osteoarthritis | Most common; mechanical stress; hands, hips, and knees most common |
| | | Secondary osteoarthritis | Degenerative joint disease (DJD) secondary to prior trauma, or avascular necrosis |
| | | Charcot arthropathy | Fragmentation; joint destruction; sclerosis; most often secondary to diabetes |
| | | CPPD | Chondrocalcinosis; DJD in unusual sites |
| **Erosive arthritis** | Erosions | Rheumatoid | Carpals, metacarpal-phalangeal joints, proximal interphalangeal joints of hands; osteoporosis; soft-tissue swelling |
| | | Gout | Juxta-articular erosions with overhanging edges; long-latency; metatarsal-phalangeal joint of big toe; no osteoporosis |
| | | Psoriatic | Juxta-articular erosions of distal interphalangeal joints of hands; pencil-in-cup deformity; enthesophytes |
| | | Hemophilia | Remodeling from hemarthroses and hyperemia; if you see the same changes in the knee in female patients—think of juvenile rheumatoid arthritis |
| | | Ankylosing spondylitis | `HLA antigen B27 positive; bilateral sacroiliac (SI) joints; syndesmophytes |
| | | Seronegative spondyloarthropathies | Rheumatoid factor negative; HLA antigen B27 positive; SI joints; syndesmophytes; reactive arthritis; psoriasis |
| **Infectious arthritis** | Osteopenia and soft-tissue swelling; early and marked destruction of most or all of the articular cortex | Pyogenic | Early destruction of articular cortex; marked osteoporosis |

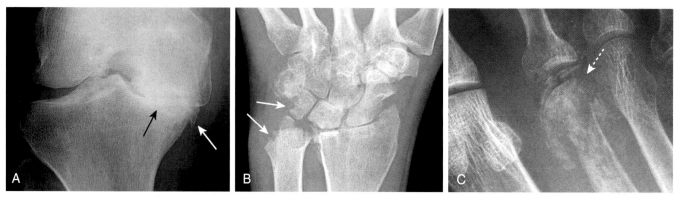

**Fig. 21.26** Imaging Hallmarks of the Three Major Categories of Arthritis. (A) **Hypertrophic arthritis** features subchondral sclerosis *(black arrow)* and marginal osteophyte production *(white arrow)*. (B) **Erosive (inflammatory) arthritis** displays characteristic marginal, lytic erosions *(arrows)*. (C) **Infectious arthritis** features destruction of the articular cortex *(arrow)*.

the parent bone *(subchondral sclerosis)* or protrude from the parent bone *(osteophyte)* (Fig. 21.26A).

- *Erosive arthritis* indicates underlying inflammation and is characterized by tiny, marginal, irregularly shaped lytic lesions in or around the joint surfaces called *erosions* (Fig. 21.26B).
- *Infectious arthritis* is characterized by joint swelling, osteopenia, and **destruction of long, contiguous segments of the articular cortex** (Fig. 21.26C).
- Within each of these three main categories, we will look at a few of the more common types of arthritis that also have characteristic imaging findings.

> ## » IMPORTANT POINTS
>
> - **The imaging findings of primary osteoarthritis** (Fig. 21.27):
>   - *Marginal osteophyte formation* is a hallmark of hypertrophic arthritis. Osseous transformation of cartilaginous excrescences and metaplasia of synovial lining cells leads to the production of these **bony protrusions at or near the joint.**
>   - *Subchondral sclerosis.* This is a reaction of the bone to the mechanical stress to which it is subjected when its protective cartilage has been destroyed.
>   - *Subchondral cysts.* As a result of chronic impaction, necrosis of bone, and/or imposition of synovial fluid into the subchondral bone, cysts of varying sizes form in the subchondral bone.
>   - **Narrowing of the joint space.** Seen in all forms of arthritis.

## Hypertrophic Arthritis

- **Hypertrophic arthritis is characterized by bone formation,** either **subchondral sclerosis** or **osteophytes.**
- **Hypertrophic** arthritides are classified in Table 21.6.

## Primary Osteoarthritis

- *Primary osteoarthritis,* also known as **primary degenerative arthritis** or **degenerative joint disease (DJD),** is the **most**

**common form of arthritis,** estimated to affect over 20 million Americans. It results from **intrinsic degeneration** of the **articular cartilage,** mostly from the mechanical stress of **excessive wear and tear** in weight-bearing joints.

- It mostly involves the **hips, knees,** and **hands** and increases in prevalence with increasing age.
- **What joints are involved?**
  - In osteoarthritis, destruction of the cartilaginous buffer between the apposing bones of a joint leads to narrowing of the joint space, most often on the **weight-bearing** side of the joint (i.e., **hip [superior and lateral] and knee [medial])** (Fig. 21.28).

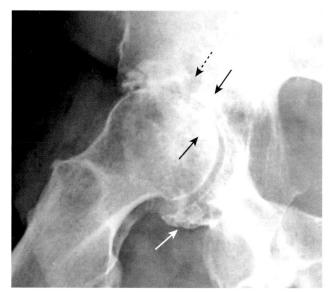

**Fig. 21.27** Primary Osteoarthritis. The hallmarks of osteoarthritis are demonstrated in this patient's right hip. There is **marginal osteophyte formation** *(white arrow)*, **subchondral sclerosis** *(solid black arrows)*, and **subchondral cyst formation** *(dashed black arrow)*.

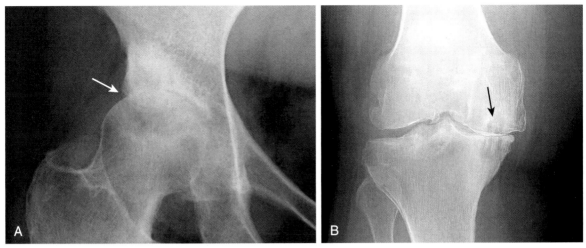

**Fig. 21.28** Osteoarthritis. (A) In the hip, the superior and lateral surfaces *(arrow)* are the weight-bearing aspects and most affected by osteoarthritis, while in the knee (B) the medial compartment bears the most weight and is more affected *(arrow)*.

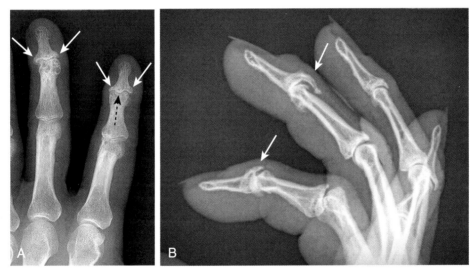

**Fig. 21.29** Osteoarthritis of the Hands. (A) There are osteophytes at the distal interphalangeal joints *(white arrows)* along with narrowing of the joint spaces *(dashed black arrow)*. (B) Large osteophytes are seen at the distal interphalangeal joints of the fingers *(arrows)* in another patient, an 87-year-old female with joint pain.

- In most patients with osteoarthritis of the interphalangeal joints of the hands, the first carpometacarpal joint (**base of thumb**) **is also affected.** It is also common for osteoarthritis to affect the **distal interphalangeal joints**, especially in older women (Fig. 21.29).

## Secondary Osteoarthritis (Secondary Degenerative Arthritis)

- *Secondary osteoarthritis* is a form of degenerative arthritis of synovial joints that occurs because of an underlying, predisposing condition, **most frequently trauma**, that damages or leads to damage of the articular cartilage.

### ▶ IMPORTANT POINTS

- The radiographic findings of **secondary osteoarthritis** are the same as those for the primary form, with several special clues to help suggest secondary osteoarthritis:
  - It **occurs at an atypical age** for primary osteoarthritis (e.g., a 30-year-old with osteoarthritis) (Box 21.3).
  - It has an **atypical appearance for primary osteoarthritis,** e.g., primary osteoarthritis is usually bilateral and often symmetric. Severe osteoarthritic changes of one hip while the opposite appears perfectly normal suggests the possibility of secondary osteoarthritis (Fig. 21.30).
  - It may **appear in an unusual location** for primary arthritis, (e.g., the elbow joint).
- **Eventually any arthritis that affects the articular cartilage, no matter what the etiology, can lead to the changes of secondary osteoarthritis.**

## BOX 21.3 Some Causes of Secondary Osteoarthritis

- Trauma
- Infection
- Avascular necrosis
- Calcium pyrophosphate deposition disease
- Rheumatoid arthritis

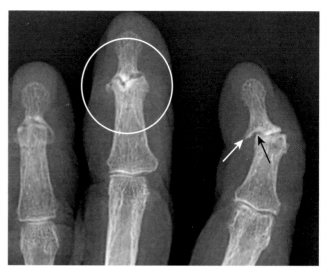

**Fig. 21.31** Erosive Osteoarthritis. This a close-up of the fingers of a 51-year-old female with marked swelling, redness, and tenderness of the distal interphalangeal joints. There are central erosions *(black arrow)* and marginal osteophytes *(white arrow)* that produce a pattern called a ***gull-wing deformity*** *(circle),* consistent with erosive osteoarthritis.

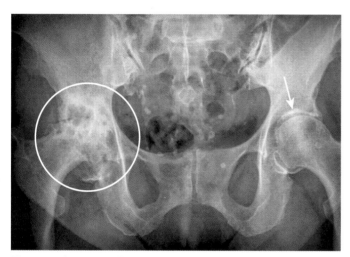

**Fig. 21.30** Secondary Osteoarthritis. There is a marked discrepancy in the appearance of each hip with advanced osteoarthritis and fusion of the right hip joint *(circle)* but a relatively normal left hip *(arrow).* Many times, the severity of the findings in secondary arthritis leave little clue as to the original, inciting cause. This patient had hip trauma on the right as a child.

### Erosive Osteoarthritis

- *Erosive osteoarthritis* is a type of **primary osteoarthritis** characterized by more **severe inflammation** and by the development of **erosive joint changes.** It occurs most often in **perimenopausal women.**
- Erosive osteoarthritis may feature bilaterally symmetric changes like the osteophytes of primary osteoarthritis but with **marked inflammation (swelling and tenderness)** and **erosions** at the affected joints.
  - The **erosions are typically centrally located within the joint** and, combined with the small osteophytes associated with the disease, may produce the so-called ***gull-wing deformity*** (Fig. 21.31).
- Erosive osteoarthritis most commonly occurs at the **proximal and distal interphalangeal joints of the fingers, first carpal-metacarpal, and the interphalangeal joint of the thumb.**

- **Bony ankylosis may occur,** an uncommon finding in primary osteoarthritis.

### Charcot Arthropathy (Neuropathic Joint)

- *Charcot arthropathy* develops from a **disturbance in sensation** that leads to **multiple microfractures** as well as an autonomic imbalance that leads to hyperemia, **bone resorption,** and **fragmentation of bone.**
- Even though the joint lacks sensory feedback, almost three of four patients with a Charcot joint **complain of some degree of pain,** although it is usually far less than would be expected for the degree of joint destruction present.
- **Soft-tissue swelling is a prominent feature.**
- The **most common cause** of a Charcot joint today is **diabetes** and most Charcot joints are found in the **lower extremities,** particularly in the **feet and ankles.**
- Causes of Charcot joints by location:
  - **Shoulders:** syrinx, spinal tumor, and syphilis
  - **Hips:** tertiary syphilis, diabetes
  - **Ankles and feet:** diabetes (common) and syphilis (uncommon)

### ▶▶ IMPORTANT POINTS

- **Radiographic findings of Charcot arthropathy:**
  - As a hypertrophic arthritis, a Charcot joint will demonstrate **extensive subchondral sclerosis.**
  - The **hallmark findings of a Charcot joint** are:
    - ***Fragmentation*** of the bones surrounding the joint, which produces numerous small bony densities within the joint capsule. Sometimes,

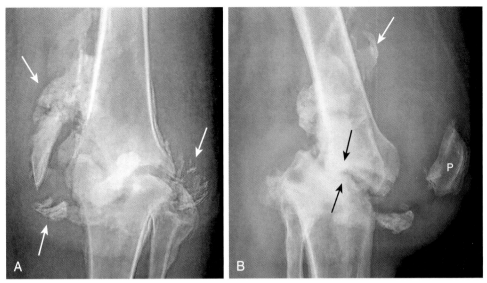

**Fig. 21.32 Charcot Arthropathy, Frontal and Lateral Knee.** A Charcot joint is a form of hypertrophic arthritis. The hallmark findings of a Charcot joint are fragmentation of the bones surrounding the joint *(white arrows in A and B)* as well as marked joint space destruction *(black arrows in B)*. There is a large joint effusion that is displacing the patella (P) forward. The most common cause of a Charcot joint of the knee is now diabetes.

## ▶▶ IMPORTANT POINTS—cont'd

> **many—if not all—of the fragments may be resorbed** and no longer be visible (Fig. 21.32).
> - Eventual *destruction of the joint.* Charcot neuropathy is responsible for some of the **most dramatic examples of total joint destruction of any arthritis** (Fig. 21.33).
> - A Charcot joint shares findings with osteomyelitis, and the two diseases may mimic each other in that they both produce **bone destruction** and **periosteal reaction (from fracture healing).** A radioisotope-tagged, white-cell bone scan can help to differentiate infection from Charcot joint.

## Calcium Pyrophosphate Deposition Disease (Pyrophosphate Arthropathy)

- *Calcium pyrophosphate deposition disease* is an arthropathy resulting from the deposition of **calcium pyrophosphate dihydrate (CPPD)** crystals in and around joints, **mostly in hyaline cartilage and fibrocartilage.** This is especially common in the **triangular fibrocartilage of the wrist** and the **menisci of the knee.**
- The terminology associated with describing this disease can be confusing.
  - *Chondrocalcinosis* refers primarily to **calcification** of the articular cartilage or fibrocartilage and is seen in about 50% of adults over the age of 85, most of whom are **asymptomatic.** Chondrocalcinosis can occur in other

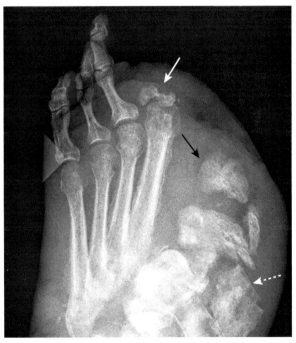

**Fig. 21.33 Charcot Arthropathy, Foot.** This patient had previously undergone an amputation of the phalanges of the second toe *(solid white arrow)* for diabetic gangrene but the destruction and marked fragmentation of the remaining portion of the great toe *(black arrow)* and tarsal bones *(dashed arrow)* are manifestations of diabetic neuropathy.

diseases besides CPPD, such as hyperparathyroidism or hemochromatosis (Fig. 21.34).

- *Pseudogout (also known as **acute CPPD crystal arthritis**)* is a **clinical syndrome** consisting of an **acute, monoarticular arthropathy** characterized by **redness, pain, and swelling** of the affected joint (most commonly the knee) from which **calcium pyrophosphate dihydrate** crystals can be aspirated. Clinical attacks resemble those of gout, except the knee and joints of the arm are most commonly affected in pseudogout.

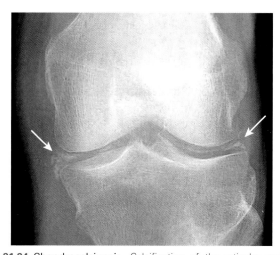

**Fig. 21.34 Chondrocalcinosis.** Calcification of the articular cartilage *(arrows)* is quite common with advanced age and may be present without symptoms. If this same patient presented with inflammatory symptoms and signs about the knee and crystals of calcium pyrophosphate dihydrate in the joint, it would be called ***pseudogout***. Changes of pyrophosphate arthropathy are shown in Fig. 21.35.

- *Pyrophosphate arthropathy* is a radiologic diagnosis confirmed by identification of calcium pyrophosphate crystals in synovial fluid and the most common form of CPPD.

> ### ▶▶ IMPORTANT POINTS
>
> - **Pyrophosphate arthropathy** may be indistinguishable from other forms of osteoarthritis, but it does differ from them in several important respects:
>   - Pyrophosphate arthropathy affects joints not **usually affected by primary osteoarthritis** such as the **patellofemoral joint space of the knee,** the **radiocarpal joint,** the **metacarpophalangeal joints of the hands,** and the joints of the **wrist.**
> - **Chondrocalcinosis is usually present** in pyrophosphate arthropathy but is not required for the diagnosis (Fig. 21.35A).
> - **Subchondral cysts** are **more common, larger, more numerous,** and more widespread than in primary osteoarthritis.
> - **Hook-shaped bony excrescences** along the second and third metacarpal heads are a common finding in this form of CPPD (Fig. 21.35B).
> - **In the wrist,** characteristic findings include **calcification of the triangular fibrocartilage,** narrowing of the radiocarpal joint, separation of the scaphoid and the lunate by more than 3 mm *(**scapholunate dissociation**),* and collapse of the distal carpal row toward the radius *(**scapholunate advanced collapse**)* (Fig. 21.35C).

## Erosive Arthritis

- *Erosive arthritis* is composed of a large number of arthritides, all of which are associated with some degree of **inflammation** and **synovial proliferation** *(**pannus formation**)* that participates in the production of **lytic lesions in or near the joint** called *erosions,* especially in the small joints of the hands and feet.

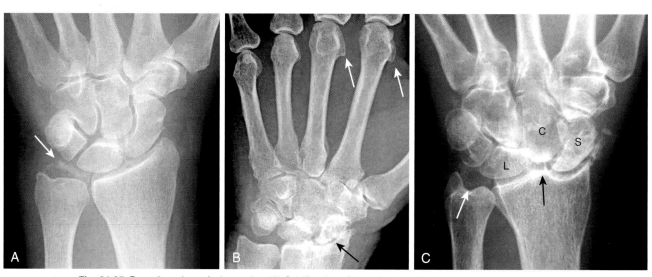

**Fig. 21.35 Pyrophosphate Arthropathy.** (A) Calcification of the triangular fibrocartilage *(arrow)* is due to the deposition of calcium pyrophosphate (CPP) crystal and is a common finding in pyrophosphate arthropathy. (B) Hook-shaped bony excrescences along the second and third metacarpal heads are also a common finding *(white arrows)*. Note that the radiocarpal joint is narrowed *(black arrow)*. (C) Other characteristic findings in the wrist besides calcification of the triangular fibrocartilage *(white arrow)* include separation of the scaphoid (S) and the lunate (L) *(**scapholunate dissociation**)* and collapse of the capitate (C) toward the radius *(black arrow)*, called ***scapholunate advanced collapse (SLAC)***.

- **Pannus** acts like a mass of growing and enlarging synovial tissue that leads to **marginal erosions** of the **articular cartilage and underlying bone.**
- Box 21.4 lists some of the many causes of erosive arthritis. We discuss four of the more common, which are **bolded** in the box.

| BOX 21.4  **Some Causes of Erosive Arthritis** | |
|---|---|
| • **Rheumatoid arthritis** | • Rheumatoid variants |
| • **Gout** | • Reactive arthritis |
| • **Psoriatic arthritis** | • Sarcoid |
| • **Ankylosing spondylitis (spine)** | • Hemophilia |

## Rheumatoid Arthritis (RA)

- *Rheumatoid arthritis* is **more common in female patients,** frequently involving the **proximal joints of the hands and wrists.** It is **usually bilateral** and **symmetric.**
- Conventional radiographs remain the study of first choice in imaging RA.

### » IMPORTANT POINTS

- The **earliest** radiographic changes are **soft-tissue swelling** of the affected joints and osteoporosis, which tends to be most severe on both sides of the joint space (*periarticular osteoporosis* or *periarticular demineralization*).

- **In the hand,** the erosions tend to involve the **proximal joints:** the carpal-metacarpal joints, metacarpal-phalangeal, and proximal interphalangeal joints (Fig. 21.36).

- **Late findings in the hands** include deformities such as **ulnar deviation of the fingers at the metacarpophalangeal (MCP) joints, subluxation of the MCP joints,** and ligamentous laxity leading to deformities of the fingers *(swan-neck* and *boutonnière deformities).*
- In the **wrist,** erosions of the **carpals, ulnar styloid,** and **narrowing of the radiocarpal joint** space are frequently seen.
- Elsewhere in the body, the **larger joints usually show no erosions,** but there may be **marked uniform narrowing of the joint space with little or no subchondral sclerosis** (Fig. 21.37).

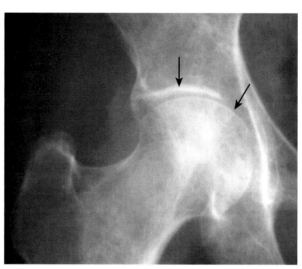

**Fig. 21.37 Rheumatoid Arthritis, Hip.** There is marked uniform narrowing of the hip joint with little or no subchondral sclerosis *(arrows).* Erosions are not present. If this were primary osteoarthritis, you should expect far more subchondral sclerosis and osteophyte production for this degree of joint space narrowing.

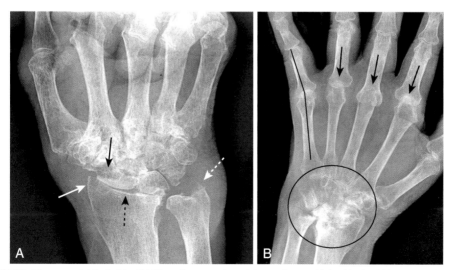

**Fig. 21.36 Rheumatoid Arthritis.** (A) There is narrowing of the radiocarpal joint *(dashed black arrow),* erosion of the radial styloid *(solid white arrow),* and a large erosion in the scaphoid *(solid black arrow).* The ulnar styloid is also eroded *(dashed white arrow).* (B) The radiocarpal and intercarpal joints *(circle)* along with the metacarpal-phalangeal joints (MCP) *(arrows)* tend to be the most involved in the hand. There is also evidence of ulnar deviation of the fifth finger at the MCP joint *(black line).*

- In the spine, RA tends to involve the **cervical spine** by producing **ligamentous laxity,** which can lead to forward subluxation of C1 on C2 *(atlantoaxial subluxation).* Atlantoaxial subluxation can produce cord compression if severe (Fig. 21.38).
  - **RA may also cause narrowing, sclerosis, and eventual fusion of the facet joints in the cervical spine.**

## Gout

- *Gouty arthritis* represents the **inflammatory changes incited by the deposition of calcium urate crystals** in the joint. There is characteristically an **extremely long latent period (5 to 7 years)** between the onset of symptoms and the visualization of bone changes, so **gout is usually a clinical and not a radiologic diagnosis** (see Table 21.5).
- Gout tends to be **monoarticular** at its onset and **asymmetric later** in its course.
- It is **more common in male patients** and **most commonly affects the metatarsal-phalangeal joint of the great toe** at the time of symptom onset.

> ## ▶ IMPORTANT POINTS
>
> - **Imaging findings of gout:**
>   - As an erosive arthritis, the hallmark of gout is the **sharply marginated, juxta-articular erosion that tends to have a sclerotic border.** The appearance of the overhanging edges of gouty erosions have been called **rat-bites.**
>   - **Joint space narrowing may be a late finding** in the disease and there is **characteristically little or no periarticular osteoporosis** (Fig. 21.39).
>   - **Tophi,** collections of urate crystals in the soft tissues, are a late finding in gout and, when present, **rarely calcify.**
>   - **Olecranon bursitis is common** (Fig. 21.40).

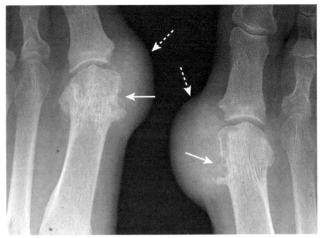

**Fig. 21.39 Gout, Both Great Toes.** Gout is an erosive arthritis and displays sharply marginated, juxta-articular erosions (called **rat-bites**) *(solid arrows)*. There are **tophi** *(dashed arrows)*, soft-tissue nodules containing urate crystals that incite a foreign body reaction, that can be associated with chronic gout. As expected in gout, the metatarsophalangeal joint space is not particularly narrowed and there is no periarticular osteoporosis.

## Psoriatic Arthritis

- **Most patients** with psoriatic arthritis **also have skin and nail changes of psoriasis** for many years, although for some the joint manifestations may be the initial presentation of the disease. About 25% of patients with long-standing psoriasis develop psoriatic arthritis. It is **usually polyarticular.**
- Psoriatic arthritis typically involves the **small joints of the hands, especially the distal interphalangeal (DIP) joints.**

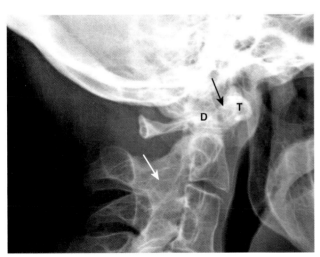

**Fig. 21.38 Rheumatoid Arthritis, Cervical Spine.** The distance between the anterior border of the dens (D) and the posterior border of the anterior tubercle of C1 (T) is called the **predentate space** and is normally no more than 3 mm. This patient's predentate space measured 8 mm *(black arrow)* because of laxity of the atlantoaxial ligaments leading to **atlantoaxial subluxation.** Rheumatoid arthritis may also cause fusion of the facet joints of the cervical spine *(white arrow).*

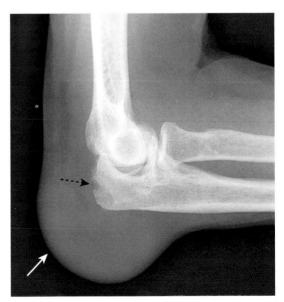

**Fig. 21.40 Olecranon Bursitis in Gout.** Olecranon bursitis is a relatively common manifestation of gout (large soft-tissue mass around elbow shown by *white arrow*) and its presence alone should call attention to the possibility of underlying gout. This patient also displays erosions adjacent to the elbow joint *(black arrow).*

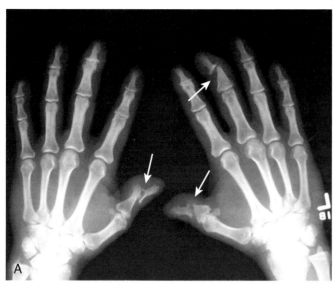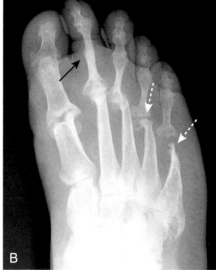

**Fig. 21.41 Psoriatic Arthritis, Hand and Foot.** (A) The distal interphalangeal (DIP) joints of both hands *(arrows)* are narrowed and eroded leading to telescoping of one phalanx into another *(pencil-in-cup deformity)*. (B) In the foot of another patient with psoriasis, there is ankylosis (fusion) of the joints of the second toe *(black arrow)* and additional pencil-in-cup deformities *(white arrows)*.

- In the **sacroiliac joints,** psoriasis can produce **bilateral, but asymmetric, sacroiliitis. The sacroiliac joints do not usually completely fuse as they do in ankylosing spondylitis** (see Chapter 22).

## Infectious Arthritis

- *Infectious arthritis* (also called *septic arthritis*) usually occurs as a result of **hematogenous seeding of the synovial membrane from an infected source elsewhere in the body,** such as a wound infection or **from direct, contiguous extension from osteomyelitis** adjacent to the joint.
- It is usually subdivided into *pyogenic (septic) arthritis,* mostly caused by *Staphylococcal* and *Gonococcal* organisms, and *nonpyogenic arthritis,* due mostly to infection with *Mycobacterium tuberculosis.*
- **Risk factors** include intravenous drug use, steroids either injected or orally administered, joint prostheses, and recent joint trauma, including joint surgery.
- **In children and adults, the knee is frequently affected; in children, the hip is** another **common** site of infection. Hands may be infected from human bites and the feet from diabetes.
- Although **conventional radiographs** are obtained as the initial study, they are **relatively insensitive** to the early

findings of the disease except for soft-tissue swelling and osteopenia.

- If septic arthritis is strongly suspected, aspiration of the joint will usually confirm the diagnosis.

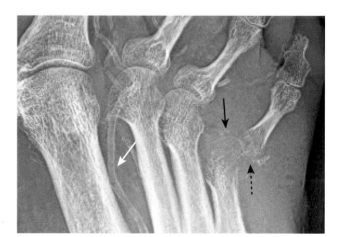

**Fig. 21.42 Septic Arthritis and Osteomyelitis.** This patient has destruction of the metatarsal-phalangeal joint *(solid black arrow)* that has extended to and destroyed the adjacent bone as osteomyelitis *(dashed black arrow)*. There is extensive vascular calcification secondary to the patient's advanced atherosclerosis from diabetes *(white arrow)*. Notice there are only four toes—the fifth toe was previously amputated because of osteomyelitis.

- Because of its sensitivity, MRI is now used extensively in diagnosing septic joints. **Enhancement of the synovium** and the **presence of a joint effusion** have the best correlation with the clinical diagnosis of a septic joint.
- *Nonpyogenic infectious arthritis* is most often caused by *M. tuberculosis*, which **spreads via the bloodstream from lung.**

- Unlike pyogenic arthritis, **tuberculous arthritis** has an **indolent and protracted course,** resulting in **gradual loss of the joint space** and **late destruction of the articular cortex.**
- Nonpyogenic infectious arthritis is **usually monoarticular. Severe osteoporosis is a common finding.** In children, the spine is most often affected; in adults, the knee.
- Healing with fibrous and bony ankylosis occurs in both pyogenic and nonpyogenic infectious arthritis.

## CASE QUIZ 21 ANSWER

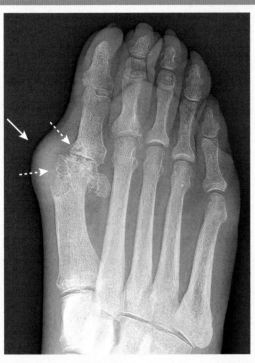

A soft-tissue mass *(solid arrow)* representing a ***tophus*** is seen at the junction of the metatarsal-phalangeal joint of the great toe that, by itself, is pathognomonic of chronic gouty arthritis in this location. Additionally, there are juxta-articular erosions *(dashed arrows)*, particularly on the head of the first metatarsal. The findings are classic for chronic tophaceous gout.

## TAKE HOME POINTS

- Long bones consist of a **cortex** of compact bone surrounding a **medullary cavity** containing cancellous bone arranged as trabeculae, separated by blood vessels, hematopoietic cells, and fat.
- Conventional radiography relies on two views taken 90 degrees from each other to help localize findings **(orthogonal views).**
- On conventional radiographs, the cortex is best seen in tangent. On CT, the entire cortex is visualized. MRI is particularly sensitive to assessment of the marrow. Both CT and MRI are superior to conventional radiographs in evaluating soft tissues.
- Bone is undergoing continuous change from a combination of biochemical and mechanical forces.
- Abnormalities in bone density can arbitrarily be divided into those that **increase density** and those that **decrease density**, either **focally or diffusely.**
- **Osteoblastic metastases,** especially from carcinoma of the prostate and breast, can produce focal or generalized increases in bony density.
- The **radionuclide bone scan** is the modality of choice in screening for skeletal metastases. MRI is used primarily to solve specific questions related to a lesion's composition and extent.

- Other diseases that can increase bone density include avascular necrosis of bone and Paget disease.
- **Avascular necrosis** of bone usually involves bones with poor collateral blood supply, such as the femoral head, and is most readily detected by MRI.
- Hallmarks of **Paget disease** include thickening of the cortex, accentuation of the trabecular pattern, and enlargement and increased density of the affected bone.
- Examples of diseases that can cause a **generalized decrease in bone density** include osteoporosis and hyperparathyroidism.
- **Osteoporosis** is characterized by low bone mineral density and is most often either postmenopausal or age-related. Osteoporosis predisposes to pathologic fractures.
- **Hyperparathyroidism** is caused by excessive parathormone secretion, which leads to increased stimulation of osteoclastic activity. Its diagnosis is based on clinical and laboratory findings.
- **Osteolytic metastases,** especially from lung, renal, thyroid, and breast cancer, can produce focal areas of decreased bone density as can solitary plasmacytomas. **Plasmacytomas** are considered to be a precursor to multiple myeloma, the most common primary tumor of bone.

- **Osteomyelitis** is frequently caused by *Staphylococcus aureus* and more often spreads to an adjacent joint space in adults rather than in children.
- An **arthritis** is a disease of a joint that invariably leads to joint space narrowing and changes to the bones on both sides of the joint.
- Arthritides can be roughly divided into hypertrophic, erosive (inflammatory), and infectious categories.
- **Hypertrophic arthritis** features subchondral sclerosis, marginal osteophyte production, and subchondral cyst formation.
- **Primary osteoarthritis,** the most common form of arthritis, is a type of hypertrophic arthritis. It typically occurs on weight-bearing surfaces of the hip and knee as well as the distal interphalangeal joints of the fingers.
- Other hypertrophic arthritides include erosive osteoarthritis, Charcot joints, and CPPD. **Secondary osteoarthritis** may occur from either prior trauma or avascular necrosis or be superimposed on another underlying arthritis.
- **Erosive osteoarthritis** has findings similar to primary osteoarthritis, but tends to feature more inflammatory changes. The erosions are typically centrally located within the joint.
- **Charcot or neuropathic joints** feature fragmentation, sclerosis, and soft-tissue swelling. Diabetes is the most frequent cause of a Charcot joint today.
- **Pyrophosphate arthropathy** occurs with the deposition of calcium pyrophosphate crystals (chondrocalcinosis). It can produce multiple, large sub-chondral cysts, narrowing of the patellofemoral joint space, metacarpal "hooks," and proximal migration of the distal carpal row.
- **Erosive (or inflammatory) arthritis**, which is associated with inflammation and synovial proliferation (pannus formation), produces lytic lesions called **erosions** in or near the joint.
- Rheumatoid arthritis, gout, and psoriasis are three examples of erosive arthritis; the site of involvement is helpful in differentiating among the causes of erosive arthritides.
- **Rheumatoid arthritis** affects the carpals and proximal joints of the hand; it can widen the predentate space in the cervical spine and can lead to fusion of the posterior elements in the cervical spine.
- **Gout** most often affects the metatarsal-phalangeal joint of the great toe with juxta-articular erosions and little or no osteoporosis. Tophi, which are late manifestations of the disease, usually do not calcify.
- **Psoriatic arthritis** usually occurs in patients with known skin changes of psoriasis; it affects the distal joints, primarily in the hands, and produces characteristic erosions that may resemble a pencil-in-cup.
- **Infectious arthritis** features soft-tissue swelling and osteopenia and, in the case of pyogenic arthritis, relatively early and marked destruction of most or all of the articular cortex. It is mostly caused by *Staphylococcal* and *Gonococcal* organisms.

 Additional content is available online including chapters on Nuclear Medicine, Artificial Intelligence, Radiation Dose and Safety, an Early History of Radiology, and a compendium of 200 Diagnostic Radiology Signs.

# Recognizing Nontraumatic Abnormalities of the Spine

*William Herring, MD, FACR*

Back pain, particularly low back pain, is the leading cause of years lived with a disability worldwide, a measure reflecting the impact an illness has on quality of life. In 2017, studies estimated that at any given moment 577 million people were suffering with low back pain globally, making it the world's leading cause of limitation of activity and absenteeism from work.

### CASE QUIZ 22 QUESTION

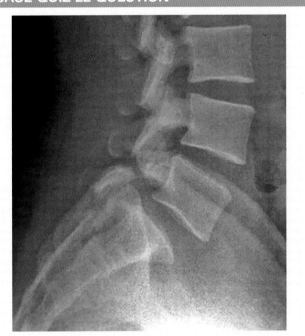

This is a close-up conventional radiograph of the lumbosacral junction in a 28-year-old male with back pain. The cause of his back pain is revealed in the radiograph. What is it? The answer is at the end of this chapter.

- **Magnetic resonance imaging**, with its superior soft-tissue differentiation, is the **study of choice** for most diseases of the spine because of its ability to visualize and detect abnormalities in **soft tissues,** such as bone marrow, the spinal cord, and the intervertebral disks, along with its ability to display images in **any plane** and the **lack of exposure to radiation.**
- MRI studies **remain relatively expensive** and their **availability is not as widespread** as CT or conventional radiographs, **patients with pacemakers** and certain internal

ferromagnetic materials (e.g., certain aneurysm clips) **are not able to be scanned**, the procedure **takes more time** to complete, and some patients cannot tolerate the **claustrophobia** they experience in some of the high-field-strength MRI scanners (see **Chapter 20**).

## THE NORMAL SPINE (FIG. 22.1)

### Vertebral Body

- Almost every vertebra has a **body** composed of inner cancellous bone and marrow and **posterior elements** made of

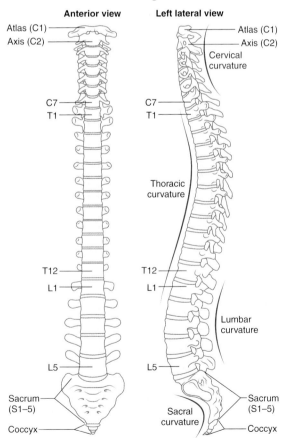

**Fig. 22.1 Normal Spine.** This illustration depicts the entire spine consisting of 7 cervical vertebra, 12 thoracic vertebra—all of which normally bear ribs—5 lumbar vertebra, and 5 fused sacral vertebrae. The curvature of the cervical and lumbar spines is called *lordotic,* and the curvature of the thoracic spine is *kyphotic.*

compact dense bone consisting of the pedicles, laminae, facets, transverse processes, and a spinous process (Fig. 22.2A).

- From the level of **C3** through the level of **L5** the vertebral bodies are more or less **rectangular in shape** and of about equal height posteriorly as anteriorly.
- The **endplates of contiguous vertebral bodies** are roughly **parallel** to each other.
- The **articular facets** of the **superior** and **inferior articular processes** are lined with cartilage and these facet joints are **true synovial joints.**
- In the frontal projection, each vertebral body displays two ovoid **pedicles** visible on each side of the vertebral body. The pedicles of L5 are frequently difficult to visualize, even in normal individuals, because of the lordosis of the lumbar spine (Fig. 22.2B).
- On conventional radiographs of the **lumbar spine** performed in the **oblique** projection, the anatomic structures normally superimpose to produce a shadow that resembles the front end of a Scottish terrier, the *Scottie dog* sign (Fig. 22.3).

## Intervertebral Disks

- The intervertebral disks have a central gelatinous **nucleus pulposus** surrounded by an outer **annulus fibrosus** that is, in turn, made up of inner fibrocartilaginous fibers and

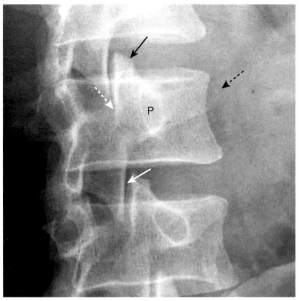

**Fig. 22.3 Normal Scottie Dog.** This is a left posterior oblique view of the lumbar spine (the patient is turned about halfway toward her own left). The **Scottie dog** is made up of the following: the **ear** *(solid black arrow)* is the superior articular facet, the **leg** *(solid white arrow)* is the inferior articular facet, the **nose** *(dashed black arrow)* is the transverse process, the **eye** (P) is the pedicle, and the **neck** *(dashed white arrow)* is the **pars interarticularis.** All of these structures are paired—an identical set should be visible on the patient's other side.

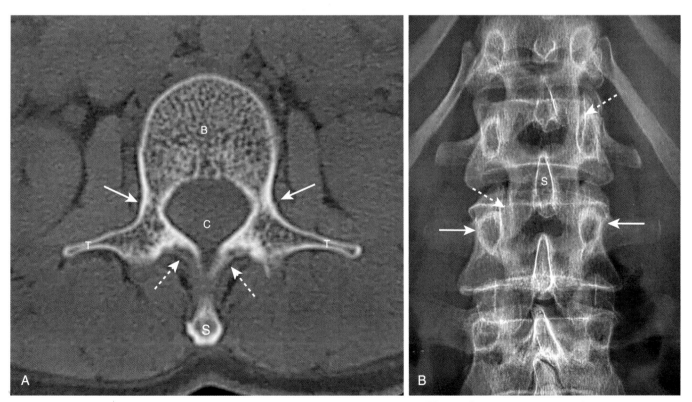

**Fig. 22.2 Normal Spine, Axial CT and Frontal Radiograph.** (A) In this CT scan of a "typical" vertebral body, we see the body (B), pedicles *(solid arrows)*, laminae *(dashed arrows)*, transverse processes (T), spinal canal (C) and spinous process (S). (B) Each vertebral body has two pedicles that project as small ovals on either side of the vertebral body *(solid arrows)*. The spinous process (S) may be visualized slightly above the body to which it is attached. Facet joints are seen here *en face (dashed arrows)*.

outer cartilaginous fibers *(Sharpey's fibers)*. The nucleus pulposus is located near the posterior aspect of the disk (Fig. 22.4).

## Spinal Ligaments

- Several ligaments traverse the spine (Table 22.1) (see Fig. 22.4).

## Spinal Cord and Spinal Nerves

- The spinal cord extends from the medulla oblongata to the level of L1-L2, ending as the **conus medullaris.** The **cauda equina** extends inferiorly from that point as a collection of nerve roots, with each root exiting **below** its respectively numbered vertebral body.
- Each of the paired **neural foramina** of the spine contains a **spinal nerve, blood vessels,** and **fat.**
- **Spinal nerves** are named and numbered **according to the site they exit** from the spinal canal. **From C1-C7,** nerves exit **above** their respective vertebrae. The **C8** nerve exits **between the seventh cervical and first thoracic** vertebrae. The remaining nerves exit **below** their respectively numbered vertebrae.

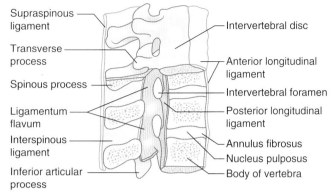

**Fig. 22.4 Normal Spine and Soft Tissues.** A partial cross-section illustration of the spine depicts the normal bony and ligamentous structures.

### TABLE 22.1   Ligaments of the Spine

| Ligament | Connects |
| --- | --- |
| **Anterior longitudinal ligament** | Anterior surfaces of vertebral bodies |
| **Posterior longitudinal ligament** | Posterior surfaces of vertebral bodies |
| **Ligamentum flavum** | Laminae of adjacent vertebral bodies; lies in posterior portion of spinal canal |
| **Interspinous ligament** | Between spinous processes |
| **Supraspinous ligament** | Tips of spinous processes |

> ## ▶▶ IMPORTANT POINTS
>
> - The **relative height of the disk space varies in each part of the spine.**
>   - In the **cervical spine,** the disk spaces are about **equal** to each other in height.
>   - In the **thoracic spine,** they are usually slightly **decreased** in size **from the cervical spine,** but **equal** in height to each other.
>   - In the **lumbar spine,** the disk spaces progressively **increase** in height with each successive interspace, **except for L5-S1,** which can be equal to or slightly less than the height of L4-L5 on conventional radiographs.

## NORMAL MRI APPEARANCE OF THE SPINE

> ## ▶▶ IMPORTANT POINTS
>
> - On **T1-weighted** sagittal MRI images of the spine, the **vertebral bodies,** containing bone marrow, will normally be of **high signal intensity** (bright); the **disks** will be **lower in signal intensity,** and **cerebrospinal fluid (CSF)** in the thecal sac will have a **low signal intensity** (dark) (Fig. 22.5A).

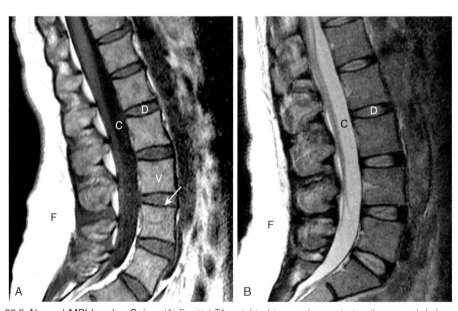

**Fig. 22.5 Normal MRI Lumbar Spine.** (A) Sagittal T1-weighted image demonstrates the normal dark appearance of the disk (D) relative to the vertebral body (V). The CSF in the spinal canal (C) is dark, and the subcutaneous fat of the back (F) is bright. Cortical bone has a low signal *(arrow)*. (B) Sagittal T2-weighted image demonstrates the normal appearance of the disk (D), which is slightly higher intensity (brighter) than the vertebral bodies. The CSF (C) in the spinal canal is now bright, and the subcutaneous fat (F) of the back remains bright.

## BACK PAIN

- It has been estimated that **almost 80% of all Americans will have some episode of back pain** during their lifetime. The causes of back pain are numerous and the anatomic and physiologic interrelationships that produce it are still not known in many cases.
- Some causes of back pain are:
  - Herniation of an intervertebral disk
  - Degeneration of an intervertebral disk
  - Arthritis involving the synovial joints of the spine
  - Diffuse idiopathic skeletal hyperostosis
  - **Compression fractures,** usually from osteoporosis
  - **Spinal stenosis**
  - Malignancy involving the spine
  - Infection of the spine
  - Ankylosing spondylitis
  - Trauma to the spine
  - Muscle and ligament strain
- In this chapter we discuss all of these (in bold) except muscle and ligament strains. Spinal trauma appears in **Chapter 23.**

### Herniated Disks

- Only about 2% of patients with acute low back pain have a herniated disk. In the **lumbar region,** disk herniation may lead to **back pain** and **sciatica,** whereas herniation of a **cervical disk** may produce **radiculopathy** and **myelopathy. MRI is the study of choice for evaluating herniated disks.**
- In the **cervical spine,** disk herniations occur most frequently at **C4-C5, C5-C6,** and **C6-C7** (Fig. 22.6).

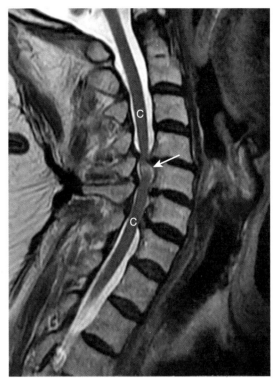

**Fig. 22.6 Herniated Cervical Disk, MRI.** The spinal cord (C) is dark relative to the high-intensity (whiter) signal surrounding it, which is the cerebrospinal fluid in the spinal canal. A herniated disk *(arrow)* extends posteriorly from the disk space and compresses the cord.

- Compared with the cervical and lumbar spine, **thoracic disks are very stable,** in part because they are protected by the rib cage that surrounds them.
- **Degeneration** of the outer annular fibers of the disk or **trauma** can lead to an interruption in those fibers and allow the disk material to *bulge,* which may or may not be associated with back pain.
- When the annular fibers rupture, the **nucleus pulposus** may *herniate* (usually posterolaterally) through a **weakened** area of the **posterior longitudinal ligament.**
- The herniated material may *protrude* but remain in contact with the parent disk from which it originated, or it may be completely *extruded* into the spinal canal.
- Symptoms are caused by acute **compression** of the **nerve root.**
- Disk herniations can be visualized on both **CT** and **MRI.** CT shows disk material compressing nerve roots or the thecal sac. On MRI, the herniated disk material is usually a **focal, asymmetric protrusion of hypointense disk material** that

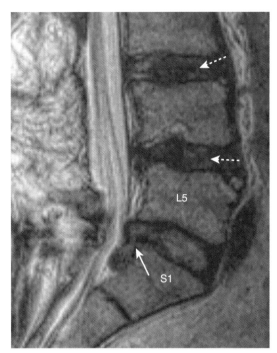

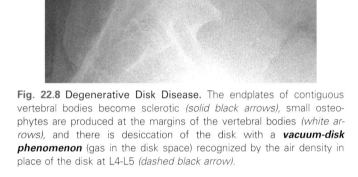

**Fig. 22.7 Disk Herniation, L5-S1.** Sagittal T2-weighted image of the lower lumbar spine shows disk material *(solid arrow)* beyond the confines of the L5-S1 intervertebral disk space representing a disk herniation extending posteriorly and inferiorly. Notice that degeneration and desiccation of the other disks has led them to become darker than normal on this T2-weighted image *(dashed arrows)*.

**Fig. 22.8 Degenerative Disk Disease.** The endplates of contiguous vertebral bodies become sclerotic *(solid black arrows)*, small osteophytes are produced at the margins of the vertebral bodies *(white arrows)*, and there is desiccation of the disk with a **vacuum-disk phenomenon** (gas in the disk space) recognized by the air density in place of the disk at L4-L5 *(dashed black arrow)*.

extends beyond the confines of the annulus fibrosus (Fig. 22.7).

- *Postlaminectomy syndrome* is persistent pain in the back or legs following spine surgery. In some studies, it has been estimated to occur in 40% of postoperative patients. Gadolinium-enhanced MRI studies of the spine are useful in differentiating persistent or recurrent **disk herniation** from **scar formation** as a cause of the pain.

## Degenerative Disk Disease (DDD)

- With increasing age, the normally gelatinous nucleus pulposus becomes dehydrated and degenerates. This gradually leads to **progressive loss of the height of the intervertebral disk space.** At times, desiccation of the disk leads to **release of nitrogen** from tissues surrounding the disk resulting in the appearance of **air density in the disk space,** which is called a *vacuum-disk phenomenon.* A vacuum-disk appearance represents a **late sign** of a degenerated disk (Fig. 22.8).
- **Degenerative disk disease on MRI**
  - The decrease in water content of the nucleus pulposus results in a lower signal intensity of the disk on T2-weighted images (see Fig. 22.7).
- **Degenerative disk disease on conventional radiographs**
  - There is **disk-space narrowing** and also changes in the vertebral bodies themselves.

- The **endplates** of contiguous vertebral bodies become *eburnated* or **sclerotic. Small osteophytes** are produced at the margins of the vertebral bodies at each disk space (see Fig. 22.8).
- At the same time, there is typically degeneration of the outer annulus fibrosus. This can lead to the production of **larger marginal osteophytes** at the endplates than those seen with degeneration of the nuclear material.
- It should be noted that osteophytes are an **extremely common** finding, increasing in prevalence with increasing age, and that most patients with osteophytes of the spine are **asymptomatic.**

## Osteoarthritis of the Facet Joints

- The *facet joints* (also known as the *apophyseal joints*) are **true joints** in that they have cartilage, a synovial lining, and synovial fluid. As such, they are subject to an arthritis, such as **osteoarthritis,** similar to true joints in the appendicular skeleton.
- Some consider the small joint-like structures at the lateral edges of C3 to T1, called the **uncovertebral joints** or the *joints of Luschka,* to be true joints, whereas others do not.
  - In either case, the uncovertebral joints are frequent sites of osteophyte formation. **Osteophytes** at the **uncovertebral joints** are **frequently associated** with both **degenerative disk disease** and osteophytes of the **facet joints.**

- In the **cervical spine, osteophytes that develop** at the **uncovertebral joints** can produce **protrusions of bone into** the normally oval-shaped **neural foramina,** which can be visualized on conventional radiographs taken in the oblique projection (Fig. 22.9A).

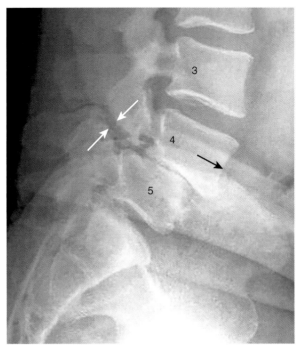

- There is usually a **complex interrelationship between degenerative disk disease and facet arthritis** such that the two frequently occur together. The osteophytes formed by osteoarthritis of the facet joints may also encroach on the neural foramina and produce radicular pain.
- In the **lumbar spine,** facet osteoarthritis may cause **narrowing** and **sclerosis of the facet joints,** best seen on oblique views of the spine (Fig. 22.9B). Facet arthritis is easier to visualize on CT scans of the spine than on conventional radiographs, and actual nerve compression is easier to visualize on MRI of the spine.

## Spondylolysis and Spondylolisthesis

- *Spondylolysis* is a unilateral or bilateral break in the ***pars interarticularis,*** most commonly at L5-S1, believed to be mainly due to repetitive microtrauma. The pars interarticularis connects each vertebral body's paired **superior articulating facets** with their corresponding **inferior articulating facets** (see Fig. 22.3).
- **Conventional radiographs** of the lumbar spine are usually the **initial imaging study.** If further imaging is warranted, either **CT or MRI** may be performed.
- If the break in the pars interarticularis is bilateral, it can lead to *spondylolisthesis*—slippage (typically forward) of one

**Fig. 22.10** Spondylolysis and Spondylolisthesis. This lateral view of the lower lumbar spine demonstrates bilateral breaks in the pars interarticularis ***(spondylolysis)*** at L4-L5 *(white arrows)* allowing L4 and the spine above it to slip forward on L5 *(black arrow),* producing ***spondylolisthesis***.

vertebral body on another, called ***spondylolytic spondylolisthesis*** (Fig. 22.10).
- Forward slipping spondylolisthesis is also called ***anterolisthesis.*** Posterior slipping is called ***retrolisthesis.***

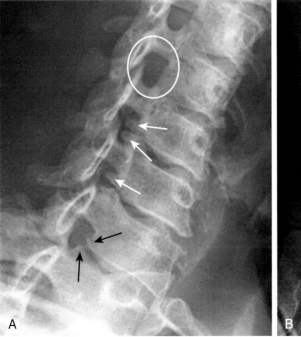

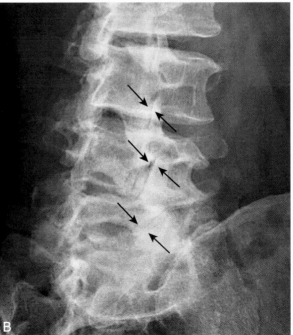

**Fig. 22.9** Uncovertebral and Facet Arthritis. (A) In the cervical spine, osteophytes may develop at the uncovertebral joints *(black arrows)* producing bony protrusions *(white arrows)* into the normally oval-shaped neural foramina *(circle),* as shown in this radiograph taken in the oblique projection. (B) There is narrowing and sclerosis involving all of the lower facet joints of the lumbar spine *(arrows).*

- *Degenerative spondylolisthesis,* in which there is no break in the pars interarticularis, can occur with **facet arthritis,** especially in females.
- The overwhelming number of those with spondylolysis and/or spondylolisthesis are asymptomatic. The most common symptom is back pain.

## Diffuse Idiopathic Skeletal Hyperostosis (DISH)

- DISH is a common disorder characterized by bone or calcium excrescences at the sites of ligamentous insertions. The excrescences are called *enthesophytes* and the conditions in which they form (of which DISH is only one) are called *enthesopathies.*
- DISH usually affects **men** over the age of **50**; it can occur anywhere in the spine, but **most often** affects the **lower thoracic and/or lower cervical spine.**
- Frequently patients with DISH complain of back stiffness, but may have **no pain** or **mild back pain.**
- **Conventional radiographs** of the spine are **sufficient** to make the diagnosis of DISH.
- Unlike ankylosing spondylitis, which may radiographically resemble DISH in the spine, the **sacroiliac joints are normal in DISH.**
- *Ossification of the posterior longitudinal ligament* (OPLL), which is often present with DISH, is better visualized on CT and MRI than on conventional radiographs. It may cause compression of the spinal cord, especially in the cervical spine, because of narrowing of the spinal canal (Fig. 22.11B).

> **IMPORTANT POINTS**

- DISH is manifest by **thick bridging or flowing calcification/ossification** of the **anterior** or, sometimes, **posterior longitudinal ligaments.**
- This ossification is visualized along the anterior or anterolateral aspects of at least **four contiguous vertebral bodies.** Unlike degenerative disk disease, the **disk spaces** and (usually) the **facet joints** are **preserved.** The flowing ossification seen in DISH is **separated slightly from the vertebral body** (Fig. 22.11A).

## Compression Fractures of the Spine

- Vertebral compression fractures are **common,** affecting **women more than men,** and typically occur secondary to **osteoporosis.** They may be **asymptomatic** or they may produce **pain** in the mid-thoracic or upper lumbar area that typically disappears in 4 to 6 weeks. Sometimes they are first noticed because of increasing **kyphosis** or **loss of overall body height.**
- **Conventional spine radiographs are usually the study of first choice.** MRI can be utilized for differentiating **osteoporotic** compression fractures from compression fractures caused by **malignancy.** Both MRI and nuclear bone scans can help in establishing the **age** of a compression abnormality, which might be impossible on conventional radiographs alone.

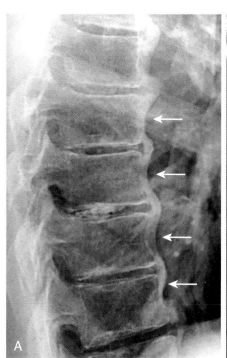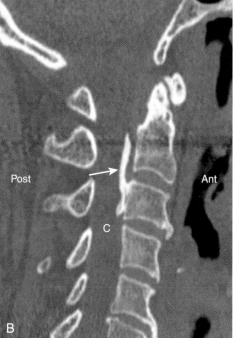

**Fig. 22.11** Diffuse Idiopathic Skeletal Hyperostosis (DISH) and Ossification of the Posterior Longitudinal Ligament (OPLL). (A) DISH is manifest by thick bridging or flowing calcification/ossification of the **anterior** longitudinal ligaments of at least four contiguous vertebral bodies *(arrows).* (B) Ossification of the **posterior** longitudinal ligament *(arrow)* can be seen on this sagittal CT of the cervical spine and may contribute to the production of spinal stenosis. *Ant,* Anterior; *C,* spinal canal; *Post,* posterior.

## IMPORTANT POINTS

- **Osteoporotic compression fractures** usually involve the **anterior and superior** aspects of the vertebral body, **sparing the posterior aspect.** This will lead to a difference in the height between the **anterior and posterior** aspects of the same vertebral body **in excess of 3 mm.** Alternatively, the compressed body is typically more than 20% shorter than the body above or below it.
  - This compression pattern produces a **wedge-shaped deformity** that leads to accentuation of the normal kyphosis in the thoracic spine (the so-called **Dowager's hump**) (Fig. 22.12).

- **Usually no neurologic deficit** is associated with an osteoporotic compression fracture because the fracture involves the anterior part of the vertebral body, away from the spinal cord.

## Spinal Stenosis

- Spinal stenosis refers to **narrowing of the spinal canal** or the neural foramina secondary to **soft-tissue or bony abnormalities,** either on an **acquired or congenital** basis. Acquired etiologies, such as those from **degenerative changes,** are more common than congenital causes.
- **Soft-tissue abnormalities** that can lead to **spinal stenosis** include hypertrophy of the ligamentum flavum, bulging disk(s), and ossification of the posterior longitudinal ligament (see Fig. 22.11B).
- **Bony abnormalities** that can lead to **spinal stenosis** include a congenitally narrow spinal canal, osteophytes, facet osteoarthritis, or spondylolisthesis. A spinal canal that was borderline normal in size may become stenotic when any of these processes superimpose to further narrow the canal.

## IMPORTANT POINTS

- Spinal stenosis is **most common in the cervical and lumbar areas;** it can lead to radicular pain, myelopathy, or, in the lumbar region, neurogenic claudication. **Neurogenic claudication** is intermittent pain and paresthesias radiating down the leg worsened by standing or walking and relieved by flexing the spine when lying supine or squatting.

- **Conventional radiographs are usually obtained first** in evaluating for spinal stenosis. **CT** provides an excellent method of demonstrating bony abnormalities, but **MRI is the study of choice** because the bony dimensions alone do not account for the soft tissues that can produce the stenosis (Fig. 22.13).

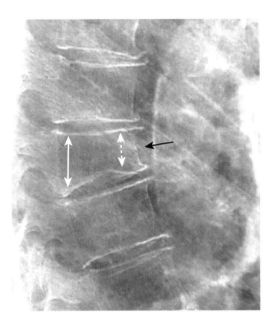

**Fig. 22.12 Compression Fracture Secondary to Osteoporosis.** There is compression of a lower thoracic vertebral body *(black arrow).* The anterior *(dashed double arrow)* and superior aspects of the vertebral body are most often involved, frequently sparing the posterior aspect *(solid double arrow).* Progressive loss of overall height of the person is a common finding with compression fractures in the elderly.

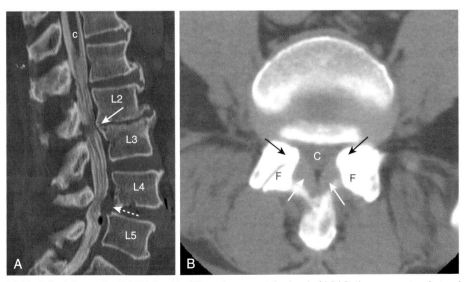

**Fig. 22.13 Spinal Stenosis, CT.** (A) On this CT myelogram, at the level of L2-L3, there are osteophytes *(solid arrow)* that narrow the canal (C). There is a protruding disk *(dashed arrow)* at L4-L5 that reduces the size of the spinal canal at this level. (B) The canal (C) is narrowed by thickening of the ligamenta flava *(white arrows)* and by bony overgrowth *(black arrows)* from osteoarthritis of the facet joints (F).

- **Conventional radiographic** findings may include an **anteroposterior diameter of the spinal canal of 10 mm or less, facet joint arthritis,** and **spondylolisthesis.**

## Malignancy Involving the Spine

- **Metastases** to bone are 25 times more common than **primary** bone tumors. Metastases usually occur where **red marrow** is found, with 80% of metastatic bone lesions occurring in the **axial skeleton** (i.e., spine, pelvis, skull, and ribs) because this is where the red marrow exists with normal aging.
- Because of the rich blood supply in the **posterior** portion of vertebral bodies, hematogenous **metastatic deposits to that part of the spine are common**, especially from **lung** and **breast** carcinoma.
- In the spine, metastases may lead to **compression fractures.** Metastases tend to **destroy the whole vertebral body,** including and especially the posterior aspect and the pedicles, which is different from **osteoporotic compression fractures** in which **the posterior vertebral body and pedicles remain intact** (see Fig. 22.12).
- As discussed in **Chapter 21, metastatic disease** can either be mostly bone-producing (i.e., *osteoblastic*) or mostly bone-destroying (i.e., *osteolytic*). Metastases that contain both osteolytic and osteoblastic processes occurring simultaneously are called **mixed metastatic lesions.**
- **Prostate cancer** is the prototype example of a primary malignancy that produces **osteoblastic metastases;** the prototype primary malignancy for the origin of osteoblastic metastatic disease in a **female** patient is **breast cancer.** The most common causes of primary malignancies that produce **osteolytic** metastatic lesions are **lung** and **breast** cancer. **Thyroid** and **renal** carcinomas may produce **osteolytic** lesions that are also expansile (see Fig. 21.20).
- The spine is also a frequent site of **multiple myeloma,** the most common primary malignancy of bone. Multiple myeloma is known for its tendency to produce almost **totally lytic lesions.** One of the hallmarks of multiple myeloma is **osteoporosis,** so that myeloma may be associated with **diffuse spinal osteoporosis** and **multiple compression fractures** (Fig. 22.14).

> ▶▶ **IMPORTANT POINTS**
>
> - The current **screening study of choice** for the detection of spinal metastases is a **technetium-99m (Tc-99m) bone scintiscan** (radionuclide bone scan). The technetium radioisotope is most commonly bound to **methylene diphosphonate (MDP)** that transports the Tc-99m to bone. A radionuclide bone scan is relatively inexpensive, widely available, and screens the entire body. Although bone scans are **highly sensitive** to the presence of metastatic deposits, they are **not very specific.** In many cases a confirmatory study, usually a conventional radiograph, is needed to exclude other causes of abnormal radio-tracer uptake, such as fractures, infection, and arthritis (Fig. 22.15).

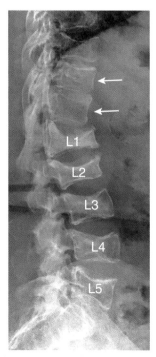

**Fig. 22.14 Multiple Myeloma of the Spine.** There are multiple compression fractures of the vertebral bodies (L1-L5) from the osteoporosis produced by multiple myeloma. The T11 and T12 vertebral bodies are osteoporotic *(arrows)* but not yet as compressed as the lumbar vertebrae. Notice how the posterior aspects of the vertebral bodies remain essentially normal in height in osteoporotic fractures while the central and anterior aspects collapse.

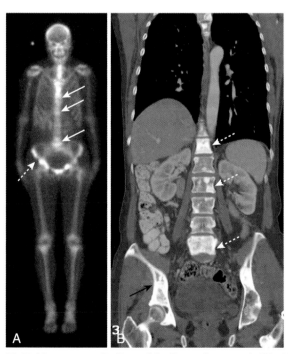

**Fig. 22.15 Metastases, Radionuclide Bone Scan and CT.** (A) A Technetium-99m methylene diphosphonate (MDP) bone scan demonstrates abnormal tracer uptake in numerous areas including the spine *(solid arrows)* and pelvis *(dashed arrow).* Because of the nonspecific nature of positive bone scans, a confirmatory study, usually conventional radiography, is obtained as well. In this case the patient had undergone a CT scan, and the coronal reformatted image (B) shows numerous osteoblastic lesions in the spine *(white arrows)* and the pelvis *(black arrow)* corresponding to the lesions seen on bone scan. This patient had known breast carcinoma.

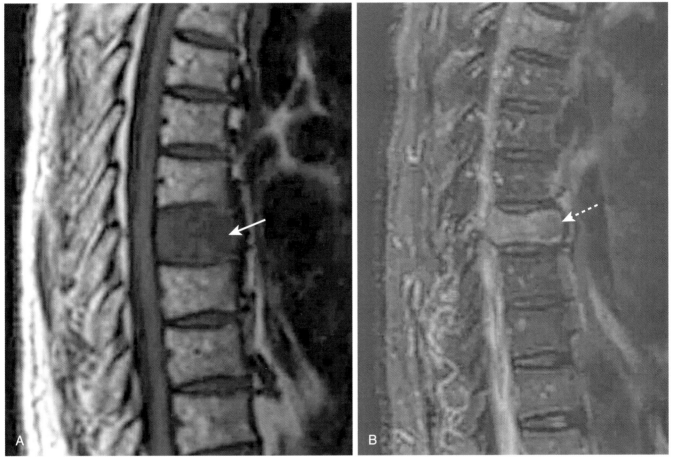

**Fig. 22.16** Metastases to the Spine, MRI. (A) T1-weighted sagittal MRI of the thoracic spine shows marrow replacement in the T8 vertebral body *(arrow)*. The signal is decreased compared to the normal bodies above and below it. (B) T2-weighted sagittal MRI shows abnormally high signal in the compressed vertebral body *(arrow)*. The patient had primary breast carcinoma.

## MRI in Metastatic Spine Disease

- MRI can detect changes of osseous metastases even **earlier than a radionuclide scan** and techniques have been described that may allow for **whole-body screening** utilizing MRI, similar to radionuclide bone scanning.

> ▶ **IMPORTANT POINTS**
>
> - With neoplastic infiltration of the bone marrow, there is a **decrease** in the normally high signal of the vertebrae on **T1-weighted images** and there is usually a **high signal on T2-weighted** images (Fig. 22.16).

## Diskitis/Osteomyelitis of the Spine

- **Infection of the disk (*diskitis* or *discitis*) is almost al-ways associated with osteomyelitis of the contiguous vertebrae,** and it almost always spreads **hematogenously** from infection in another organ (e.g., urinary tract or soft tissues). The **lumbar region** is most commonly involved, and *Staphylococcus aureus* is most often the pathogen. **Back pain** and **tenderness** are presenting symptoms.

- Because of the blood supply, children are more likely to start with diskitis, which then spreads to the adjacent vertebrae, whereas adults more frequently develop vertebral osteomyelitis that spreads to the disk.

> ▶ **IMPORTANT POINTS**
>
> - **Diskitis/osteomyelitis** should be considered any time there are abnormalities of a disk space **(narrowing, irregularity)** and **destruction of the adjacent vertebral body endplates**. Findings on conventional radiographs may take weeks or months to manifest. CT is more sensitive and can also detect extra-spinal disease, such as an abscess. MRI is most sensitive (Fig. 22.17).

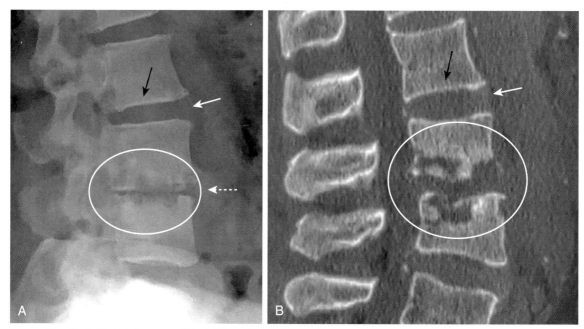

**Fig. 22.17** Diskitis/Osteomyelitis. (A) There is destruction of the endplates of L4 and L5 *(oval)* with narrowing of the intervening disk space at L4-L5 *(dashed arrow)*. Notice, for comparison, a normal endplate *(black arrow)* and disk space *(solid white arrow)* in both (A) and (B). (B) Sagittal CT in another patient shows destruction of the endplates and subchondral destruction at L3-L4 *(oval)* consistent with diskitis with osteomyelitis.

- Treatment is antibiotics, sometimes along with surgery.

## Ankylosing Spondylitis

- Ankylosing spondylitis is a chronic and progressive arthritis characterized by **inflammation** and eventual **fusion of the sacroiliac joints** along with the spinal facet joints and involvement of the paravertebral soft tissues.
- More **common in young males**, the disease characteristically **ascends the spine starting in the sacroiliac joints** and moves to the lumbar, thoracic, and finally cervical spine.
- Almost all patients with ankylosing spondylitis test **positive** for the **human leukocyte antigen B27 (HLA-B27)** as opposed to only about 5% to 10% of the general population.
- Conventional radiographs of the affected areas are the usual studies performed for diagnosis and follow-up of patients with ankylosing spondylitis.
- Like DISH, ankylosing spondylitis is an *enthesopathy.* There is inflammation, with subsequent **calcification** and **ossification** at and around the *entheses*, which are the insertion **sites of tendons, ligaments,** and **joint capsules.**

> ## ▶▶ IMPORTANT POINTS
>
> - *Sacroiliitis* is the hallmark of ankylosing spondylitis. It is usually **bilaterally symmetric** and **eventually leads to bony fusion** or *ankylosis* of these joints such that they appear either as a thin white line (instead of a joint space) or they disappear altogether (Fig. 22.18).

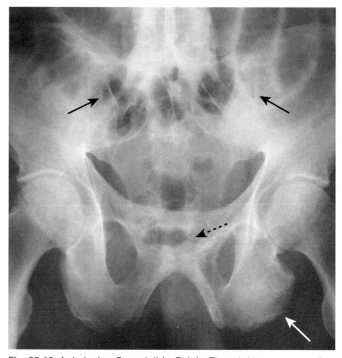

**Fig. 22.18** Ankylosing Spondylitis, Pelvis. There is bony overgrowth at the ischial tuberosity, the insertion point of the hamstring muscles *(white arrow)*. Bilaterally symmetric sacroiliitis eventually leads to bony fusion or ankylosis of the SI joints until they disappear as joints altogether *(solid black arrows)*. The symphysis pubis is also ankylosed *(dashed black arrow)*.

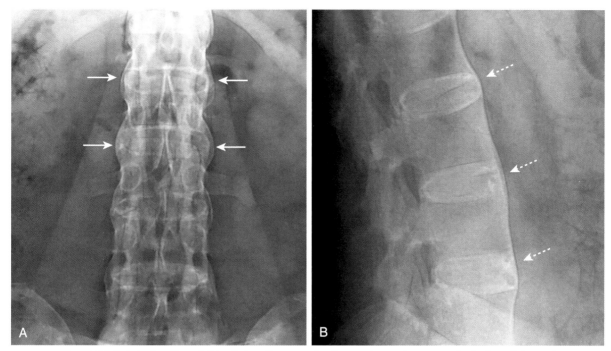

**Fig. 22.19 Ankylosing Spondylitis, Spine.** There are flowing syndesmophytes seen in the frontal *(arrows)* and lateral views *(arrows)* of the lumbar spine. Progressive ossification connecting adjacent vertebral bodies produces the ***bamboo-spine*** appearance characteristic of ankylosing spondylitis.

- In the spine, there is **ossification of the outer fibers of the annulus fibrosis** producing **thin bony bridges** joining the corners of one vertebra to another, called *syndesmophytes.*

Progressive syndesmophyte production connecting adjacent vertebral bodies produces a ***bamboo-spine*** appearance (Fig. 22.19).

## CASE QUIZ 22 ANSWER

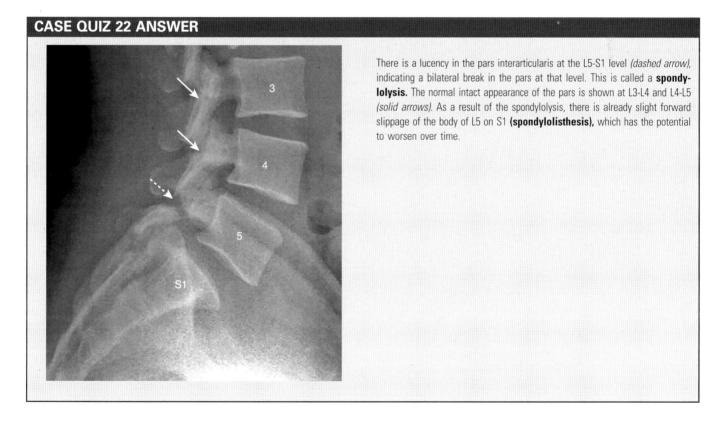

There is a lucency in the pars interarticularis at the L5-S1 level *(dashed arrow)*, indicating a bilateral break in the pars at that level. This is called a **spondylolysis.** The normal intact appearance of the pars is shown at L3-L4 and L4-L5 *(solid arrows)*. As a result of the spondylolysis, there is already slight forward slippage of the body of L5 on S1 **(spondylolisthesis),** which has the potential to worsen over time.

## TAKE HOME POINTS

- Conventional radiographs, CT, and MRI are all used to evaluate the spine, but MRI is the study of choice for most diseases of the spine because of its superior ability to display soft tissues.
- Normal features of the vertebral bodies, intervertebral disks, the spinal cord, spinal nerves, and spinal ligaments are described.
- Some of the more **common causes of back pain** are muscle and ligament strain, herniation of an intervertebral disk, degeneration of an intervertebral disk, arthritis involving the synovial joints of the spine, diffuse idiopathic skeletal hyperostosis, and spinal stenosis.
- Most **herniated disks** occur posterolaterally in the lower cervical or lower lumbar spine and are best evaluated with MRI.
- **Postlaminectomy syndrome** is persistent pain in the back or legs following spine surgery. Gadolinium-enhanced MRI can be very helpful in its detection.
- With increasing age, the nucleus pulposus becomes dehydrated and degenerates, leading to changes of **degenerative disk disease,** such as progressive loss of the height of the disk space, marginal osteophyte production, sclerosis of the endplates of the vertebral bodies, and, occasionally, the appearance of a vacuum disk.
- The facet joints are true joints and so are subject to changes of osteoarthritis; **facet osteoarthritis,** which is frequently associated with degenerative disk disease, can lead to radicular pain.
- **Spondylolysis** is a unilateral or bilateral break in the pars interarticularis. Bilateral spondylolysis can lead to forward slippage of one body on the next, called **spondylolisthesis.**

- **Diffuse idiopathic skeletal hyperostosis** is manifest by thick, bridging, or flowing calcification/ossification of the anterior longitudinal ligaments, usually occurring in men over the age of 50. The disk spaces and the facet joints are most often preserved.
- **Compression fractures** of the spine, which are most often secondary to osteoporosis, are seen more commonly in women. They can be seen on conventional radiographs and, because they usually disproportionately involve the anterior portion of the body, can produce an exaggerated kyphosis in the thoracic spine.
- **Spinal stenosis** is a narrowing of the spinal canal or the neural foramina secondary to soft-tissue or bony abnormalities, either on an acquired (more common) or congenital basis; it is most common in the cervical and lumbar regions.
- **Metastatic lesions to the spine** occur mostly in the blood-rich, posterior aspect of the vertebral body, including the pedicles. Lung (mixed), breast (mixed), and prostate (osteoblastic) metastases are the most common primary sites.
- **Multiple myeloma** also frequently involves the spine, with either severe osteoporosis which can produce compression fractures, or lytic destruction of the vertebral body.
- **Ankylosing spondylitis** is a chronic and progressive arthritis characterized by symmetric fusion of the sacroiliac joints and ascending involvement of the spine, eventually producing a bamboo-spine appearance.

 Additional content is available online including chapters on Nuclear Medicine, Artificial Intelligence, Radiation Dose and Safety, an Early History of Radiology, and a compendium of 200 Diagnostic Radiology Signs.

# Recognizing Trauma to the Bony Skeleton

*William Herring, MD, FACR*

## RECOGNIZING AN ACUTE FRACTURE

Recognizing a fracture seems to hold a certain attraction for many. They are a favorite among those learning radiology, perhaps because of how common and seemingly straightforward they are. In this chapter we tell you how to recognize a fracture, describe it, name it, and avoid overlooking it.

- A fracture is a **disruption in the continuity of all or part of the cortex of a bone.**
  - If the **cortex** is **broken through and through,** the fracture is called *complete.*
  - If only a **part of the cortex** is fractured, it is called *incomplete.* Incomplete fractures tend to occur in bones that are more elastic, such as those normally seen in children or abnormally in adults with bone-softening diseases, such as Paget disease (see Chapter 21).
- Examples of **incomplete** fractures in children are the *greenstick fracture,* which involves only one part of, but not the entire, cortex and the *torus fracture (buckle fracture),* which represents compression of the cortex (Fig. 23.1).

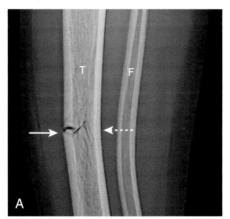
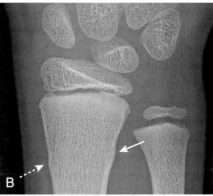

**Fig. 23.1** Greenstick and Buckle (Torus) Fractures. (A) There is a greenstick fracture *(solid arrow)* that involves only the convex cortex of the tibia, but not the entire cortex *(dashed arrow).* The fibula is **bowed** medially, but there is no cortical break identified. (B) A buckle fracture is characterized by bulging of the cortex *(arrows). F,* Fibula; *T,* tibia.

### CASE QUIZ 23 QUESTION

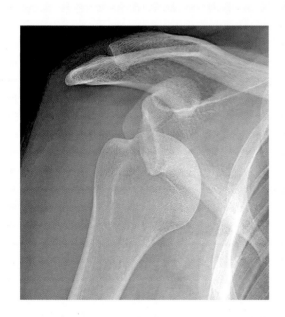

This is a frontal view of the right shoulder in a 23-year-old male who was injured playing football. He complains of severe pain in the shoulder and has a reduced range of motion. What is the diagnosis? The answer is at the end of this chapter.

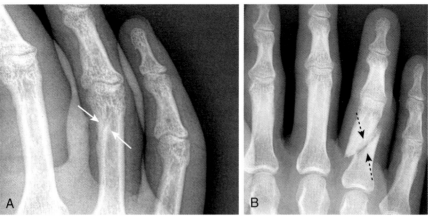

**Fig. 23.2 Nutrient Canal Versus Fracture.** (A) This is a nutrient canal *(arrows)*. Notice how the nutrient canal has a sclerotic (whiter) margin as it passes through the cortex. (B) This is a true fracture *(arrows)* seen in another patient. Fracture lines are blacker and traverse the cortex and medullary cavity. The edges of a fracture tend to be jagged and rough.

- Radiologic features of acute fractures
  - **Fracture lines**, when viewed in the optimum orientation, tend to be **blacker (more lucent)** than other lines normally found in bones, such as **nutrient canals** (Fig. 23.2A).
  - There may be an **abrupt discontinuity of the cortex**, sometimes associated with abrupt **angulation** of the normally smooth contour of bone (Fig. 23.2B).
  - Fracture lines tend to be relatively **straight** but where they change their course, the changes are **more acute in their angulation** than any naturally occurring lines (such as **growth plates**) (Fig. 23.3).
  - The **edges** of a fracture may be **jagged** or **irregular**.

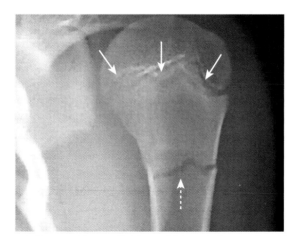

**Fig. 23.3 Fracture Versus Epiphyseal Plate.** A fracture line *(dashed arrow)* tends to be more linear and acute in its angulation than any naturally occurring line, such as the **growth plate** in the proximal humerus *(solid arrows)*. Because the top of the humeral metaphysis has irregular hills and valleys, the growth plate has an undulating contour that allows you to see it on both the anterior and posterior margins of the humeral head, leading to the appearance that there is more than one growth plate.

---

## ⚠ DIAGNOSTIC PITFALLS

- **Sesamoids, accessory ossicles, and unhealed fractures** (Table 23.1)
  - **Sesamoids** are bones that form normally in a tendon as it passes over a joint. The **patella** is the largest and most famous sesamoid bone (Fig. 23.4A).
  - **Accessory ossicles** are accessory epiphyseal or apophyseal ossification centers that fail to fuse with their parent bone (Fig. 23.4B).
  - **Apophyses** are growth centers that add to the **shape** of a bone on which a tendon or ligament inserts. Epiphyses add to the **length** of bones and form parts of a joint. Apophyses can be confused for fractures (Fig. 23.4C).
  - **Old, unhealed fracture fragments** can sometimes mimic acute fractures (Fig. 23.4D).
  - Unlike fractures, almost all of these small bones are **corticated** (i.e., there is a white line that completely surrounds the bony fragment) and their edges are usually **smooth.**
  - In the case of **sesamoids, accessory ossicles,** and **unfused apophyses**, they are **usually bilaterally symmetric** so that a view of the opposite extremity will usually demonstrate the same bone in the same location. Many also **occur at anatomically predictable sites.**
    - Sesamoids are almost always present in the thumb, posterolateral aspect of the knee (**fabella**), and great toe (see Fig. 23.4A).
    - Accessory ossicles are most common in the **foot** (see Fig. 23.4B).

---

## TABLE 23.1 Differentiating Fractures, Ossicles, and Sesamoids

| Feature | Acute Fracture | Sesamoids and Accessory Ossicles |
|---|---|---|
| Abrupt disruption of cortex | Yes | No |
| Bilaterally symmetrical* | Almost never | Almost always |
| "Fracture line" | Sharp, jagged | Smooth |
| Bony fragment has a cortex completely around it | No | Yes |

*Old, unhealed fractures will not be bilaterally symmetric.

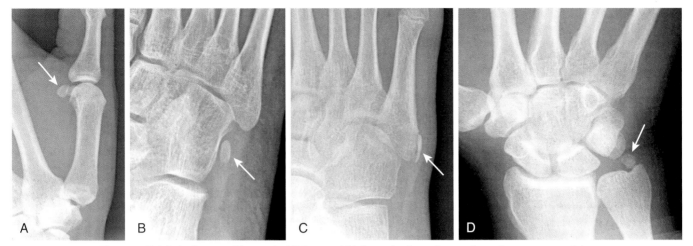

**Fig. 23.4** Pitfalls in Fracture Diagnosis. (A) **Sesamoid** (a bone that forms in a tendon as it passes over a joint, in this case the thumb) *(arrow)*; (B) **accessory ossicles** like this *os peroneum* in the foot *(arrow)*; (C) **apophyseal** ossification centers that have not fused with their parent bone *(arrow)*; and (D) old, **unhealed fracture fragments** or an **unfused ossification center** *(arrow)*—all can sometimes mimic acute fractures.

# RECOGNIZING DISLOCATIONS AND SUBLUXATIONS

- In a *dislocation,* the bones that originally formed the two components of a joint are no longer in apposition to each other. Dislocations can only occur at joints (Fig. 23.5A).
- In a *subluxation,* the bones that originally formed the two components of a joint are in **partial contact** with each other. Subluxations also occur only at joints (Fig. 23.5B).

# DESCRIBING FRACTURES

- There is a common lexicon used in describing fractures to facilitate a reproducible description and to assure reliable and accurate communication.

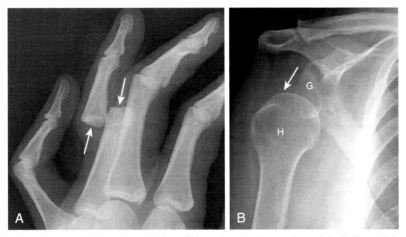

**Fig. 23.5** Dislocation and Subluxation. (A) In a **dislocation,** the bones that originally formed the two components of the proximal interphalangeal joint of the 4th finger are no longer in apposition to each other *(arrows)*. (B) In a **subluxation,** the bones that originally formed the two components of the shoulder joint are in partial contact with each other. The humeral head (H) is subluxed inferiorly *(arrow)* in the glenoid (G) because of flaccid right-sided paralysis in this patient with a history of a previous stroke.

- Fractures are usually described using four major parameters (Table 23.2):
  - The **number** of fragments
  - The **direction** of the **fracture line**
  - The spatial **relationship** of the **fragments** to each other
  - Whether the fracture communicates **with the outside atmosphere**

## Describing Fractures: Number of Fragments

- If the fracture divides a single bone into **two fragments**, it is called a *simple fracture.*
- If the fracture produces **more than two** fragments, it is called a **comminuted fracture.** Some comminuted fractures have special names.
  - A *segmental fracture* is a comminuted fracture in which a portion of the shaft exists as an **isolated fragment** (Fig. 23.6A).
  - A *butterfly fragment* is a comminuted fracture in which the central fragment has a triangular shape (Fig. 23.6B).

## Describing Fractures: Fracture Line Direction (Table 23.3)

- In a *transverse fracture,* the fracture line is perpendicular to the long axis of the bone. Transverse fractures are caused by a force directed **perpendicular to the shaft** (Fig. 23.7A).
- In a *diagonal or oblique fracture,* the fracture line is diagonal in orientation relative to the long axis of the bone. Diagonal or oblique fractures are caused by a force usually applied in the **same direction as the long axis** of the affected bone (Fig. 23.7B).
- With a *spiral fracture,* a twisting force or torque produces a fracture like those that might be caused by planting the foot in a hole while running. Spiral fractures are usually **unstable** and often associated with soft-tissue injuries such as **tears** in **ligaments** or **tendons** (Fig. 23.7C).

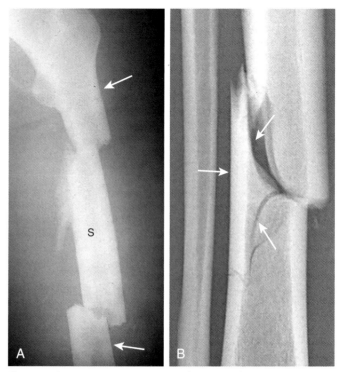

**Fig. 23.6 Segmental Fracture and Butterfly Fracture.** (A) There is a **segmental fracture** in which a portion of the shaft of the femur exists as an isolated fragment. Notice how the femur has a central fragment (S) and two additional segments, one on either side *(arrows)*. (B) A **butterfly fragment**, here shown in the tibia, is a comminuted fracture in which the central fragment has a triangular shape *(arrows)*.

| TABLE 23.2 **How Fractures Are Described** | |
|---|---|
| **Parameter** | **Terms Used** |
| **Number of fracture fragments** | Simple or comminuted |
| **Direction of fracture line** | Transverse, oblique (diagonal), spiral |
| **Relationship of one fragment to another** | Displacement, angulation, shortening, and rotation |
| **Open to the atmosphere (outside)** | Closed or open (compound) |

| TABLE 23.3 **Direction of Fracture Line and Mechanism of Injury** | |
|---|---|
| **Direction of Fracture Line** | **Mechanism** |
| **Transverse** | Force applied perpendicular to long axis of bone; fracture occurs at point of impact |
| **Diagonal (also known as oblique)** | Force applied along the long axis of bone; fracture occurs somewhere along shaft |
| **Spiral** | Twisting or torque injury |

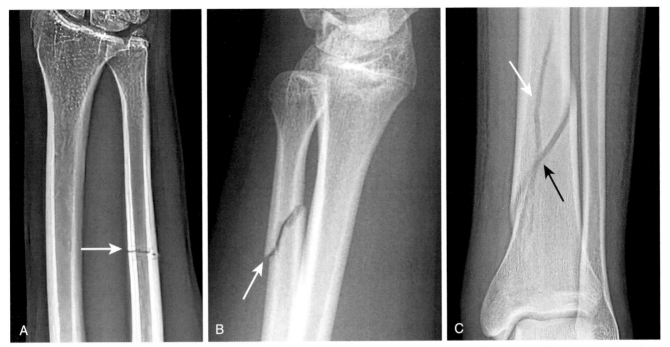

**Fig. 23.7** Direction of Fracture Lines. (A) In a **transverse fracture** *(arrow)*, the fracture line is perpendicular to the long axis of the bone. (B) Diagonal or **oblique fractures** *(arrow)* are diagonal in orientation relative to the normal axis of the bone. (C) **Spiral fractures** *(arrows)* are usually caused by twisting or torque injuries.

## Describing Fractures: Relationship of One Fragment to Another

> ### ▶ IMPORTANT POINTS
>
> - By convention, abnormalities of the position of bone fragments secondary to fractures describe **the altered relationship of the distal fracture fragment relative to the proximal fragment.** These descriptions are based on the expected position the distal fragment would normally have occupied assuming the bone had not been fractured.

- There are four major parameters most commonly used to **describe the spatial relationship** of **fracture fragments.** Some fractures display more than one of these abnormalities of position. The four parameters are:
  - Displacement
  - Angulation
  - Shortening/distraction
  - Rotation
- *Displacement* describes **the amount by which the distal fragment is off-set,** front to back and side to side, from the proximal fragment. Displacement is most often described either in terms of **percent** (e.g., *The distal fragment is displaced by 50% of the width of the shaft*) or by **fractions** (e.g., *The distal fragment is displaced ½ the width of the shaft of the proximal fragment*) (Fig. 23.8A).

- *Angulation* describes **the angle between the distal and proximal fragments** as a function of the degree to which the distal fragment is **deviated** from the position it would have assumed were it in its **normal** position. Angulation is described in degrees and by position (e.g., *The distal fragment is angulated 15° anteriorly relative to the proximal fragment*) (Fig. 23.8B).
- *Shortening* describes how much, if any, **overlap** there is of the **ends of the fracture fragments,** which translates into how much shorter the length of the fractured bone is than it would have been had it not been fractured (Fig. 23.8C).
  - The opposite term from shortening is *distraction*, which refers **to the longitudinal distance the bone fragments are separated from each other** (Fig. 23.8D).
  - Shortening (overlap) or distraction (lengthening) are usually described by a number of centimeters *(e.g., There are 2 cm of shortening of the fracture fragments).*

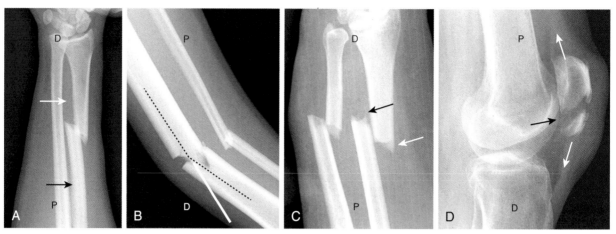

**Fig. 23.8 Fracture Orientation Parameters.** (A) **Displacement** describes the amount by which the distal fragment *(white arrow)* is off-set, front to back and side-to-side, from the proximal fragment *(black arrow)*. (B) **Angulation** describes the angle between the distal and proximal fragments *(dashed black line)* as a function of the degree to which the distal fragment is deviated from its normal position *(solid white line)*. (C) **Shortening** describes how much, if any, overlap occurs at the ends of the fracture fragments *(arrows)*. (D) The opposite of shortening is **distraction,** which refers to the distance the bone fragments are separated from each other *(white arrows* show pull of tendons on fracture fragments of patella; *black arrow* points to fracture). *D,* Distal; *P,* proximal.

- *Rotation* is an unusual abnormality in fracture positioning almost always involving the **long bones,** such as the femur or humerus. Rotation describes the orientation of the **joint** at **one end** of the fractured bone relative to the orientation of the **joint** at the **other end** of the **same bone.**
  - Normally, for example, when the hip joint is pointing forward, the knee joint is also pointing forward. If there is **rotation** at the site of a fracture of the femoral shaft, the hip joint could be pointing forward while the knee joint is oriented in a different direction (Fig. 23.9). To appreciate rotation radiographically, both the joint above and the joint below a fracture should be visualized, preferably on the same radiograph.

## Describing Fractures: Relationship to the Atmosphere

- A *closed fracture* is the **more common** type of fracture in which there is **no communication** between the fracture fragments and the outside air/atmosphere.
- In an *open* or *compound fracture,* there is **communication between the fracture and the outside** atmosphere (e.g., a fracture fragment penetrates the skin) (Fig. 23.10). Compound fractures have implications regarding the way in which they are treated in order to avoid the complication of **osteomyelitis.** Whether a fracture is open or not is best diagnosed **clinically.**

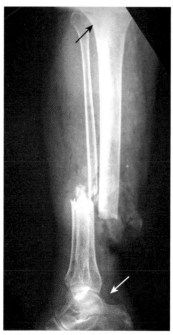

**Fig. 23.9 Rotation.** To appreciate rotation, which usually occurs in long bones, both the joint above and the joint below a fracture must be visualized, preferably on the same radiograph. In this patient, the proximal tibia *(black arrow)* is oriented in the frontal plane while the distal tibia and ankle *(white arrow)* are rotated and oriented laterally.

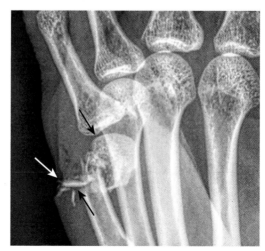

**Fig. 23.10 Open (Compound) Fracture.** Open or compound fractures *(black arrows)* have an open wound or break in the skin allowing the bone to communicate with the outside *(white arrow)*. Whether a fracture is open or not is best evaluated clinically.

## AVULSION FRACTURES

- *Avulsion* is a **common mechanism** of fracture production in which the fracture fragment (called the ***avulsed fragment***) is torn from its parent bone usually by **the** forceful **pull of a tendon** or **ligament.**
- Although avulsion fractures can and do occur at any age, they are **particularly common in younger individuals** engaging in athletic endeavors; in fact, they derive many of their names from the **type** of athletic activity that produces them (e.g., ***dancer's fracture, skier's fracture,*** and ***sprinter's fracture***).
- They **occur in anatomically predictable locations** because tendons insert on bones in known locations (Table 23.4) and the avulsed fragment is **typically small** (Fig. 23.11).
- They sometimes **heal with such abundant (*exuberant*) callus formation** that they might subsequently appear tumor-like (Fig. 23.12).

## SALTER-HARRIS FRACTURES: GROWTH PLATE FRACTURES IN CHILDREN

- Salter-Harris fractures are discussed in **Chapter 27** on pediatrics.

## CHILD ABUSE

- Child abuse is discussed in **Chapter 27** on pediatrics.

## STRESS FRACTURES

- *Stress fractures* occur as a result of numerous microfractures in which bone is subjected to repeated stretching and compressive forces, the cumulative effect of which eventually causes the fracture.

> ### ⟫ IMPORTANT POINTS
>
> - Although **conventional radiographs are usually the study first obtained**, they may **initially appear normal in as many as 85%** of stress fractures, so it is common for a patient to complain of pain yet have a normal-appearing radiograph at first.
> - With conventional radiographs the **fracture may not be diagnosable** until after **periosteal new bone formation** occurs days or weeks later (Fig. 23.13) or, in the case of a **healing** stress fracture of cancellous bone, **the appearance of a thin, dense zone of sclerosis across the medullary cavity.**

### TABLE 23.4 Avulsion Fractures Around the Pelvis

| Avulsed Fragment | Muscle That Inserts on That Fragment |
| --- | --- |
| **Anterior, superior iliac spine** | Sartorius muscle |
| **Anterior, inferior iliac spine** | Rectus femoris muscle |
| **Ischial tuberosity** | Hamstring muscles |
| **Lesser trochanter of femur** | Iliopsoas muscle |

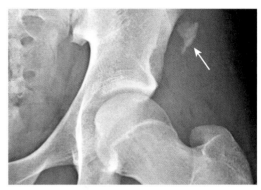

**Fig. 23.11 Avulsion Fracture.** There is an avulsion of the **anterior superior iliac spine (ASIS)** *(arrow)*, which is the site of the origin of the sartorius muscle. The patient was a recreational soccer player.

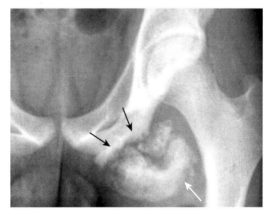

**Fig. 23.12 Healing Avulsion Fracture.** There is a healing fracture *(black arrows)* of the ischial tuberosity that had been caused by forceful contraction of the hamstring muscles. There is a large amount of external callus present, called ***exuberant callus*** *(white arrow)*.

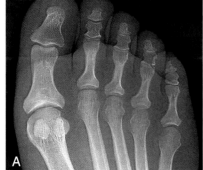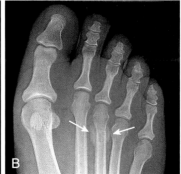

**Fig. 23.13 Stress (March) Fracture.** (A) Although conventional radiographs are the study of first choice, they may initially appear normal, as in this patient 2 days after pain began in the 3rd toe. (B) Four weeks after the original radiograph, there is periosteal new bone formation demonstrating healing of a stress fracture *(arrows)*.

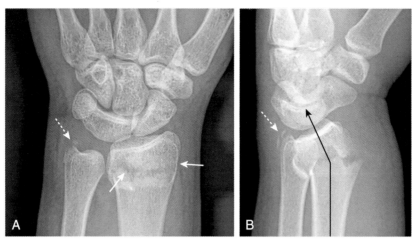

**Fig. 23.14  Colles Fracture.** (A) Frontal view displays a fracture of the distal radius *(solid arrows)* caused by a fall on the outstretched hand. There is frequently an associated fracture of the ulnar styloid *(dashed arrows in A and B)*. (B) Posterior (dorsal) angulation of the distal fragment is seen on the lateral view *(black arrow)*.

- **MRI** has the ability to detect a stress fracture **as soon as it happens.** In fact, MRI can detect bone **contusions** before an actual fracture occurs. Radionuclide **bone scan** will usually be positive for a stress fracture much earlier than conventional radiographs—**within 6 to 72 hours** after the injury. Compared with MRI or bone scans, the sensitivity of CT scanning in stress fractures is rather low.
- Some **common locations for stress fractures** are the **shafts of long bones,** such as the proximal femur or proximal tibia, as well as the calcaneus and the second and third metatarsals.

## COMMON FRACTURE EPONYMS

- There are almost as many fracture eponyms as there are types of fractures. If you entertained a desire to have a fracture named after you some day, then you are probably too late. We will focus on six of the most commonly used eponyms.

- *Colles fracture* (named after Abraham Colles who described it 80 years **before** x-rays were discovered) is a **fracture of the distal radius with dorsal angulation** of the distal radial fracture fragment caused by a **fall on the outstretched hand** (sometimes abbreviated as *FOOSH)*. There is frequently an associated fracture of the ulnar styloid (Fig. 23.14).
- *Smith fracture* is a fracture of the distal radius with **palmar angulation** of the distal radial fracture fragment (in effect, it is a **reverse** Colles fracture). It is caused by a fall on the back of the flexed hand (Fig. 23.15).
- *Jones fracture* is a transverse fracture of the fifth metatarsal about 2 cm from its base, caused by plantar flexion of the foot and inversion of the ankle. A Jones fracture may take longer to heal than the more common avulsion fracture of the tuberosity of the fifth metatarsal (Fig. 23.16).
- *Boxer's fracture* is a fracture of the neck of the fifth metacarpal with palmar angulation of the distal fracture

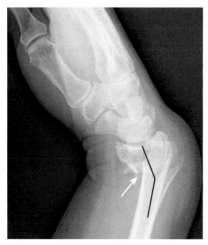

**Fig. 23.15  Smith Fracture.** A Smith fracture is a fracture of the distal radius *(arrow)* with palmar angulation of the distal radial fracture fragment *(black lines)*, the reverse of a Colles fracture. It is caused by a fall on the back of the flexed hand.

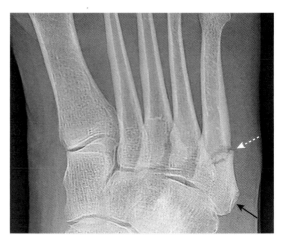

**Fig. 23.16  Jones Fracture.** A Jones fracture is a transverse fracture of the base of the 5th metatarsal *(white arrow)* that occurs about 1 to 2 cm from the tuberosity of the 5th metatarsal *(black arrow)* in an area of poorer blood supply that may affect healing. A Jones fracture can be either a stress fracture from repetitive injury or an acute break.

fragment. Sometimes the fourth metacarpal may be involved. It is most often the result of punching a person or wall (Fig. 23.17).

- *March fracture* is a type of *stress fracture* caused by microfractures to the foot from repetitive trauma (such as marching) most often affecting the **shafts of the second and third metatarsals** (see Fig. 23.13).

- *Lisfranc fracture-dislocations* (named after Jacques Lisfranc de St. Martin, a French surgeon) are relatively uncommon and most often result from either athletic injuries or motor vehicle collisions/industrial accidents. They may be obvious, as in the example shown (Fig. 23.18), or inapparent on conventional radiographs. CT or MRI may be needed to demonstrate the injury.

## SOME SUBTLE FRACTURES OR DISLOCATIONS

- Look at these areas carefully when evaluating for a possible fracture; then look a second and third time.
- **Scaphoid fractures**
  - Scaphoid (navicular) fractures are common injuries clinically suspected if there is tenderness in the

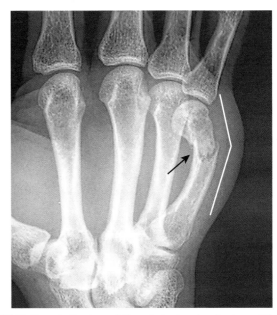

**Fig. 23.17** Boxer's Fracture. A Boxer's fracture is a fracture of the neck of the 5th metacarpal *(arrow)* with palmar angulation of the distal fracture fragment *(white lines)*. Despite its name, it is **not** a fracture commonly sustained by professional boxers whose 2nd and 3rd metacarpals and radius assume the brunt of the force.

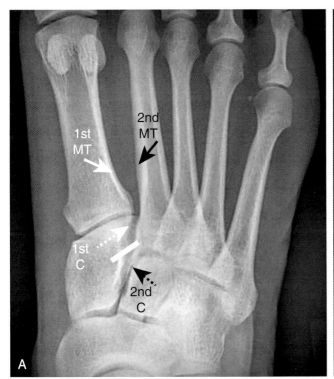

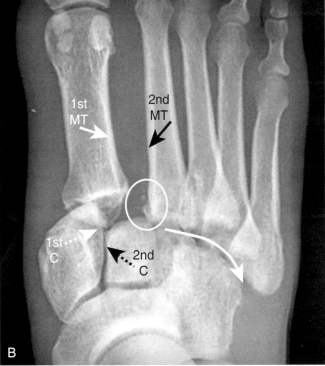

**Fig. 23.18** Lisfranc Fracture-Dislocation. (A) is a close-up view of a **normal** right foot. Notice how the lateral border of the **1st MT** *(solid white arrow)* aligns with the lateral border *(dashed white arrow)* of the 1st or medial cuneiform (**1st C**) and the medial border of the **2nd MT** *(solid black arrow)* lines up with the medial border of the 2nd or middle cuneiform (**2nd C**) *(dashed black arrow)*. The Lisfranc ligament is depicted by the *white bar* that joins the 1st C with the base of the 2nd MT. (B) This is a Lisfranc fracture-dislocation. The lateral border of the **1st MT** *(solid white arrow)* no longer aligns with the lateral border of the **1st C** *(dashed white arrow)*, and the medial border of the **2nd MT** *(solid black arrow)* no longer aligns with the **2nd C** *(dashed black arrow)*. There is a fracture at the base of the **2nd MT** *(circle)*. All of the metatarsals are dislocated laterally *(curved arrow)*, called a **homolateral** dislocation. *C*, Cuneiform; *MT*, metatarsal.

*anatomic snuff box* after a fall on an outstretched hand. Look for **hairline-thin radiolucencies** in the scaphoid (Fig. 23.19).

- Because of peculiarities of vascularization, a fracture through the midportion (*waist*) of the scaphoid may **interrupt blood supply to the proximal pole,** leading to *avascular necrosis* of the proximal pole. Because the remainder of the bones of the wrist continue to undergo the process of bone turnover, the result is an apparent relative **increase in the density** of the **devascularized part compared** with the **remainder of the bone** (Fig. 23.20).
- **Buckle fractures of radius and/or ulna in children**

- These are common fractures in children. Look for **acute and sudden angulation of the cortex,** especially near the wrist (see Fig. 23.1B). These are impacted fractures and usually heal quickly with no deformity.
- **Radial head fracture**
- A fracture of the radial head is the **most common fracture of the elbow in an adult.** On the lateral view, look for a crescentic lucency of fat along the posterior aspect of the distal humerus produced by normally invisible **intracapsular, extrasynovial fat** that is lifted away from the bone by swelling of the joint capsule due to a *traumatic hemarthrosis*—called a *positive posterior fat-pad sign* (Fig. 23.21).

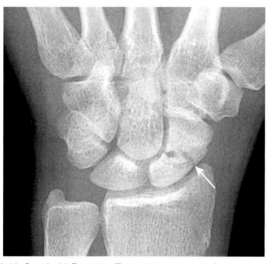

**Fig. 23.19 Scaphoid Fracture.** There is a transverse fracture across the waist of the scaphoid *(arrow)*. Fractures across the waist of the scaphoid can lead to avascular necrosis of the proximal pole of that bone (see Fig. 23.20).

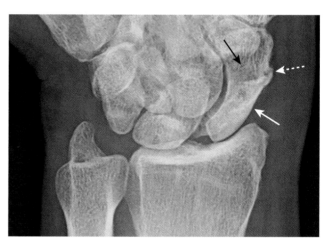

**Fig. 23.20 Avascular Necrosis of the Scaphoid.** A close-up scaphoid view of the wrist demonstrates that the proximal pole of the scaphoid *(solid white arrow)* appears denser than the distal pole *(black arrow)* due to avascular necrosis of the proximal pole. The fracture had occurred a year earlier through the waist of the scaphoid *(dashed white arrow)*.

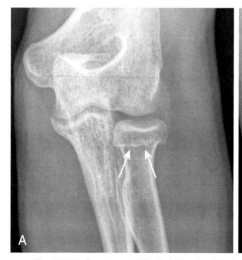
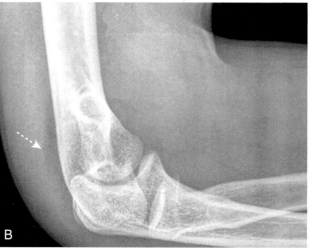

**Fig. 23.21 Fracture of Radial Head with Joint Effusion.** (A) Radial head fractures *(arrows)* are the most common fractures of the elbow in an adult. (B) There is a crescentic lucency along the dorsal aspect of the distal humerus *(arrow)*—the *positive posterior fat-pad sign*. Virtually all studies of bones will include at least two views at 90° angles to each other called **orthogonal views.** Many protocols call for two additional oblique views that enable visualization of more of the cortex in tangent.

- **Supracondylar fracture of the distal humerus in children**
  - This is the **most common fracture of the elbow in a child.** Most of these fractures produce **posterior displacement** of the distal humerus and they can be quite subtle (Fig. 23.22).
- **Dislocations of the shoulder**
  - *Anterior dislocations* of the shoulder are more common than posterior dislocations and easier to recognize radiographically (Fig. 23.23A and B). They are caused by a combination of abduction, external rotation, and extension.
  - In a *posterior dislocation,* the humeral head is fixed in internal rotation and looks like a *light bulb* in all views of the shoulder. Look at a view like the **axillary** or **"Y"** view

to see if the humeral head still lies within the glenoid fossa. On the "Y" view (an oblique view of the shoulder), the head will lie **lateral to the glenoid** in a posterior dislocation (Fig. 23.23C and D).
- **Hip fractures in the elderly**
  - Hip fractures are common, especially in the elderly, and frequently related to osteoporosis. If possible, conventional radiographs of the femoral neck should be performed with the patient's leg in internal rotation so as to display the femoral neck in profile. Look for sharp **angulation of the cortex** or zones of **increased density** indicating **impaction** (Fig. 23.24).
  - Hip fractures can be subtle radiographically and require an MRI or radionuclide bone scan for diagnosis.

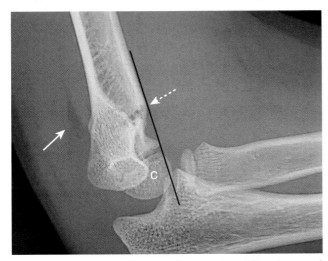

**Fig. 23.22 Supracondylar Fracture.** On a true lateral film, the **anterior humeral line** (a line drawn tangential to the anterior humeral cortex and shown here in black) should bisect the **middle-third** of the ossification center of capitellum (C). When there is a supracondylar fracture, this line will usually pass through the capitellum more anteriorly, as it does here. More importantly, the fracture in the distal humerus itself is visible *(dashed arrow).* There is a positive **posterior fat-pad sign** present *(solid arrow).*

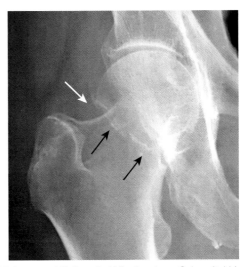

**Fig. 23.24 Impacted Subcapital Hip Fracture.** Subcapital hip fractures occur at the junction between the femoral head and neck. Most hip fractures in the elderly (90%) occur as a result of a fall, frequently a minor fall such as from the standing position. Look for a step-off of the cortex *(white arrow)* and evidence of overlapping impacted fragments *(black arrows).*

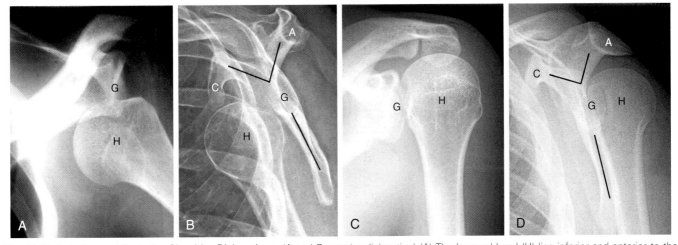

**Fig. 23.23 Anterior and Posterior Shoulder Dislocations.** (A and B anterior dislocation) (A) The humeral head (H) lies inferior and anterior to the glenoid (G). (B) The head (H) is in a subcoracoid (C) location on this angled "Y-view *(black lines)."* (C and D posterior dislocation) (C) In a posterior dislocation, the humeral head (H) is persistently fixed in internal rotation and resembles a **lightbulb** no matter how the patient turns the arm. There is also an increased distance between the head (H) and the glenoid (G). (D) On the angled Y-view of the shoulder *(black lines)* in a posterior dislocation, the head (H) will lie under the acromion (A), a posterior structure of the scapula. *A,* Acromion; *C,* coracoid process; *G,* glenoid; *H,* humeral head.

## Indirect Signs of a Possible Fracture

- Look also for **soft-tissue abnormalities** or **indirect signs** indicating the possibility of an underlying fracture (Table 23.5, Fig. 23.25).

# FRACTURE HEALING

- Fracture healing is determined by many factors, including the **age of the patient,** the **fracture site,** the **position of the fracture fragments**, the degree of **immobilization,** and the **blood supply** to the fracture site (Table 23.6).
- Immediately following a fracture, there is hemorrhage into the fracture site.
- Over the next several weeks, osteoclasts act to remove the diseased bone. The fracture line may **minimally widen** at this time.
- Then, over the course of several more weeks, **new bone (callus)** begins to bridge the fracture gap (Fig. 23.26).

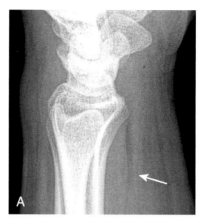
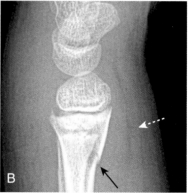

**Fig. 23.25** Pronator Quadratus Fat Plane. (A) This is an example of a normal fascial plane produced by the pronator quadratus *(arrow points to lucency)* on the volar aspect of the wrist compared to the bulging fascial plane *(white arrow)* in (B), which has occurred because of soft-tissue swelling accompanying a fracture of the distal radius *(black arrow)*.

### TABLE 23.5  Indirect Signs of Possible Fracture

| Sign | Remarks |
|---|---|
| **Soft-tissue swelling** | Frequently accompanies a fracture but does not necessarily mean that a fracture is present. |
| **Disappearance of normal fat stripes** | The **pronator quadratus fat stripe** on the volar aspect of the wrist, for example, may be displaced with a fracture of the distal radius (Fig. 23.25). |
| **Joint effusion** | The **positive posterior fat-pad sign** seen on the dorsal aspect of the distal humerus from a traumatic joint effusion is an example (see Fig. 23.21B). |
| **Periosteal reaction** | Sometimes the healing of fractures will be the first manifestation that a fracture was present, especially with stress fractures of the foot (see Fig. 23.13). |

### TABLE 23.6  Factors that Affect Fracture Healing

| Accelerate Fracture Healing | Delay Fracture Healing |
|---|---|
| Youth | Old age |
| Early immobilization | Delayed immobilization |
| Adequate duration of immobilization | Too short a duration of immobilization |
| Good blood supply | Poor blood supply |
| Physical activity after adequate immobilization | Steroids |
| Adequate mineralization | Osteoporosis, osteomalacia |

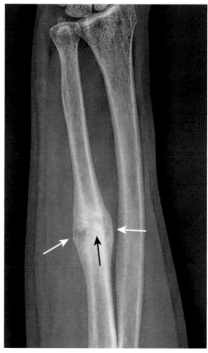

**Fig. 23.26** Healing Ulnar Fracture. Internal, endosteal healing occurs several weeks after a fracture and is demonstrated by indistinctness of the fracture line *(black arrow)* eventually leading to obliteration of that line. External, periosteal healing is manifest by external callus formation *(white arrows)* leading to bridging of the fracture site.

## ⟫ IMPORTANT POINTS

- *Internal endosteal healing* is manifest by **indistinctness of the fracture line** leading to eventual obliteration of the fracture line, in most cases.
- *External periosteal healing* is manifest by external callus formation eventually leading to **bridging of the fracture site.**

- *Remodeling* of bone **begins at about 8 to 12 weeks** postfracture as mechanical forces, in part, begin to adjust the bone to its original shape.
  - In **children, this occurs much more rapidly** and usually leads to a bone that will eventually appear normal. In adults, this process may take much longer and the healed fracture may never assume a completely normal shape.
- Complications of the healing process
  - *Delayed union.* **The fracture does not heal in the expected time** for a fracture at that particular site (e.g., longer than 6 to 8 weeks for a fracture of the shaft of the radius). **Most** cases of **delayed union** will eventually **progress** to **complete healing** with further immobilization.
  - *Malunion.* Healing of the fracture fragments occurs in a **mechanically** or **cosmetically unacceptable position.**
  - *Nonunion.* This implies that **fracture healing will never occur.** It is characterized by **smooth** and **sclerotic fracture margins** with **distraction of the fracture fragments** (Fig. 23.27). A *pseudarthrosis,* complete with a synovial lining, may form at the fracture site.
    - **Motion at the fracture site** may be demonstrated under fluoroscopic manipulation or on stress views.

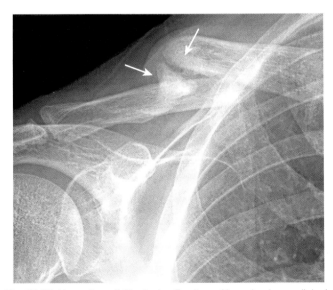

**Fig. 23.27 Nonunion of Clavicular Fracture.** Nonunion is a radiologic diagnosis that implies fracture healing is not likely to occur as the processes leading to the repair of bone have probably ceased. It is characterized by smooth and sclerotic fracture margins with distraction of the fracture fragments *(arrows).* A *pseudarthrosis,* complete with a synovial lining, may form at the fracture site.

## SPINAL TRAUMA

- Fractures of the spine are infrequent compared with fractures of other parts of the skeleton. When they occur, they have particular importance because of the implications for associated spinal cord injury.
- CT, with its ability to reformat images in different planes and provide additional information about the soft tissues, now supplements and, in most cases, **has replaced conventional radiography in the evaluation of spinal trauma.** CT is utilized to determine **the extent of the injury** in any patient in whom a traumatic spinal injury has already been demonstrated by conventional radiographs.
- CT is also utilized to **detect bony lesions not visible on conventional radiographs** and to **evaluate soft-tissue abnormalities** in patients who are unable to undergo an MRI examination.
- Most spinal fractures occur in the **thoracic** and **lumbar spines.** The **most commonly fractured vertebrae are L1, L2, and T12,** accounting for more than half of all thoracolumbar spine fractures. **Compression fractures** are the most common type of spinal fracture.
- **The three cervical lines** (Fig. 23.28).

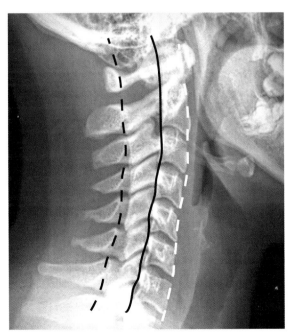

**Fig. 23.28 The Three Cervical Lines.** Three parallel arcuate lines should smoothly join three sets of structures in the cervical spine. Most posterior are the **spinolaminar white lines** that occur at the junctions between the laminae and the spinous processes *(dashed black line).* The second line should join all of the **posterior aspects of the vertebral bodies** *(solid black line).* The most anterior line should join all of the **anterior aspects of the vertebral bodies** *(dashed white line).*

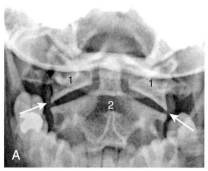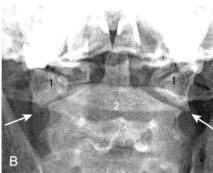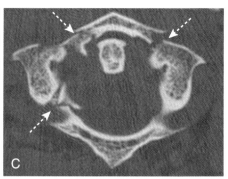

**Fig. 23.29** Normal Open-mouth View and Jefferson Fracture. (A) A normal "open-mouth" view of C1 and C2 demonstrates that the lateral margins of C1 *(1)* line up with the lateral margins of C2 *(2) (arrows)*. (B) The hallmark of a Jefferson fracture is bilateral, lateral offset of the lateral masses of C1 *(1) (arrows)* relative to C2 *(2)*. (C) The fracture is better shown on CT, which displays fractures of both the right and left anterior arches and the right posterior arch of C1 *(arrows)*.

- Many trauma protocols include a **cross-table lateral view** of the cervical spine (the patient's neck is immobilized, the patient remains on the stretcher or examining table, and the x-ray beam is directed **horizontally** so that the patient's **head is not moved**).
- This view enables a **quick assessment for spinal fracture/subluxation** before further studies that might involve motion of the patient's neck are performed.
- Three smooth, parallel, arcuate lines should be envisioned on the lateral spine radiograph. Deviation from the normal parallel curvature of these lines should suggest a subluxed and/or fractured vertebral body.
- Some of the more **common spinal fractures** described below are:
  - **Jefferson fracture**
  - **Hangman's fracture**
  - **Burst fracture**
  - **Chance fracture**
  - **Compression fractures** (discussed in **Chapter 22**).

## Jefferson Fracture

- A *Jefferson fracture* is a **fracture of C1** usually involving both the anterior and posterior arches. In its classical presentation, there are **bilateral fractures of both the anterior and posterior arches of C1,** producing four fractures in all.
- The fracture is **caused by an axial-loading injury** (e.g., diving into a swimming pool and hitting one's head on the bottom).

### ▶▶ IMPORTANT POINTS

- On **conventional radiographs,** the hallmark of a Jefferson fracture is bilateral, *lateral* offset of the lateral masses of C1 relative to C2 as seen on the *open-mouth view* (atlantoaxial view) of the cervical spine. When an open-mouth view can not be obtained, the fracture is **visualized utilizing CT** (Fig. 23.29).

- A Jefferson fracture is a **self-decompressing** fracture in that the spinal canal at the level of the fracture is usually wide enough to accommodate any swelling of the cord. There is typically **no neurologic deficit** associated with this type of fracture.

## Hangman's Fracture

- A *Hangman's fracture* is a **fracture of the posterior elements of C2.** Hangman's fractures **result from a hyperextension-compression injury** typically occurring in an unrestrained occupant in a motor vehicle accident who strikes their forehead on the windshield with the neck extended.
- They are **best evaluated on the lateral view** of the cervical spine on conventional radiography and the **sagittal view** on CT.

### ▶▶ IMPORTANT POINTS

- The fracture effectively **separates** the **posterior aspect** of the **C2** vertebral body from the **anterior** aspect of **C2,** allowing the anterior aspect of C2 to **sublux forward** on the body of C3 (Fig. 23.30).

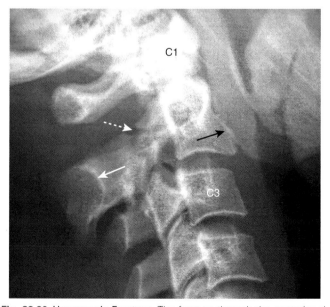

**Fig. 23.30** Hangman's Fracture. The fracture through the posterior elements of C2 *(dashed white arrow)* effectively separates the posterior aspect of the C2 vertebral body from the anterior aspect of C2 allowing the anterior aspect to sublux forward on the body of C3 *(black arrow)*. Notice that the spinolaminar line of C2 *(solid white arrow)* lies abnormally posterior to the spinolaminar lines of the other vertebral bodies.

- Some Hangman's fractures have so little displacement that CT is required for their detection.
- Because Hangman's fractures lead to overall **widening** of the **spinal canal**, they are usually **not associated with neurologic deficits.** This is in contradistinction to the intended injury after which this fracture is named, the fracture incurred during a **judicial hanging** in which there was **hyperextension** leading to a fracture of C2 and **marked distraction** of C2 from C3 with distraction of the **spinal cord** itself.

## Burst Fractures

- *Burst fractures* occur most commonly in the **cervical spine, thoracic spine, and upper lumbar spine.**
- They are high-energy, **axial-loading injuries,** typically secondary to motor vehicle accidents or falls, in which the intervertebral disk above is driven into the vertebral body below and the vertebral body bursts. This in turn drives bony fragments **posteriorly** into the **spinal canal** (*retropulsed fragments*), whereas the anterior aspect of the vertebral body is displaced **forward.**
- Because these fractures involve bony incursion on the spinal canal, the **majority of burst fractures are associated** with a **neurologic deficit.**

> ⏩ **IMPORTANT POINTS**
>
> - Findings of burst fractures include a **comminuted compression fracture** of the **vertebral body** in which the **posterior aspect** of the **body** is **bowed backward toward** the **spinal canal. CT** is the **best imaging modality** for identifying **bony fragments** in the spinal canal (Fig. 23.31).

## Chance Fracture

- *Chance fractures* (named after George Q. Chance, a British radiologist who first described them) are **transverse fractures** through the **entire vertebral body, pedicles, and spinous process,** frequently occurring as a result of a fall or motor vehicle accident in which the occupant was using only a lap seatbelt. They typically occur in the **upper lumbar-lower thoracic spine** and are associated with a relatively **high incidence** of associated **intraabdominal visceral injuries,** especially to the duodenum, pancreas, and mesentery (Fig. 23.32).

> ⏩ **IMPORTANT POINTS**
>
> - Radiographic findings include a **horizontal fracture** that shears through the vertebral body, pedicles, and spinous process. The vertebral body component may not be as obvious as the fractures through the posterior elements (Video 23.1).

## Locked Facets

- Bilateral *locking of the facets* in the cervical spine can occur as a result of a **hyperflexion injury** in which the **inferior facets** of one vertebral body **slide over** and **in front of** the **superior facets** of the **body below.** In this position, the slipped facets **cannot return** to their normal position without medical intervention— thus the term **locked facets.**

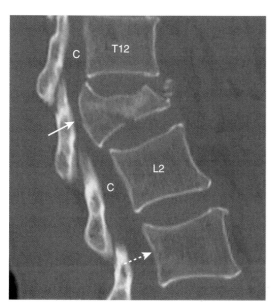

**Fig. 23.31 Burst Fracture.** There is a burst fracture of L1. Findings include a comminuted compression fracture of the L1 vertebral body in which the posterior aspect of the body is propelled dorsally **(retropulsed)** *(solid arrow)* into the spinal canal (C). Notice how the posterior aspects of the normal vertebral bodies are usually concave inward *(dashed arrow).*

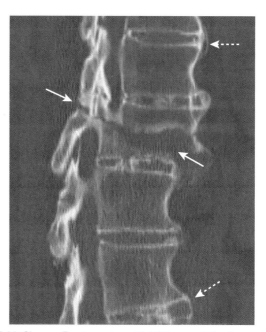

**Fig. 23.32 Chance Fracture.** A sagittal CT scan at the thoracolumbar junction displays a linear fracture that traverses the entire vertebral body from front to back *(solid arrows).* This patient had underlying ankylosing spondylitis *(dashed arrows).* The rigid and osteoporotic spine in ankylosing spondylitis is more susceptibe to fractures, even after a relatively minor trauma.

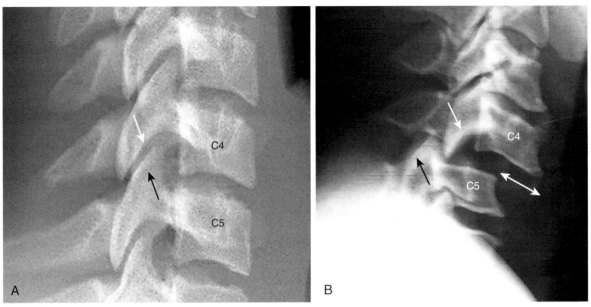

**Fig. 23.33 Normal and Bilateral Locked Facets.** (A) Normally, the inferior articular facet of the body above (in this case C4, *white arrow*) covers and lies **posterior** to the superior articular facet of the body below (in this case C5, *black arrow*). (B) The inferior articulating facet of C4 *(white arrow)* lies **anterior** to the superior articular facet of C5 *(black arrow)*, the reverse of normal. Locking of the facets in the cervical spine can occur as a result of a hyperflexion injury which results in forward slippage of the affected vertebral body on the body below it by at least 50% of its AP diameter *(double white arrow)*.

- Locked facets occur with **forward slippage** of the affected vertebral body on the body below it **by at least 50% of its anteroposterior diameter.**
- This injury virtually **always results in neurologic impairment.**

>> **IMPORTANT POINTS**

- On **lateral (sagittal) imaging** of the cervical spine, the **inferior articular facet will lie in front of the superior facet** of the body below. This is the **reverse** of the **normal** anatomic relationship between adjacent facets (Fig. 23.33).
  - Because the superior articular facet is no longer "covered" by the inferior facet above it, this appearance was described on CT as the **naked facet sign.**

## PATHOLOGIC FRACTURES

- Pathologic fractures are those that occur in **bone with a pre-existing abnormality.** Pathologic fractures tend to occur with **minimal** or **no trauma.**
  - *Insufficiency fractures* are a type of pathologic fracture (Box 23.1, Fig. 23.34).
- Diseases that produce either an **increase** or a **decrease** in bone density tend to **weaken the normal architecture** of bone and predispose to pathologic fractures.
- Diseases that predispose to pathologic fractures may be **local** (e.g., metastasis) or **diffuse** (e.g., osteoporosis). In general, pathologic fractures occur more often in the **ribs, spine, and proximal appendicular skeleton** (especially the humerus and femur).

**BOX 23.1   Insufficiency Fractures**

- Insufficiency fractures are a form of pathologic fracture in which mechanically weakened bone fractures from a normal or physiologic stress.
- They are most common in postmenopausal women secondary to osteoporosis.
- Common sites include the pelvis, thoracic spine, sacrum, tibia, and calcaneus.
- Unlike other fractures that manifest themselves by a lucency in the bone, most insufficiency fractures display a **sclerotic band** (representing healing) on conventional radiographs.
- CT, MRI, or nuclear medicine bone scans are more sensitive than conventional radiographs in detecting insufficiency fractures (Fig. 23.34).

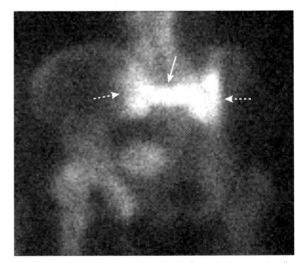

**Fig. 23.34 Sacral Insufficiency Fractures.** There is increased radiotracer uptake in vertical fractures through the sacral ala *(dashed arrows)* and a horizontal fracture through the body of the sacrum *(solid arrow)*. This has been called the **Honda sign** because it resembles the carmaker's insignia. The sacrum is a common site for such fractures from osteoporosis.

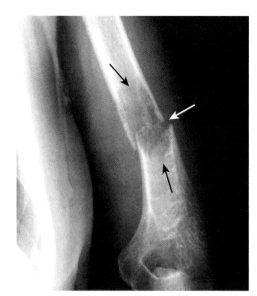

**Fig. 23.35** Pathologic Fracture. In this patient with metastatic renal cell carcinoma to the humerus, there is a geographic, lytic lesion seen in the distal humerus *(black arrows)* through which a transverse, pathologic fracture has occurred *(white arrow)*.

- **Recognizing pathologic fractures** (Fig. 23.35).
  - First, there has to be a fracture present.
  - The bone surrounding the fracture should demonstrate abnormal density or architecture (i.e., the underlying disease that allowed the fracture to occur).
- Attempts to predict "impending" fractures in diseased bone have, by and large, proved to be unreliable.

- The treatment of a pathologic fracture depends in part on successful treatment of the underlying condition that produced it.
  - **Delayed healing** is **common** in pathologic fractures.

**CASE QUIZ 23 ANSWER**

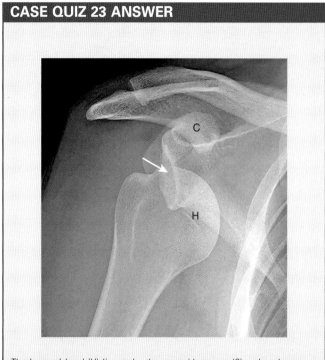

The humeral head (H) lies under the coracoid process (C) and no longer articulates with the glenoid *(arrow)*. These are findings of an **anterior, subcoracoid shoulder dislocation.** Almost all shoulder dislocations are anterior in location. Most occur in younger males or older females.

## TAKE HOME POINTS

- A **fracture** is described as a disruption in the continuity of all or part of the cortex of a bone.
- **Complete fractures** involve the entire cortex, are more common, and typically occur in adults. **Incomplete fractures** involve only a part of the cortex and typically occur in bones that are softer, such as those of children. **Torus** and **greenstick fractures** are incomplete fractures.
- **Fracture lines** tend to be blacker, more sharply angled, and more jagged than other lucencies in bones such as nutrient canals or growth plates.
- Sesamoids, accessory ossicles, apophyseal ossification centers, and unhealed fractures may mimic acute fractures, but most all will have smooth and corticated margins.
- **Dislocation** is present when two bones that originally formed a joint are no longer in contact with each other; **subluxation** is present when two bones that originally formed a joint are in partial contact with each other.
- Fractures are described in many ways, including the number of fracture fragments, direction of the fracture line, spatial relationship of the fragments to each other, and whether or not they communicate with the outside atmosphere.
- **Simple fractures** have two fragments; **comminuted fractures** have more than two fragments; segmental and butterfly fractures describe two types of comminuted fracture.
- The direction of fracture lines is described as **transverse, diagonal, or spiral.**
- The relationships of the fragments of a fracture are described by four parameters: **displacement, angulation, shortening/distraction, and rotation.**
- **Closed fractures** are those in which there is no communication between the fracture and the outside atmosphere; they are much more common than **open or compound fractures** in which there is a communication with the outside atmosphere.
- **Avulsion fractures** are produced by the forceful pull of a tendon or ligament; they can occur at any age but are particularly common in younger, athletic individuals.
- **Stress fractures**, such as march fractures in the metatarsals, occur as a result of numerous microfractures and frequently are not visible on conventional radiographs taken when the pain first begins; after some time, bony callus formation and/or a dense zone of sclerosis becomes visible.
- Some common, named fractures are **Colles fracture** (of the radius), **Smith fracture** (of the radius), **Jones fracture** (of the base of the fifth metatarsal), **Boxer's fracture** (of the neck of the fifth metacarpal), **march fracture,** and the **Lisfranc fracture-dislocation** of the foot.
- Some fractures are more difficult to detect than others; the **more subtle fractures** include scaphoid fractures, buckle fractures of the radius and ulna, radial head fractures, supracondylar fractures, posterior dislocations of the shoulder (which are uncommon), and hip fractures.
- Soft-tissue swelling, the disappearance of normal fat stripes and fascial planes, joint effusions, and periosteal reaction are **indirect signs** that should alert you to the possibility of an underlying fracture.
- **Fractures heal** with a combination of endosteal callus, recognized by a progressive indistinctness of the fracture line, and external callus that bridges the fracture site; many factors affect fracture healing, including the age of the patient, the degree of mobility of the fracture, and its blood supply.
- **Delayed union** refers to a fracture that is taking longer to heal than is usually required for that site; **malunion** means the fracture is healing, but in a mechanically or cosmetically unacceptable way; **nonunion** is a radiologic diagnosis that implies there is little if any likelihood the fracture will heal.
- **Spinal fractures** are less common than fractures of the appendicular skeleton, but they have important implications because of the possibility of spinal cord injury. CT has replaced conventional radiography as the modality of choice for imaging most cases of spinal trauma.
- The findings in a Jefferson fracture, hangman's fracture, burst fracture, Chance fracture, and locked facets are discussed; the first two are self-decompressing injuries that are usually not associated with neurologic deficit.
- **Pathologic fractures** are those that occur with minimal or no trauma in bones that had a preexisting abnormality.

 Additional content is available online including chapters on Nuclear Medicine, Artificial Intelligence, Radiation Dose and Safety, an Early History of Radiology, and a compendium of 200 Diagnostic Radiology Signs.

# Recognizing the Imaging Findings of Trauma to the Chest

*William Herring, MD, FACR*

Trauma is the leading cause of death, hospitalization, and disability in Americans from the age of 1 year through age 45. The major imaging findings of chest trauma will be discussed in this chapter. Table 24.1 summarizes some of the traumatic injuries that are discussed in other chapters.

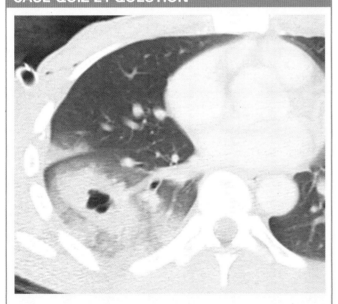

This is an image from an axial CT scan of the chest in a 31-year-old male who sustained significant blunt trauma to the right side of his thorax. He has hemoptysis. There are **two** manifestations of pulmonary trauma demonstrated here. What are they? See the answer at the end of this chapter.

### TABLE 24.1 Other Manifestations of Trauma

| Injury | Discussed in |
| --- | --- |
| **Pleural effusion/hemothorax** | Chapter 7 |
| **Aspiration** | Chapter 8 |
| **Fractures and dislocations** | Chapter 23 |
| **Spinal trauma** | Chapter 23 |
| **Abdominal and pelvic trauma** | Chapter 25 |
| **Head trauma** | Chapter 26 |

- Trauma-related injuries can be divided by the two major mechanisms that produce them.
  - **Blunt trauma** is usually the result of motor vehicle accidents and is the more common of the two.
  - **Penetrating trauma** is usually the result of accidental or criminal stabbings and gunshot wounds.
  - Table 24.2 is an overview of the initial imaging workup for **penetrating** injuries to various body parts.
- In this chapter, we will discuss various manifestations of chest trauma, starting from the periphery (chest wall) and progressing centrally (aorta).
- Chest injuries in trauma patients are **very common** and are responsible for one out of four of the trauma-related deaths. The overwhelming majority of chest trauma is the result of motor vehicle accidents.

## CHEST WALL TRAUMA

### Rib Fractures

- **Rib fractures are a common** result of blunt chest trauma and the associated morbidity and mortality from such trauma increases as the **number** of rib fractures increases. The severity of underlying visceral injury is usually more

### TABLE 24.2 Initial Imaging Workup of Penetrating Trauma

| Body Part | Studies of Choice |
| --- | --- |
| **Head** | CT scan of the head without and then possibly with contrast. |
| **Neck** | CT angiogram of head and neck if damage to the vessels is suspected. |
| **Chest** | Chest radiographs are obtained first; ultrasound FAST scan of chest, abdomen, and pelvis; then a contrast-enhanced CT scan of the chest in almost all patients unless hemodynamically unstable. |
| **Abdomen** | Ultrasound FAST scan of chest, abdomen, and pelvis; contrast-enhanced CT scan of abdomen and pelvis and possibly chest. |

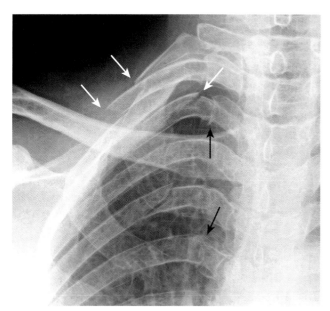

**Fig. 24.1** Rib Fractures. Fractures present as linear lucencies in the ribs and are easier to detect when the fracture ends are displaced *(white arrows)*. Don't mistake the normal costovertebral junctions *(black arrows)* near the spine for a fracture.

important than the rib fractures themselves, but their presence might provide clues to unsuspected pathology.

> ⟫ **IMPORTANT POINTS**
>
> • Fractures of the **first three ribs** are relatively **uncommon** and, if they occur following blunt trauma, **indicate a sufficient amount of force** to produce other internal injuries (Fig. 24.1).

• Fractures of **ribs 4 to 9 are common** and especially important if they are **displaced** (they can produce a pneumothorax) or if there are two fractures seen radiographically in each of three or more contiguous ribs *(flail chest).*
  • **Flail chest** is almost always accompanied by a **pulmonary contusion** (see later). Partly because of the severity of the injuries with which it is usually associated, a flail chest has a significant mortality (Fig. 24.2).
• Fractures of **ribs 10 to 12** may indicate the presence of **underlying trauma** to the **liver** (right side) or the **spleen** (left side), especially if they are displaced (Video 24.1).
• In cases of minor trauma, it is **not unusual for rib fractures to be undetectable on the initial examination** but to become visible in several weeks after callus begins to form.

## Subcutaneous Emphysema

• **Air** can **extend into the soft tissues** of the **neck, chest, and abdominal walls** from the mediastinum, or it can dissect in the subcutaneous tissues from a thoracotomy drainage tube or a penetrating injury to the chest wall.
• **Air dissecting along muscle bundles** produces a **characteristic comb-like, striated appearance** that superimposes on the underlying lung, sometimes making it difficult to evaluate the lungs by conventional radiography (Fig. 24.3).

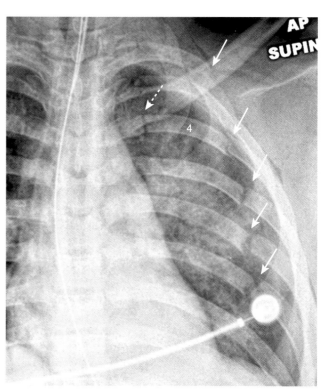

**Fig. 24.2** Flail Chest. There were two or more fractures *(dashed arrow demonstrates second fracture in rib 4)* present in more than three contiguous ribs *(solid arrows)* in this patient struck by an automobile. The airspace disease in the left lung is a pulmonary contusion, which almost always accompanies a flail chest.

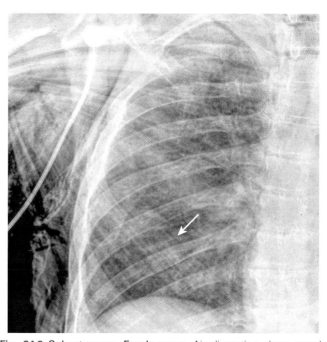

**Fig. 24.3** Subcutaneous Emphysema. Air dissecting along muscle bundles produces this characteristic striated appearance *(arrow)*. Although dramatic radiographically, subcutaneous emphysema usually produces no serious clinical effects by itself.

- Even though it may present a striking imaging appearance, **subcutaneous emphysema usually produces no serious clinical effects by itself.**
- Depending on the volume of subcutaneous air present, it may require **several days** to **a week** or longer for the air to reabsorb.

# PLEURAL ABNORMALITIES: PNEUMOTHORAX

## Causes of a Pneumothorax

- **Spontaneous**
  - **Spontaneous pneumothoraces** are common and often develop from **rupture of an apical, subpleural bleb** or bulla. They **characteristically occur in tall, thin males between 20 to 40 years of age.** Trauma is not a prerequisite for a spontaneous pneumothorax.
- **Traumatic**
  - Trauma is the **most common cause** of a **pneumothorax, either accidental or iatrogenic.** The trauma may be:
    - Through the chest wall, e.g., stab wound
    - Internal, e.g., rupture of a bronchus from a motor vehicle collision
    - Iatrogenic, e.g., following an attempt at central venous catheter insertion
- **Diseases that decrease lung compliance**
  - Chronic fibrotic disease, e.g., eosinophilic granuloma of the lung, or diseases like neonatal respiratory distress syndrome (hyaline membrane disease) in infants.
- **Rupture of an alveolus or bronchiole**, e.g., asthma

## Types of Pneumothoraces

### Simple Pneumothorax

- Pneumothoraces can be categorized as *primary*, i.e., occurring in what appears to have been normal lung (*spontaneous pneumothorax* being an example) or *secondary*, i.e., those that occur in diseased lung (as in **chronic obstructive pulmonary disease**).
- Pneumothoraces have also been classified based on the presence or absence of a **shift of the mobile mediastinal structures,** like the heart and trachea.
- In a **simple pneumothorax,** there is **no shift of the mediastinal structures** (Fig. 24.4). Simple pneumothoraces have a better prognosis and lower mortality than tension pneumothoraces.

### Tension Pneumothorax

- With a **tension pneumothorax,** there is **a shift of the mediastinal structures away from the side of the pneumothorax** frequently associated with cardiopulmonary compromise (Fig. 24.5).
- Progressive accumulation of air in the pleural space through a one-way, check-valve mechanism may cause a shift of the heart and mediastinal structures **away** from

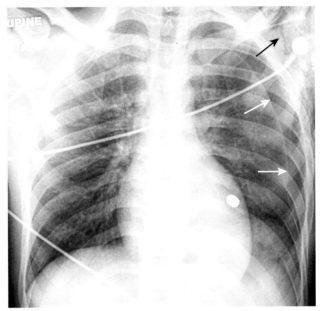

**Fig. 24.4** Simple Pneumothorax. There is a large, left-sided pneumothorax *(white arrows)* with no shift of the heart or trachea to the right. There is subcutaneous emphysema in the region of the left shoulder *(black arrow)*. Can you detect why the patient had all of these findings? There is a bullet superimposed on the heart (but on CT it was actually posterior to the heart in the left lower lobe).

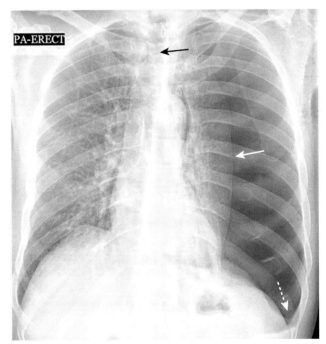

**Fig. 24.5** Tension Pneumothorax. In this patient with a spontaneous pneumothorax, the left lung is almost totally collapsed *(solid white arrow)* and there is a shift of the trachea *(black arrow)* and heart to the right side. The left hemidiaphragm is depressed because of the elevated left intrathoracic pressure *(dashed white arrow)*.

the side of the pneumothorax. The air may enter through a rent in the parietal pleura, visceral pleura, or from the tracheobronchial tree.

- The continuously **increasing intrathoracic pressure may lead to cardiopulmonary compromise** by **impairing venous return to the heart.**
- Besides a shift of the mobile mediastinal structures **away** from the side of the pneumothorax, there may be **inversion of the hemidiaphragm** (especially on the left side) and there may be **flattening of the heart contour on the side under tension.**
- There should **never** be a shift of the heart or mediastinal structures **toward** the side of a pneumothorax.
- The question "**How large is the pneumothorax?**" is an oft-repeated question but the actual issue is "Does this patient require an intervention to drain the pneumothorax?" Box 24.1 summarizes the answer.

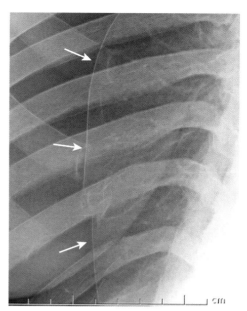

Fig. 24.6 Visceral Pleural Line in a Pneumothorax. You should be able to see the visceral pleural line to make the definitive diagnosis of a pneumothorax *(arrows)*. The visceral and parietal pleurae are normally not visible, both normally lying adjacent to the chest wall.

---

**BOX 24.1    How Large Is the Pneumothorax?**

- Size measurements of pneumothoraces on conventional radiographs correlate poorly with CT scans of their actual size.
- There is also poor correlation between the size of the pneumothorax and the degree of clinical impairment.
- **The 2 cm rule:** If the distance between the lung margin and the chest wall at the apex is <2 cm, intervention with a catheter or chest tube is usually not needed; a distance >2 cm usually requires such an intervention.
- Assessment of the patient's clinical status is the most important determinant in deciding whether chest tube drainage is required.

---

## Imaging Modalities Used to Diagnose a Pneumothorax
### Conventional Radiographs

- A **pneumothorax occurs when air enters the pleural space.**
  - The negative pressure normally present in the pleural space rises higher than the intraalveolar pressure and the lung collapses.
  - The parietal pleura remains on the inner surface of the chest wall but the visceral pleura retracts toward the hilum attached to the collapsing lung.
    - The **visceral pleura becomes visible as a thin white line** outlined by air in the lung on one side and air in the pleural space on the other side. The visible visceral pleura is called the *visceral pleural white line* or simply the *visceral pleural line.*

> ▶ **IMPORTANT POINTS**
>
> - You should be able to **identify the visceral pleural line** (Fig. 24.6) in order **to make the definitive diagnosis of a pneumothorax.**

- Even as the lung collapses, it tends to maintain its usual lung-like shape so that the curvature of **the visceral pleural line parallels the curvature of the chest wall**; that is, the visceral pleural line is **convex outward toward the chest wall** (Fig. 24.7).

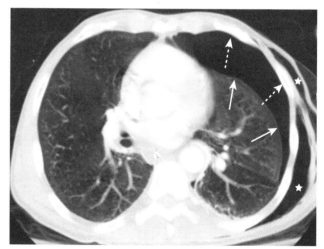

Fig. 24.7 Pneumothorax, CT. As the lung collapses, it tends to maintain its usual shape so that the curvature of the visceral pleural line *(solid arrows)* parallels the curvature of the chest wall *(dashed arrows)*. This patient also has **subcutaneous emphysema** (air in the soft tissues) of the left lateral chest wall *(stars)*. The patient had been stabbed by a former friend.

- Most other linear densities that **mimic** a pneumothorax **do not** demonstrate this spatial relationship with the chest wall.
- There is usually, but not always, an **absence of lung markings peripheral to the visceral pleural line.**
  - **Pleural adhesions** may keep part, but not all, of the visceral pleura adherent to the parietal pleura, even in the presence of a pneumothorax. On conventional radiographs, it therefore may be possible to visualize lung markings in front or in back of the pneumothorax and

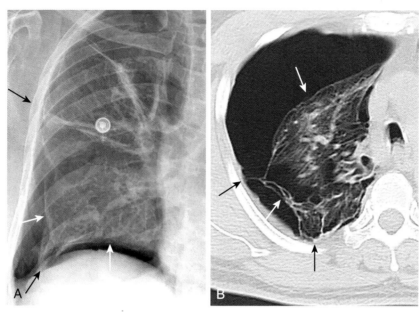

**Fig. 24.8** Pneumothorax with Pleural Adhesions. (A) There is a pneumothorax *(white arrows),* but the lung is prevented from collapsing by pleural adhesions *(black arrows)* affixing parts of the visceral to the parietal pleura. (B) On a CT scan, the pleural adhesions *(black arrows)* are seen tethering the partially collapsed lung *(white arrows)* to the parietal pleura. Adhesions most frequently result from prior infection or blood in the pleural space.

to overlook the presence of a pneumothorax because lung markings appear to extend to the chest wall (Fig. 24.8).

- **Absence** of lung markings **alone** is **not sufficient** for the **diagnosis of a pneumothorax nor** is the **presence** of lung markings **distal** to the **visceral pleural line** sufficient to eliminate the possibility of a pneumothorax.
- The **presence of an air-fluid interface in the pleural space** is, by definition, an indication that there is a pneumothorax present (see Fig. 7.15).
  - For more about recognizing a **hydropneumothorax**, see **Chapter 7.**
- Many times an **upright** view of the chest is impossible to obtain in the traumatized patient or those in intensive care.
  - In the **supine position**, air in a relatively large pneumothorax may collect anteriorly and inferiorly in the thorax and manifest itself by **displacing the costophrenic sulcus inferiorly** while, at the same time, producing **increased lucency of that costophrenic sulcus.** This is called the *deep sulcus sign,* and it is presumptive evidence for the presence of a pneumothorax on a supine chest radiograph (Fig. 24.9).
- The key signs for recognizing a pneumothorax are summarized in Box 24.2.

**BOX 24.2   Recognizing a Pneumothorax: Signs to Look for**

- Visualization of the **visceral pleural line**—a must for the diagnosis
- Convex curve of the visceral pleural line paralleling the contour of the chest wall
- Absence of lung markings peripheral to the visceral pleural line (almost always)
- The **deep sulcus sign** of an inferiorly displaced costophrenic sulcus seen on a supine chest radiograph
- The presence of an air-fluid interface in the pleural space

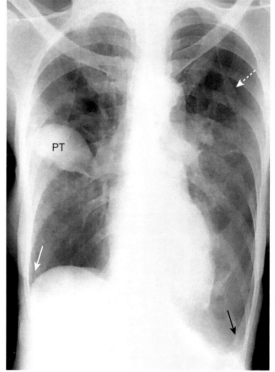

**Fig. 24.9** Deep Sulcus Sign. In the supine position, air in a relatively large pneumothorax *(dashed white arrow)* may collect anteriorly and inferiorly in the thorax depressing the lateral costophrenic sulcus *(black arrow).* This is called the *deep sulcus sign* and is a sign of a pneumothorax on a supine radiograph. Notice how much lower the left costophrenic sulcus appears than the right sulcus *(solid white arrow).* An unrelated finding in this patient is a **pseudotumor** (PT) in the minor fissure from congestive heart failure (see Fig. 7.13).

- For additional ways to diagnose a pneumothorax, see page 307.

## Pitfalls in Diagnosing a Pneumothorax

- Several pitfalls can lead to the mistaken diagnosis of a pneumothorax.

- **Pitfall 1: Absence of lung markings mistaken for the presence of a pneumothorax.**
  - The simple absence of lung markings is not sufficient to warrant the diagnosis of a pneumothorax, as there are other diseases that produce such a finding.
  - These diseases include:
    - **Bullous disease of the lung** (Fig. 24.10).
    - **Large cysts in the lung**
    - **Pulmonary embolism,** which can lead to a lack of perfusion and hence a decrease, but not a complete absence of, the number of vessels in a particular part of the lung *(**Westermark sign of oligemia**)*.
  - In none of these diseases would the treatment ordinarily include the insertion of a chest tube and, in fact, insertion of a chest tube into a bulla might actually **produce** an intractable pneumothorax.
  - **Solution:** Look at the contour of the structure you believe is the visceral pleural line. Unlike the margin of a bulla, the **visceral pleural line** will be **convex outward** toward the chest wall and will **parallel the curve of the chest wall** (Fig. 24.11). If in doubt, consider CT of the chest.
- **Pitfall 2: Mistaking a skin fold for a pneumothorax**
  - When the patient lays directly on the radiographic cassette (as for a portable supine radiograph), a **crease of the patient's skin** may become trapped between the patient's back and the surface of the cassette. This produces a *skin fold.*
  - A skin fold can produce an **edge** in the expected position of the visceral pleural line that **may, in fact, parallel the chest wall** just as you would expect the visceral pleural line in a pneumothorax (Fig. 24.12).
  - **Solution:** Unlike the thin, discrete white line of the visceral pleura, **skin folds produce a relatively thick band of increased density.**
- **Pitfall 3: Mistaking the medial border of the scapula for a pneumothorax**
  - Ordinarily, the patient is positioned for an **upright** frontal chest radiograph in such a way that the scapulae are retracted lateral to the outer margins of the rib cage, thus preventing the medial borders of the scapulae from overlapping the lung fields.
  - Most trauma patients, however, undergo supine chest radiographs. With **supine** radiographs, the **medial border of the scapula may superimpose on the upper lobe** and **mimic the visceral pleural line** of a pneumothorax (Fig. 24.13).
  - **Solution:** Before diagnosing a pneumothorax, make sure you can **trace the outlines of the scapula** on the side in question and identify its medial border as being distinct from the suspected pneumothorax.

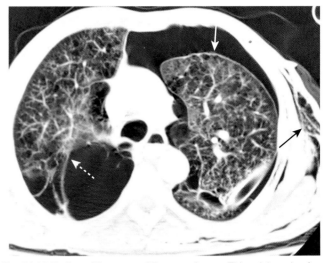

**Fig. 24.11 Bullous Disease and Pneumothorax.** This axial section from a chest CT demonstrates the different appearances between bullous disease, seen on the right as a rounded, cystic lucency with a concave arc with reference to the adjacent chest wall *(dashed white arrow)*, and a pneumothorax seen on the left with its border convex, paralleling the chest wall *(solid white arrow)*. This patient also has subcutaneous emphysema on the left *(black arrow)*.

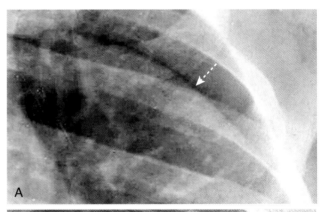

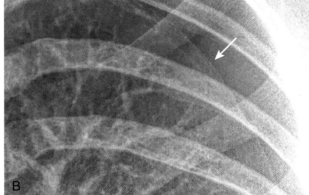

**Fig. 24.12 Skin Fold Mimicking a Pneumothorax; True Pneumothorax.** (A) When patients lay directly on the radiographic cassette as they might for a portable supine radiograph, a **fold** of the patient's skin may produce an **edge** *(arrow)* in the expected position of a pneumothorax and that edge may, in fact, parallel the chest wall just as you would expect a pneumothorax to appear. (B) While skin folds produce relatively thick, white bands of density, another patient demonstrates the thin, white line of the visceral pleura *(arrow)* seen with a pneumothorax. A skin fold is an **edge;** the visceral pleura produces a **line.**

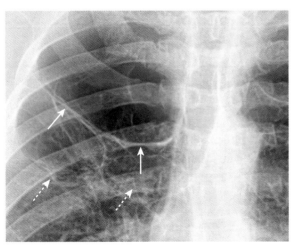

**Fig. 24.10 Bullous Disease.** There is a thin white line *(solid arrows)* visible on this close-up of the right upper lobe. Unlike the visceral pleural line of a pneumothorax, this white line is **concave** with reference to the chest wall and does **not** parallel the curvature of the chest wall as a pneumothorax usually does. This is the classical appearance of a **bulla** in a patient with emphysema. The walls of several other bullae are visible in this patient *(dashed arrows)*. On rare occasions, bullae can grow so large as to render the hemithorax seemingly devoid of any visible lung tissue *(**vanishing lung syndrome**)*.

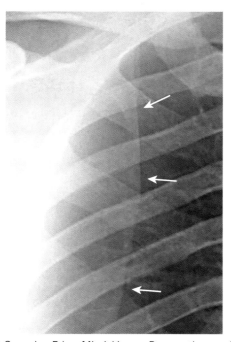

**Fig. 24.13 Scapular Edge Mimicking a Pneumothorax.** On supine radiographs, the medial border of the scapula *(arrows)* will frequently superimpose on the upper lung field and may mimic the visceral pleural line of a pneumothorax. Before diagnosing a pneumothorax, make sure you can identify the medial border of the scapula as being separate from the suspected pneumothorax.

## Pneumothorax: CT of the Chest

- Today, CT of the chest has essentially replaced conventional radiography alone if there is a strong clinical suspicion of a pneumothorax that is not demonstrated on conventional radiographs. **CT is able to detect extremely small amounts of air in the pleural space** (Fig. 24.14).

## Pneumothorax: Other Imaging Techniques

- **Ultrasound** (see Chapter 19)
- **Decubitus chest x-rays**
    - Because air rises to the highest point in the body, lateral decubitus films of the chest with the affected side "up" and the x-ray beam directed horizontally (parallel to the floor) may detect a small pneumothorax not seen in the supine position. This method may be helpful in demonstrating a pneumothorax in an infant.
- **Delayed films** are sometimes obtained about **6 hours after a penetrating injury** to the chest in patients in whom no pneumothorax is visible on the initial examination because of the occasional appearance of a delayed traumatic pneumothorax.

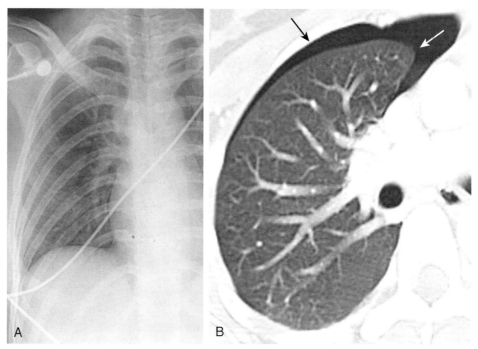

**Fig. 24.14 Pneumothorax Visible Only on CT.** (A) A view of the right lung shows no evidence of a pneumothorax. (B) CT scan in the same patient displays air in the pleural space *(black arrow)* and the partially collapsed lung retracted from the chest wall *(white arrow)* from a small pneumothorax. Smaller pneumothoraces may be visible only on CT scans of the chest.

# TRAUMATIC PARENCHYMAL ABNORMALITIES

## Pulmonary Contusions

- Pulmonary contusions are the **most frequent** complications of **blunt chest trauma.** They represent **hemorrhage into the lung,** usually occurring at the point of impact.
- The **history of trauma** is of **paramount importance** as contusions present as **airspace disease** that can be **indistinguishable from other airspace diseases** like pneumonia or aspiration.

> ### ▶▶ IMPORTANT POINTS
>
> - **Recognizing a pulmonary contusion:**
>   - Contusions tend to be **peripherally placed** and **frequently occur at the point of maximum impact. Air bronchograms** are usually **not present** in the contusion because blood fills the bronchi as well as the airspaces (Fig. 24.15).

- Classically, they **appear within 6 hours after the trauma** and, because blood in the airspaces tends to be reabsorbed quickly, **disappear within 72 hours,** often sooner.

- Airspace disease that **lingers more than 72 hours** should **raise suspicions** of another process such as **aspiration, pneumonia,** or a **pulmonary laceration.**

## Pulmonary Lacerations

- **Pulmonary lacerations** result from a **tear of the lung parenchyma** and, as such, may accompany more severe **blunt trauma** or **penetrating chest trauma.**
- A pulmonary laceration can also be called a *traumatic pneumatocele* (when it contains primarily air) or a *pulmonary hematoma* (when it contains primarily blood).
- On conventional radiographs, they are often **masked** by the airspace disease from a surrounding pulmonary contusion, at least for the first few days until the contusion resolves.
- Unlike pulmonary contusions that clear rapidly, **pulmonary lacerations,** especially if they are blood filled, **may take weeks or months to completely clear.**

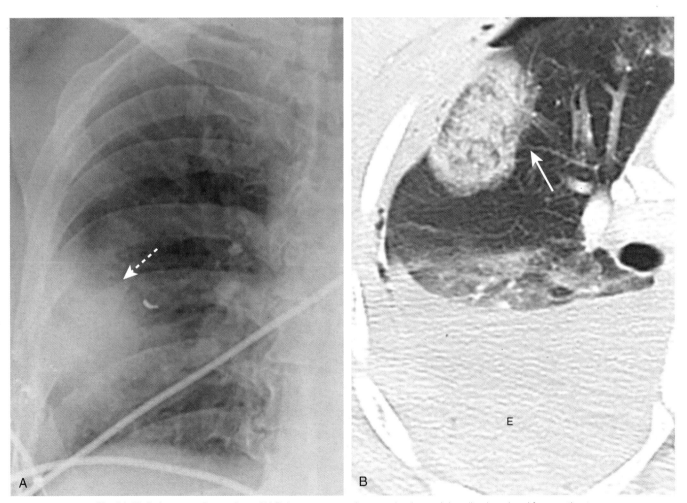

**Fig. 24.15 Pulmonary Contusions.** (A) Pulmonary contusions tend to be peripherally placed and frequently at the point of maximum impact *(arrow)*. They do not usually contain air bronchograms. (B) CT scan of the chest on another patient, who was an unrestrained passenger in an automobile accident, also displays a pulmonary contusion *(arrow)* with an associated large effusion (E).

## Pulmonary Interstitial Emphysema

- When the pressure or volume in the alveolus becomes sufficiently elevated, the **alveolus may rupture**, leading to **extraalveolar air.**
- This extraalveolar air may take one of two main paths:
  - If the alveolus is in proximity to a pleural surface, the air may burst **outward** into the pleural space and create a **pneumothorax.**
  - Alternatively, the air can **track backward along the bronchovascular bundles** in the lung **to the mediastinum,** then into the **neck** and out to the **subcutaneous tissues** of the chest and abdominal wall. Occasionally, the air can track downward into the abdomen as well as retroperitoneum.
- It is also possible for air to dissect **both** into the **pleural space** and backward along the **bronchovascular bundles** at the same time.
- The air that tracks backward toward the hilum does so along the **perivascular connective tissue of the lung** forming **small, cystic collections** of extraalveolar air that **dissect retrograde through the bronchovascular sheaths** to the hila. When the extraalveolar air is confined to the interstitial network of the lung, it is called *pulmonary interstitial emphysema* or *perivascular interstitial emphysema (PIE).*
- Presumably because of the looser connective tissue in the lungs of children and young adults, pulmonary interstitial emphysema is **more likely to occur** in those **under the age of 40.**
- **Assisted, mechanical ventilation increases the risk** of developing pulmonary interstitial emphysema, and its formation can **herald a significant risk for the imminent appearance of a pneumothorax,** frequently within a matter of a few hours or days.
- Other causes of increased intraalveolar pressure and rupture include asthma and barotrauma.

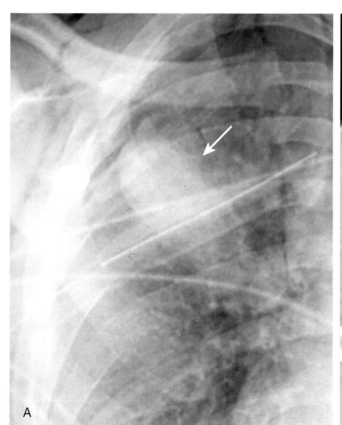
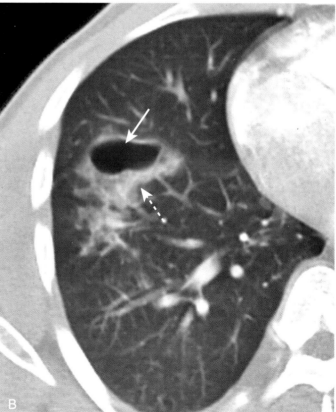

**Fig. 24.16 Pulmonary Lacerations.** (A) If lacerations are completely filled with blood, they will appear as an ovoid mass *(arrow).* (B) On CT, another pulmonary laceration is air-filled *(solid arrow)* and is surrounded by airspace disease, representing a pulmonary contusion *(dashed arrow).*

- **Pulmonary interstitial emphysema may not be recognizable** on conventional radiographs because the air **collections are small** and because there is usually a **considerable amount of coexisting disease** in the lung that obscures it. It may, however, be more visible on CT scans of the chest (Fig. 24.17).

## Pneumomediastinum

- About **one in three patients** with **pulmonary interstitial emphysema** will develop *pneumomediastinum* (more often it leads to a pneumothorax). Pneumomediastinum can occur in trauma because the air tracks backward along the bronchovascular bundles until it enters the mediastinum.
- Pneumomediastinum may also develop when there is **perforation** of an **air-containing viscus** that lies **within the mediastinum,** such as the **esophagus** or **tracheobronchial tree.**
  - **Rupture of the distal esophagus,** usually the left posterolateral wall, can occur with increased intraesophageal pressure from retching or vomiting in *Boerhaave syndrome.*
- **Rupture of the tracheobronchial tree** is most often **secondary to significant trauma,** either **iatrogenic** such as during a traumatic **intubation** or **accidental,** such as from a penetrating wound or severe blunt trauma.

> ## IMPORTANT POINTS
>
> - **Radiographic findings of pneumomediastinum:**
>   - **Linear, streak-like lucency** associated with a **thin white line paralleling the left heart border.**
>   - **Streaky air outlining the great vessels** (aorta, superior vena cava, carotid arteries).
>   - Linear streaks of air **parallel to the spine** in the upper thorax extending into the neck and surrounding the esophagus and trachea (Fig. 24.18).
>   - *Continuous diaphragm sign.* With pneumomediastinum, air can outline the central portion of the diaphragm beneath the heart, producing an unbroken superior surface of the diaphragm which extends from one lateral chest wall to the other (Fig. 24.19).

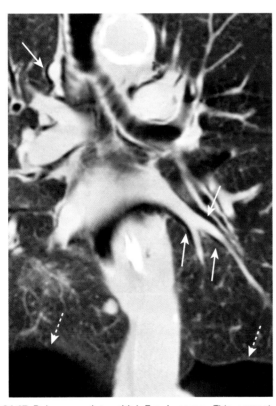

**Fig. 24.17 Pulmonary Interstitial Emphysema.** This coronal, reformatted CT scan of the chest demonstrates air *(solid arrows)* surrounding the pulmonary arteries (white branching structures) in the lung. This air arose from a ruptured alveolus in a patient with asthma and is tracking back to the hilum where it also produced pneumomediastinum and subcutaneous emphysema. The patient also has bilateral, basilar pneumothoraces *(dashed arrows).*

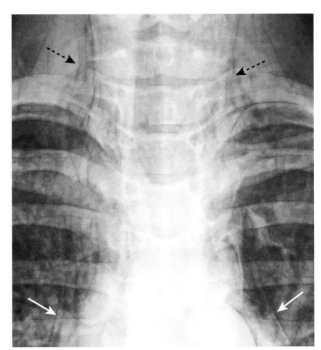

**Fig. 24.18 Pneumomediastinum and Subcutaneous Emphysema.** This patient with asthma developed spontaneous pneumomediastinum, most likely from rupture of an alveolus followed by formation of pulmonary interstitial emphysema. The air tracked back to the hila, then into the mediastinum where it produced streaky white, linear densities *(white arrows)* extending to the neck. In the neck, there is subcutaneous emphysema *(black arrows).*

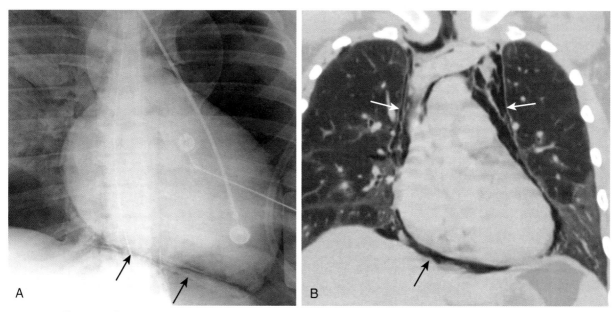

**Fig. 24.19 Continuous Diaphragm Sign of Pneumomediastinum.** (A) The central portion of the diaphragm is usually not visible because it is silhouetted by the heart, which has the same soft-tissue density as the diaphragm on radiographs. When air enters the mediastinum, the entire diaphragm under the heart may become visible *(arrows)*. This is called the **continuous diaphragm sign.** (B) A coronal reformatted CT scan of the chest in another patient shows pneumomediastinum outlining the central portion of the diaphragm *(black arrow)* and the remainder of the pneumomediastinum extending superior to the great vessels *(white arrows)*.

## Pneumopericardium

- **Pneumopericardium is usually due to direct penetrating injuries** to the pericardium **either caused iatrogenically** (during cardiac surgery) **or accidentally** (from penetrating trauma). Pneumopericardium is **more common in pediatric patients** than adults and may develop in neonates with **neonatal respiratory distress syndrome** (hyaline membrane disease, surfactant deficiency disorder).
- It is **rare for air in the pleural space to enter the pericardium,** except in those who have a pericardial defect, such as a surgical *window* incised in the pericardium that allows free exchange between the pleural and pericardial spaces.

> ## ▶▶ IMPORTANT POINTS
>
> - **Pneumopericardium** produces a **continuous** band of **lucency that encircles the heart** bound by the parietal pericardial layer, **which extends no higher than the root of the great vessels** (corresponding to the level of the main pulmonary artery) (Fig. 24.20).
>   - **Pneumomediastinum,** in contrast, **does extend** above the root of the great vessels into the uppermost thorax.
> - **CT is usually necessary to demonstrate the findings of pneumopericardium.**

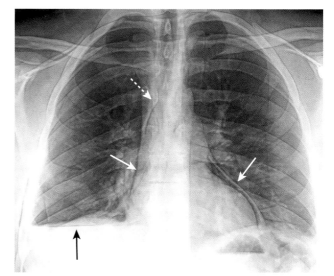

**Fig. 24.20 Pneumopericardium.** This patient sustained penetrating chest trauma. There is a pneumopericardium as shown by the visible parietal pericardium *(solid white arrows)* outlined by air around the heart in the pericardial space. Notice how the air does not extend above the reflection of the aorta and main pulmonary artery *(dashed white arrow)* as it would in a pneumomediastinum. There is also a right-sided hemopneumothorax as evidenced by the air-fluid level in the right hemithorax *(black arrow)*.

## AORTIC TRAUMA

- Trauma to the aorta is most frequently the result of **deceleration injuries** in **motor vehicle accidents.** Although the survival rates are improving, **most patients** with rupture of the thoracic aorta **die before reaching the hospital** and, of those who survive an aortic injury, the likelihood of death increases the longer the abnormality remains untreated. Frequently, only those with **incomplete** tears in which the **adventitial lining prevents exsanguination** (producing a *pseudoaneurysm*) survive to be imaged.
- Only emergency surgery will prevent approximately 50% of patients with blunt aortic injuries from dying within the first 24 hours if left untreated.

» **IMPORTANT POINTS**

- The most common site of injury is the **aortic isthmus**, which is the portion of the **aorta just distal to the origin of the left subclavian artery.** Seat-belt injuries may involve the abdominal aorta but such injuries are far less common than the deceleration injuries to the thoracic aorta.

## Recognizing Aortic Trauma

- **Findings seen on conventional radiographs of the chest** are the same as those discussed under **Aortic Dissection** in Chapter 11. A **completely normal chest radiograph** has a relatively **high negative predictive value** for aortic injury, but chest radiographs are sufficiently insensitive as to require another study to rule out an aortic injury.
  - There may be **loss of the normal shadow of the aortic knob, a left apical pleural cap** of fluid or blood, a **left pleural effusion,** or **deviation of the trachea or esophagus to the right** (Fig. 24.21).
- Under most circumstances, suspected aortic injuries are now studied using **CT** that allows for rapid image acquisition in one breath-hold and appropriately timed contrast delivery to the aorta (**CT-angiography**). Most experts agree that a negative CT angiogram obviates the need for angiography. The findings of aortic injury are **frequently subtle** and require experience to recognize, as those patients with the more obvious findings may not have survived to be imaged.
- **Findings on contrast-enhanced CT scans of the aorta** (Fig. 24.22):
  - *Aortic intimal flap.* A linear, lucent defect in the contrast column of the aorta arising from a **tear** in the intima and media.
  - *Contour or caliber abnormalities.* Abrupt change in the smooth contour or size of the aorta at the point of injury.

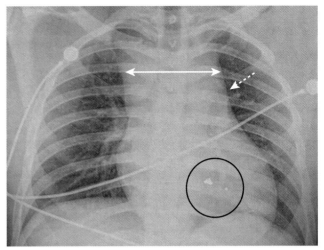

**Fig. 24.21 Mediastinal Hematoma.** There is "widening of the mediastinum" *(double arrow)*, an inexact finding on an anteroposterior, supine, portable chest radiograph. More importantly, the normal shadow of the aortic knob is obscured by something of similar soft-tissue density *(dashed arrow)*. Because the patient had been shot (bullet fragments in the *circle*), these findings did lead to a suggestion for a CT angiogram that demonstrated a large mediastinal hematoma.

- *Periaortic hematoma.* Delineation of a **contrast-filled collection outside of the normal confines of the aorta** representing pseudoaneurysm or extravasation.
- *Mediastinal hematoma.* Increased attenuation in the mediastinum from an admixture of blood and normal fat. This may occur in the absence of an aortic injury, presumably due to small vessel trauma.
- *Hemopericardium.* Fluid of high-attenuation (i.e., blood) in the pericardial sac indicates a significant injury to the aorta or heart itself.
- Patients with **equivocal** CT findings may go on to a catheter study of the aorta (**aortography**).

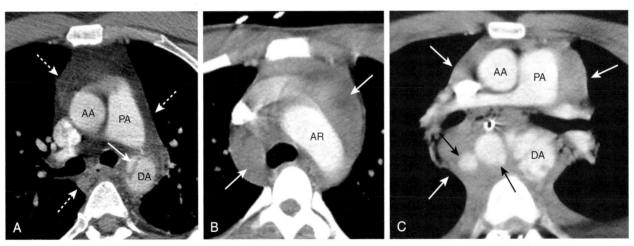

**Fig. 24.22 Aortic Trauma, Three Different Patients.** (A) There is a tear at the level of the aortic isthmus represented by the linear defect in the wall of the descending aorta *(solid arrow)*. A mediastinal hematoma is also present *(dashed arrows)*. (B) There is a large mediastinal hematoma *(solid arrows)*. (C) There are periaortic hematomas containing extravasated blood *(black arrows)* and a large mediastinal hematoma *(white arrows)*. (*AA*, Ascending aorta; *AR*, aortic arch; *DA*, descending aorta; *PA*, pulmonary artery).

## CASE QUIZ 24 ANSWER

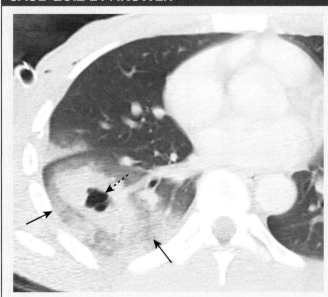

There is a **pulmonary laceration** present *(dashed arrow)*. Surrounding the laceration is airspace disease representing a **pulmonary contusion** *(solid arrows)*. It is not unusual for a pulmonary contusion to *mask* the presence of an underlying pulmonary laceration, particularly on conventional radiographs.

## 🏠 TAKE HOME POINTS

- Trauma is generally divided into **blunt** and **penetrating** trauma. Most trauma-related injuries are due to blunt trauma, with motor vehicle accidents contributing the majority.
- **Rib fractures** may herald more serious internal injuries, such as lacerations of the liver or spleen or pneumothoraces. Most rib fractures occur in ribs 4 to 9.
- A **flail chest** is defined radiographically as one in which at least two fractures occur in each of three contiguous ribs. It is associated with significant morbidity and mortality.
- **Subcutaneous emphysema** may produce dramatic, but largely clinically insignificant, findings. It heralds the presence of an underlying abnormality, but usually does not require treatment itself.
- There is normally no air in the pleural space; air in the pleural space is called a **pneumothorax.** The visceral pleural white line must be identified to diagnose a pneumothorax.
- Beware of the pitfalls that resemble pneumothoraces: **bullae, skin folds,** and the medial border of the **scapula.**
- **Simple pneumothoraces** are those with no shift of the heart or mobile mediastinal structures; most pneumothoraces are simple.
- **Tension pneumothoraces** (frequently associated with cardiorespiratory compromise) produce a shift of the heart and mediastinal structures **away** from the side of the pneumothorax by virtue of a check-valve mechanism that allows air to enter the pleural space but not leave.
- Most pneumothoraces are **traumatic** in etiology, either accidental or iatrogenic.
- Conventional chest radiographs are poor at estimating the size of a pneumothorax; CT is better; the most important assessment to be made regarding intervention for a pneumothorax is the clinical status of the patient.

- Besides the conventional upright chest radiograph, other ways to diagnose a pneumothorax include ultrasound, decubitus views, and delayed images. CT remains the mainstay for detecting small pneumothoraces.
- **Pulmonary contusions** are the most common lung manifestation of blunt chest trauma and represent hemorrhage into the lung, usually at the point of impact. They classically clear in a few days.
- **Pulmonary lacerations** are tears in the lung parenchyma that may be fluid and/or air-containing. Their presence may be hidden by a surrounding contusion, and they typically take longer than a contusion to clear.
- **Pulmonary interstitial emphysema** results from an increase in the intraalveolar pressure that, in turn, leads to rupture of an alveolus and dissection of air back toward the hila along the bronchovascular bundles; it is frequently difficult to visualize.
- **Pneumomediastinum** can occur when air tracks back to the mediastinum from a ruptured alveolus or from perforation of an air-containing viscus, such as the esophagus or trachea; it can produce the **continuous diaphragm sign** on a frontal chest radiograph.
- **Pneumopericardium** usually requires direct penetration of the pericardium rather than dissection of air from a pneumomediastinum; it can be difficult to differentiate from a pneumomediastinum, but a key is that pneumopericardium does not extend above the roots of the great vessels, whereas pneumomediastinum does.
- **Aortic injuries** usually occur at the isthmus, require rapid recognition for optimum survival, and may appear on contrast-enhanced CT as intimal flaps, contour abnormalities, or hematomas.

🛜 Additional content is available online including chapters on Nuclear Medicine, Artificial Intelligence, Radiation Dose and Safety, an Early History of Radiology, and a compendium of 200 Diagnostic Radiology Signs.

# Recognizing the Imaging Findings of Trauma to the Abdomen and Pelvis

*William Herring, MD, FACR*

## ABDOMINAL TRAUMA

The role of advanced imaging techniques deserves special mention in abdominal trauma. Radiology has made a significant impact on the lives of traumatized patients by distinguishing those patients who can be managed conservatively from those who need surgical or other interventions and by helping to direct the most appropriate intervention for those who need it.

### CASE QUIZ 25 QUESTION

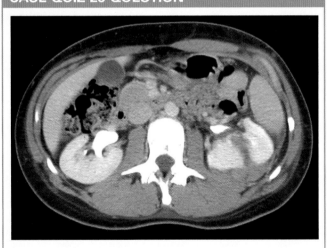

This is a contrast-enhanced axial CT image at the level of the kidneys in a 25-year-old male pedestrian struck by a motor vehicle. His vital signs are stable but he complains of low back pain. The scan shows a traumatic abdominal injury. What is it? The answer is at the end of the chapter.

### ▶▶ IMPORTANT POINTS

- **CT is the study of choice in abdominal trauma.**
  - **Intravenous contrast is always used** (unless contraindicated) to identify devascularized areas, hematomas, active extravasation of blood or extraluminal urine (after contrast has passed through the kidneys) (Box 25.1).
    - If a **head CT is to be done** as well, it should be **done first before** contrast is injected for the abdomen.

### BOX 25.1   Contrast Reactions and Renal Insufficiency

- Intravenous contrast materials available today are **nonionic, low osmolar solutions** containing a high concentration of iodine that circulate through the bloodstream, opacify those tissues and organs with **high blood flow,** are absorbed by x-ray (and therefore appear *whiter* on images), and are finally **excreted in the urine by the kidneys.**
- In some patients (e.g., those with a personal history of chronic kidney disease) who have an eGFR less than 30 mL/min/1.73 m$^2$, the intravenous administration of iodinated contrast may be associated with acute kidney injury. Though usually reversible, in a small number of patients with underlying renal disease, renal dysfunction may permanently worsen. When the eGFR is lower than 30 mL/min/1.73m$^2$ and intravenous contrast is deemed necessary, prophylaxis may be indicated through the administration of **isotonic volume expansion with normal saline.**
- Iodinated contrast agents can sometimes produce **mild side effects,** including a feeling of warmth, nausea, and vomiting, local irritation at the site of injection, and itching and hives; these side effects usually require no treatment. Occasional idiosyncratic reactions include itching, hives, and laryngeal irritation.
- Asthmatics and those with a history of severe allergies or prior reactions to IV contrast have a higher likelihood of contrast reactions (but still very low overall) and may benefit from steroids or diphenhydramine (Benadryl™) administered prior and/or after injection. **Prior shellfish allergy** bears absolutely **no relationship** to iodinated contrast reactions.
- In about 0.01% to 0.04% of all patients, severe and idiosyncratic reactions to contrast can occur that can produce intense bronchospasm, laryngeal edema, circulatory collapse, and, very rarely, death (1 in 200,000 to 300,000).

- **Oral contrast** is usually not given. **Rectal contrast** is occasionally administered in penetrating trauma to search for a bowel laceration.
- It is always best to consult with the radiologist so as to tailor the best study to fit the patient's needs.
- In some emergency settings, a quick abdominal ultrasound is used in unstable trauma patients to evaluate for hemoperitoneum (FAST scan, see Chapter 19).
- The most commonly affected solid organs in **blunt** abdominal trauma (in order of decreasing frequency) are the **spleen, liver, kidney, and urinary bladder.** Traumatic injuries to each of them will be discussed under each organ.

# LIVER

- The liver is discussed first because it is actually the **most frequently injured organ** if **both penetrating and blunt trauma** are included together. The liver is the largest intraabdominal organ and is fixed in position, making it especially susceptible to injury. Injuries to the liver account for the **majority of deaths from abdominal trauma.**
- The posterior aspect of the **right lobe** is injured most frequently. Most hepatic injuries are associated with blood in the peritoneal cavity *(hemoperitoneum).*
- **Contrast-enhanced CT is the study of choice** and, because of its ability to demonstrate both the nature and extent of the trauma, the overwhelming majority of patients with liver trauma are now managed conservatively and do not require surgery.

>> **IMPORTANT POINTS**

- **CT findings in hepatic trauma:**
  - *Subcapsular hematoma.* Lenticular fluid collections that conform to the shape of the **outer** contour of the liver but frequently **flatten** the adjacent liver parenchyma. Most occur anterolaterally over the right hepatic lobe (Fig. 25.1A).
  - *Lacerations.* Most common finding. Irregularly marginated, low attenuation, linear or branching defects, usually at the periphery. *Fracture* is a term that has been used to describe a laceration that avulses a section of the liver (Fig. 25.1B).

>> **IMPORTANT POINTS—cont'd**

- *Intrahepatic hematomas.* Focal, high-attenuation lesions first caused by blood, hematomas may progress to become low attenuation, mass-like lesions filled with serous fluid (Fig. 25.1C).
- *Wedge-shaped defects.* Devascularized sections of liver parenchyma that do not contrast-enhance.
- *Contusions.* A term used to describe an area of minimal parenchymal hemorrhage; they are lower in attenuation than the surrounding liver and have indistinct margins.
- *Pseudoaneurysms and acute hemorrhages.* Irregular collections of high-attenuation, extravasated contrast that often require angiography with embolization and/or surgery.

# SPLEEN

- Splenic trauma is usually caused by **deceleration injuries** in unrestrained occupants of motor vehicle collisions, by a fall from a height, or by being struck by a motor vehicle as a pedestrian. The spleen is affected in about 1/3 of patients with traumatic abdominal injuries.
- Because the **spleen is the most highly vascular intraabdominal organ**, **hemorrhage** represents the most serious complication of trauma. Despite its vascular nature and the delayed presentation of many splenic injuries, **most splenic trauma is treated conservatively** (nonsurgically). However, the presence of hypotension in a patient with a suspected splenic injury can be a critical sign and a surgical emergency.

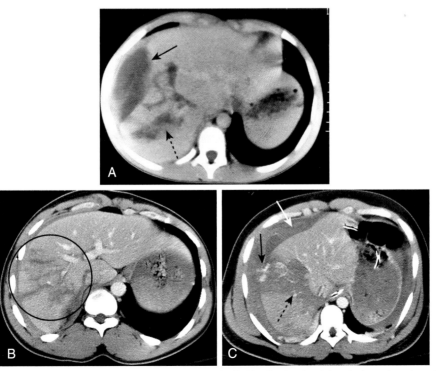

**Fig. 25.1 Hepatic Trauma, Three Different Patients.** (A) There is a lenticular fluid collection involving the lateral portion of the right lobe of the liver that represents a **subcapsular hematoma** *(solid arrow)*. There is also a **laceration** of the right lobe *(dashed arrow)*. (B) There are multiple **lacerations** of the right lobe of the liver *(circle)*. (C) There is active **extravasation** of contrast-enhanced blood *(solid black arrow)* from a large intrahepatic laceration with **hematoma** *(dashed black arrow)* and both **subcapsular** blood and hemoperitoneum *(white arrow)*.

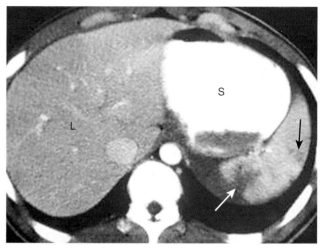

**Fig. 25.3 Splenic Contusions.** There are several low-attenuation lesions in the spleen *(arrows)* in this patient who fell from a ladder. The treatment for splenic contusions is usually conservative. *L,* Liver; *S,* stomach (containing oral contrast).

## KIDNEYS

- Motor vehicle accidents are the most common cause of blunt abdominal trauma to the kidneys in the United States. In the pediatric age group, falls are the most common cause. Both kidneys are affected equally. Increasing emphasis has been placed on nonsurgical management when clinically appropriate. Almost all patients with renal trauma will have **hematuria.**

- **Contrast-enhanced CT is the study of first choice** and has almost completely replaced the intravenous urogram and standard cystogram.

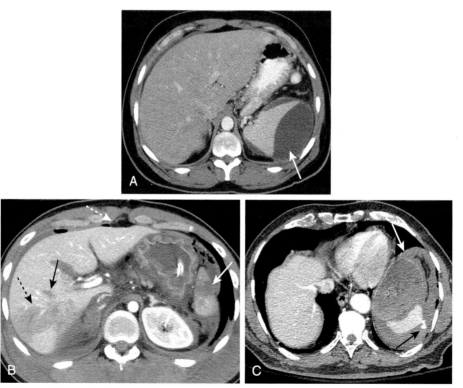

**Fig. 25.2 Splenic Trauma, Three Different Patients.** (A) There is a crescent-shaped collection of fluid in the subcapsular space that compresses the normal splenic parenchyma representing **subcapsular hematoma** *(arrow)*. (B) This patient has a splenic *(solid white arrow)* and hepatic *(solid black arrow)* **laceration** and a large **hepatic contusion** *(dashed black arrow)*. There is also pneumoperitoneum *(dashed white arrow)*. (C) This patient has active **extravasation** of contrast-enhanced blood *(black arrow)* and a large **intrasplenic hematoma** *(white arrow)*.

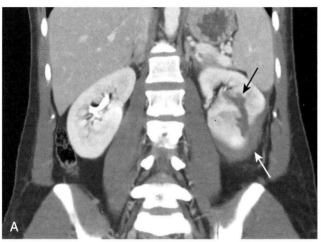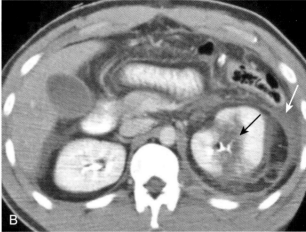

**Fig. 25.4** Renal Trauma, Two Different Patients. (A) Coronal-reformatted, contrast-enhanced CT scan shows a low-attenuation linear defect representing a **renal laceration** *(black arrow)* and a **subcapsular hematoma** *(white arrow)*. (B) Axial CT scan on another patient also displays a renal laceration *(black arrow)* and a **perinephric hematoma** *(white arrow)*.

---

### ▶▶ IMPORTANT POINTS

- **CT findings in renal trauma:**
  - **Contusion.** Ill-defined, patchy, low-attenuation areas in the contrast-enhanced kidney.
  - **Subcapsular hematoma.** Crescentic or elliptical densities that compress the denser underlying renal parenchyma (Fig. 25.4A).
  - **Perinephric hematoma.** Ill-defined fluid collection surrounding the kidney confined by Gerota's fascia (Fig. 25.4B).
  - **Laceration.** Low-attenuation linear or branching defects in the renal parenchyma. More severe lacerations may extend through the renal hilum into the collecting system, renal artery, or vein. **Fracture** is a term that may be used when the laceration connects the hilum with the cortex (see Fig. 25.4B).
  - **Vascular injuries.** If arterial, there may be no flow to the kidney and hence no contrast-enhancement. They may also produce wedge-shaped defects in the kidney.
  - **Injuries to the collecting system.** Extraluminal contrast arising from the renal pelvis or ureter (Fig. 25.5).

## CT HYPOPERFUSION COMPLEX/SHOCK BOWEL

- The *CT hypoperfusion complex,* including changes in the bowel *(shock bowel),* can occur with **blunt abdominal trauma** in which there is severe **hypovolemia** and profound **hypotension.** The findings can be completely reversed following resuscitation. The small bowel is more affected than the large bowel.
- Besides trauma, the hypoperfusion complex can be seen with severe head injury, cardiac arrest, or septic shock.

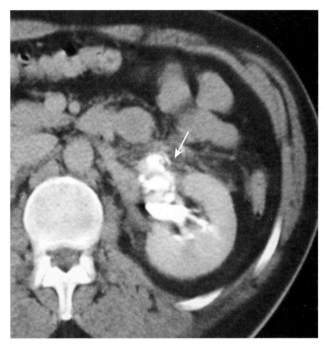

**Fig. 25.5** Tear of Proximal Ureter. There is a tear of the ureter at the level of the left ureteropelvic junction demonstrated by extraluminal contrast *(arrow)* representing contrast-containing urine that is leaking from the collecting system. The patient was an unrestrained driver in a motor vehicle accident.

- **Recognizing the CT hypoperfusion complex** (not all findings may be present):
  - Diffuse **thickening** of the **small bowel wall** with **increased enhancement**
  - Fluid-filled and **dilated loops** of bowel

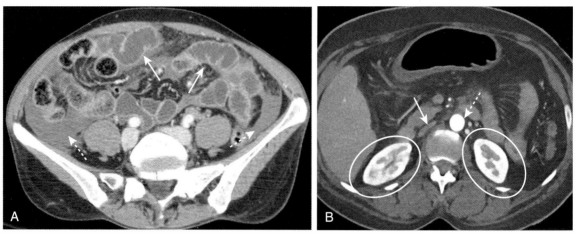

**Fig. 25.6 CT Hypoperfusion Complex.** (A) There is marked enhancement of the bowel wall accompanied by multiple dilated and fluid-filled loops *(solid arrows)* in this patient with bowel changes of hypotension (shock bowel). There is also peritoneal fluid present *(dashed arrows)*. (B) In another patient, additional signs of the *CT hypoperfusion complex* are seen, including a small caliber aorta *(dashed arrow)*, a flattened inferior vena cava *(solid arrow)*, and hyperintense kidneys *(ovals)*.

- Ascites (Fig. 25.6A)
- **Small** calibers of the **aorta** and **inferior vena cava**
- **Hyperenhancement** of the kidneys *(white kidney sign)* (Fig. 25.6B)
- **Hypoenhancement** of the **liver** and **spleen**

## PELVIC TRAUMA

- Pelvic injuries are usually the result of high-energy trauma. There is a potential for hemorrhage with associated shock, a major cause of morbidity and mortality. **Urogenital lesions** make up over 40% of associated injuries. Gross blood on rectal examination or blood at the urethral meatus could be signs of gastrointestinal or urethral injuries, respectively.

### Rupture of the Urinary Bladder

- About **70% of bladder ruptures** occur with **pelvic fractures** and about 10% of patients with pelvic fractures have an associated rupture of the bladder.

- Bladder ruptures are best demonstrated by a **CT cystogram** in which contrast is infused under gravity through a Foley catheter into the bladder, but they can also be well-demonstrated by antegrade filling of the bladder from renal excretion of intravenously injected contrast.
- There are **two major types** of bladder rupture (Fig. 25.7):
  - *Extraperitoneal* bladder rupture is more common (80%) and usually the **result of a pelvic fracture** with **direct puncture** of the bladder. Extraluminal contrast **remains around the bladder**, especially the retropubic space (Fig. 25.7A).
  - *Intraperitoneal* bladder rupture is less common and usually the **result of a forceful blow to the pelvis with a distended bladder,** especially in children. Rupture usually occurs at the **dome** of the bladder adjacent to the peritoneal cavity. Contrast runs freely through the **peritoneal cavity, surrounds the bowel, and may extend into the paracolic gutters** (Fig. 25.7B).

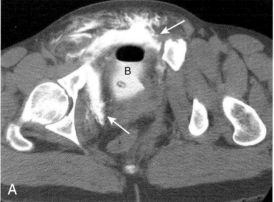
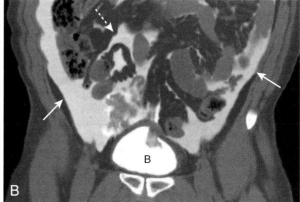

**Fig. 25.7 Bladder Ruptures, Extraperitoneal and Intraperitoneal.** (A) Contrast-containing urine *(arrows)* has leaked into the **extraperitoneal** spaces from a perforated bladder following pelvic fractures. Intravenous contrast, the tip of a Foley catheter, and air are seen inside of the partially filled urinary bladder (B). (B) **Intraperitoneal** bladder ruptures are less common and may occur with blunt trauma. The contrast flows freely away from the bladder (B) up the paracolic gutters *(solid arrows)* and outlines loops of bowel *(dashed arrow)*.

## Urethral Injuries

- Urethral injuries are associated with significant pelvic trauma in **males,** and occur most often from **blunt trauma.**
- Urethral injuries should be considered especially when there are *straddle fractures* of the pelvis or **penetrating injuries** in the region of the **urethra.** Hematuria, blood at the urethral meatus, and inability to void are suggestive clinical findings.
  - A **straddle fracture** involves both superior and both inferior pubic rami and is an **unstable** pelvic fracture.
- Imaging is done most often using **retrograde urethrography (RUG)** in which contrast is instilled at the urethral meatus and there is retrograde filling of the urethra. This is usually done before insertion of a Foley catheter into the bladder.
  - The **most common injury** is a rupture of the **posterior urethra** through the urogenital diaphragm into the proximal bulbous urethra. Extraluminal contrast can be seen outside of the urethra in the pelvis and perineum (Fig. 25.8).

## LESS COMMON ABDOMINAL INJURIES

### Diaphragm

- Diaphragmatic injuries are estimated to occur in up to 5% of trauma patients. They can be the result of either **blunt** (motor vehicle accidents) or **penetrating** (knife wound) injuries. The **left hemidiaphragm** is involved more than the right and the **posterolateral** portion of the diaphragm is affected most often. The diaphragm is rarely injured in isolation of injury to other organs, especially in blunt trauma.
- It is easier to visualize defects in the diaphragm on the left than the right. There may be **herniation** of abdominal contents into the thorax. The intraabdominal contents may be **constricted** where they pass through the diaphragmatic rent, producing the *collar sign* (Fig. 25.9).

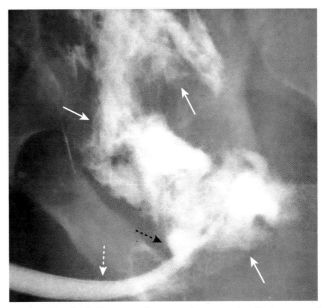

**Fig. 25.8 Urethral Trauma.** Contrast that was instilled retrograde through the penile urethra *(dashed white arrow)* is seen to leak from the posterior urethra secondary to a perforation *(dashed black arrow)* and collects outside of the urinary system in the perineum and extraperitoneal bladder spaces *(solid white arrows).* The patient had pelvic fractures secondary to a fall.

- There may be **delayed presentation** of a ruptured diaphragm months or years after the initial trauma either from **delayed rupture** of the diaphragm or **delayed detection** of a diaphragmatic rupture.

### Pancreas

- Pancreatic injury is relatively uncommon but occurs more frequently with **penetrating trauma** than with blunt trauma. It is almost always accompanied by injuries to other organs no matter what the cause.

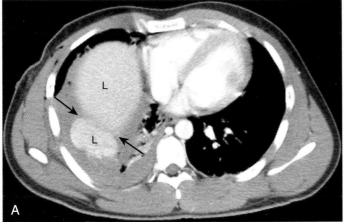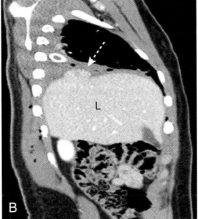

**Fig. 25.9 Ruptured Diaphragm.** (A) There is a rent in the right hemidiaphragm that allows a portion of the liver (L) to extrude through the rupture. Where the organ passes through the rupture, a constricted zone called the *collar sign* is seen *(arrows).* (B) The sagittal view demonstrates the small, extruded portion *(arrow)* of the liver (L). *HL,* Herniated portion of liver.

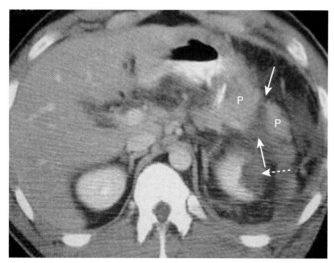

**Fig. 25.10** Pancreatic Laceration. There is a laceration (transection) of the tail of the pancreas (P) *(solid arrows)* with an associated left renal injury *(dashed arrow)*. There is a high likelihood of damage to the pancreatic duct in such injuries, a finding that would increase morbidity and mortality. The patient had been stabbed in the abdomen.

- CT is the imaging study of choice. The CT findings may be subtle, including **peripancreatic fluid** and diffuse **enlargement** of the pancreas. The most obvious finding is a **fracture** through the pancreas (Fig. 25.10). Magnetic resonance cholangiopancreatography (MRCP) may be used to visualize the pancreatic duct.
- The changes of **posttraumatic pancreatitis** may not be visualized for some time following trauma and delayed diagnosis

of pancreatic injury can considerably increase morbidity and mortality.
- Complications can include pancreatic pseudocysts, recurrent pancreatitis, or fistula formation.

## CASE QUIZ 25 ANSWER

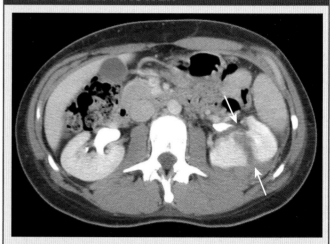

There is disruption of the renal parenchyma of the left kidney due to a renal laceration *(arrows)* that additional study indicated did not extend into the collecting system. The anatomic structure of the kidney, its location in a closed retroperitoneal compartment that retards bleeding, and the increased use of CT imaging allow many more patients with renal trauma to be managed without operative intervention

## 🏠 TAKE HOME POINTS

- CT has had a profound impact on traumatized patients by distinguishing those patients who can be managed conservatively from those who need surgical or other interventions.
- The most commonly affected solid organs in **blunt** abdominal trauma (in order of decreasing frequency) are the spleen, liver, kidney, and urinary bladder.
- The **liver** is commonly injured in **both blunt and penetrating trauma** and its injuries account for the majority of the deaths from abdominal trauma. The liver may demonstrate lacerations, hematomas, wedge-shaped defects, pseudoaneurysms, and acute hemorrhage.
- Because the **spleen** is highly vascular, hemorrhage is the most serious sequela of splenic trauma whose other findings include hematomas, lacerations, and contusions.
- Patients who have had **renal trauma** almost always have hematuria and may show contusions, lacerations, hematomas, or vascular pedicle injuries on CT. They may also demonstrate extraluminal contrast from an injury to the renal pelvis or ureter.

- **CT hypoperfusion complex** is a consequence of profound hypotension and demonstrates diffuse small bowel wall thickening with enhancement of dilated and fluid-filled loops along with possible changes in the aorta, inferior vena cava, liver, kidneys, and spleen.
- **Bladder ruptures** may be either extraperitoneal (more common) or intraperitoneal, the former demonstrating extraluminal contrast surrounding the bladder and the latter displaying contrast that flows freely in the peritoneal cavity.
- **Urethral injuries** occur almost exclusively in males, are frequently associated with pelvic fractures, and usually involve the posterior urethra where extraluminal contrast may be seen in the perineum or extraperitoneally in the pelvis.
- **Diaphragmatic rupture** usually occurs on the left side and requires forceful blunt trauma. It is almost always associated with other traumatic abdominal lesions.
- **Pancreatic injuries** are relatively uncommon, almost always associated with other abdominal trauma, and may have a significant morbidity and mortality.

 Additional content is available online including chapters on Nuclear Medicine, Artificial Intelligence, Radiation Dose and Safety, an Early History of Radiology, and a compendium of 200 Diagnostic Radiology Signs.

# 26

# Recognizing Some Common Causes of Intracranial Pathology

*William Herring, MD, FACR*

Advances in neuroimaging have had a remarkable impact on the diagnosis and treatment of neurologic diseases ranging from earlier detection and treatment of stroke to a more timely diagnosis of dementia, from the rapid detection and treatment of cerebral aneurysms to the ability to diagnose multiple sclerosis after a single attack.

## CASE QUIZ 26 QUESTION

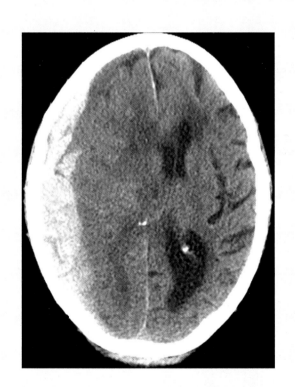

This is an image from an unenhanced head CT on a 68-year-old male who fell and struck his head earlier in the same day and has become progressively disoriented. Pertinent clinical history is the current use of anticoagulants for heart disease. What is the diagnosis? See the answer at the end of this chapter.

- Both CT and MRI are utilized for studying the brain and spinal cord, but MRI is the study of first choice in most clinical scenarios (Table 26.1). Conventional radiography has no significant role in imaging intracranial abnormalities.

**TABLE 26.1  Imaging Studies of the Brain for Selected Abnormalities**

| Abnormality | Study of First Choice | Other Studies |
|---|---|---|
| Acute stroke | Diffusion-weighted imaging (see Table 26.8) for acute or small strokes, if available | Noncontrast CT can differentiate hemorrhagic from ischemic infarct |
| Headache, acute and severe | Noncontrast CT to detect subarachnoid hemorrhage | MR angiography (MRA) or CT angiography (CTA) if subarachnoid hemorrhage is found in order to detect aneurysm |
| Headaches, chronic (with new features) | MRI, without and with contrast, or MRI without contrast | CT, without and with contrast |
| Seizures | MRI, without and with contrast. Add thin section images through hippocampi in patients with history of childhood seizures | CT, without and with contrast, can be substituted if MRI not available |
| Blood | Noncontrast CT | Ultrasound for infants |
| Head trauma | Nonenhanced CT is readily available and the study of first choice in head trauma | MRI is better at detecting diffuse axonal injury but requires more time and is not always available |
| Extracranial carotid disease | Doppler ultrasonography | MRA excellent study; CTA best for preoperative stenosis evaluation |
| Hydrocephalus | MRI as initial study | CT for follow-up |
| Vertigo and dizziness | Contrast-enhanced MRI | MRA if needed and/or thin section images through internal auditory canals as needed |
| Masses | MRI, without and with contrast | Contrast-enhanced CT if MRI not available |
| Change in mental status | MRI, without or with contrast | CT without contrast |

# NORMAL ANATOMY (FIG. 26.1)

- We will look at the normal anatomy of the brain using CT.
- In the posterior fossa, the **fourth ventricle** appears as an inverted U-shaped structure. Like all cerebrospinal fluid-containing structures on CT, it normally appears black. Posterior to the fourth ventricle are the **cerebellar hemispheres,** anteriorly lie the **pons** and **medulla oblongata.** The **tentorium cerebelli** separates the **infratentorial** components of the posterior fossa (cerebellum and fourth ventricle) from the **supratentorial** compartment.

- The **interpeduncular cistern** lies in the midbrain and separates the paired **cerebral peduncles** (which emerge from the superior surface of the pons). The **suprasellar cistern** is anterior to the interpeduncular cistern and usually has a five- or six-point star-like appearance.
- The **Sylvian fissures** are bilaterally symmetric and contain cerebrospinal fluid (CSF). They separate the temporal from the frontal and parietal lobes.
- The **lentiform nucleus** is composed of the **putamen** (laterally) and **globus pallidus** (medially). The **third ventricle** is slit-like and midline. At the posterior aspect of the third ventricle is the **pineal gland.** Farther posterior is the **quadrigeminal plate cistern.**

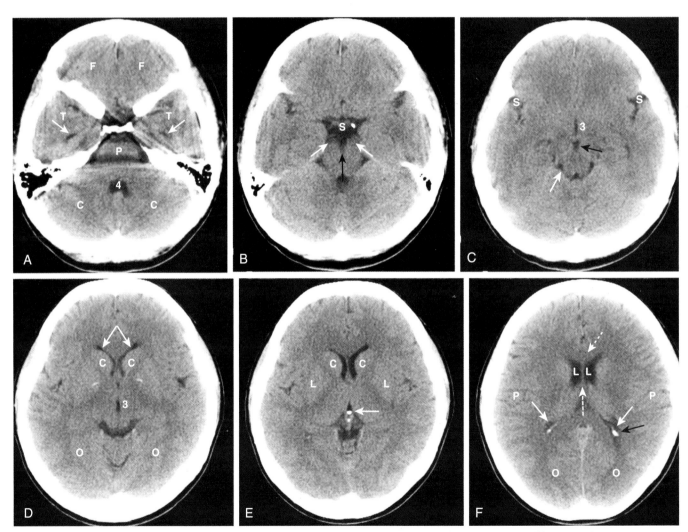

**Fig. 26.1 Normal Unenhanced CT Scans of the Head.** (A) Frontal lobes (F); temporal lobes (T); temporal horns *(arrows);* fourth ventricle (4); cerebellum (C); pons (P). (B) Suprasellar cistern (S); cerebral peduncles *(white arrows);* interpeduncular cistern *(black arrow).* (C) Sylvian fissures (S); third ventricle (3); interpeduncular cistern *(black arrow);* quadrigeminal plate cistern *(white arrow).* (D) Frontal horns of the lateral ventricles *(white arrows);* caudate nuclei (C); third ventricle (3); occipital lobes (O). (E) Caudate nuclei (C); lentiform nuclei (L); calcified pineal gland *(arrow).* (F) Genu of corpus callosum *(dashed arrow);* lateral ventricles (L); septum pellucidum *(dashed arrow);* parietal lobes (P); occipital horn *(black arrow);* calcified choroid plexus *(solid white arrows);* occipital lobes (O).

- The **corpus callosum** connects the right and left cerebral hemispheres and forms the roof of the lateral ventricle. The anterior end is called the **genu** and the posterior end is called the **splenium.**
- The **basal ganglia** are represented by the **subthalamic nucleus** and the **substantia nigra, globus pallidus, putamen, and caudate nucleus.** The putamen and caudate nucleus are called the **striatum.**
- The **frontal** (also known as **anterior**) **horns** of the **lateral ventricles** hug the head of the **caudate nucleus.** The two

frontal horns are separated by the midline **septum pellucidum.** The **temporal horns,** which are normally very small, are more inferior and contained in the t**emporal lobes.** The posterior horns (**occipital horns**) of the lateral ventricle lie in the occipital lobes. The most superior portion of the ventricular system are the **bodies** of the lateral ventricles.

- The **falx cerebri** lies in the **interhemispheric fissure,** which separates the two **cerebral hemispheres,** and is frequently calcified in adults.
- The surface or **cortex** of the brain is composed of **gray matter** convolutions made up of **sulci** (grooves) and **gyri** (elevations). The medullary **white matter** lies below the cortex.

### TABLE 26.2 CT Densities

| Hypodense (Dark) | Isodense | Hyperdense (Bright) |
|---|---|---|
| Fat (not usually present in the head) | Normal brain | Metal (e.g., aneurysm clips or bullets) |
| Air (e.g., sinuses) | Some forms of protein (e.g., subacute subdural hematomas) | Iodine (after contrast administration) |
| Water (e.g., CSF) | | Calcium |
| Chronic subdural hematomas/hygromas | | Hemorrhage (high protein) |

>> **IMPORTANT POINTS**

- On an unenhanced CT scan of the brain, anything that appears *white* will generally either be **bone (calcium)** density or **blood,** in the absence of a metallic foreign body (Table 26.2).

- **Physiologic calcifications that may be seen on CT of the brain:**
  - Pineal gland (Fig. 26.2A)
  - Basal ganglia (see Fig. 26.2A)
  - Choroid plexus (see Fig. 26.2A)
  - Falx and tentorium (Fig. 26.2B)

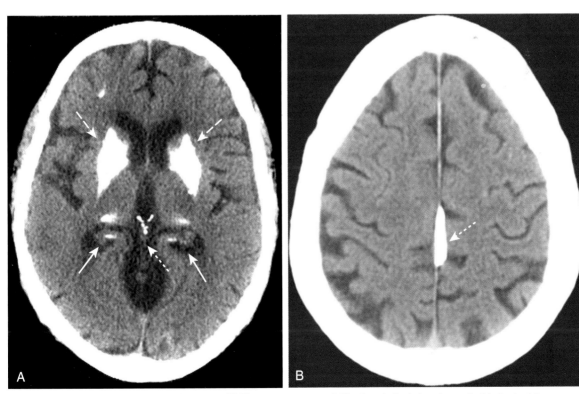

**Fig. 26.2 Physiologic Calcifications.** (A) There are coarse calcifications in both basal ganglia *(dashed white arrows),* choroid plexus *(solid white arrows),* and pineal gland *(dotted white arrow).* (B) There is calcification of the falx cerebri *(arrow).* Physiologic calcifications tend to increase in incidence with advancing age.

- **Normal structures** that can **enhance** after administration of iodinated intravenous contrast:
  - **Venous sinuses**
  - **Choroid plexus**
  - **Pituitary gland and stalk**
- **Metallic densities** in the head can cause artifacts on CT scans. Dental fillings, aneurysm clips, and bullets can all cause *streak artifacts.*

## MRI AND THE BRAIN

- In general, **MRI is the study of choice** for detecting and staging intracranial and spinal cord abnormalities. It is usually more sensitive than CT because of its **superior contrast** and **soft-tissue resolution.** It is, however, **less sensitive** to CT in detecting **calcification** in lesions or in evaluating **cortical bone**, which appear as signal voids with MR. It may be contraindicated in some patients with pacemakers.
- MRI is more difficult to interpret in part because the same structure or abnormality may appear differently on the same study, depending on the pulse sequence, the scan parameters, and the fact that MRI is more variable in its depiction of differences that occur over the **time course of some abnormalities** (e.g., hemorrhage) than is CT.
- **Initial evaluation of an MRI of the brain** might start with a T1-weighted sagittal sequence of the brain. On this sequence, the brain looks more like the anatomic specimens or diagrams that you are more accustomed to seeing

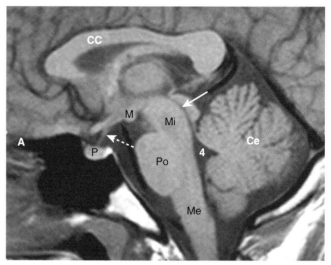

**Fig. 26.3 Normal Midline MRI.** Sagittal, T1-weighted, close-up image demonstrates the midline structures of the brain. For orientation purposes, anterior is to your left (A). The corpus callosum (CC) is located superiorly. The pituitary gland (P) sits in the sella turcica and connects to the hypothalamus via the pituitary stalk or infundibulum *(dashed arrow).* The mamillary bodies (M) are located anterior to the brainstem. The cerebral aqueduct *(solid arrow)* is superior to the midbrain. The brainstem is composed of the midbrain (Mi), the pons (Po), and the medulla (Me). The fourth ventricle (4) communicates with the cerebral aqueduct and lies between the cerebellum (Ce) and the brainstem.

(Fig. 26.3). Many structures in the brain are **paired**, so remember to compare one side with the other on axial scans of the brain (Fig. 26.4).

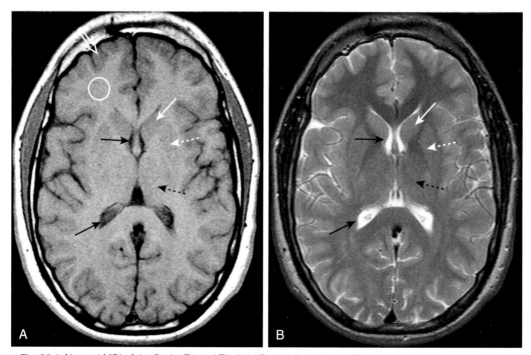

**Fig. 26.4 Normal MRI of the Brain, T1 and T2.** Axial T1-weighted (A) and T2-weighted (B) images of the brain demonstrate that CSF in the lateral ventricles is dark on T1 and bright on T2 *(solid black arrows).* Gray matter, which contains the neuronal cell bodies, is actually gray on T1-weighted images *(open white arrow),* and white matter, which contains myelinated axon tracts, is whiter *(circle).* The caudate nuclei *(solid white arrows)* and lentiform nucleus *(dashed white arrows)* together form the basal ganglia. The thalamus *(dashed black arrows)* is located posterior to the basal ganglia.

**TABLE 26.3   Signal Characteristics of Various Tissues Seen on T1-Weighted and T2-Weighted MRI Scans**

| Bright on T1 | Dark on T1 | Bright on T2 | Dark on T2 |
|---|---|---|---|
| Fat | Calcification | Water (edema, CSF) | Fat |
| Gadolinium | Air | | Calcification |
| High protein | Chronic hemorrhage | Hyperacute hemorrhage | Air |
| Subacute hemorrhage | Acute hemorrhage is isointense to hypointense on T1 | Late subacute hemorrhage | Early subacute hemorrhage |
| Melanin | Water (edema, CSF) | | Chronic hemorrhage |
| | | | Acute hemorrhage |
| | | | High protein |

- Table 26.3 summarizes the signal characteristics of various tissues seen on MRI.

# HEAD TRAUMA

- *Traumatic brain injuries* extract a huge cost to the patient and society, not only as a result of the acute injury but for the long-term disability they produce. In the United States, motor vehicle accidents account for nearly half of traumatic brain injuries.
- **Unenhanced CT is the study of choice in acute head trauma.** The primary goal in obtaining the scan is to determine whether there is a life-threatening, but treatable, lesion. One of the principle advances in the advent of CT scanning of the head was its ability to detect surgically amenable lesions in a timely fashion.
- **Initial CT evaluation of the brain** in the emergency setting focuses on whether there is (1) **mass effect** and (2) **blood.**

- To determine whether there is **mass effect,** look for a **displacement or compression** of key structures from their normal positions by analyzing the location and appearance of the **ventricles, basal cisterns,** and the **sulci.**
- **Blood** will usually be hyperattenuating (bright) and might collect in the **basal cisterns, Sylvian** and **interhemispheric fissures, ventricles, subdural** or **epidural spaces,** or in the **brain parenchyma (intracerebral).**

## Skull Fractures

- Skull fractures are usually produced by **direct impact** to the skull, and they most often occur at the point of impact. They are important primarily because their presence implies a **force substantial enough to cause intracranial injury.**
- In order to visualize skull fractures, you must view the CT scan using the *bone window* settings that optimize visualization of the osseous structures (Fig. 26.5).
- Skull fractures can be described as **linear, depressed, or basilar.**

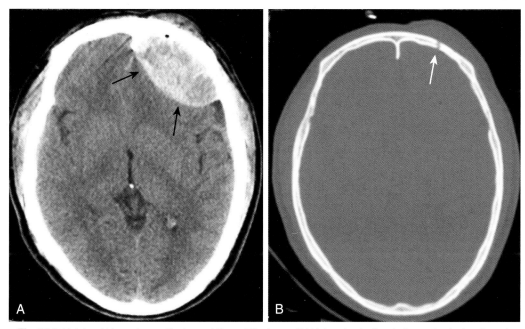

**Fig. 26.5 Epidural Hematoma, Brain and Bone Windows.** (A) Using the *brain window,* a lenticular-shaped, hyperintense lesion is seen in the left frontal region, displaying the typical appearance of an epidural hematoma *(arrows).* (B) In order to optimally visualize skull fractures, a head CT scan is best viewed using the *bone windows.* Viewing the same scan at the bone window setting demonstrates a linear skull fracture *(arrow)* of the left frontal bone at the site of the epidural hematoma.

## Linear Skull Fractures

- *Linear skull fractures* are the most common, and their primary importance lies in the intracranial abnormalities that may have occurred at the time of the fracture, such as an epidural hematoma. Fractures of the cranial vault most likely occur in the **temporal** and **parietal bones** (see Fig. 26.5B).

## Depressed Skull Fractures

- *Depressed skull fractures* are more likely to be associated with **underlying brain injury.** They result from a high-energy blow to a small area of the skull (e.g., from a hammer), most often in the **frontoparietal region,** and are **usually comminuted.** They may require **surgical elevation** of the depressed fragment when the fragment lies deeper than the inner table adjacent to the fracture (Fig. 26.6A).

## Basilar Skull Fractures

- *Basilar fractures* are the **most serious** and consist of a linear fracture at the base of the skull. They can be associated with tears in the dura mater with subsequent **CSF leak,** which can lead to CSF rhinorrhea and otorrhea. They can be suspected if there is air seen in the brain *(traumatic pneumocephalus),* **fluid in the mastoid air cells,** or an **air-fluid level** in the **sphenoid sinus** (Fig. 26.6B).

## Facial Fractures

- **CT is the imaging study of choice** for evaluating **facial fractures.** Multislice scanners allow for reconstruction of the images in the sagittal and coronal planes so the patient does not have to be repositioned in the scanner.
- The most common **orbital fracture** is the *blow-out fracture,* which is produced by a **direct impact on the orbit** (e.g., a ball strikes the eye). The impact causes a sudden increase in intraorbital pressure leading to a fracture of the **inferior orbital floor** (into the maxillary sinus) or the **medial wall of the orbit** (into the ethmoid sinus). Sometimes the **inferior rectus muscle** can be trapped in the fracture, leading to **restriction of upward gaze** and **diplopia** as presenting symptoms.

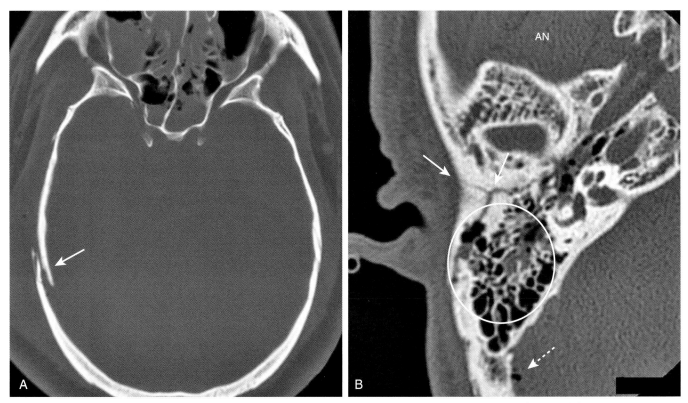

**Fig. 26.6 Skull Fractures.** (A) There is a depressed fracture of the right parietal bone with the fragment lying deeper than the inner table of the adjacent bone *(arrow).* Depressed skull fractures occur more often in the frontoparietal region. (B) A comminuted fracture of the right temporal bone *(solid arrows)* is seen, there is fluid in some of the mastoid air cells *(circle),* and there is air in the brain *(pneumocephalus) (dashed arrow).* Basilar skull fractures can be associated with tears in the dura mater with subsequent CSF leak *(AN, Anterior).*

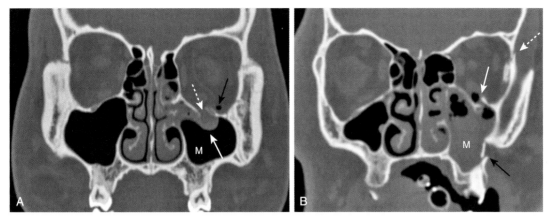

**Fig. 26.7** Facial Bone Fractures. (A) **Blow-out fracture**. Air is seen in the left orbit representing *orbital emphysema (black arrow)*. A fracture of the floor of the orbit *(dashed arrow)* is present and soft tissue (in this case, fat) extends inferiorly into the top of the maxillary sinus *(white arrow)*. (B) **Tripod fracture**. There is diastasis of the frontozygomatic suture on the left *(dashed white arrow)*, a fracture of the floor of the orbit with orbital emphysema *(solid white arrow)*, and a fracture *(black arrow)* through the lateral wall of the maxillary sinus, which is filled with blood. *M*, Maxillary sinus.

- **Recognizing a blow-out fracture of the orbit** (Fig. 26.7A).
  - *Orbital emphysema.* Air in the orbit from communication with one of the adjacent, air-containing sinuses, either the ethmoid or maxillary sinus.
  - **Fracture** through either the medial wall or floor of the orbit.
  - **Entrapment of fat and/or extraocular muscle** that projects downward as a soft-tissue mass into the top of the maxillary sinus.
  - **Fluid (blood)** in the maxillary sinus.
- A *tripod fracture,* usually a result of blunt force to the cheek, is another relatively common facial fracture. This fracture involves **separation of the zygoma** from the remainder of the facial bones through the combination of **separation of the frontozygomatic suture, fracture of the floor of the**

orbit, and fracture of the **lateral wall of the ipsilateral maxillary sinus** (Fig. 26.7B).

## INTRACRANIAL HEMORRHAGE

- Skull fractures may be accompanied by **intracranial hemorrhage** and/or **diffuse axonal injury.**
- There are **four types of intracranial hemorrhages** that can be **associated with head trauma** (Fig. 26.8):
  - *Epidural hematoma*
  - *Subdural hematoma*
  - *Intracerebral hemorrhage*
  - *Subarachnoid hemorrhage* (discussed with aneurysms)

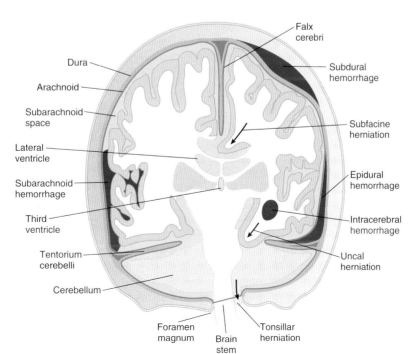

**Fig. 26.8** Hemorrhages and Herniations. This illustration is a coronal composite illustration showing the meninges, several types of intracranial hemorrhages, and several of the most common types of brain herniation.

### TABLE 26.4  The Meninges

| Layer | Comments |
|---|---|
| **Dura mater** | Composed of two layers, an **outer periosteal layer** that cannot be separated from the skull and an **inner meningeal layer;** the inner meningeal layer enfolds to form the tentorium and falx. |
| **Arachnoid** | The avascular middle layer is separated from the dura by a potential space known as the **subdural space.** |
| **Pia mater** | Closely applied to the brain and spinal cord, the pia mater carries blood vessels that supply both; separating the arachnoid from the pia is the **subarachnoid space;** together the **pia and arachnoid** are called the **leptomeninges.** |

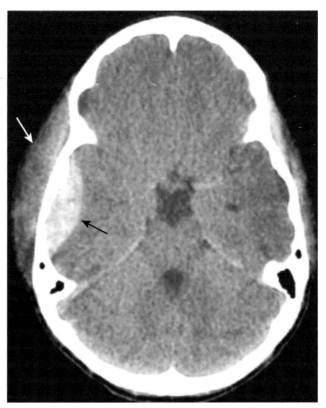

**Fig. 26.9 Epidural Hematoma.** Findings of an epidural hematoma include a high-density, extraaxial, biconvex, lens-shaped mass-like lesion often found in the temporal-parietal region of the brain *(black arrow).* There is a scalp hematoma also present *(white arrow).* The patient had a temporal bone skull fracture seen on bone windows.

## Epidural Hematoma (Extradural Hematoma)

- Epidural hematomas represent **hemorrhage** into the potential space **between the dura mater** and the **inner table of the skull** (Table 26.4).
- Most cases are due to injury to the **middle meningeal artery or vein** from blunt head trauma, typically from a motor vehicle accident.
- Almost all epidural hematomas (95%) have an associated skull fracture, frequently in the temporal bone. Epidural hematomas may also be caused by disruption of the dural venous sinuses adjacent to a skull fracture.
- Recognizing an epidural hematoma:
  - They appear as a **hyperintense, extraaxial, biconvex, lens-shaped density** most often found in the **temporoparietal region** of the brain (Fig. 26.9).
  - Because the dura is normally fused to the calvarium at the margins of the sutures, it is **impossible for an epidural hematoma to cross suture lines (subdural hematomas can cross sutures).**
    - Epidural hematomas can cross the tentorium, but subdural hematomas do not.

## Subdural Hematoma (SDH)

- *Subdural hematomas* are more common than epidural hematomas and are usually **not associated with a skull fracture.** They are most commonly a result of **deceleration injuries** in motor vehicle or motorcycle accidents (younger patients) **or secondary to falls** (older patients).
- Subdural hematomas are usually produced by **damage to the bridging veins** that cross from the cerebral cortex to the venous sinuses of the brain. SDH represents hemorrhage into the potential space **between the dura mater and the arachnoid.**

> ### ⟫ IMPORTANT POINTS
>
> - **Acute subdural hematomas** frequently herald the presence of more severe parenchymal brain injury as well as increased intracranial pressure and are associated with a **higher mortality rate.**

- Recognizing an acute subdural hematoma:
  - On CT, acute subdural hematomas are **crescent-shaped, extracerebral bands of high attenuation** that may **cross suture lines** and **enter the interhemispheric fissure.** They **do not cross the midline.**
  - Typically, an SDH is **concave inward** toward the brain (epidural hematomas are convex inward) (Fig. 26.10A).
  - As time passes and they become subacute, or if the subdural blood is mixed with lower attenuating CSF, they may appear *isoattenuating (isodense)* to the remainder of brain, in which case they may cause **compressed or absent sulci** or sulci **displaced away from the inner table** as signs of SDH (Fig. 26.10B).
  - Subdural collections may demonstrate a **fluid-fluid level** after 1 week, as the cells settle under serum.
- **Chronic subdural hematoma**
  - Chronic subdural hematomas are those present **more than 3 weeks after injury.**
  - Chronic subdural hematomas are usually **low density** compared with the remainder of the brain (Fig. 26.10C).

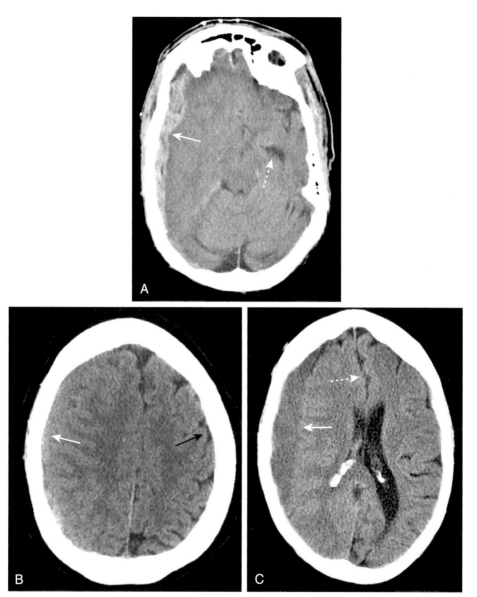

**Fig. 26.10 Acute, Isodense, and Chronic Subdural Hematomas.** (A) A crescent-shaped band of high-density blood concave inward toward the brain *(solid arrow)* represents the **acute** subdural collection of blood. There is associated mass effect with herniation of the brain as indicated by the dilated, contralateral temporal horn *(dashed arrow)*. (B) As they become **subacute,** subdural hematomas become less dense and may be the same density (isodense) as the normal brain tissue *(white arrow)*. At this stage, they can be recognized by the unilateral absence or displacement of the sulci away from the inner table of the skull compared to the normal opposite side *(black arrow)*. (C) **Chronic** subdural hematomas (more than 3 weeks old) are usually of low density *(solid arrow)* compared to the remainder of the brain. There is still mass effect demonstrated by displacement of the interhemispheric fissure *(dashed arrow)* and compression of the lateral ventricle.

## Intracerebral Hematoma (Intracerebral Hemorrhage)

- Trauma is only one of the mechanisms that can lead to intracerebral hemorrhage. Intracerebral hematomas can also occur from ruptures of **aneurysms, atheromatous disease in small vessels, vasculitis, vascular malformations (e.g., arteriovenous malformations, arteriovenous fistulae),** and **amyloid.** Venous thrombosis can also cause parenchymal hemorrhage.

- Injuries occurring at the **point of impact** (called *coup injuries)* and injuries occurring **opposite the point of impact** (called *contrecoup injuries*) are most common following trauma. **Coup** injuries are most often due to *shearing* of small intracerebral vessels. **Contrecoup** injuries are **acceleration/deceleration injuries** that occur when the brain is propelled in the opposite direction, striking the inner surface of the skull.

- Either of these mechanisms can produce a *cerebral contusion.*
  - **Hemorrhagic contusions** are hemorrhages with **associated edema** usually found in the **inferior frontal lobes and anterior temporal lobes on or near the surface of the brain.** Trauma can also produce **nonhemorrhagic** contusions as well.
- CT findings of intracerebral hemorrhage change over time and **may not be immediately evident on the initial scan.** MRI typically demonstrates the lesions, such as small contusions and subdural hematomas, from the time of injury, but may not be available on an emergency basis.
- **Recognizing traumatic intracerebral hemorrhage on CT:**
  - Hemorrhagic cerebral contusions may appear as multiple, small, well-demarcated areas of **high attenuation** within the brain parenchyma (Fig. 26.11A).
  - They may be surrounded by a **hypodense rim** from **edema** (Fig. 26.11B).
  - **Intraventricular blood** may be present (Fig. 26.12).
  - **Mass effect is common.** The mass effect may produce **compression** of the **ventricles** and **displacements of the third ventricle** and **septum pellucidum** to the **opposite** side.
    - These shifts or displacements of brain tissue from their normal location into an adjacent space are called *herniations.* Herniations may lead to brain damage, compression of cranial nerves and/or vessels producing hemorrhage or ischemia, or obstruction to the normal flow of cerebrospinal fluid, producing hydrocephalus.

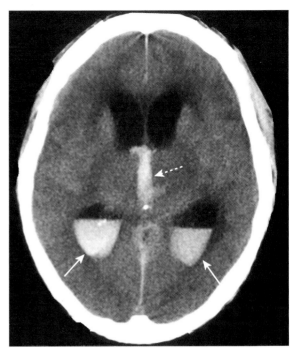

**Fig. 26.12 Intraventricular Hemorrhage.** Intraventricular hemorrhage in adults is frequently the result of breakthrough bleeding from a hypertensive basal ganglia hemorrhage, brain contusion, or subarachnoid hemorrhage. It is typically associated with severe brain damage, results in communicating hydrocephalus, and has a poor prognosis. In this unenhanced CT image, blood is seen in the 3rd ventricle *(dashed arrow)* and the occipital horns of the lateral ventricles *(solid arrows).*

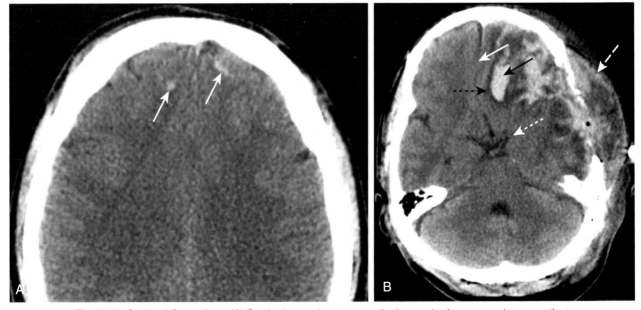

**Fig. 26.11 Cerebral Contusions.** (A) Cerebral contusions are usually the result of trauma and can manifest with multiple areas of high attenuation hemorrhage within the brain parenchyma on CT *(arrows).* (B) A contusion *(solid black arrow)* is frequently surrounded by a rim of hypoattenuation from edema *(dashed black arrow)* and mass effect is common, as is demonstrated here by amputation of the ipsilateral basilar cisterns *(dotted white arrow)* and midline displacement *(solid white arrow)* representing **subfalcine herniation.** A portion of the left side of the skull has been surgically removed and there is a large scalp hematoma present *(dashed white arrow).*

- Patients with sufficient mass effect are at risk for *transtentorial* and *subfalcine brain herniation* and death (see Fig. 26.10).
- **The types of brain herniation are described in** Table 26.5 (Fig. 26.13).

## DIFFUSE AXONAL INJURY

- Diffuse axonal injury is **responsible for the prolonged coma following head trauma** and is the head injury with the poorest prognosis.
- Acceleration/deceleration forces **diffusely injure axons deep to the cortex,** producing unconsciousness from the moment of injury. This occurs most often as a result of a motor vehicle accident.
- The **corpus callosum is most commonly affected,** and the initial CT scan may be normal or underestimate the degree of injury. CT findings may be similar to those described for intracerebral hemorrhage following head trauma.

| TABLE 26.5 | Common Types of Brain Herniation |
|---|---|
| **Type** | **Remarks** |
| **Subfalcine herniation (Fig. 26.13A)** | The supratentorial brain, along with the lateral ventricle and septum pellucidum, herniates beneath the falx and shifts across the midline toward the opposite side (Fig. 26.13A). This is the most common type of brain herniation. |
| **Transtentorial herniation (e.g., uncal herniation) (Fig. 26.13B)** | In the second most common type of herniation, the medial portion of the temporal lobe (uncus) is displaced downward through the tentorial notch compressing the ipsilateral temporal horn and causing dilatation of the contralateral temporal horn (see Fig. 26.10A). |
| **Tonsillar herniation (see Fig. 26.8)** | Infratentorial brain is displaced downward through the foramen magnum. |

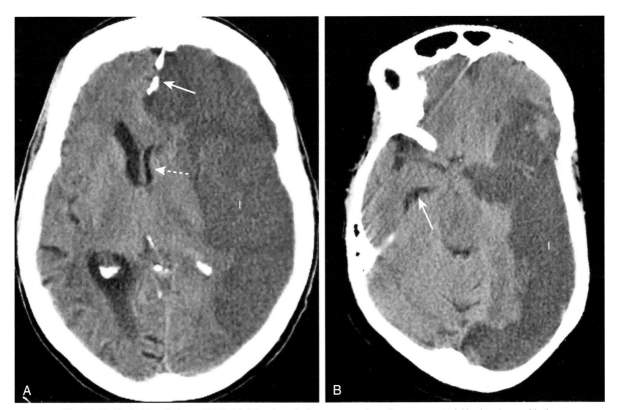

**Fig. 26.13** Brain Herniations. (A) **Subfalcine herniation** occurs when the supratentorial brain, along with the lateral ventricle and septum pellucidum, herniate beneath the falx *(solid arrow)* and shift across the midline toward the opposite side *(dashed arrow)*. (B) **Transtentorial herniation** usually occurs when the cerebral hemispheres are displaced downward through the incisura beneath the tentorium, compressing the ipsilateral temporal horn and causing dilatation of the contralateral temporal horn *(arrow)*. Both patients had large cerebral infarcts (I) with cytotoxic edema.

# INCREASED INTRACRANIAL PRESSURE

- Some of the clinical signs of **increased intracranial pressure** are **papilledema, headache,** and **diplopia.**
- In general, increased intracranial pressure is caused by either *cerebral edema,* which leads to increased **volume of the** brain, or *hydrocephalus,* which is **increased size of the ventricles.**

## Cerebral Edema

- In adults, **trauma, hypertension** (associated as it is with **intracerebral bleeds** and **stroke**), and **masses** are the most common causes of brain edema.
  - Cerebral edema is divided into **two major types: vasogenic** and **cytotoxic.**
    - *Vasogenic edema* represents extracellular accumulation of fluid and is the type that is associated with **malignancy** and **infection.** It is due to **abnormal permeability of the blood-brain barrier.** It predominantly affects the **white matter** (Fig. 26.15A).
    - *Cytotoxic edema* represents cellular edema and is associated with **cerebral ischemia.** It is due to **cell death.** It **affects both the gray and white matter** (Fig. 26.15B).

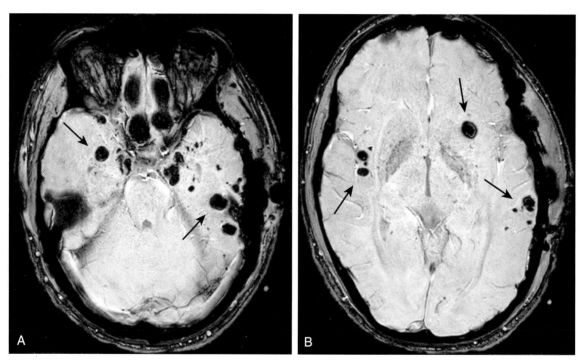

**Fig. 26.14 Diffuse Axonal Injury, MRI.** These images were obtained using a pulse sequence extremely sensitive to bleeding at the gray/white matter boundary, facilitating visualization of very small lesions. It is particularly helpful for evaluation of the small hemorrhages present in diffuse axonal injury (DAI) not routinely visible on CT or conventional MR imaging sequences. (A) and (B) are axial images demonstrating innumerable foci of abnormally decreased signal *(arrows)* in a patient with diffuse axonal injury.

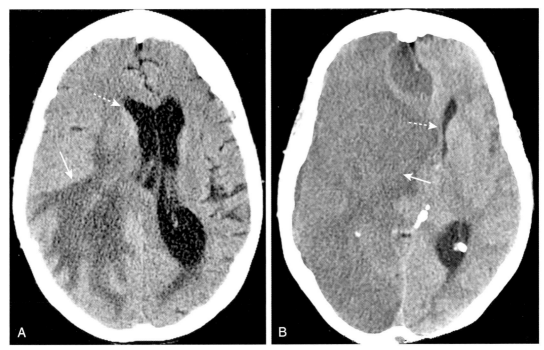

**Fig. 26.15 Vasogenic and Cytotoxic Edema.** In both of these patients, there is increased intracranial pressure as manifest by the herniation of brain to the contralateral side *(dashed arrows)*. (A) **Vasogenic edema** *(solid arrow)* is the type that occurs with infection and malignancy, as in this unenhanced scan of a patient with a glioma. It predominantly affects the white matter. (B) **Cytotoxic edema** *(solid arrow)* affects both the gray and white matter. Cytotoxic edema is associated with cerebral ischemia, as in this patient with a very large ischemic infarct on the right.

- **Recognizing cerebral edema:**
  - There is a **loss** of the **normal differentiation between gray and white matter** in cytotoxic edema, whereas it is retained in vasogenic edema (see Fig. 26.15).
  - There may be **effacement** (compression or obliteration) of the normal **sulci.**
  - The **ventricles** may be **compressed** (Fig. 26.16).
  - **Herniation** of the brain may manifest, in part, by **effacement of the basal cisterns** (see Fig. 26.11B).
- Increased intracranial pressure secondary to an increase in the size of the ventricles is discussed later in this chapter under Hydrocephalus.

# STROKE

## General Considerations

- Stroke is a nonspecific term that usually denotes an **acute loss of neurologic function** that occurs when the blood supply to an area of the brain is lost or compromised.
- The diagnosis of stroke is usually made clinically. Patients with suspected stroke are imaged to (1) determine if there is **another cause of the neurologic impairment** besides a stroke (e.g., a brain tumor); (2) **identify the presence of blood** so as to distinguish **ischemic** from **hemorrhagic** stroke, which may determine what additional therapy will be instituted; and (3) **identify** the **cerebral infarct** and **characterize it.**
- **Most strokes are** *embolic* **in origin**, the emboli often arising from the **internal carotid artery** or the common

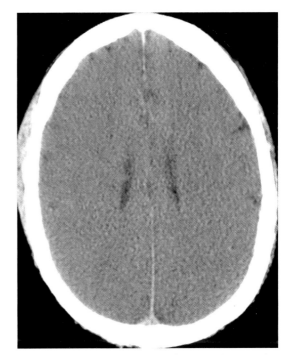

**Fig. 26.16 Diffuse Cerebral Edema, CT.** Cerebral edema produces loss of normal differentiation between gray and white matter, effacement (narrowing or obliteration) of the normal sulci, and ventricular compression, all of which are present in this patient with anoxic encephalopathy.

carotid bifurcation. Emboli can also arise in the heart and aortic arch.

- The other common cause of stroke is ***thrombosis,*** representing *in situ* **occlusion** of the carotid, vertebrobasilar, or intracerebral circulations from **atheromatous lesions.** Thrombosis of the **middle cerebral artery** is particularly common.

> ▶▶ **IMPORTANT POINTS**
>
> - Strokes are divided into two large groups: ***ischemic*** or ***hemorrhagic.*** **Ischemic** strokes are much **more common.** The classification is important because rapid reperfusion of ischemic stroke with ***recombinant tissue plasminogen activator (rt-PA)*** in the first 4 hours after onset and/or **mechanical thrombectomy** within 24 hours may substantially improve the prognosis. Not all patients may qualify for a mechanical thrombectomy due to the location of the occlusion or the availability of the procedure.

- Most **acute strokes** are **initially imaged** by obtaining a **noncontrast CT scan of the brain** (within 24 hours of the onset of symptoms), mostly because of its availability and its significant ability to show acute hemorrhage that might affect therapeutic choices.
- CT findings may be present immediately after a hemorrhagic stroke and within hours after the onset of symptoms from ischemic stroke.
- MRI has become more widely used for early diagnosis. **Diffusion-weighted MRI** is more sensitive and relatively specific for detecting early infarction with the capacity to detect changes within 20 to 30 minutes of the onset of the event (Fig. 26.17).

- On MRI, the temporal staging of hemorrhage can be conducted based on chemical changes that occur in the hemoglobin molecule as the hemorrhage evolves.

## Ischemic Stroke

- **Thromboembolic disease** as a consequence of **atherosclerosis** is the **most common cause of an ischemic stroke.** The source of the emboli can be from atheromatous debris, arterial stenosis and occlusion, or from emboli arising from the left side of the heart (e.g., atrial fibrillation).

> ▶▶ **IMPORTANT POINTS**
>
> - ***Vascular watershed*** areas are the distal arterial territories that represent the **junctions between areas served by the major intracerebral vessels,** such as the region between the anterior cerebral artery distribution and the middle cerebral artery distribution. **Reduction in blood flow,** whatever its cause, **affects these sensitive and susceptible watershed areas the most.**

- The most common finding of an acute, nonhemorrhagic stroke is a normal CT scan (<24 hours old). If multiple vascular distributions are involved, emboli or **vasculitis** should be thought of as the cause. If the **stroke crosses or falls between vascular territories,** then hypoperfusion owing to hypotension *(watershed infarcts)* should be considered.

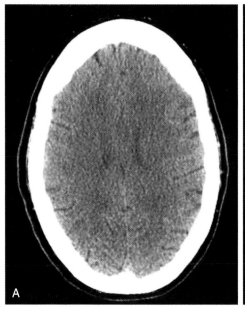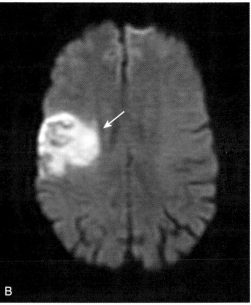

**Fig. 26.17 CT and Diffusion-weighted MRI in Acute Stroke.** (A) The CT scan in this patient with stroke symptoms for 2 hours prior to the study is normal. (B) A diffusion-weighted MRI scan on the same patient a few minutes later shows an area of abnormally bright signal intensity in the right frontoparietal region *(arrow)*. Diffusion-weighted imaging (DWI) is an MRI sequence that can be rapidly acquired and that is extremely sensitive to detecting abnormalities in normal water movement in the brain so that it can identify a stroke within 20 to 30 minutes after the event.

## TABLE 26.6   Vascular Distribution Territories of Stroke

| Circulation | Anatomy Affected | Signs and Symptoms |
|---|---|---|
| **Anterior cerebral artery (uncommon)** | Supplies all of the frontal and parietal lobes (medial surfaces), the anterior four-fifths of the corpus callosum, the frontobasal cerebral cortex, and the anterior diencephalon. | Can result in disinhibition with perseveration of speech; produces primitive reflexes (e.g., grasping or sucking), altered mental status, impaired judgment, contralateral weakness (greater in legs than arms). |
| **Middle cerebral artery (common)** | Supplies almost the entire convex surface of the brain, including the frontal, parietal, and temporal lobes (laterally), insula, claustrum, and extreme capsule. Lenticulostriate branches supply the basal ganglia, including the head of the caudate nucleus, and the putamen, including the lateral parts of the internal and external capsules. | Produces contralateral hemiparesis or hypesthesia, ipsilateral hemianopsia, and gaze preference toward the side of the lesion; agnosia is common; receptive or expressive aphasia may result if the lesion occurs in the dominant hemisphere; weakness of the arm and face is usually worse than that of a lower limb. |
| **Posterior cerebral artery** | Supplies portions of the midbrain, subthalamic nucleus, basal nucleus, thalamus, mesial inferior temporal lobe, and occipital and occipitoparietal cortices. | Occlusions affect vision, producing contralateral homonymous hemianopsia, cortical blindness, visual agnosia, altered mental status, and impaired memory. |
| **Vertebrobasilar system** | Perfuses the medulla, cerebellum, pons, midbrain, thalamus, and occipital cortex. | Occlusion of large vessels in this system usually leads to major disability or death; small lesions usually have a benign prognosis; may cause a wide variety of cranial nerve, cerebellar, and brainstem deficits; a hallmark of posterior circulation stroke is crossed findings: i.e., ipsilateral cranial nerve deficits and contralateral motor deficits (in contrast to an anterior circulation stroke). |

- Table 26.6 briefly summarizes the four major vascular distribution patterns of strokes and some of the symptoms associated with each.
- **Recognizing ischemic stroke:**
  - On CT the findings of an ischemic stroke will depend on the amount of time that has elapsed since the original event.
  - **12 to 24 hours:** Indistinct area of low attenuation in a vascular distribution.

- **>24 hours:** Better circumscribed lesion with mass effect that peaks at 3 to 5 days and usually disappears by 2 to 4 weeks (Fig. 26.18A).
- **72 hours:** Although contrast is rarely used in the initial setting of acute stroke, contrast enhancement typically occurs when the mass effect is waning or has disappeared.
- **>4 weeks:** Mass effect disappears; there is now a well-circumscribed low attenuation lesion with no contrast enhancement (Fig. 26.18B).

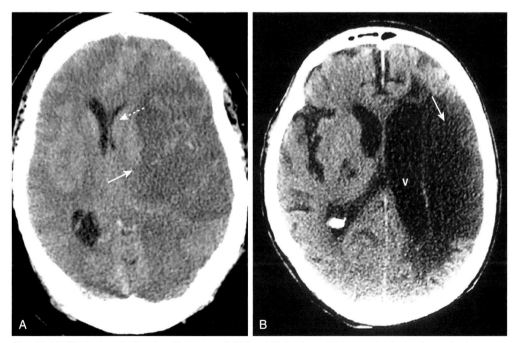

**Fig. 26.18** CT, Ischemic Stroke, Newer and Older. (A) At about 24 hours, the ischemic stroke becomes relatively well-circumscribed *(solid arrow)* with mass effect evidenced by a shift of the ventricles *(dashed arrow)* that will peak at 3 to 5 days and disappear by about 2 to 4 weeks. (B) As the stroke matures, it loses its mass effect, tends to become an even more sharply marginated low-attenuation lesion *(arrow)*, and may be associated with enlargement of the adjacent ventricle *(V)* due to loss of brain substance in the infarcted area.

- *Lacunar strokes* are a type of ischemic stroke that are small and located in noncortical areas (Box 26.1, Fig. 26.19).

---

### BOX 26.1   Lacunar Infarcts

- Small ischemic cerebral infarcts produced by occlusion of small end arteries account for up to 20% of all cerebral infarctions.
- They have a predilection for the basal ganglia, internal capsule, and pons and occur in association with hypertension, atherosclerosis, and diabetes.
- The term **lacunar infarct (lacune)** is reserved for low-density cystic lesions, about 5 to 15 mm in size (Fig. 26.19).

---

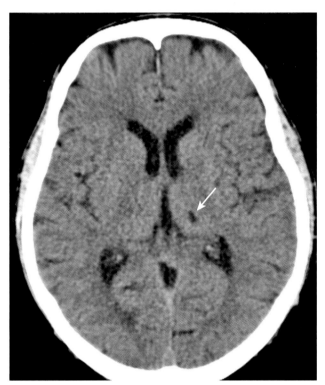

**Fig. 26.19 Lacunar Infarct.** A lacunar infarct, or **lacune**, is a small cerebral infarct produced by occlusion of an end artery. The term **chronic lacunar infarct** is reserved for low-density, cystic lesions, 5 to 15 mm in size *(arrow)*.

## Hemorrhagic Stroke

- Hemorrhage **occurs in about 15%** of strokes. Hemorrhage is **associated with a higher morbidity and mortality** than ischemic stroke. Hemorrhage from stroke can occur into the brain parenchyma or the subarachnoid space.
- In the majority of cases, there has been preceding **hypertension. About 60% of hypertensive hemorrhages occur in the basal ganglia.** Other areas commonly involved are the thalamus, pons, and cerebellum (Fig. 26.20).
- The decision to utilize **thrombolytic** or another **intraarterial recanalization therapy** has been based on algorithms formulated by the initial nonenhanced CT scan findings. The **more rapidly treatment is initiated** (usually <4 to 5 hours after the onset of symptoms), the **greater its potential benefit.**
- **Recognizing intracerebral hemorrhage (in general):**
  - Freshly extravasated whole blood in people with a normal hematocrit will be visible as **increased density** on

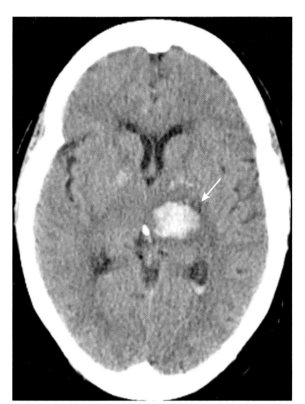

**Fig. 26.20 Intracerebral Hemorrhage, Acute.** Freshly extravasated whole blood, such as this bleed into the thalamus *(arrow)*, will be visible as increased density on nonenhanced CT scans of the brain due primarily to the protein in the blood (mostly hemoglobin). The clot will usually become invisible over the next several weeks.

nonenhanced CT scans of the brain immediately after the event (see Fig. 26.20). This is due to the protein in the blood (mostly hemoglobin).
- **Dissection** of blood into the **ventricular system** can occur in hypertensive intracerebral bleeds and has a poorer prognosis (see Fig. 26.12).
- As the clot begins to form, the **blood becomes denser for about 3 days** because of dehydration of the clot.
- **After the third day**, the **clot decreases in density** and becomes invisible over the next several weeks. The clot loses density from the **outside in** so that it appears to **shrink.**
- **After about 2 months, only a small hypodensity may remain.**
- On MRI the changes in the appearance of hemorrhage over time are more dramatic. MRI is sensitive to changing effects in both the **iron** and **protein** portions of the **hemoglobin molecule** in the days and weeks following an acute bleed. Table 26.7 summarizes those changes.

---

### TABLE 26.7   Changes in the Appearance of Blood Over Time on MRI

| Phase | Time | T1 | T2 |
| --- | --- | --- | --- |
| **Hyperacute** | <24 hours | Isointense | Bright |
| **Acute** | 1–3 days | Isointense | Dark |
| **Early subacute** | 3–7 days | Bright | Dark |
| **Late subacute** | 7–14 days | Bright | Bright |

# RUPTURED ANEURYSMS

- The most frequent central nervous system aneurysm is the *berry aneurysm,* which develops from a **congenital weakening in the arterial wall**, usually at the sites of vessel branching in the **Circle of Willis** at the base of the brain. They can be familial (about 10% of cases) or associated with connective tissue diseases. They are called berry aneurysms because of their shape.
- **Hypertension** and **aging** play a role in the growth of aneurysms. **Larger aneurysms bleed more frequently** than do smaller ones.
- The aim is to discover and treat the aneurysm **before** it has undergone a major bleed. In some studies, **10 mm was found to be the critical size for rupture.**
- The classic history a patient who has had a ruptured aneurysm describes is "the worst headache of my life."
- When aneurysms rupture, the **blood usually enters the subarachnoid space.** Rupture of an aneurysm is the **most common nontraumatic cause of a subarachnoid hemorrhage** (80%) but not the only cause. Arteriovenous malformations, breakthrough of an intraparenchymal bleed, or amyloid angiopathy (Box 26.2) can also produce subarachnoid hemorrhage.
- Today most aneurysms are detected by **either CT angiography (CTA) or MR angiography (MRA).** Computerized

postprocessing of the imaging can generate 3D reconstructions.

- **CT angiography** is performed using a power injector to deliver a rapid bolus intravenous injection of iodinated contrast, a CT scanner capable of rapid acquisition of data, and special computer algorithms and postprocessing techniques that can highlight the vessels and, if desired, display them in three dimensions (Fig. 26.21).
- **Magnetic resonance angiography (MRA)** is routinely done without contrast, using a time-of-flight technique. This technique displays flowing blood within the arteries as white.

---

## BOX 26.2  Amyloid Angiopathy

- **Cerebral amyloid-β** is a proteinaceous material that can be deposited with increasing age in the media and adventitia of small- and medium-sized intracranial vessels, mostly involving the frontal and parietal lobes.
- This deposit produces a loss of elasticity of the vessels and increases their fragility.
- Amyloid angiopathy plaques may be visible on a special MR gradient sequence. They are too small to see on routine CT or most MR sequences.
- Hemorrhages from amyloid angiopathy are usually large, involving an entire lobe; they may be multiple and occur in several areas simultaneously. They can also present as subarachnoid hemorrhage.

---

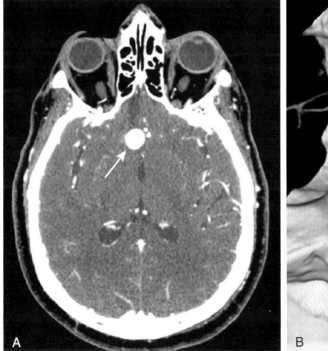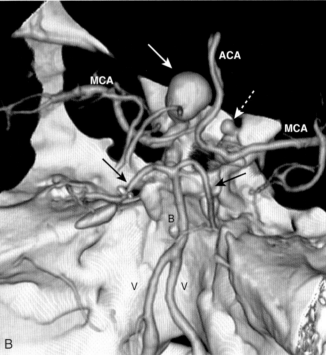

**Fig. 26.21 Berry Aneurysm, Axial CT and 3D Reconstruction.** (A) There is a 2 cm focal collection of contrast *(arrow)* consistent with an aneurysm in the region of the right internal carotid artery (ICA) on this contrast-enhanced CT of the brain. (B) A 3D reconstruction of the Circle of Willis from a CT angiogram demonstrates the aneurysm *(solid white arrow)* arising from the supraclinoid segment of the right ICA and another smaller aneurysm *(dashed white arrow)* arising from the supraclinoid segment of the left ICA. *ACA,* Anterior cerebral arteries; *B,* basilar artery; *MCA,* middle cerebral arteries; *V,* vertebral arteries. *Black arrows* point to posterior cerebral arteries.

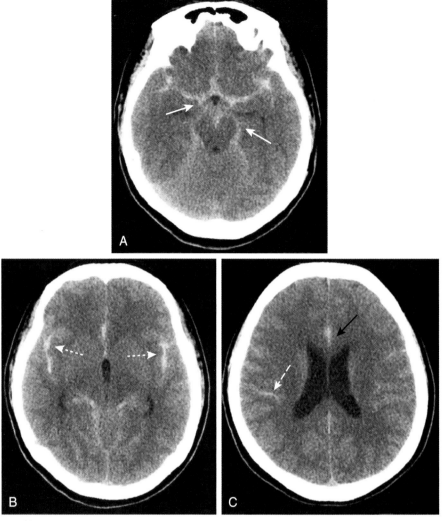

**Fig. 26.22** Subarachnoid Hemorrhage, Unenhanced CT Scans. (A) Subarachnoid blood is most easily visualized within the basal cisterns *(arrows)*, (B) in the fissures *(arrows)*, and (C) interdigitated in the subarachnoid spaces of the sulci *(white arrow)*. The region of the falx may become hyperdense, widened, and irregularly marginated *(black arrow)*.

- **Recognizing a subarachnoid hemorrhage (from a ruptured aneurysm):**
  - On **CT, acute blood** is **hyperdense** and may be visualized **within the sulci and basal cisterns** (Fig. 26.22A and B).
  - The region of the **falx may become hyperdens**e, widened, and irregularly marginated (Fig. 26.22C).
  - Generally the **greatest concentration of blood indicates the most likely location of the ruptured aneurysm.**

## HYDROCEPHALUS

- *Hydrocephalus* is defined as an expansion of the ventricular system on the basis of an increase in the volume of CSF contained within it (Box 26.3).
- Follow-up studies to evaluate the status of hydrocephalus are usually conducted with CT scans, although MRI may be preferred for pediatric patients.
- Hydrocephalus may be caused by several factors:
  - Underabsorption of CSF (**communicating hydrocephalus**)
  - Restriction of the outflow of CSF from the ventricles (**noncommunicating hydrocephalus**)

---

**BOX 26.3  Normal Flow of Cerebrospinal Fluid**

- Most cerebrospinal fluid is produced by the choroid plexuses in the ventricles, primarily the lateral and fourth ventricles.
- The direction of flow is from the lateral ventricles through the Foramina of Monro to the third ventricle, then through the Aqueduct of Sylvius to the fourth ventricle, and then into the basilar subarachnoid cisterns through the two lateral Foramina of Luschka and the medial Foramen of Magendie.
- CSF can then take one of two paths. It can pass upward over the convexities of the brain to be reabsorbed into the bloodstream at the arachnoid villi.
- Or, CSF can also pass inferiorly down the spinal subarachnoid space where it is either reabsorbed directly or ascends back to the brain to the arachnoid villi.

---

- Overproduction of cerebrospinal fluid (rare)
- With hydrocephalus, the **ventricles** are usually **disproportionately dilated** compared to the **sulci**, whereas **both the ventricles and sulci** are **proportionately enlarged** in *cerebral atrophy.*
- The **temporal horns are particularly sensitive** to increases in CSF pressure. In the absence of hydrocephalus, the **temporal**

**horns are barely visible.** With **hydrocephalus** the temporal horns may be greater than 2 mm in size (Fig. 26.23).

## Obstructive Hydrocephalus

- Obstructive hydrocephalus is divided into two major categories: **communicating (extraventricular obstruction)** and **noncommunicating (intraventricular obstruction).**

- *Communicating hydrocephalus* is due to abnormalities that **inhibit the resorption of CSF,** most often at the level of the arachnoid villi (Fig. 26.24).
  - **CSF flow** through the **ventricles** and **over the convexities** normally occurs **unimpeded.** Reabsorption of CSF through the arachnoid villi can become restricted by such things as **subarachnoid hemorrhage** or **meningitis.**

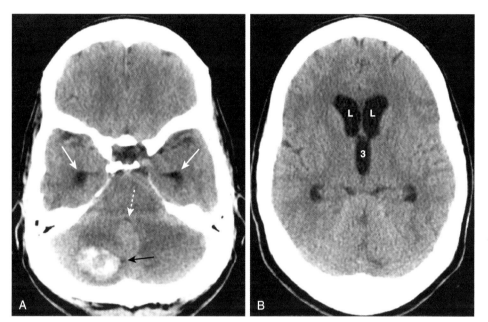

**Fig. 26.23 Noncommunicating Hydrocephalus.** (A) There is dilatation of the temporal horns *(solid white arrows)*, and the 4th ventricle is compressed and nearly invisible *(dashed white arrow)*. There is a hemorrhagic metastatic lesion *(black arrow)* that is obstructing the 4th ventricle. (B) The frontal horns of the lateral ventricles (L) and 3rd ventricle (3) are dilated, but note that the sulci are not dilated. This form of hydrocephalus is the result of obstruction to the outflow of cerebrospinal fluid from the ventricles.

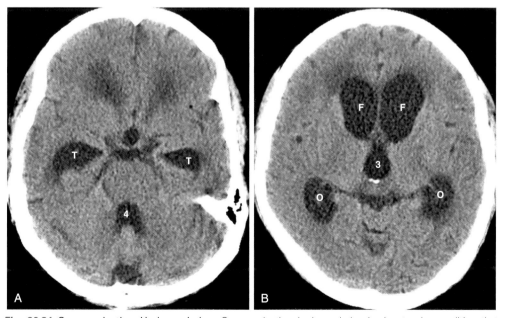

**Fig. 26.24 Communicating Hydrocephalus.** Communicating hydrocephalus is due to abnormalities that inhibit the resorption of cerebrospinal fluid, most often at the level of the arachnoid villi. (A) Classically, the 4th ventricle (4) is dilated (as it is here) in communicating hydrocephalus but normal in size in noncommunicating hydrocephalus. The temporal horns (T) are particularly sensitive to increases in intraventricular volume or pressure and are dilated. (B) The frontal horns (F), occipital horns (O), and third ventricle (3) are markedly dilated. There is a disproportionate dilatation of the ventricles compared to the sulci, which are normal to small here. Communicating hydrocephalus is usually treated with a ventricular shunt.

## ▶ IMPORTANT POINTS

- Classically the fourth ventricle is **dilated** in **communicating hydrocephalus** and **normal** in size in **noncommunicating** hydrocephalus.

- Communicating hydrocephalus is **usually treated with a ventricular shunt.**
- *Noncommunicating hydrocephalus* occurs as a result of **tumors, cysts,** or other physically obstructing lesions that **do not allow CSF to exit from the ventricles.**
  - Congenital hydrocephalus is often produced by a blockage between the third and fourth ventricles at the level of the **Aqueduct of Sylvius (aqueductal obstruction).**
  - When the obstruction is caused by a tumor or a cyst, noncommunicating hydrocephalus is **usually treated by surgically** removing the obstructing lesion (Fig. 26.25).

- **Nonobstructive hydrocephalus** from overproduction of CSF is rare and can occur with a *choroid plexus papilloma.*

## Normal-Pressure Hydrocephalus (NPH)

- *Normal-pressure hydrocephalus* is a form of **communicating hydrocephalus** characterized by a classical **triad of clinical symptoms,** including **abnormalities of gait, dementia,** and **urinary incontinence.** The age of onset is typically between 60 and 70 years old.
- Its recognition is important because it is usually amenable to treatment using a one-way **ventriculoperitoneal shunt** that allows the CSF to exit the ventricles and drain into the peritoneal cavity where the CSF is reabsorbed.
- Imaging findings are similar to other forms of communicating hydrocephalus and include **enlarged ventricles,**

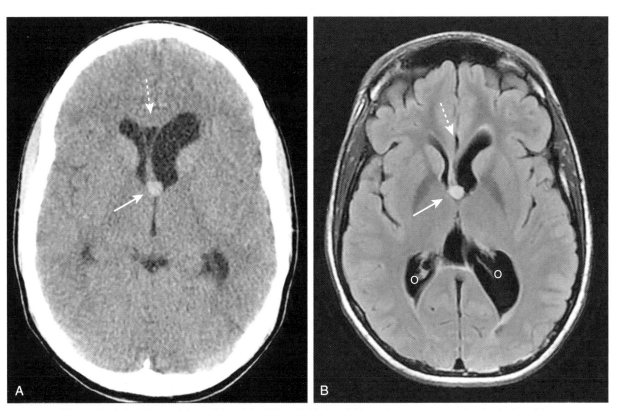

**Fig. 26.25 Colloid Cyst of the 3rd Ventricle, CT and MRI.** A colloid cyst is an uncommon, benign lesion of the 3rd ventricle that can cause obstructive hydrocephalus. (A) There is a hyperdense mass in the anterior aspect of the third ventricle *(solid arrow)* causing asymmetric obstruction of the left foramen of Monro compared to the right *(dashed arrow).* (B) On this MRI T2 FLAIR sequence, the lesion has increased signal *(solid arrow)* and is causing dilatation of the left frontal *(dashed arrow)* and occipital (O) horns of the lateral ventricle.

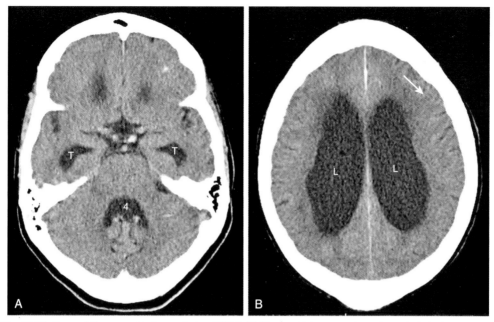

**Fig. 26.26 Normal-Pressure Hydrocephalus (NPH).** (A) The ventricles are enlarged, particularly the temporal horns (T) as well as the 4th ventricle (4). (B) The bodies of the lateral ventricles (L) are also markedly enlarged but the sulci are normal or flattened *(arrow)*. The patient had gait disturbances.

particularly the temporal horns, with **normal or flattened sulci** (Fig. 26.26).

## CEREBRAL ATROPHY

- Disorders associated with **gross cerebral atrophy** are also associated with **dementia, Alzheimer's disease** being one of the most common. Atrophy implies a loss of both gray and white matter.

- A major finding in patients with Alzheimer's disease (though not specific) is **diffuse cortical atrophy**, especially in the **temporal lobes.**
- As in hydrocephalus, the **ventricles dilate** in cerebral atrophy, but do so because a loss of normal cerebral tissue produces a vacant space that is filled passively with CSF. **Unlike hydrocephalus,** the **dynamics of CSF** production and absorption are **normal** in **cerebral atrophy.**
- In general, cerebral atrophy leads to **proportionate enlargement** of both the **ventricles** and the **sulci** (Fig. 26.27).

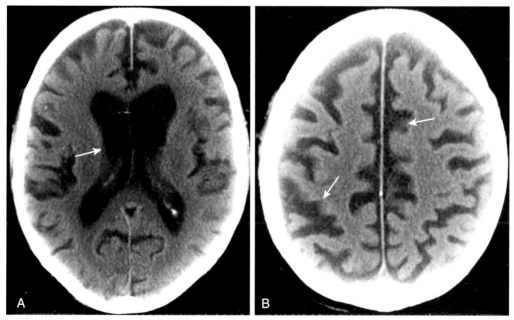

**Fig. 26.27 Diffuse Cortical Atrophy.** Disorders that cause gross cerebral atrophy are also associated with dementia, Alzheimer's disease being one of the most common. (A) The lateral ventricles *(arrow)* are enlarged. (B) Unlike hydrocephalus, the sulci are also enlarged *(arrows)*.

# BRAIN TUMORS

## Gliomas of the Brain

- *Gliomas* are a **common, primary supratentorial intraaxial mass in an adult.** They account for **30% of all brain tumors** and 80% of all malignant **primary** brain tumors (**metastases** to the brain from other organs are the most common **malignant** tumors in the brain **overall**).
- *Glioblastoma multiforme* accounts for more than half of all gliomas, astrocytomas for about 20%, and the remainder split between **ependymoma, oligodendroglioma, and mixed glioma** (e.g., oligoastrocytoma).
- Glioblastoma multiforme occurs **more commonly in males** between 65 and 75 years of age, especially in the **frontal and temporal lobes.** It has the **worst prognosis** of all gliomas. Today, **tumor biomarkers** play an important role in aiding **diagnosis,** suggesting **prognosis** including the likelihood of recurrence, and for their **predictive value** suggesting whether the disease is likely to respond to new drugs.
  - The tumor **infiltrates** adjacent areas of the brain along **white matter tracts** making it difficult to resect but, like most brain tumors, it **does not produce extracerebral metastases.**

- Recognizing **glioblastoma multiforme:**
  - Because of its aggressive growth, glioblastoma multiforme frequently demonstrates **necrosis** within the tumor.
  - The tumor **infiltrates** the surrounding brain tissue, frequently **crossing** the white matter tracts of the **corpus callosum** to the **opposite** cerebral hemisphere, producing a pattern called a *butterfly glioma.*
  - It tends to produce considerable **vasogenic edema** and **mass effect** and **enhances with contrast,** at least in part (Fig. 26.28).

## Metastases

- About **40% of all intracranial neoplasms** are metastases. **Lung, breast, and melanoma** are the most common primary malignancies to produce brain metastases.
- **Recognizing metastases to the brain:**
  - Metastases to the brain are frequently **well-defined, round masses near the gray-white junction.**
  - They are **usually multiple but can be solitary.**
  - They are **typically hypodense or isodense on nonenhanced CT.**

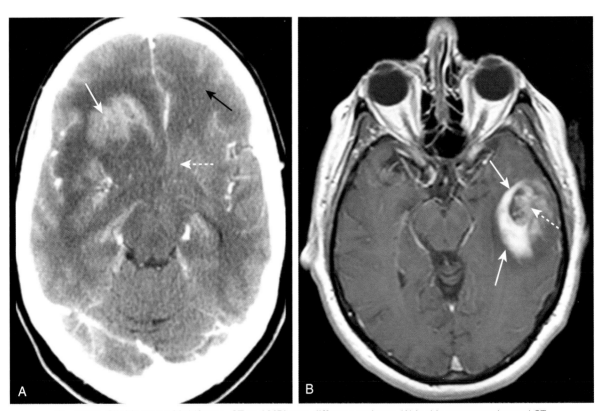

**Fig. 26.28** Glioblastoma Multiforme, CT and MRI, two different patients. (A) In this contrast-enhanced CT, the tumor enhances *(solid white arrow)*, produces considerable vasogenic edema *(dashed white arrow)*, and infiltrates the surrounding brain tissue. There is either edema or tumor that has crossed-over to the left frontal lobe *(black arrow)*. (B) Axial, T1-weighted, postgadolinium image in another patient demonstrates an enhancing mass in the left temporal lobe *(solid arrows)*. The internal enhancement of the mass is somewhat heterogeneous *(dashed arrow)*, which implies intratumoral necrosis or cystic change.

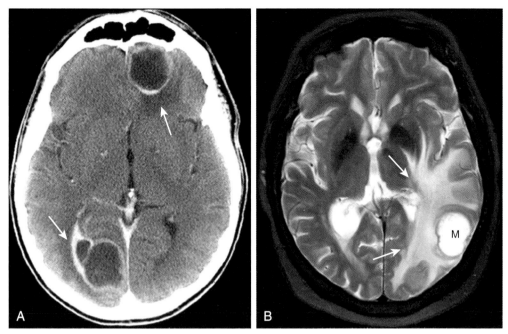

**Fig. 26.29 Metastases, Contrast-enhanced CT and MRI.** (A) With intravenous contrast, metastases can enhance as solid masses or show ring-like enhancement *(arrows)*. Lung, breast, and melanoma are the most common primary malignancies to produce brain metastases. (B) In another patient, MRI shows the characteristic pattern of vasogenic edema *(arrows)* surrounding a large, metastatic lesion (M). Both patients had lung cancer.

- With intravenous contrast, they can **enhance,** sometimes with a pattern of **ring-enhancement** (Fig. 26.29A).
- Most evoke some **vasogenic edema,** frequently disproportionately large compared to the size of the mass (Fig. 26.29B).

## Meningioma

- *Meningiomas* are **the most common primary brain tumor (benign and malignant) and the most common extraaxial mass.** They most commonly occur in middle-aged women. Their most frequent locations are **parasagittal,** over the **convexities,** the **sphenoid wing,** and the **cerebellopontine angle** cistern, in decreasing frequency.
- They tend to be **slow-growing** with an **excellent prognosis** if surgically excised.
- When **multiple,** they may have an association with *neurofibromatosis type 2.*
- Recognizing a meningioma on CT scan of the brain:
  - On **unenhanced CT,** over half of meningiomas are **hyperdense** to normal brain and about **20% contain calcification** (Fig. 26.30).
  - On contrast-enhanced studies, **meningiomas enhance markedly.**
  - They **may induce vasogenic edema in the adjacent brain parenchyma.**

## Vestibular Schwannoma (Acoustic Neuroma)

- *Vestibular schwannomas* are the most common schwannomas of all of the cranial nerves. Their most frequent symptom is **hearing loss,** but they also produce **tinnitus** and disturbances in **equilibrium.**

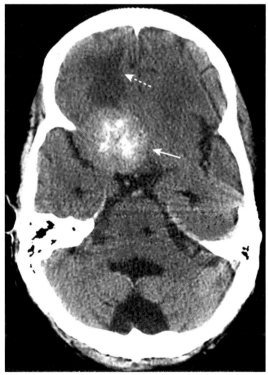

**Fig. 26.30 Meningioma, Unenhanced CT.** This meningioma *(solid arrow)* is arising from the right sphenoid wing, a relatively common site of origin. On unenhanced CT, over half are hyperdense to normal brain and about 20% contain calcification, as does this lesion. There is vasogenic edema associated with the mass *(dashed arrow).*

- They usually occur along the **course of the eighth cranial nerve** within the **internal auditory canal** at the **cerebellopontine angle** (Fig. 26.31).
- Like meningiomas, when they are multiple (i.e., **bilateral**) they are usually associated with **neurofibromatosis type 2.**

- **Contrast-enhanced MRI** is the **most sensitive** imaging study for detecting vestibular schwannomas that virtually **always enhance**, usually **homogeneously.**

## OTHER DISEASES

### Multiple Sclerosis (MS)

- *Multiple sclerosis* is considered to be **autoimmune** in origin and is the **most common demyelinating disease.** Any neurologic function can be affected by the disease, with some patients having mostly cognitive changes, whereas others present with ataxia, paresis, or visual symptoms.
- Characterized by a **relapsing and remitting course**, there are specific clinical criteria that must be met to establish this diagnosis, but imaging by MRI along with ancillary tests now permit the diagnosis to be made after a single clinical episode.
- MS characteristically affects **myelinated (white matter) tracts** with lesions known as *plaques.* Lesions of MS have a predilection for the **periventricular area, corpus callosum,** and **optic nerves.**

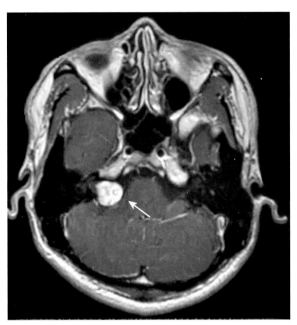

**Fig. 26.31** Vestibular Schwannoma, T1-weighted MRI with contrast. There is a homogeneously enhancing soft-tissue mass at the right cerebellopontine angle *(arrow)*, classical for a vestibular schwannoma. These tumors occur most commonly along the course of the 8th nerve. Hearing loss is the most common presenting symptom.

> ## ⟫ IMPORTANT POINTS
>
> - **MRI is the study of choice** in imaging MS because of its greater sensitivity than CT in demonstrating plaques, both in the brain and in the spinal cord.
>   - The lesions produce **discrete globular foci of high-signal intensity (brighter) on T2-weighted images.**
>   - On T1-weighted nonenhanced images, they are isointense to hypointense, but in **acute MS, the lesions enhance with gadolinium on T1-weighted images.**
>   - The lesions tend to be oriented with their long axes perpendicular to the ventricular walls (Fig. 26.32).

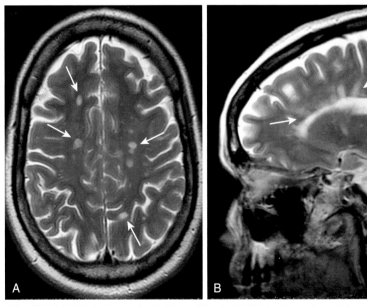

**Fig. 26.32** Multiple Sclerosis, Axial and Sagittal MRI. Lesions of multiple sclerosis have a predilection for the periventricular area, corpus callosum, and optic nerves. (A) The lesions produce discrete, globular foci of high-signal intensity *(arrows)* on T2-weighted images. (B) Ovoid lesions seen in multiple sclerosis with their long axes perpendicular to the ventricular surface are called ***Dawson's finger's*** *(arrows)*. MRI is the study of choice in imaging multiple sclerosis because of its greater sensitivity than CT in demonstrating plaques both in the brain and spinal cord.

# TERMINOLOGY

- Table 26.8 defines some of the terms used in this chapter.

## TABLE 26.8  Terminology

| | |
|---|---|
| **Intraaxial/extraaxial** | Intraaxial lesions originate in the brain parenchyma and extraaxial lesions originate outside of the brain substance (i.e., meninges, intraventricular). |
| **Infratentorial** | Beneath the tentorium cerebelli, which includes the cerebellum, brainstem, fourth ventricle, and cerebellopontine angles. |
| **Supratentorial** | Above the tentorium cerebelli, which includes the cerebral hemispheres (frontal, parietal, occipital, and temporal lobes) and the sella. |
| **Transient ischemic attack (TIA)** | Sudden neurologic loss that persists for a short time and resolves within 24 hours. |
| **Open versus closed head injuries** | ***Open*** = communication of intracranial material outside of the skull. ***Closed*** = no external communication. |
| **Increased attenuation/hyperattenuation/ hyperdense/hyperintense** | On CT, tissue that is of increased attenuation, hyperattenuates, or hyperdense is **whiter** than surrounding tissues. Hyperintense refers to **increased signal** on MRI imaging. |
| **Decreased attenuation/hypoattenuation/ hypodense/hypointense** | On CT, tissue that is of decreased attenuation, hypoattenuates, or hypodense is **darker** than surrounding tissues. Hypointense refers to **decreased** signal on MRI imaging. |
| **Diffusion-weighted imaging (DWI)** | An MRI sequence that can be rapidly acquired and that is extremely sensitive to detecting abnormalities in normal water movement in the brain so that it can identify a stroke within minutes after the event. DWI also helps differentiate acute infarction from more chronic infarction. |

## CASE QUIZ 26 ANSWER

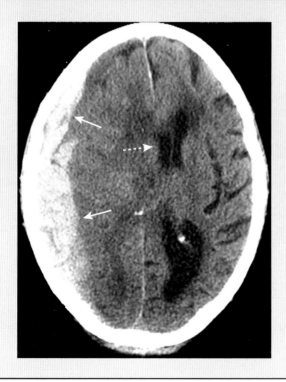

A crescent-shaped, high-density lesion is seen on the right consistent with an **acute subdural hematoma** *(solid arrows)*. There is a subfalcine herniation of the lateral ventricles to the opposite side due to mass effect *(dashed arrow)*. The CT findings are consistent with the patient's history of a fall, progressive disorientation, and use of anticoagulants. Frequently, patients with subdural hematomas fall comatose at the time of their injury but a subgroup remain conscious while still others worsen in a delayed manner as the hematoma enlarges.

## 🏠 TAKE HOME POINTS

- The anatomy of the brain can be demonstrated on either CT or MRI scans, although MRI is generally the study of choice for detecting and staging intracranial and spinal cord abnormalities because of its superior contrast and soft-tissue resolution.
- Unenhanced CT is usually the study of first choice in acute head trauma. The search for findings should initially focus on finding mass effect or blood.
- **Linear skull fractures** are important mainly for the intracranial abnormalities that may have occurred at the time of the fracture; **depressed skull fractures** can be associated with underlying brain injury and may require elevation of the fragment; **basilar skull fractures** are more serious and can be associated with CSF leaks.
- **Blow-out fractures** of the orbit result from a direct blow and may present with orbital emphysema, fracture through either the floor or medial wall of the orbit, and entrapment of fat and/or extraocular muscles in the fracture.
- There are four types of intracranial hemorrhages that may be associated with trauma: epidural hematoma, subdural hematoma, intracerebral hemorrhage, and subarachnoid hemorrhage.
- **Epidural hematomas** represent hemorrhage into the potential space between the dura mater and the inner table of the skull and are usually due to injuries to the middle meningeal artery or vein from blunt head trauma; almost all (95%) have an associated skull fracture. When acute, epidural hematomas appear as hyperintense collections of blood that typically have a lenticular shape.
- **Subdural hematomas** most commonly result from deceleration injuries or falls; acute subdural hematomas portend the presence of more severe brain injury. They are crescent-shaped bands of blood that may cross suture lines and enter the interhemispheric fissure, although they do not cross the midline.
- Traumatic **intracerebral hematomas** are frequently from shearing injuries and present as petechial or larger hemorrhages in the frontal or temporal lobes; they may be associated with increased intracranial pressure and brain herniation.
- **Brain herniations** include subfalcine, transtentorial, foramen magnum/tonsillar, sphenoid, and extracranial herniations.
- **Diffuse axonal injury** is a serious consequence of trauma in which the corpus callosum is most commonly affected; CT findings are similar to those for intracerebral hemorrhage following head trauma; MRI is the study of choice in identifying diffuse axonal injury.
- In general, **increased intracranial pressure** is due to either increased volume of the brain (cerebral edema) or increased size of the ventricles (hydrocephalus).
- There are two major categories of **cerebral edema:** vasogenic and cytotoxic.
- **Vasogenic edema** represents extracellular accumulation of fluid and is the type that occurs with malignancy and infection and affects the white matter more.
- **Cytotoxic edema** represents cellular edema, is due to cell death, and affects both the gray and white matter; cytotoxic edema is associated with cerebral ischemia.

- **Stroke** denotes an acute loss of neurologic function that occurs when the blood supply to an area of the brain is lost or compromised. MRI is more sensitive to the early diagnosis of stroke than CT.
- Strokes are usually due to **embolic** (more common) or **thrombotic** events and are typically divided into **ischemic** (more common) and **hemorrhagic** varieties (poorer prognosis); hypertension is frequently associated.
- **Intracerebral hemorrhage** will display as increased density on non-enhanced CT scans of the brain; after about 2 months, only a small hypo-density may remain.
- **Berry aneurysms** are usually formed from congenital weakening in the arterial wall; when they rupture, the blood typically enters the subarachnoid space appearing in the basilar cisterns and in the sulci. The aneurysm itself can be detected on either CTA or MRA.
- **Hydrocephalus** represents an increased volume of CSF in the ventricular system and may be due to overproduction of CSF (rare), underabsorption of CSF at the level of the arachnoid villi (**communicating**), or obstruction of the outflow of CSF from the ventricles (**noncommunicating**).
- **Normal-pressure hydrocephalus** is a form of communicating hydrocephalus characterized by a classical triad of symptoms that include abnormalities of gait, dementia, and urinary incontinence, which may be improved by insertion of a ventricular shunt.
- **Cerebral atrophy** is a loss of both gray and white matter that may resemble hydrocephalus, except that the CSF fluid dynamics are normal in atrophy and, in general, cerebral atrophy produces proportionate enlargement of both the ventricles and the sulci.
- **Glioblastoma multiforme** is a highly malignant glioma that occurs most commonly in the frontal and temporal lobes, producing a very aggressive infiltrating, partially-enhancing, sometimes necrotic mass, which may cross the corpus callosum to the opposite cerebral hemisphere.
- **Metastases to the brain** are frequently well-defined round masses near the gray-white junction and are usually multiple, typically hypodense or isodense on nonenhanced CT that can enhance with contrast; they can provoke vasogenic edema out of proportion to the size of the mass. Lung, breast, and melanoma are the most frequent sources of brain metastases.
- **Meningiomas** usually occur in middle-aged women in a parasagittal location; they tend to be slow-growing with an excellent prognosis if surgically excised; on CT they characteristically can be dense without contrast because of calcification within the tumor and may enhance dramatically.
- **Vestibular schwannomas** occur most commonly along the course of the eighth cranial nerve within the internal auditory canal at the cerebellopontine angle and are best identified on MRI, where they homogeneously enhance.
- **Multiple sclerosis** is the most common demyelinating disease, characterized by a relapsing and remitting course and a predilection for the periventricular area, corpus callosum, and optic nerves; it is best visualized on MRI and produces discrete globular foci of high-signal intensity (white) on T2-weighted images.

 Additional content is available online including chapters on Nuclear Medicine, Artificial Intelligence, Radiation Dose and Safety, an Early History of Radiology, and a compendium of 200 Diagnostic Radiology Signs.

# 27

# Recognizing Pediatric Diseases

*William Herring, MD, FACR*

Children differ physiologically from adults and are susceptible to abnormalities in development and maturation not seen in adults. They differ in anatomy (e.g., the thymus) and are more susceptible to the harmful effects of ionizing radiation. This chapter will highlight some of the more common pediatric diseases associated with imaging findings.

## CASE QUIZ 27 QUESTION

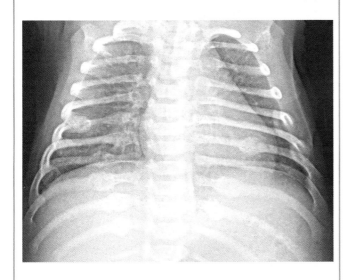

This is a frontal view of the thorax and upper abdomen in a 6-month-old infant with bruises on the back. Because of a clinical suspicion, a skeletal survey was ordered. What is the most likely diagnosis? See the correct answer at the end of this chapter.

## DISEASES DISCUSSED IN THIS CHAPTER

- **Newborn respiratory distress**
  - Transient tachypnea of the newborn
  - Neonatal respiratory distress syndrome
  - Meconium aspiration syndrome
  - Chronic lung disease of infancy
- **Childhood lung disease**
  - Reactive airways disease/bronchiolitis
  - Asthma
  - Pneumonia
- **Soft tissues of the neck**
  - Enlarged tonsils and adenoids

- Epiglottitis
- Croup (laryngotracheobronchitis)
- Ingested foreign bodies
- **Other diseases**
  - Cardiomegaly in infants
  - Salter-Harris growth plate fractures
  - Child abuse
  - Necrotizing enterocolitis (see also Chapter 19)
  - Esophageal atresia with/without trachea-esophageal fistula
  - Hypertrophic pyloric stenosis (Chapter 19)
  - Intussusception (Chapter 19)
  - Developmental dysplasia of the hips (Chapter 19)

## NEWBORN RESPIRATORY DISTRESS

- Respiratory distress is one of the **most common** presenting problems of **newborns.** Clues to its etiology include the infant's **gestational age**, the severity and the progression of symptoms, and the appearance of the chest radiograph. There are many etiologies of respiratory distress including those produced by cardiac, metabolic, hematologic, and anatomic causes. Four pulmonary causes will be discussed but first, a word about names.
- Pediatric diseases, like many other diseases, adjust their names over time. Table 27.1 contains the term we will use in this chapter and other names by which the disease has been or may be known.

### TABLE 27.1   Coming to Terms

| Used in the Chapter | Other Terms by which the Disease May Be Known |
|---|---|
| **Transient tachypnea of the newborn (TTN)** | Retained fetal fluid |
| **Neonatal respiratory distress syndrome (NRDS)** | Surfactant deficiency disorder<br>Infantile respiratory distress syndrome<br>Respiratory distress syndrome of newborn<br>Hyaline membrane disease |
| **Meconium aspiration syndrome** | Neonatal aspiration of meconium |
| **Chronic lung disease of infancy (CLD)** | Chronic lung disease of prematurity<br>Bronchopulmonary dysplasia |
| **Growth plate fractures** | Salter-Harris fractures<br>Epiphyseal plate fractures<br>Physeal plate fractures |

## Transient Tachypnea of the Newborn (TTN)

- Occurring in infants born by Caesarian or precipitous vaginal delivery, **transient tachypnea of the newborn is the most common cause of respiratory distress in the newborn.** It is thought to be due to delay in the resorption of fetal lung fluid.
- Clinically, TTN is marked by the **immediate onset** of tachypnea and mild respiratory distress. Intubation is usually not required. Infants typically **improve over several hours** with noninvasive oxygen supplementation and supportive therapy and completely recover by 48 hours.

---

>> **IMPORTANT POINTS**

- **Imaging findings of TTN:**
  - The lungs are often **hyperinflated,** though less so in premature infants.
  - There can be **streaky, perihilar linear densities.**
  - There also may be **fluid in the fissures** and/or **laminar pleural effusions** (Fig. 27.1).

---

## Neonatal Respiratory Distress Syndrome

- **Neonatal respiratory distress syndrome (NRDS)** is a disease of **premature infants,** usually less than 34 weeks of gestation. The incidence and severity of the disease often worsens with increasing prematurity. There are numerous risk factors, including perinatal asphyxia, hypoxia, and maternal diabetes.
- The major cause of this disorder is **surfactant deficiency.** Without surfactant, the alveolar sacs have an increased tendency to collapse, leading to widespread atelectasis.
- Typically, these premature infants have severe respiratory distress **after birth that progressively worsens.** Clinical findings include cyanosis, grunting, nasal flaring, intercostal and subcostal retractions, and tachypnea.

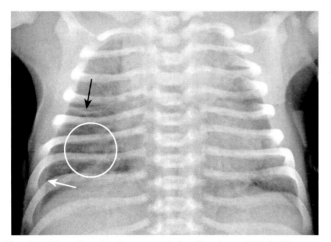

**Fig. 27.1** Transient Tachypnea of the Newborn (TTN). There are streaky, perihilar linear densities *(circle)* as well as fluid in the fissures *(black arrow)* and a laminar pleural effusion *(white arrow)*. The lungs are often hyperinflated.

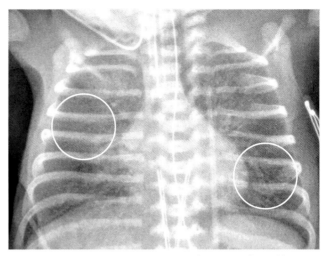

**Fig. 27.2** Neonatal Respiratory Distress Syndrome (NRDS). There is a diffuse **ground-glass** or finely granular appearance *(circles)* in a bilateral and symmetric distribution.

---

>> **IMPORTANT POINTS**

- **Imaging findings of NRDS** (Fig. 27.2):
  - There is typically a diffuse **ground-glass** or **finely granular** appearance to the lungs in a **bilateral** and **symmetric** distribution. The granularity seen in the lungs is the interplay of air-distended bronchioles and ducts against a background of atelectatic alveoli.
  - **Air bronchograms are common and extensive,** especially extending peripherally.
  - **Hypoaeration** is seen in nonmechanically ventilated lungs. **Hyperinflation** in nonintubated patients **excludes NRDS.**

---

- **Oxygen requirements progressively increase** over the first few hours after birth. The treatment of NRDS generally includes **positive-pressure ventilation** and may include **intratracheal surfactant replacement.**
- Infants who are very premature (23 to 27 weeks gestation) may require positive-pressure respiratory support for several weeks. The ductus arteriosus may fail to close, leading to **patent ductus arteriosus,** and **pulmonary edema or hemorrhage** can occur. They are at increased risk for the development of **chronic lung disease of infancy.**
- The **mortality rate** from NRDS in the newborn varies by country and is dependent, in part, on the rate of premature births and the availability of appropriate treatment interventions in those who develop the disease. In the United States, the mortality rate has declined dramatically in the last several decades.

## Meconium Aspiration Syndrome

- Meconium aspiration syndrome is **most common in postmature infants.**
- Meconium is found in the amniotic fluid in approximately 15% to 20% of all pregnancies. As a consequence, **meconium aspiration** as such is considered to be a **relatively common event.** Meconium products produce bronchial obstruction, air trapping, and a chemical pneumonitis.
- There is **severe respiratory distress almost immediately,** differentiating it from neonatal respiratory distress syndrome, whose onset is usually delayed by hours to a few days. However, whereas many infants with meconium aspiration have the

onset of symptoms at birth, some infants have an asymptomatic period of several hours and then worsen over time.

- Clinically, there may be tachypnea, hypoxia, and hypercapnia. Small airway obstruction may produce a ball-valve effect, leading to **air trapping, overdistension,** and **air leaks.**
- Treatment is **supportive,** consisting of **antibiotics** and **oxygen,** inhaled nitric oxide, or extracorporeal membrane oxygenation (ECMO), if needed.

> ## IMPORTANT POINTS
>
> - **Imaging findings of meconium aspiration** (Fig. 27.3):
>   - The lungs are hyperinflated with diffuse *ropey* densities (similar in appearance, but not in timing, to chronic lung disease of infancy).
>   - There may be patchy areas of **atelectasis** and **emphysema** from air trapping.
>   - Spontaneous **pneumothorax** and **pneumomediastinum** occur in 25% (Fig. 27.4).
>   - There may be an associated **pneumonia**, usually without air bronchograms.
>   - Small **pleural effusions** may be present in 20%.

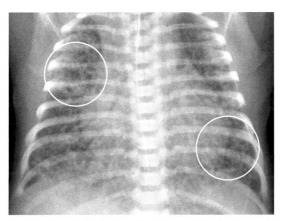

**Fig. 27.3 Meconium Aspiration Syndrome.** The lungs are hyperinflated with diffuse *rope-like* densities *(circles)*. The patchy pattern is a mosaic of areas of atelectasis along with emphysema from air trapping. This is a baby of 40+ weeks gestation with meconium staining.

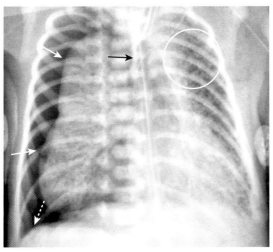

**Fig. 27.4 Meconium Aspiration Syndrome with Pneumothorax.** Spontaneous pneumothorax and pneumomediastinum occur in 25% of babies with meconium aspiration syndrome. The lungs show a coarse interstitial pattern *(circle)*. There is a large right pneumothorax *(solid white arrows)*. A *deep sulcus sign* (see Chapter 24) is also present *(dashed white arrow)*. This is a tension pneumothorax, because the heart and trachea *(black arrow)* are pushed to the left.

## Chronic Lung Disease of Infancy (CLD)

- Chronic lung disease of infancy is a **consequence of early, acute lung disease,** frequently **neonatal respiratory distress syndrome.** CLD may also complicate meconium aspiration syndrome and neonatal pneumonia.
- It is a clinical diagnosis with recently updated definitions including a degree of oxygen dependence at certain corrected gestational ages as well as abnormal lung parenchyma on chest radiograph.
- Associated with most cases of CLD is the **prior use of oxygen,** which was administered under positive pressure.
- Clinically, infants with CLD have **oxygen dependence,** hypercapnia, and a compensatory metabolic alkalosis. They may develop pulmonary arterial hypertension and right-sided heart failure.
- CLD more often manifests in a milder form now than the severe manifestations of the disease when it was first described in 1967.

> ## IMPORTANT POINTS
>
> - **Imaging findings of CLD** (Fig. 27.5):
>   - It may be impossible to distinguish early stages of chronic lung disease of infancy from later stages of NRDS.
>   - The lungs are usually **hyperaerated** overall.
>   - They may contain **coarse, irregular, rope-like, linear densities** representing **atelectasis** or, later, **fibrosis.**
>   - These areas of atelectasis may be intermixed with **lucent, cyst-like** foci representing hyperexpanded areas of **air trapping.** Together, these processes give the lung a *sponge-like* appearance.

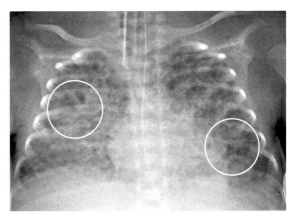

**Fig. 27.5 Chronic Lung Disease of Infancy (CLD).** The lungs in this radiograph have a typical *sponge-like* appearance *(circles)*. They contain coarse, linear densities representing atelectasis intermixed with lucent, cyst-like foci from areas of air trapping.

- Infants with CLD may require mechanical ventilation for months. Changes of CLD will revert to normal on the chest radiograph in most patients after the age of 2 years although abnormalities may still remain visible on CT of the chest.

• In any of these conditions (TTN, NRDS, meconium aspiration, and CLD), sudden worsening in the patient's symptoms suggests the possibility of an **air leak**—a complication of positive-pressure ventilation in relatively noncompliant lungs. There are four manifestations of an air leak discussed in Table 27.2, Figs. 27.6, 27.7, 27.8, and 27.9.

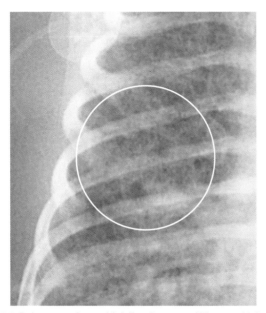

**Fig. 27.6 Pulmonary Interstitial Emphysema.** When multiple, small collections of air *(circle)* are seen in the interstitial tissues of the lung, it is called **pulmonary interstitial emphysema**. This is most likely the result of an alveolus rupturing and the air tracking back along the bronchovascular bundles of the lung. This baby has underlying neonatal respiratory distress syndrome.

| TABLE 27.2 | Complications of Treatment-Barotrauma |
|---|---|
| Assisted ventilation with high peak inspiratory pressures and positive end-expiratory pressures may cause overdistension and rupture of alveoli | |
| **Complication** | **Remarks** |
| **Pulmonary interstitial emphysema** | Rupture of an alveolus with dissection of the air back along the bronchovascular and perilymphatic interstitium may produce multiple small pockets of air in the lung called **pulmonary interstitial emphysema**. (Fig. 27.6) |
| **Pneumothorax** | Rupture of an alveolus adjacent to the visceral pleural surface of the lung may dissect outward into the pleural space producing a **pneumothorax**. (Fig. 27.7) |
| **Pneumomediastinum** | Air leaks along the bronchovascular bundles of the lung will eventually reach the mediastinum and may produce a **pneumomediastinum**. (Fig. 27.8) |
| **Pneumopericardium** | In infants, there may be connections between the mediastinum and the pericardial sac. Air that surrounds the heart but does not extend above the level of the great vessels may be a sign of **pneumopericardium**. (Fig. 27.9) |

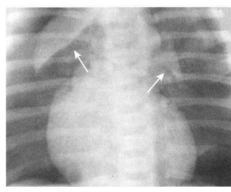

**Fig. 27.8 Spinnaker Sail Sign from Pneumomediastinum.** Air leaks may produce a pneumomediastinum. The right and left lobes of the thymus normally rest on the base of the heart. When pneumomediastinum forces the thymic lobes upward and outward, they can form a characteristic appearance, shown here, that has been likened to the **spinnaker sail** on a boat *(arrows).*

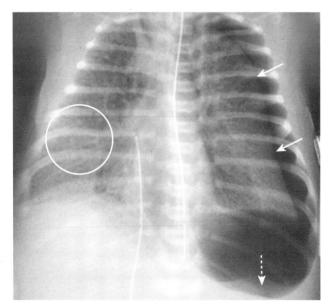

**Fig. 27.7 Neonatal Respiratory Distress Syndrome with Pneumothorax.** Rupture of an alveolus adjacent to the visceral pleural surface of the lung may dissect outward into the pleural space producing a pneumothorax. There is a ground-glass appearance to the lungs *(circle).* A left-sided pneumothorax is present *(solid arrows),* producing a deep sulcus sign from the pneumothorax *(dashed arrow).*

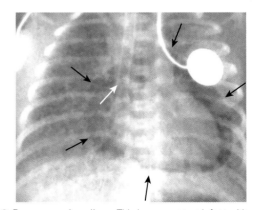

**Fig. 27.9 Pneumopericardium.** This is a premature infant with underlying neonatal respiratory distress syndrome who is on a ventilator. There is a lucency surrounding the heart *(black arrows)* representing air in the pericardial space. Notice how the air does not extend above the reflection of the aorta and main pulmonary artery. The tip of the endotracheal tube extends too far and is in the right main bronchus *(white arrow).*

# CHILDHOOD LUNG DISEASE

## Reactive Airways Disease/Bronchiolitis

- This is a general term for a group of diseases in the pediatric population featuring **wheezing, shortness of breath,** and **coughing.** Initial episodes are frequently referred to as *bronchiolitis.* Unlike asthma, which is chronic, reactive airways disease is usually **transient,** although it can progress over time to asthma
  - The **clinical findings** of reactive airways disease/bronchiolitis are tachypnea, retractions, cough, fever, and rhinorrhea.

---

### » IMPORTANT POINTS

- **Imaging findings of reactive airways disease** (Fig. 27.10):
  - *Peribronchial thickening,* which involves primarily the lobar or segmental bronchi and is detectable by **visualization of the walls of the bronchi on conventional radiographs.**
  - Bronchi viewed on end appear as **small, doughnut-like** densities.
  - Peribronchial thickening may also produce *tram-track* linear densities in the lungs from the thickened bronchial walls visualized in profile.
  - There may be **hyperinflation** of the lungs.
  - **Atelectasis** from mucus plugging may be present.

---

- **Treatment** for reactive airways disease includes bronchodilators, steroids, and oxygen.

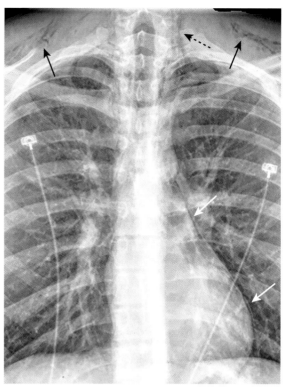

**Fig. 27.11 Asthmatic with Pneumomediastinum.** There is a thin white line *(white arrows)* visible because there is now air in the mediastinum. The air extends into the neck *(dashed black arrow)* and out to the subcutaneous tissues of the shoulders *(solid black arrows).*

## Asthma

- **Asthma** is a clinical, not a radiologic, diagnosis. Chest radiographs can help in determining either the **cause** or the **complications** of an asthmatic episode.
- Inciting events include **pneumonia,** usually accompanied by a fever that provides a clue to its presence. Complications include **atelectasis** secondary to plugging by mucus, **pneumothorax,** and **pneumomediastinum** (Fig. 27.11).
- During or after an acute attack, the lungs may be **overaerated** with **flattening of the diaphragm.** There may be **peribronchial thickening** as is seen with reactive airways disease.

## Pneumonia

- Age is a determining factor in both the etiology and clinical presentation of childhood pneumonia.
- In **neonates,** group B beta hemolytic streptococcus is the most common cause of pneumonia. Its imaging appearance can mimic neonatal respiratory distress syndrome.
- In **older infants,** the most common causes are **respiratory viruses** (RSV, parainfluenza, influenza, and adenoviruses) **and *Mycoplasma pneumoniae*** in children **older than five.**
- Clinically, neonates may exhibit only a fever. In older infants and children, **bacterial** pneumonia tends to produce **fever, chills, tachypnea, cough, pleuritic chest pain, and shortness of breath.** Viral pneumonia is more often associated with cough, wheezing, and stridor than fever.
- **Treatment** is supportive with antibiotics, as needed.

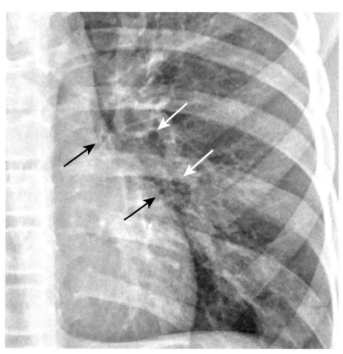

**Fig. 27.10 Reactive Airways Disease.** There is peribronchial thickening that involves primarily the lobar and segmental bronchi and is recognizable by visualization of the walls of the bronchi on conventional radiographs. Here they are seen as small circles or doughnuts near the hilum of a child *(arrows).* Adults may normally demonstrate bronchi on end in the hilar regions, but children usually do not.

## SOFT TISSUES OF THE NECK

### Enlarged Tonsils and Adenoids

- **Newborns do not have visible adenoids,** even though the adenoids are present at birth. They are usually not visible radiographically **until 3 to 6 months** (Fig. 27.12). The adenoids can grow until about age 6 years. They then involute through adulthood. **Adults normally do not have visible adenoids.**
- The **palatine tonsils and adenoids** frequently enlarge at the same time. As with enlarged adenoids, the significance of enlarged tonsils is best made in light of clinical symptoms and compression of the airway.
- **Clinical findings** of enlarged tonsils and adenoids include nasal congestion, mouth-breathing, chronic or recurrent

otitis media due to their proximity to the eustachian tubes, painful swallowing, and sleep apnea.

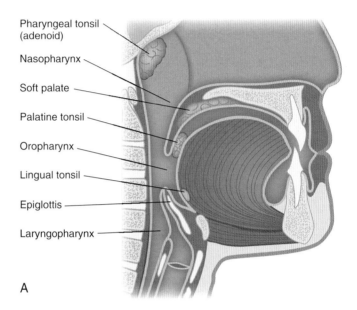

Pharyngeal tonsil (adenoid)
Nasopharynx
Soft palate
Palatine tonsil
Oropharynx
Lingual tonsil
Epiglottis
Laryngopharynx

A

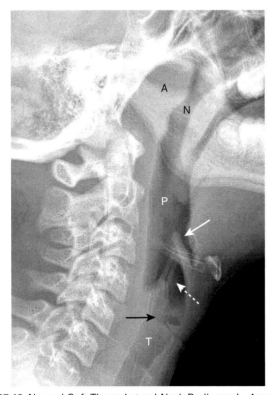

**Fig. 27.12 Normal Soft-Tissue Lateral Neck Radiograph, 4-year-old.** The adenoids (A) are seen at the base of the skull and are adjacent to the nasopharyngeal airway (N). More distally is the pharynx (P). The epiglottis *(solid white arrow)* is bounded superiorly by air in the vallecula. The aryepiglottic folds are thin, paired structures *(dashed white arrow)*. The normal-sized laryngeal ventricle *(solid black arrow)* separates the false vocal cords above from the true cords below. The trachea (T) begins below the true cords.

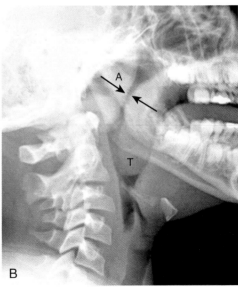

B

**Fig. 27.13 Illustration of Normal Tonsils and Adenoids and Enlarged Adenoids.** (A) The illustration demonstrates the normal relationships between the tonsils, adenoids, pharynx, and epiglottis. (B) There is marked narrowing of the nasopharynx *(arrows)* due to posterior incursion by enlarged adenoids (A). The palatine tonsils (T) are also enlarged. The tonsils and adenoids frequently enlarge at the same time.

## Epiglottitis

- **Acute bacterial epiglottitis** can be a **life-threatening, medical emergency** leading to airway obstruction due to infection with edema of the epiglottis and aryepiglottic folds.
- The most frequent causative organism had been *Haemophilus influenzae* type B, but introduction of the vaccine in 1985 has led to a marked decrease in the number of cases of epiglottitis. *H. influenzae* **still remains the most common cause,** although it may also be caused by pneumococcus, streptococcus group A, viral infection, such as herpes simplex 1, parainfluenza and thermal injury, or angioneurotic edema. Chemical irritation has also been reported from the ingestion of laundry detergent pods.
- Epiglottitis typically has a **peak incidence from about 3 to 6 years of age.**
- **Clinically,** epiglottitis resembles **croup**, but the clinician should think of epiglottitis if the child cannot breathe unless **sitting up,** what appears to be "croup" seems to be **worsening,** or if the child cannot swallow saliva and **drools.** Cough is rare in epiglottitis. The classical triad of epiglottitis is: **drooling, severe dysphagia, and respiratory distress with inspiratory stridor.**
- The patient should be accompanied everywhere by someone experienced in endotracheal intubation. Imaging studies are not always necessary for the diagnosis and may be falsely negative in early stages.
- The imaging study of choice is the **lateral neck radiograph,** which should be exposed in the **upright position only,** as the supine position may close off the airway.

> ## ▶▶ IMPORTANT POINTS
>
> - **Imaging findings of the epiglottitis:**
>   - **Enlargement of the epiglottis**: The epiglottis should not be "larger than your thumb," no matter what the size of your thumb. There is **thickening of the** *aryepiglottic folds* (which is an important component of airway obstruction and the true cause of stridor) and, sometimes, circumferential **narrowing of the subglottic portion of the trachea** during inspiration (Fig. 27.14).

- **Treatment** includes securing the airway, which may require intubation or emergency tracheostomy. Some treatment protocols call for administering intravenous steroids and starting empiric antibiotic therapy.

## Croup (Laryngotracheobronchitis)

- Croup is usually **viral in etiology,** the most common causes being parainfluenza viruses (types 1, 2, and 3). Respiratory syncytial virus, influenza, and mycoplasma are other common causes. It typically occurs from age **6 months to 3 years,** which is a younger age range than epiglottitis. It **frequently follows a common cold.**
- The diagnosis of croup usually is made on the basis of **clinical findings.** It may be difficult to distinguish from early retropharyngeal abscess; the differential diagnosis can be aided by imaging.
- There is characteristically a **harsh cough** described as *barking* or *brassy,* associated with hoarseness, inspiratory stridor, low-grade fever, and respiratory distress.
- **Treatment** can consist of steroids, aerosolized epinephrine, and humidification.

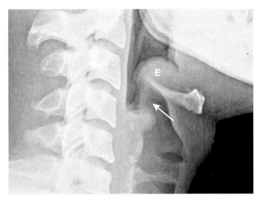

**Fig. 27.14** Epiglottitis. The epiglottis (E) should **not** be thumb-like in appearance (see Fig. 27.12). It is very enlarged in this case. The aryepiglottic folds are thickened *(arrow)*. Care must be taken to protect the airway from complete closure in any patient with epiglottitis.

> ## ▶▶ IMPORTANT POINTS
>
> - **Imaging findings of croup** (Fig. 27.15):
>   - The three key findings, seen on the lateral soft-tissue neck radiograph, are (1) **distension of the hypopharynx, (2) distension of the laryngeal ventricle,** and (3) haziness and/or **narrowing of subglottic trachea.** The *steeple sign,* which may be seen on the frontal radiograph of the neck is, by itself, an **unreliable** sign of croup.

## INGESTED FOREIGN BODIES

- The majority of foreign body ingestions occur between **6 months and 6 years.** Over **80% pass spontaneously.** Food or true foreign body ingestions include coins, toys, chicken bones (opaque), and fish bones (nonopaque).
- Most often the foreign body impacts at a point at which the esophagus naturally narrows—**just below** the **cricopharyngeus** at the level of C5-C6 (70%), at the level of the **thoracic inlet,** at the **aortic arch** (20%), or at the level of the **esophagogastric junction** (10%). Once past the esophagus, most foreign bodies will pass through the gastrointestinal tract.

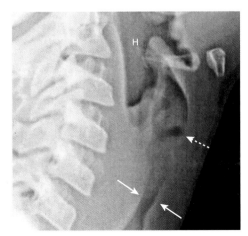

**Fig. 27.15** Laryngotracheobronchitis (Croup). There is distension of the hypopharynx (H), distension of the laryngeal ventricle *(dashed arrow)*, and haziness with narrowing of subglottic space, which is the proximal trachea *(solid arrows)*. This child had the characteristic barking cough of croup.

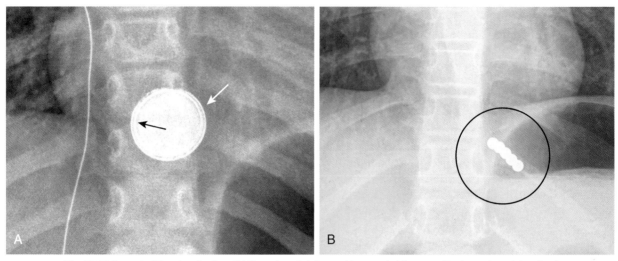

**Fig. 27.16 Ingested Foreign Bodies.** (A) There is a disk (button) battery *(white arrow)* in the region of the distal esophagus. It has distinctive linear dark bands around its perimeter *(black arrow)*. (B) Multiple small, ingested magnets are seen in the region of the distal esophagus *(circle)*. Both disk batteries and small magnets pose unique risks among ingested foreign bodies.

- The **major complications** of ingested foreign bodies are perforation, obstruction, or stricture formation.
- **Disk (button) batteries** and **magnets** pose **particular hazards.**
  - Button batteries should be removed from the esophagus **emergently** because of their ability to produce perforation (Fig. 27.16).
  - Multiple small magnets also pose the risk of perforation by drawing apposing loops of bowel together and should be removed, if possible. Lack of magnet movement on serial radiographs suggests bowel entrapment and can be an indication for surgical intervention.
- **Clinical findings** of an impacted esophageal foreign body most commonly include **dysphagia** and **odynophagia.** Even after the foreign body passes, many complain of pain occurring in the cervical esophagus regardless of the actual site of impaction.

> **》 IMPORTANT POINTS**
>
> - **Imaging findings of an impacted foreign body:**
>   - The imaging findings will depend on whether the foreign body is opaque or not. **Conventional radiographs** of the **neck** and **chest** are usually obtained **first.** If no foreign body is visualized, the abdomen may also be radiographed.
>   - A coin may appear differently on conventional radiographs depending on whether it is impacted in the **esophagus** or in the **trachea** (Fig. 27.17).
>   - If conventional radiographs are negative and there is still a very high suspicion for a nonopaque, ingested foreign body, then either contrast esophagram or CT may be considered.

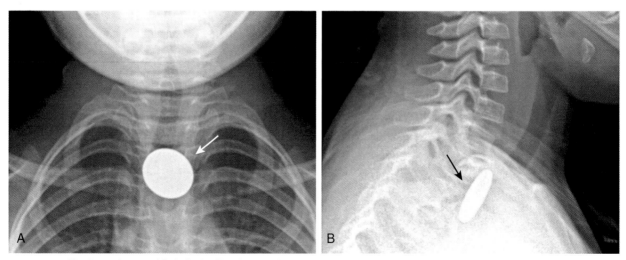

**Fig. 27.17 Ingested Coin in the Esophagus.** A coin impacted in the esophagus will usually appear **round** on the (A) frontal view *(arrow)* and **flat** on the (B) lateral view *(arrow)* because of its orientation in the esophagus. A coin in the **trachea** will more likely appear on end on the frontal view and round on the lateral view because of the shape of the trachea. This coin was a US nickel and it passed uneventfully a day later.

- Because children who ingest foreign bodies may also be predisposed to eating **other foreign material** *(pica)* such as paint, **always look for** dense lines in the metaphyses of visible bones on any foreign body study, a sign of **lead poisoning.**
- **Treatment**
  - Under most circumstances, **watchful waiting** will result in elimination of the foreign body. Endoscopy is performed if removal is considered clinically necessary (e.g., sharp objects, disk batteries, magnets).

## OTHER DISEASES

### Recognizing Cardiomegaly in Infants

- In **newborns and infants,** it is important to remember that the **heart will normally appear larger** relative to the size of the thorax than it does in adults. Whereas a cardiothoracic ratio greater than 50% is considered abnormal in adults, the **cardiothoracic ratio may reach up to 65% in infants and still be normal** because newborns cannot take as deep an inspiration as adults and the relative proportions in the size of their abdomen to chest are not the same as for adults (Fig. 27.18).

- Any assessment of cardiac enlargement in an infant should also take into account other factors such as the appearance of the **pulmonary vasculature** and any **associated clinical signs or symptoms** (e.g., a murmur, tachycardia, or cyanosis).

> ! **DIAGNOSTIC PITFALLS**
>
> - In a child, the **thymus gland** may overlap portions of the heart and sometimes mimic cardiomegaly. The **normal thymus** may be seen on conventional chest radiographs, appearing largest up to 3 years of age but sometimes visible into the teenage years. The normal thymus gland has a somewhat **lobulated** appearance, especially where it is indented by the ribs, and tends to decrease in density toward its periphery (Fig. 27.19).

## SALTER-HARRIS FRACTURES—GROWTH PLATE FRACTURES

- In growing bone, the hypertrophic zone in the *growth plate (epiphyseal plate, physis)* is most vulnerable to shearing injuries. Growth plate fractures are **common** and account for as many as 30% of childhood fractures. By definition, because these are all fractures through an **open** growth plate, they **can only occur in skeletally immature** individuals.
- The **Salter-Harris classification of growth plate injuries** is a commonly used method of describing such injuries that

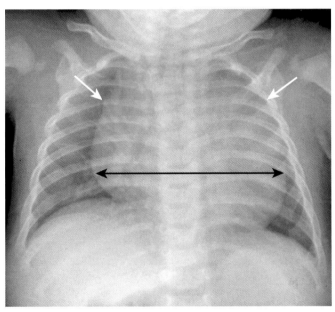

**Fig. 27.18 Normal Infant Chest.** In the normal infant, the cardiothoracic ratio may be as large as 65% (compared to 50% in adults). Here the heart appears enlarged *(double black arrow)* but is normal for a newborn. The thymus gland *(white arrows)* accounts for some of the apparent cardiomegaly.

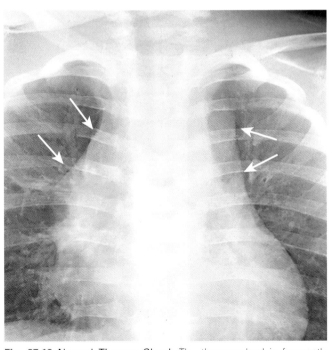

**Fig. 27.19 Normal Thymus Gland.** The thymus gland is frequently lobulated in appearance *(arrows),* an aid in identifying it on a child's chest x-ray. Although the thymus gland will usually involute with age, it may still be normally visible into the teenage years.

helps identify the type of treatment required and predicts the likelihood of complications based on the type of fracture (Fig. 27.20) (Table 27.3).

- Types I and II **heal well.**
- Type III can develop **arthritic changes** or **asymmetric growth plate fusion.**
- Types IV and V are more likely to develop **early fusion** of the growth plate with **angular deformities** and/or **shortening** of that bone.
- **Type I: fractures of the growth plate alone**
  - Salter-Harris Type I fractures can be **difficult to detect without the opposite side for comparison.** Fortunately, these fractures have a **favorable prognosis.**
  - *Slipped capital femoral epiphysis (SCFE)* is a manifestation of a Salter-Harris Type I injury.
    - Slipped capital femoral epiphysis occurs most often in **taller and/or heavier, preteen** and **teenage boys.** It can occur during periods of rapid growth, from trauma, renal osteodystrophy, and from endocrine disorders, like hypothyroidism.
    - The proximal (capital) femoral epiphysis slips **inferior, medial, and posterior** relative to the neck of the femur (Fig. 27.21).
    - It is **bilateral in about 25% of cases** and can result in **avascular necrosis** of the slipped femoral head because of interruption of its blood supply in up to 15% of cases.
- **Type II: fracture of the growth plate and fracture of the metaphysis**
  - This is the **most common type of Salter-Harris fracture (75%),** seen especially in the distal radius. Healing is

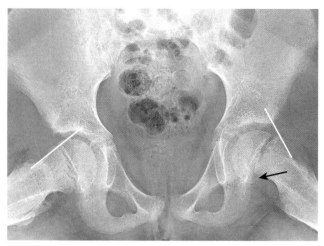

**Fig. 27.21** Slipped Capital Femoral Epiphysis (SCFE). SCFE produces inferior, medial, and posterior slippage of the proximal femoral epiphysis relative to the neck of the femur *(arrow)*. A line drawn parallel to the neck of the femur called **Klein's line** *(lines)* should normally intersect the lateral portion of the femoral head. It does so on the normal right side, but does not on the left side because the epiphysis has slipped.

typically rapid and the growth is rarely disturbed, except in the distal femur and proximal tibia where a residual deformity may occur (Fig. 27.22).

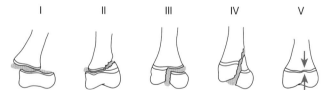

**Fig. 27.20** Salter-Harris Classification of Growth Plate Fractures. All of these fractures involve the growth plate (epiphyseal plate). **Type I** are fractures of the growth plate alone. **Type II** fractures, the most common, involve the growth plate and metaphysis. These first two types have a favorable prognosis. **Type III** are fractures of the growth plate and the epiphysis and have a less favorable prognosis. **Type IV** is a fracture of the growth plate, epiphysis, and metaphysis. It has an even less favorable prognosis. **Type V** is a crush injury of the growth plate. It has the worst prognosis.

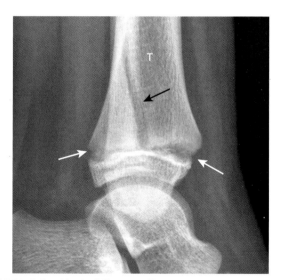

**Fig. 27.22** Salter-Harris II Fracture. This is a lateral view of the distal tibia (T). In Salter-Harris Type II fractures, there is a fracture of the growth plate *(white arrows)* and a fracture of the metaphysis *(black arrow)*.

| TABLE 27.3 | Salter-Harris Classification of Growth Plate Fractures | |
|---|---|---|
| **Type** | **What's Fractured** | **Remarks** |
| I | Growth plate (physis) | Seen in phalanges, distal radius, SCFE; good prognosis |
| II | Growth plate and metaphysis | Most common of all Salter-Harris fractures; frequently distal radius; good prognosis |
| III | Growth plate and epiphysis | Intraarticular fracture, especially distal tibia; less favorable prognosis |
| IV | Growth plate, epiphysis, and metaphysis | Seen in distal humerus and distal tibia; poor prognosis |
| V | Crush injury of growth plate | Worst prognosis; difficult to diagnose until healing begins |

- **Type III: fracture of the growth plate and the epiphysis**
  - There is a **longitudinal fracture through the epiphysis itself,** which means the fracture invariably enters the joint space and fractures the articular cartilage.
  - This type of injury can have long-term implications for the development of **secondary osteoarthritis** and can result in **asymmetric** and **premature fusion of the growth plate** with subsequent deformity of the bone (Fig. 27.23). Its treatment requires early recognition for appropriate reduction.
- **Type IV: fracture of the growth plate, metaphysis, and epiphysis**
  - Type IV fractures have a **poorer prognosis** than other Salter-Harris fractures—that is, premature and possibly asymmetric **closure of the growth plate**, especially in bones of the lower extremity, that may lead to differences in leg length, angular deformities, and secondary osteoarthritis (Fig. 27.24).
  - If the fracture is displaced, open reduction and internal fixation (ORIF) is usually performed although growth deformities can occur even with perfect reduction.
- **Type V: crush fracture of growth plate**
  - Type V Salter-Harris fractures are a **rare**, crush-type injury of the growth plate that are **associated with vascular injury** and almost always **result in growth impairment** through early focal fusion of the growth plate.

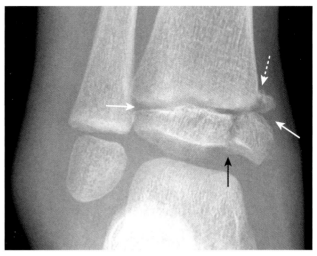

**Fig. 27.24** Salter-Harris IV Fracture. This is a frontal view of the distal tibia. In type IV fractures, there is a fracture of the growth plate *(solid white arrows)*, metaphysis *(dashed white arrow)*, and the epiphysis *(black arrow)*. These have an increased likelihood of premature and possibly asymmetric closure of the growth plate.

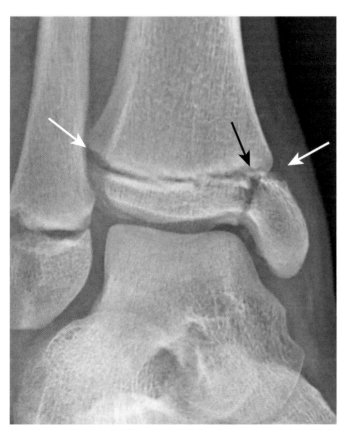

**Fig. 27.23** Salter-Harris III Fracture. This is a frontal view of the ankle in another patient. With Salter-Harris Type III fractures, there is a fracture of the growth plate *(white arrows)* as well as a longitudinal fracture through the epiphysis itself *(black arrow)*. This fracture has a poorer prognosis than types I and II.

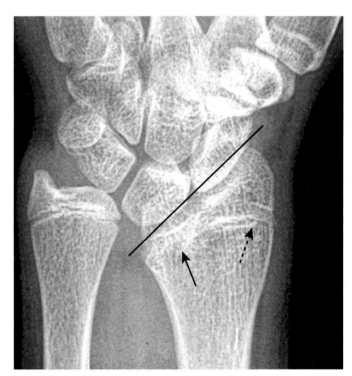

**Fig. 27.25** Salter-Harris V Fracture. Type V fractures are crush fractures of the growth plate. In this child, the medial portion of the distal radial growth plate has fused *(solid arrow)* while the lateral portion remains open *(dashed arrow)*. This premature fusion of the medial growth plate has resulted in an angular deformity of the distal radius *(line)*.

- They are **most common** in the **distal femur, proximal tibia,** and **distal tibia.** They are **difficult to diagnose** on conventional radiographs until later in their course when complications ensue (Fig. 27.25).

# CHILD ABUSE

- Salter-Harris fractures are examples of **accidental** injuries in children. The **location** or the **type** of other fractures can be highly suggestive for **nonaccidental trauma** produced by abuse. **Radiologic evaluations are key in diagnosing child abuse.**
- There are several fracture sites and characteristics that should raise the suspicion for child abuse (Table 27.4).
  - *Metaphyseal corner fractures.* These are small, shearing-type fractures of the metaphyses due to rapid rotation leading to Salter-Harris type fractures through the osteochondral junction called *corner fractures.* Corner fractures are considered **diagnostic of physical abuse.** They parallel the metaphysis and can have a *bucket-handle appearance* (Fig. 27.26A).
  - **Rib fractures,** especially multiple rib fractures and/or fractures of the posterior ribs (which rarely fracture due to accidental trauma.) (Fig. 27.26B).
  - **Head injuries** are the most common cause of death in child abuse under the age of 2 years. Findings include **subdural and subarachnoid hemorrhage** and **cerebral contusions. Skull fractures** tend to be depressed, comminuted, and bilateral and may cross suture lines.

# NECROTIZING ENTEROCOLITIS (NEC)

- **Necrotizing enterocolitis** is the **most common gastrointestinal** medical and/or surgical **emergency** occurring in **neonates.** Its etiology remains unknown, although ischemia and/or reperfusion injury have been implicated

along with poorly developed intestinal motility with resultant stasis.
- It is **more common in premature** infants but can also be seen in term babies who have undergone extreme stress (e.g., sepsis or major surgery). Usually, its **onset** occurs within the **first week** of life. Term infants have an increased risk for the disease if they have congenital heart disease or there is a history of maternal cocaine use.

| TABLE 27.4 Skeletal Trauma Suggestive of Child Abuse | |
|---|---|
| **Site(s)** | **Remarks** |
| Distal femur, distal humerus, wrist, ankle | Metaphyseal corner fractures |
| Multiple sites | Fractures in different stages of healing |
| Femur, humerus, tibia | Spiral fractures in children <1 year of age |
| Posterior ribs, avulsed spinous processes | These are unusual accidental fractures <5 years of age |
| Multiple skull fractures | Multiple fractures, especially if depressed, should suggest child abuse |
| Fractures with abundant callous formation | Implies repeated trauma and no immobilization |
| Metacarpal and metatarsal fractures | These are unusual accidental fractures in children <5 years of age |
| Sternal and scapular fractures | |
| Vertebral body fractures and subluxations | |

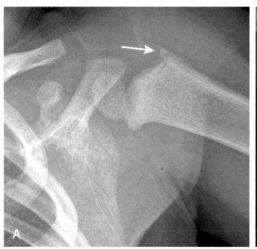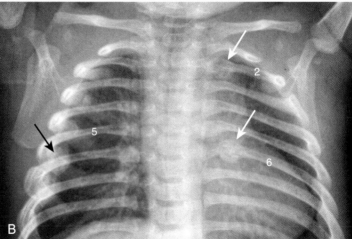

**Fig. 27.26 Child Abuse.** (A) There is metaphyseal *corner fracture* *(arrow)*, a small avulsion-type fracture of the proximal humerus that is highly suggestive of child abuse. (B) There are several healing rib fractures, as evidenced by callus formation involving the left 2nd and 6th posterior ribs *(white arrows)* and the anterolateral right 5th rib *(black arrow)*. Fractures of the posterior ribs are highly suspicious of child abuse.

- **Clinical findings** may be subtle and can include feeding intolerance, delayed gastric emptying, abdominal distension, and/or tenderness and decreased bowel sounds.
- Box 27.1 describes the imaging findings of a **normal infant abdomen** (Fig. 27.27).
- **Imaging findings of necrotizing enterocolitis**
  - **Conventional radiographs** of the abdomen remain the modality by which the disease is diagnosed most often. The acute disease **most commonly affects the terminal ileum.**
    - Early findings may be a few **distended loops of bowel.** A **persistently dilated** loop that remains **unchanged** in appearance is a nonspecific marker of ileus and it can be seen early in NEC.
    - **Thickened bowel walls** are manifest by **separation of the bowel loops.**
    - *Pneumatosis intestinalis* is **pathognomonic of NEC in the newborn.** A **linear radiolucency** within the bowel wall parallels the bowel lumen and represents **subserosal** air that has entered from the lumen (Fig. 27.28A). **Cystic** collections of air are **submucosal** in location but are also a sign of pneumatosis.
    - Abdominal **free air** is an ominous finding that usually requires emergency surgical intervention.
    - *Portal venous gas,* originally thought to be ominous, is now considered less so as it can be caused by other conditions including umbilical venous catheter placement. It appears as linear, branching, tubular structures of air density over the periphery of the liver and represents air in the portal venous system (Fig. 27.28B).

---

### BOX 27.1  Normal Infant Abdomen: Conventional Radiographs

- Almost all infants will demonstrate gas in the stomach by 15 minutes after birth and air in the rectum by 24 hours of age.
- It is virtually impossible on radiographs to differentiate small from large bowel in infants as the haustra don't develop in the colon until about 6 months of age.
- Most infants swallow a great deal of air so expect to see many air-filled, polygonal-shaped loops of bowel with walls that closely appose each other (Fig. 27.27).

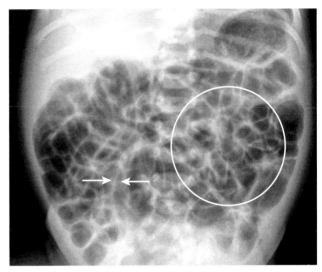

**Fig. 27.27 Normal Infant Abdomen.** Since most infants swallow a great deal of air, there are many air-filled, polygonal-shaped loops of bowel *(circle)* with walls that closely appose each other *(arrows)*.

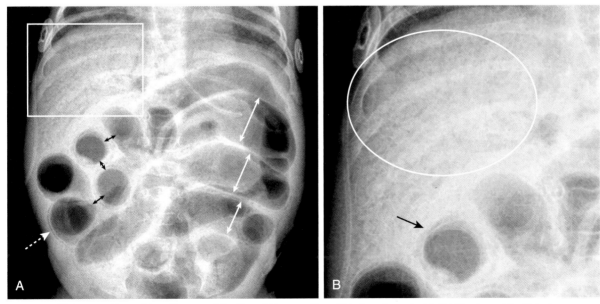

**Fig. 27.28 Necrotizing Enterocolitis, Portal Venous Gas.** This is a 1-week-old. (A) The bowel is dilated *(double white arrows)*. There is a linear radiolucency paralleling the bowel wall representing air in the bowel wall *(dashed white arrow)* and abnormal separation of the loops of bowel from wall thickening *(double black arrows)*. Numerous small, peripherally located air-containing vessels are seen in the liver (see [B] for close-up) representing portal venous gas. (B) Close-up of the liver shows multiple, tubular lucencies representing air in the portal venous system *(oval)*. There is air in the bowel wall *(arrow)*.

- **Complications**
  - Of those who survive, 50% develop a long-term complication. The two most common complications are intestinal **stricture** and **short-gut syndrome.** Mortality rates range from 10% to 44% in infants weighing less than 1500 grams.

## ESOPHAGEAL ATRESIA WITH/WITHOUT TRACHEO-ESOPHAGEAL FISTULA (TEF)

- The etiology of this complex of findings is not completely understood. By far, the most common form is a **blind-ending esophagus** *(esophageal atresia)* with a **fistulous connection between the trachea** and the **distal esophageal remnant.**
- Esophageal atresia is commonly associated with **other abnormalities of the GI tract,** including imperforate anus, duodenal atresia, or stenosis. In 25% of cases, there are 13 or more pairs of ribs or 6 or more lumbar vertebral bodies. Infants with isolated esophageal atresia have an increased incidence of trisomy 21 and duodenal atresia.
- In up to 50% of cases of esophageal atresia with/without TEF, there may be **associated congenital abnormalities** outside of the gastrointestinal tract.
  - *VACTERL* is an acronym to help recall a constellation of congenital abnormalities that may occur together and stands for **v**ertebral anomalies, **a**nal atresia, **c**ardiac abnormalities, **TE** fistula and/or **e**sophageal atresia, **r**enal agenesis or dysplasia, and **l**imb defects.
- **Clinical findings usually occur early in life** and include choking, drooling, difficulty handling secretions, regurgitation, aspiration, and respiratory distress.
- **Imaging findings** will depend on the geometry of the atresia and fistula:
  - With **esophageal atresia** and **no fistula, no air** enters the GI tract so the **abdomen is airless.** Normally, there should be air in the stomach within 15 minutes after birth.
  - In esophageal atresia with a **distal fistula** between the esophagus and trachea (the most common type), there is **gas in the bowel** that arrived via the trachea, and a radiolucent, **blind-ending, dilated pouch of upper esophagus** may be seen on chest x-ray, representing the atretic esophagus. Further imaging studies are usually not necessary, but introduction of a soft catheter into the blind-ending pouch will confirm the diagnosis (Fig. 27.29).
  - There may be **aspiration pneumonia.** Aspiration pneumonia often involves the right upper lobe when there is esophageal atresia.
  - Prenatal ultrasound can suggest the diagnosis of esophageal atresia as early as 24 weeks because of the presence of **polyhydramnios.**
- **Treatment**
  - Primary anastomosis of the proximal and distal esophagus is usually done when the infant is a few months old. Colonic interposition may be used if primary anastomosis is impossible.

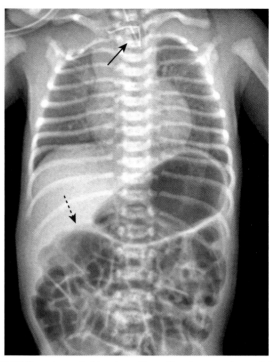

**Fig. 27.29 Esophageal Atresia with a Tracheoesophageal Fistula (TEF).** The tip of an orogastric tube is kinked in a blind-ending pouch in the upper esophagus and can pass no farther in the atretic esophagus *(solid arrow).* The air seen throughout the bowel *(dashed arrow)* arrived there **not** via the esophagus, but through a **fistula** that connected the trachea with the distal end of the esophagus (not visible on plain films).

## CASE QUIZ 27 ANSWER

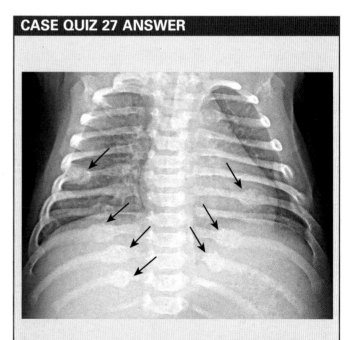

There are numerous healing rib fractures *(arrows),* all involving the posterior ribs. Studies have shown an extremely high positive predictive value between rib fractures in children less than 3 years old and **child abuse,** especially if they are multiple and the fractures are located predominantly posterior and lateral, as in this case. Rib fractures may be the only skeletal signs of child abuse in up to 1/3 of patients.

## 🏠 TAKE HOME POINTS

- **Transient tachypnea of the newborn (TTN)** is the most common cause of respiratory distress in the newborn, occurring most commonly in infants born via Caesarian section or precipitous delivery. The lungs are usually hyperinflated with streaky perihilar linear densities, fluid in the fissures, and/or laminar pleural effusions.

- **Neonatal respiratory distress syndrome (NRDS)** is a disease of premature infants. There is typically a diffuse ground-glass or finely granular appearance in a bilateral and symmetric distribution with air bronchograms. The lungs are frequently hypoaerated.

- **Meconium aspiration syndrome** is a common cause of neonatal respiratory distress in full-term/postmature infants. The lungs are hyperinflated with diffuse "ropey" densities. There may be patchy areas of atelectasis along with emphysema from air trapping.

- **Chronic lung disease of infancy (CLD)** is a consequence of early acute lung disease, frequently neonatal respiratory distress syndrome. Infants with CLD have a supplemental oxygen dependence. The lungs are usually hyperaerated and "sponge-like" in appearance, containing both coarse linear densities from atelectasis intermixed with lucent foci from hyperexpanded areas of air trapping.

- Complications of treatment of respiratory distress in the newborn are usually from **barotrauma (air leaks)** and include pulmonary interstitial emphysema, pneumomediastinum, pneumothorax, and pneumopericardium.

- **Reactive airways disease/bronchiolitis** is a general term for a group of diseases in the pediatric population featuring wheezing, shortness of breath, and coughing. There may be peribronchial thickening and hyperaeration on chest radiographs.

- **Asthma** is a clinical diagnosis. Chest radiographs can help in determining either the cause or the complications of an asthmatic episode. Pneumonia is an example of one cause and pneumothorax and atelectasis are among the complications of an asthmatic attack.

- Clinically, neonates with **pneumonia** may have only a fever. Bacterial pneumonia characteristically produces lobar consolidation or a round pneumonia, with pleural effusion in some cases. Viral pneumonia characteristically shows interstitial opacities or patchy areas of consolidation suggestive of bronchopneumonia.

- The **adenoids** can grow until about age 6 years and then involute through adulthood. The key imaging finding for enlarged adenoids is marked narrowing or obliteration of the nasopharyngeal airway on a soft-tissue lateral neck radiograph. The tonsils and adenoids frequently enlarge together.

- Acute bacterial **epiglottitis** can be a life-threatening medical emergency. The epiglottis should not normally be thumb-sized in appearance. It occurs at an older age (3 to 6 years) than croup (6 months to 3 years).

- **Croup** is usually viral in etiology and the diagnosis is most often made on the basis of clinical findings. The three key imaging findings, seen on the lateral soft-tissue neck radiograph, are distension of the hypopharynx, distension of the laryngeal ventricle, and haziness and/or narrowing of the subglottic trachea.

- Most **foreign body ingestions** occur between 6 months and 6 years of age with the vast majority passing spontaneously. They impact at several different anatomic landmarks where the esophagus naturally narrows. Disk (button) batteries and magnets pose particular hazards and should generally be removed.

- The **cardiothoracic ratio** may reach up to 65% in infants and still be normal. In a child, the thymus gland may overlap portions of the heart and sometimes mimic cardiomegaly.

- **Growth plate fractures** are common in childhood. The Salter-Harris classification of growth plate injuries is a commonly used method of describing these injuries.

- Certain kinds of fractures can be highly suggestive for nonaccidental injuries produced by **child abuse.** Included among injuries pointing to child abuse are metaphyseal corner fractures, rib fractures, and certain head injuries. Radiologic evaluations are key in diagnosing child abuse.

- **Necrotizing enterocolitis** is the most common GI medical and/or surgical emergency occurring in neonates, especially premature infants. There may be dilated loops of bowel, thickened bowel walls, pneumatosis intestinalis, and portal venous gas.

- **Esophageal atresia** may occur with or without a tracheoesophageal fistula (TEF). The most common form is a blind-ending esophagus with a fistulous connection between the trachea and the distal esophageal remnant.

- TEF may be associated with other congenital anomalies signified by the acronym VACTERL, which stands for **v**ertebral anomalies, **a**nal atresia, **c**ardiac abnormalities, **TE**F and/or esophageal atresia, **r**enal agenesis or dysplasia, and **l**imb defects.

Additional content is available online including chapters on Nuclear Medicine, Artificial Intelligence, Radiation Dose and Safety, an Early History of Radiology, and a compendium of 200 Diagnostic Radiology Signs.

# 28

# Using Image-Guided Interventions in Diagnosis and Treatment (Interventional Radiology)

*Jeffrey L. Weinstein, MD, FSIR, and Natasha Larocque, MD, FRCPC*

Interventional radiology (IR), also known as **vascular and interventional radiology (VIR),** is a medical specialty that utilizes **image guidance** to perform minimally invasive diagnostic or therapeutic procedures. Image guidance may be provided by fluoroscopy, ultrasound (US), computed tomography (CT), or magnetic resonance imaging (MRI).

## CASE QUIZ 28 QUESTION

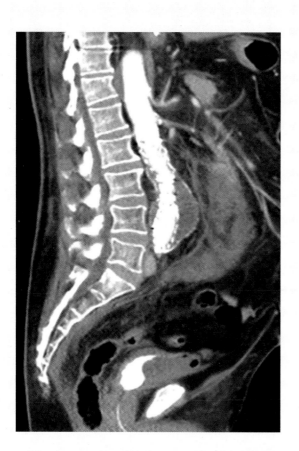

This is an image from a contrast-enhanced, sagittal CT angiogram of the abdomen in an 80-year-old male with a pulsatile abdominal mass. How might an image-guided intervention help in this case? The answer is at the end of this chapter.

- Interventional radiologists perform a wide variety of procedures that can be characterized as **vascular** or **nonvascular** and subdivided into the vascular distribution or organ system for the procedure being performed.
- This chapter will discuss the **indications, techniques, and benefits** of image-guided interventions that cover a broad gamut of interventional procedures.

## ARTERIAL ACCESS AND ARTERIOGRAPHY

- **Arterial access** and **arteriography** are fundamentals of interventional radiology, allowing for diagnostic evaluation of numerous arterial pathologies (e.g., arteriovenous fistula, aneurysm, vascular occlusion, or vascular stenosis).

> ## ⯮ IMPORTANT POINTS
>
> - The **Seldinger technique** is the basis for modern vascular access, both arterial and venous. This method, first described by Dr. Sven Seldinger (a Swedish radiologist), uses a **hollow needle** to gain entry into a blood vessel. A **wire** is then passed through this needle, which is then removed and exchanged for a **catheter** placed over the wire. This **exchange** is the basis for the initial steps in a **majority** of **endovascular interventional radiology procedures** (Fig. 28.1).

### Indications for Arterial Access

- Arterial access is used to facilitate **image-guided arterial interventions** (e.g., *embolization* for active bleeding, *angioplasty* for arterial stenosis, and *sclerotherapy* for arteriovenous malformation).

### Procedure for Arterial Access

- **Arterial access** is most commonly accomplished from a **femoral** or **radial artery approach,** though other arteries can be used. The selection depends on a number of factors, including the type of intervention, the anatomic orientation of the vasculature, and the presence of a coagulopathy.
- Arterial access is traditionally performed over a **bony landmark,** which aids in **compression** of the artery to obtain hemostasis **after** the procedure is complete. In the case of

**femoral artery** access, the segment of artery **over the femoral head** is targeted with palpatory, fluoroscopic, and/or ultrasound guidance.

- Using the Seldinger technique, an access needle is ultimately exchanged over a wire for a vascular sheath (Table 28.1).
- **Ultrasound guidance** during the arterial puncture can sometimes facilitate vascular access, especially in cases of weakly palpable pulses or challenging anatomy.
- **Radial artery** or **brachial artery** access is similar to the femoral artery approach. In the case of brachial artery access, care must be taken to choose an access site that would allow for **compression** to obtain **hemostasis after the procedure.**
- Once arterial access is obtained and a catheter or sheath is in place, the injection of iodinated contrast can be performed for *arteriography* in the desired location.

## Benefits and Potential Risks of Arterial Access

- Arterial access and arteriography allow for **diagnostic evaluation** and **localization** of abnormalities and provide a route for endovascular **treatment** by minimally invasive means.

| TABLE 28.1 | Short Glossary of Interventional Tools |
|---|---|
| **Device** | **Description** |
| **Access needle** | The entry needle used at the puncture site for percutaneous procedures; all contain a central channel for introduction of a guidewire. |
| **Guidewires** | Thin wires of varying lengths, composition, and flexibility that are fed through the channel of the access needle, and over which other devices, themselves containing a hollow channel, can be fed. |
| **Catheters** | Tubular structures usually made of some kind of plastic with varying lengths, diameters, shapes, and coatings through which substances can be either withdrawn from or introduced into the body. |
| **Sheath** | A vascular access hollow tube, usually made of plastic, which allows for the exchange of catheters during a given procedure while maintaining vascular access through the same puncture site. |
| **Dilator** | Short, tapered catheters used to increase the diameter of the hole from percutaneous access to an organ, space, or vessel to allow easier passage of a catheter, sheath, or other device; sometimes used in a serial fashion from smaller to larger. |

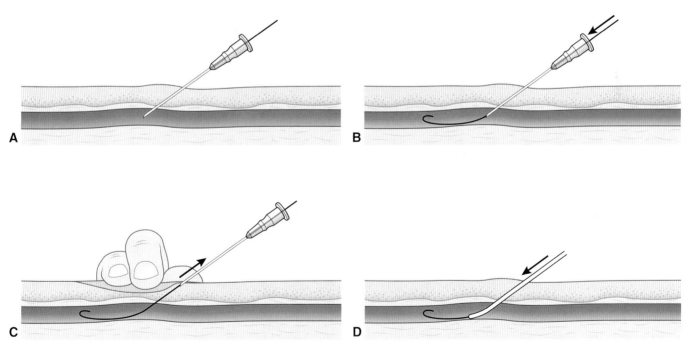

**Fig. 28.1 Seldinger Technique.** (A) Percutaneous puncture of a blood vessel with a hollow needle. (B) Introduction of an atraumatic guidewire through the needle into the blood vessel lumen. (C) Needle is removed while guidewire remains in place. Compression over the puncture secures the guidewire and prevents bleeding. (D) Angiographic catheter is advanced into vessel over the guidewire. (From Kadir S. Diagnostic Angiography. Philadelphia: WB Saunders; 1986:186.)

- **Risks** of arterial access include **bleeding** and **injury** to tissues and organs adjacent to the vessels as attempts are made to gain access, such as a ***pseudoaneurysm*** at the groin access site from puncture and arterial extravasation (see Fig. 19.6).
- Arterial access carries the further risk of **dissection**, **bleeding**, or **thrombosis** of the accessed vessel. There is a risk of **infection** and **injury** to the surrounding structures at the access site. Meticulous technique and experience can help mitigate many of these complications.

# CENTRAL VENOUS ACCESS: IMAGE-GUIDED VENOUS ACCESS

Indications for Central Venous Access
- *Central venous access* is a fundamental technique used throughout medicine that allows for entry into the venous system for:
  - **Intervention** (e.g., thrombolysis for an occlusive venous thrombus or inferior vena caval filter placement for prevention of pulmonary embolus or stenting).

- **Placement** of a port or catheter for pharmaceutical treatment for oncologic pharmacotherapy.
- **Hemodialysis/pheresis** (i.e., procedures in which blood is filtered, separated, and returned to the patient), as in ***plasmapheresis.***

## Procedure for Central Venous Access

- For venous access, **ultrasound guidance** is utilized to **locate** and **gain entry into the central veins** without injury to adjacent tissues/organs. Nearby anatomic landmarks or the relationship to a known artery may be used instead of ultrasound.
- The venous access site of choice depends on the type of procedure performed.
  - For **central venous** catheter placement, the **internal jugular, femoral,** and **subclavian veins** are commonly used as access points (Fig. 28.2).
  - **Peripherally inserted central venous catheters (PICCs)** are placed in the upper extremity veins, above the elbow, with the tip of the catheter usually located in the superior vena cava (see Fig. 9.9).

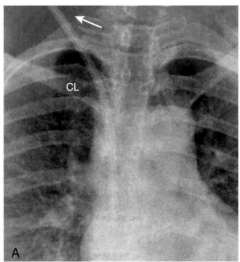

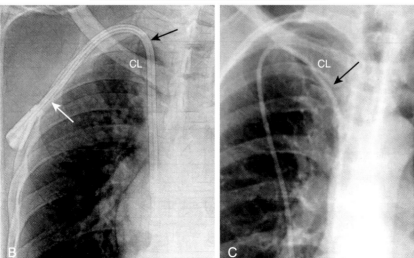

**Fig. 28.2** Central Venous Access. (A) This is a right internal jugular (IJ), nontunneled, central venous line (*arrow*). Notice its entry into the vein **above** the clavicle (CL), indicating an IJ line. (B) A tunneled hemodialysis line *(white arrow)* is seen in this image. It also enters the internal jugular vein **above** *(black arrow)* the clavicle (CL). (C) A right subclavian vein line is seen *(arrow)* that enters the subclavian vein **below** the level of the clavicle (CL).

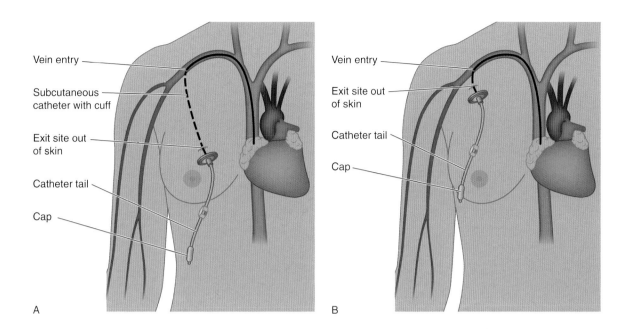

**Fig. 28.3** Tunneled and Nontunneled Access Catheters. (A) Central venous catheters can be **tunneled**, which requires an additional procedure in which a segment of the catheter is placed (tunneled) **under** the adjacent **soft tissues** *(dashed line)*. These catheters may have a segment in the subcutaneous tract wrapped in material to encourage cellular ingrowth to secure the catheter, which is referred to as a ***cuff***. They are considered to be more **resistant** to **central line infections** and are used for **long-term** hemodialysis or pharmacotherapy (e.g., chemotherapy or parenteral nutrition) (B) **A nontunneled catheter** enters the skin adjacent to or a short distance from the target vein. Nontunneled catheters are used for short-term therapy and in emergent situations.

- Most commonly, a needle is inserted into the selected vein with subsequent exchange for a catheter via a wire, using the Seldinger technique. Central venous catheters can be either *tunneled* or *nontunneled* (Fig. 28.3).

## Benefits and Potential Risks of Central Venous Access

- Central venous catheter placement allows for venous access, intervention, and pharmacotherapy. Tunneled or subcutaneous central venous access may obviate the need for repeated central access procedures if multiple treatments are necessary.
- **Risks** of venous access include **bleeding** and **injury** to tissues and organs adjacent to the vessels as attempts are made to gain entry. Access from the neck can be complicated by **pneumothorax, hemothorax,** and inadvertent subclavian and carotid **puncture. Arteriovenous fistula** formation is a rare, but reported, complication.

## PULMONARY EMBOLISM: THROMBOLYSIS

- *Massive pulmonary embolism* (**PE**) is defined as **PE with sustained hypotension.** This condition may be unrelated to the radiologic *burden of clot* in the pulmonary arterial

tree. The **burden of clot** generally refers to the qualitative assessment of thrombus in the pulmonary arteries. Quantitative scoring methods exist but are used infrequently.

> ▶▶ **IMPORTANT POINTS**
>
> - **First-line treatment** for massive PE, in the absence of a known contraindication, is **intravenous thrombolysis,** where a medication, such as **tissue plasminogen activator (tPA),** is administered in large doses to dissolve the clot.

## Indications for Catheter-Directed Pulmonary Embolism Thrombolysis

- **Indications** for catheter-directed pulmonary embolism thrombolysis include:
  - Patients who have **massive PE** and would be at high risk for developing a bleeding complication if they were to receive **systemic** intravenous thrombolytic medication.
  - Those who already have active bleeding, are perioperative from major surgery, or who have known metastatic cancer in the brain, for example, are at high risk to receive systemic thrombolytic therapy. They may be candidates for a more focal catheter-based intervention, such as

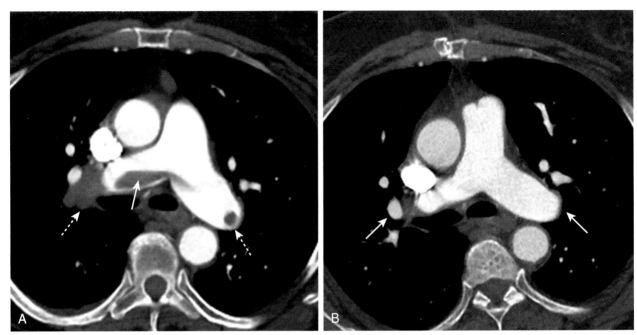

**Fig. 28.4** Pulmonary Embolism with Thrombectomy. This is a 45-year-old woman who presented with chest pain and shortness of breath. (A) CT-angiography of the chest demonstrates a saddle pulmonary embolism *(solid arrow)*, as well as bilateral lobar pulmonary emboli *(dashed arrows)*. (B) The same patient post-percutaneous mechanical thrombectomy with no residual pulmonary embolism *(arrows)*.

catheter clot fragmentation (Fig. 28.4), **aspiration** of clot, or lysis catheter placement.

- *Submassive pulmonary embolism* is defined as **PE without hemodynamic instability.** There is a wide spectrum of disease in this category, from a clinically asymptomatic subsegmental PE that was incidentally noted on chest CT to a large burden of clot in a patient who is tachycardic and may be short of breath.
  - Although the traditional treatment for submassive PE is intravenous anticoagulation, there has been research and a clinical movement toward **catheter-based therapies** for the subgroup with high-risk features for **progressing to massive PE.**
  - Among others, these risk features include **elevated biomarkers** (troponin and brain natriuretic peptide) and evidence of **right heart strain** on imaging.

## Procedure for Catheter-Directed Thrombolysis

- Under fluoroscopic guidance, a flexible catheter is inserted in the **common femoral vein** or **internal jugular vein** and threaded through the **heart** to access the **pulmonary arteries.**
- Various types of catheters with multiple holes can be placed into the **clot itself** to administer **thrombolytic medications** that can be infused over time to dissolve the clot. Other catheters that incorporate technologies to accelerate clot lysis, such as **ultrasound,** are also in use clinically. Still other devices can also be introduced that **fragment** or **aspirate** the thrombus.

## Benefits and Potential Risks of Catheter-Directed Thrombolysis

- **Catheter-based thrombolysis** or **thrombus removal** can **decrease the right heart pressure** rapidly and may prevent the patient from developing further hemodynamic compromise compared with anticoagulation alone.
- In the case of massive pulmonary embolism, catheter-based therapies may be **lifesaving** when systemic thrombolysis is contraindicated or is used but is unsuccessful in improving the patient's clinical status.
- **Risks** of catheter-based lysis include **bleeding** at **other sites** remote to the lytic infusion due to the systemic circulation of the medication after it passes through the lungs back through the heart.
- Additional risks include **arrhythmias** when passing catheters and wires through the heart and, rarely, **injury to the pulmonary artery, cardiac valves,** or **heart** itself.

## PULMONARY EMBOLISM: INFERIOR VENA CAVAL (IVC) FILTER PLACEMENT

### Indications for IVC Filter Placement

- IVC filter placement is a controversial topic but is generally accepted for the following US Food and Drug Administration–approved indications:
  - **Pulmonary thromboembolism** when **anticoagulation** is **contraindicated**

- **Progression of venous thromboembolic disease** despite use of anticoagulation
- **After massive PE** when anticipated benefits of conventional therapy are reduced
- **Chronic, recurrent PE** when anticoagulant therapy has **failed**
- Vena caval filters may be placed off-label on a case-by-case basis for other indications, such as prolonged immobility after trauma, prior to some types of surgery where the postoperative risk of PE is felt to be high, and as protection for proximal iliac or IVC deep-venous thrombosis.
- **Contraindications** to filter placement include an **inability to access the IVC** (e.g., due to thrombosis or anatomic anomalies) or a vena caval size **too large** or **too small** for a filter to deploy properly.
- IVC filters are most commonly placed in the **infrarenal IVC** in proximity to the renal vein inflow. This is felt to promote **lysis of clot** captured in the **filter** and **prevent filter thrombosis** (Fig. 28.5).
- A **suprarenal filter** is sometimes placed above the renal veins when required during **pregnancy,** when there is **insufficient room** below the renal veins to accommodate a filter, and in instances where there is **variant renal vein anatomy.**

## Procedure for IVC Filter Placement

- Central venous access is obtained via a jugular or femoral vein. The right jugular or right femoral vein is preferred given the typical rigidity of the IVC filter-delivery system, but the left common femoral vein is also commonly used

and placement via the upper extremity veins has been described.

- **IVC venography** is **first performed** with a diagnostic catheter to allow for:
  - Visualization of the **venous anatomy**, including location of the renal veins, and to see if any venous variants are present
  - Determination of the **size of the IVC,** which can affect the filter type chosen
  - Determination of **IVC patency**
- After the IVC anatomy and desired filter location have been determined, the catheter is exchanged for an **IVC filter-delivery sheath.** The filter is deployed from inside the sheath and the sheath is withdrawn.
- Postplacement venograms are sometimes performed to confirm appropriate positioning. The catheter and wire are removed. Pressure is then applied to the access site until hemostasis is achieved.

## Benefits and Potential Risks of IVC Filter Placement

- The intended benefit is to potentially **decrease** the incidence of new clinically significant **emboli to the lungs.** IVC filters **do not prevent new** deep-venous **thrombi from forming** nor do they decrease the amount of thrombus burden already present. The actual clinical benefit, which is still under investigation, is a source of debate.
- Potential **risks** include **filter migration, filter fracture,** or **filter element penetration through** the IVC wall. Caval and renal vein thrombosis are other rare, but significant,

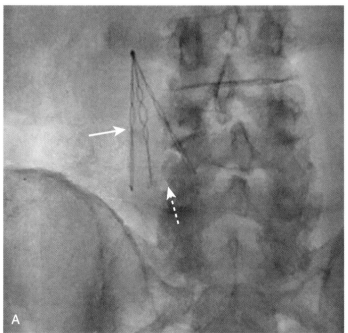
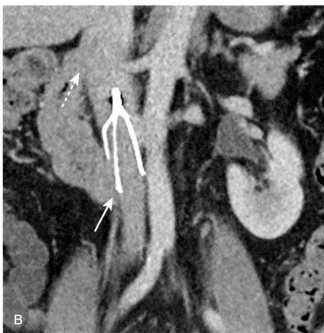

**Fig. 28.5 Inferior Vena Caval Filter.** (A) A filter (*solid arrow*) is deployed in the inferior vena cava (IVC) as seen on this close-up of a conventional radiograph of the lower abdomen. Hooks on the filter are designed to anchor it in the vena cava to prevent filter migration. The *dashed arrow* indicates the direction of blood flow in the IVC. (B) A coronal, contrast-enhanced CT shows an IVC filter (*solid arrow*) in appropriate position in the IVC below the location of the renal veins (*dashed arrow*).

complications. Some of the risks can be mitigated by retrievable filters if they are removed promptly after caval filtration is no longer medically necessary (Fig. 28.6).

- Although counterintuitive, IVC filters have been associated with an increased risk of deep vein thrombosis in the lower extremities.

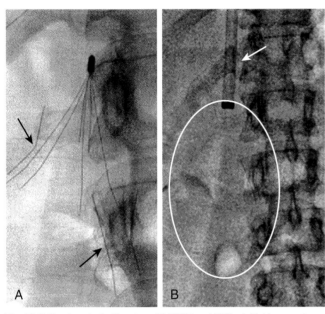

**Fig. 28.6** Retrieval of a Fractured IVC Filter. (A) The initial image shows fracture of the filter legs *(arrows)*. (B) Retrieval was attained by way of manipulations made through a vascular sheath *(arrow)*. After the filter itself was snared and removed, the fractured legs were then retrieved with no residual fragments remaining *(oval)*.

# IMAGE-GUIDED BIOPSY: GENERAL PRINCIPLES

- **Image-guided biopsy** is a means of accurately obtaining a **tissue sample** of a lesion for diagnostic analysis.
- Sampling of a lesion can determine its characteristics (benign or malignant) or provide additional information about a known lesion (cytogenetics).
- The lesion to be sampled should be reliably visualized on at least one imaging modality.

> ## ▶▶ IMPORTANT POINTS
>
> - Image-guided biopsy is indicated for the **minimally invasive sampling** of a lesion previously identified on an imaging study or when **pathology is in question** in order to aid in yielding a definitive diagnosis.

- **Sampling** of a lesion can be obtained through one of two techniques:
  - *Fine needle aspiration (FNA):* A small-gauge needle (e.g., 25 G) is inserted into the lesion under imaging guidance. The needle is then moved back and forth within the lesion to collect cells. Thyroid nodules are commonly sampled with this technique (Fig. 28.7A).
  - *Core biopsy:* A larger-gauge needle (e.g., 18 G) is inserted into the lesion under imaging guidance to remove a small piece of tissue. If the situation calls for **multiple samples** from a challenging location, a coaxial system is often used, which involves placing a **larger needle** into the lesion (called the *access needle*) and performing the biopsy using **smaller needles/devices** through the larger access needle (Fig. 28.7B).

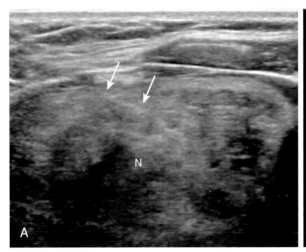 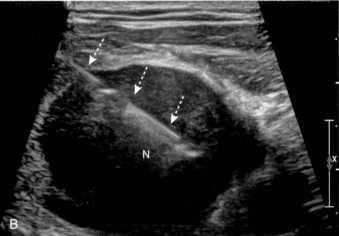

**Fig. 28.7** Fine Needle Aspiration and Core Biopsy, US. (A) Ultrasound shows a fine needle aspiration being performed using a small-gauge needle *(arrows)*, and shifting the needle back and forth within the lesion to collect cells. (B) Ultrasound image of a right neck mass shows a core biopsy being performed with a larger-gauge needle *(arrows)* in the lesion to acquire a small piece of tissue. *N,* Thyroid nodule.

## PULMONARY NODULE: IMAGE-GUIDED BIOPSY

### Indications for Pulmonary Nodule Image-Guided Biopsy

- To determine the **pathology** of a suspicious pulmonary nodule

### Procedure for Pulmonary Nodule Image-Guided Biopsy

- The modality that most reliably **demonstrates** the lesion should be used for the biopsy, if feasible; that is, if the lesion was best seen on CT, then CT localization will probably be used for the biopsy.
- A trajectory from a cutaneous entry point, along a percutaneous tract to the lesion is determined. Sometimes a course through a natural orifice may be used.
- Careful understanding of the anatomy is necessary to avoid injuring structures (e.g., blood vessels or nerves) that can lead to increased morbidity.
- A path that **limits the number of pleural surfaces crossed** by the biopsy needle and **avoids large blood vessels** is usually chosen.
- Under image guidance (CT, US, or fluoroscopy), a needle is advanced into the lesion with visual confirmation that the tip of the needle is in the lesion.
- Samples for pathology may be obtained by using a biopsy device to take pieces of tissue for analysis. Alternatively, fine needle aspiration could be performed to obtain samples for cytology (see Fig. 28.7).

- Other samples, such as for microbiology, may be taken at the same time, if clinically indicated.
- In some instances, a **fiducial marker,** which may be a small, metallic (typically gold) seed about the size of a grain of rice, can be left near the tumor to help guide future radiation therapy by providing a **standard point of reference** for localization (Fig. 28.8).

### Benefits and Potential Risks of Pulmonary Nodule Image-Guided Biopsy

- Image-guided biopsy provides a minimally invasive means of tissue sampling that can **eliminate the need for surgical biopsy** in many cases.
- **Risks** of such procedures include bleeding, infection, injury to surrounding organs and structures, and a false-negative biopsy result due to sampling error.
- In the specific case of pulmonary nodule biopsy, risks also include pneumothorax, hemothorax, pulmonary hemorrhage, chest wall hematoma, intercostal nerve injury, and even, very rarely, stroke from air embolism.

> **▶ IMPORTANT POINTS**
>
> - For **small** and **stable** pneumothoraces on serial images, the treatment is **conservative management** with observation.
> - **Chest-tube insertion** is indicated for a **large** or **symptomatic** pneumothorax or one that is **enlarging** on serial imaging studies.

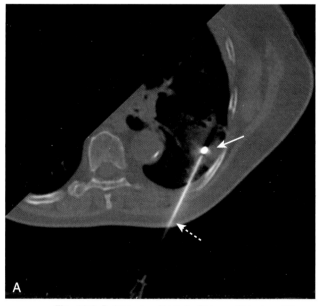 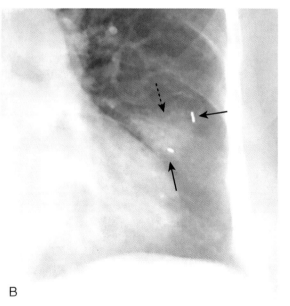

**Fig. 28.8 Pulmonary Nodule Biopsy.** This is a 76-year-old smoker with a left lower lobe nodule. (A) The biopsy needle *(dashed arrow)* traverses the nodule from a posterior approach. CT chest after biopsy of the nodule shows placement of a fiducial marker in the region of the lesion *(solid arrow)* to help facilitate future radiation therapy. The patient is lying in such a position so as to enable the biopsy needle to pass through the shortest path to reach the lesion and potentially reduce the risk of pneumothorax. This image has been reoriented to align with the orientation of panel B. (B) Chest radiograph after the procedure shows two fiducial markers *(solid arrows)* in the region of the biopsied nodule with a small amount of postbiopsy hemorrhage *(dashed arrow).*

# HEPATIC/RENAL/PULMONARY TUMORS: THERMAL ABLATION

- *Thermal ablation* is an umbrella term for tissue destruction using extreme heat or cold. Common forms of thermal ablation include *radiofrequency* and *microwave ablation* producing tissue **heating** and *cryoablation,* which has a cytotoxic effect through tissue **cooling.** Other forms of thermal ablation using laser and high-intensity, focused ultrasound are in practice at some centers.
- **Nonthermal ablation** techniques include *chemical ablation* (e.g., using acetic acid or ethanol) and newer technologies, such as irreversible *electroporation,* a process that increases the permeability of the cell membranes causing cell death.

## Indications for Thermal Ablation

- **Pulmonary tumor ablation** is indicated for **early-stage lung cancer** (usually non-small-cell lung cancer) in patients who are **not candidates for resection** or who **refuse** surgical resection. Thermal ablation using either radiofrequency or microwave is most commonly used.
  - Pulmonary tumor ablation for **metastatic disease** may be considered for small volume, limited disease to the lungs in an otherwise controlled cancer.
- **Hepatic tumor ablation** was first performed using chemical ablation but thermal means, predominately using heat in the form of radiofrequency ablation and microwave ablation, is most commonly used now. Microwave usage is newer, and its use has increased because of its ability to produce an ablation area of similar size to radiofrequency, but in less time (Fig. 28.9).
  - Hepatic tumor ablation is most efficacious in **early-stage, small, hepatocellular carcinomas** (≤3 cm); *oligometastatic disease* in patients who are not surgical candidates; or as a bridge to transplantation for patients with hepatocellular carcinoma. **Oligometastatic** is defined as a state

of highly localized and limited metastatic tumors for which local ablative therapy might be curative.
- **Renal tumor ablation** is generally performed with **radiofrequency** or **cryoablation**, with the latter more frequently used because of the ability to monitor the active ablation zone appropriate to treat the tumor while sparing as much normal kidney parenchyma as possible.
  - Renal tumor ablation is indicated for **small renal masses** in patients who have **comorbid conditions** that prevent surgery, have a condition that requires sparing of renal parenchyma (e.g., a **solitary kidney**), or who **refuse surgical** removal and desire a minimally invasive treatment.

## Procedure for Thermal Ablation

- Ablation probes can be placed using image guidance from US, CT, or MRI.
- Depending on the modality of ablation used, the type of tumor to be ablated (i.e., pulmonary, hepatic, or renal), and the morphology of the tumor, **multiple probes or multiple overlapping ablations may be used** to ablate the entire tumor effectively.
- Imaging is obtained before and during the procedure to ensure the probes are placed for effective treatment and to monitor the ablation margin, depending on the modality used.
- Adjustments in the ablation settings and duration are based on the intraprocedural imaging.
- Postablation imaging is often performed to evaluate for procedural complications (e.g., bleeding or pneumothorax) and the adequacy of ablation.

> ▶ **IMPORTANT POINTS**
>
> - An adequate margin beyond the visibly involved tissue is recommended to reduce the chance of incomplete ablation or residual tumor. In the case of hepatocellular carcinomas, a 1-cm margin or more is usually desired.

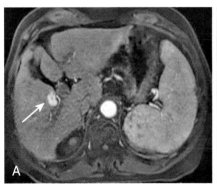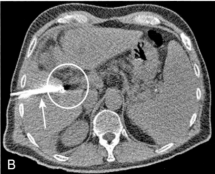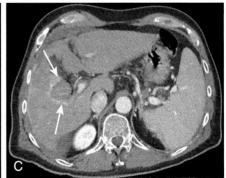

**Fig. 28.9** Pre- and Postablation of a Hepatocellular Carcinoma (HCC). (A) This 62-year-old male with history of hepatitis C presented with abdominal pain and was found to have a mass in the liver consistent with a hepatocellular carcinoma, as shown enhancing in the arterial phase of this postcontrast T1-weighted MRI image *(arrow)*. (B) This CT image was obtained for localization confirmation during the microwave ablation of the lesion seen in Fig. 28.9A. The ablation probe *(arrow)* is implanted within the tumor *(circle)*. (C) CT imaging immediately after microwave ablation of the tumor demonstrates a geographic area of hypoattenuation with a peripheral-enhancing rim *(arrows)* representing expected postablation changes.

## Benefits and Potential Risks of Thermal Ablation

- Thermal ablation provides a minimally invasive approach for treatment of primary or metastatic tumors. In the appropriate setting, ablation may **obviate the need for surgery** and reduce morbidity in patients who are not candidates for surgical treatment.
- **Risks** of thermal ablation include infection, bleeding, and injury to adjacent tissues or solid organs through unintended thermal injury, or injuries caused by the probe itself (including pneumothorax). Although controversial, a potential risk exists of spreading the tumor (i.e., *seeding*), but certain ablation techniques may mitigate such an occurrence.

## PORTAL HYPERTENSION: TRANSJUGULAR INTRAHEPATIC PORTOSYSTEMIC SHUNT (TIPS)

- **TIPS** placement (usually shortened to just TIPS) is a minimally invasive procedure for **lowering the portal pressure** by **decompression** through the creation of a **portal-hepatic venous shunt.** This shunt allows blood to **bypass the parenchyma of the diseased liver** in order to return to the heart via the systemic circulation.
- By doing so, the shunt **decreases** the pressure in the portal venous system and can help control the sequelae of sinusoidal or postsinusoidal portal hypertension, most especially **varices** (Fig. 28.10). TIPS can also act as a conduit for portal, splenic, or superior mesenteric vein thrombectomy/thrombolysis.

## Indications for TIPS

- The major indications for TIPS are the control of **recurrent variceal bleeding** refractory to endoscopic and medical management and **control of abdominal ascites** and/or

**hepatic hydrothorax** that does not respond to medical management. Additional indications include treatment of hepatic congestion from Budd-Chiari syndrome and as a means of access for portomesenteric thrombectomy/thrombolysis.

## Procedure for TIPS

- Traditionally, right-sided, internal jugular venous access is obtained with subsequent catheterization of a hepatic vein, classically the right hepatic vein (Fig. 28.11).

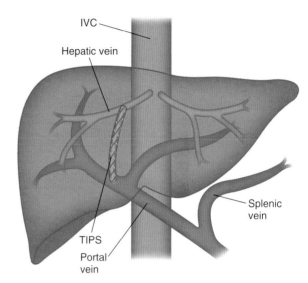

**Fig. 28.11 TIPS Illustration.** This illustration demonstrates the anatomic placement of a transjugular intrahepatic portosystemic shunt (TIPS). The shunt itself is a stent (TIPS) that connects a hepatic vein (most commonly the right hepatic vein) to the portal vein (most commonly the right branch of the portal vein), as depicted here. Blood coming toward the liver from the portal vein can bypass the resistance in the liver parenchyma, usually due to cirrhosis, and course through the stent to the hepatic vein where it returns to the IVC and right heart. This decompression procedure may reduce bleeding from varices or accumulation of ascites from portal hypertension.

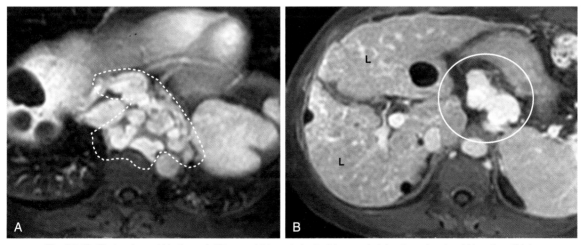

**Fig. 28.10 Cirrhosis and Varices.** A 55-year-old female had a history of cirrhosis and variceal bleeding. (A) An image from a contrast-enhanced MRI shows large paraesophageal varices *(dashed outline)* and (B) gastric varices *(circle)*, both of which are the sequelae of portal hypertension. The liver (L) displays a nodular contour consistent with cirrhosis.

- A long needle is placed through a curved cannula in the **hepatic vein** to direct the needle **through the hepatic parenchyma toward the portal vein.** From the right hepatic vein, the right portal vein is anatomically anterior and inferior.
- Gentle aspiration is performed with slow withdrawal of the needle or catheter, and blood return indicates that the needle or catheter is in a blood vessel. Contrast is then injected to confirm **portal venous** access.
- A wire is passed from the hepatic vein catheter/needle into the portal vein over which a **stent** is ultimately passed and **deployed across the tract from the portal vein back to the hepatic vein-IVC junction.** A specialized TIPS stent is available that is partially covered in a material to act as a barrier to tissue ingrowth and to line the parenchymal tract.
- Pressure measurements in the **portal vein** and **right atrium** are obtained both before and after placing the TIPS to assess for decrease in the gradient between the portal system and the systemic venous system.
    - A **reduction** in the portal pressure gradient to **<12 mm Hg** is recommended to reduce the chance of bleeding from varices.
- **Embolization** of esophageal and gastric **varices** may be performed before or after placing a TIPS stent, based on operator preference.
- Repeat venography is done to assess flow through the TIPS, which should demonstrate preferential flow **through the TIPS** as opposed to through the varices. Pressures are rechecked to confirm a reduction in the gradient between the portal pressure and right atrial pressure (Fig. 28.12).
- Usually, the TIPS is monitored with serial ultrasound to confirm patency and assess for any developing stenosis that may require intervention.

### Benefits and Potential Risks of TIPS placement

- **TIPS** can provide relief of portal hypertension and often reduce or eliminate symptoms of variceal bleeding or recurrent ascites.
- **Risks** of TIPS are generally divided into **procedural complications/risks** and **postprocedural complications/risks.**
    - **Procedural risks** include hepatic injury/infarction, hemoperitoneum, pneumothorax, skin radiation injury (from prolonged radiation exposure), hemobilia, and injury to the biliary system or adjacent organs.

> ### ▶ IMPORTANT POINTS
>
> - ***Hepatic encephalopathy*** is a **common postprocedural complication** as blood flow after TIPS is shunted through the liver without being detoxified. Although the exact cause is not well-known, increased blood ammonia levels and other byproducts are thought to play a role. Hepatic encephalopathy can often be **managed medically.**

- Additional **postprocedural complications** include **recurrent variceal bleeding** or **ascites,** as well as shunt dysfunction, including TIPS thrombosis.
- Heart failure from increased volume of blood return to the right heart and progressive liver failure from decreased perfusion are also known complications.

## ABSCESS: PERCUTANEOUS ABSCESS ASPIRATION AND DRAIN PLACEMENT

- **Abscess aspiration and drain placement** can provide definitive diagnosis and help bring curative relief for infected collections that are accessible with image guidance.

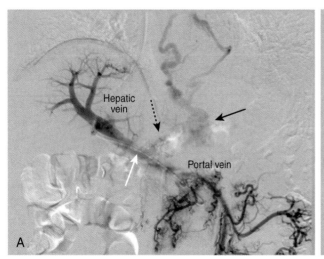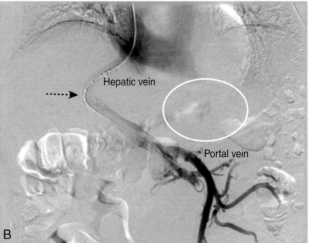

**Fig. 28.12 Transjugular Intrahepatic Portosystemic Shunt (TIPS) Procedure.** (A) A catheter (*white arrow*) has been placed through the TIPS tract connecting the hepatic vein, through the liver parenchyma, to the portal vein. Opacification of the left gastric vein (*dashed black arrow*) and gastric varices (*solid black arrow*) are secondary to elevated portal venous pressures, promoting flow through the varices. (B) A stent (*arrow*) has now been placed through the parenchymal tract connecting the hepatic and portal venous systems. The varices are no longer filling with contrast (*oval*), illustrating the desired physiologic change in the pressure gradient through the portal venous system.

- The abscess or fluid collection can be targeted for **sampling** with **aspiration** if the diagnosis is unclear, or a drain may be placed through the percutaneous tract used to access the abscess to allow for **drainage.**
- Common regions for abscess drainage include the mediastinum; abdomen (intraperitoneal and retroperitoneal); pelvis; gluteal region; and solid organs, such as the liver, kidney, and spleen.

## Indications for Abscess Aspiration and Drain Placement

- Imaging modalities used for aspiration and drain placement include ultrasound, fluoroscopy, and/or CT.

> ## IMPORTANT POINTS
>
> - In general, any complex fluid collection diagnosed as an abscess or suggestive of an abscess on imaging that includes some component that can be drained (i.e., is **liquid in character**) is a candidate for image-guided aspiration and possible drain placement.

## Procedure for Abscess Aspiration and Drain Placement

- Preprocedural imaging is reviewed to determine whether there is **enough fluid** present to place a needle and catheter into the collection for safe aspiration and drainage.
- The skin and subcutaneous tract are anesthetized and, under image guidance, a needle is passed through the tract into the collection.
- The target location is confirmed by imaging, and aspiration is performed, at which time aspirate may be sent to the laboratory for analysis, if desired.
- Once the determination has been made that a drain will be left in place, a wire is placed into the abscess cavity through the needle that was used to access it.
- A **drainage catheter** is then placed into the abscess cavity over the wire and the wire is removed, with the subsequent

creation of a **retaining loop** to keep the drainage catheter seated within the cavity (Fig. 28.13). Another technique utilizes a **trocar,** which functions as the access needle from which the drain is fed directly into the collection.
- The drainage catheter is then **anchored** in place with subcutaneous sutures and is connected to a drainage bag.
- The drain is left in place **until the infection has cleared**, as demonstrated by clinical factors (e.g., symptoms abate or patient is afebrile); laboratory values normalize; and there is no significant drainage (e.g., <10 mL/day) (see Fig. 28.13C).
- The precise drainage removal parameters are dictated by a clinical assessment of the patient on a case-by-case basis. In some centers the tube is injected under fluoroscopy to confirm patency of the drain and exclude the presence of any residual collection or fistula to adjacent structures prior to removal.

## Benefits and Potential Risks of Abscess Aspiration and Drain Placement

- Abscess aspiration and drainage provide diagnostic information and curative treatment to those affected. Percutaneous drainage can eliminate the need for surgery in many cases
- **Risks**, depending on location, include:
  - **Spread of infection**, including septic shock, peritonitis, or mediastinitis
  - **Bleeding**, hematoma, hemoperitoneum, or hemothorax
  - **Fistula formation** by forming a tract into adjacent structures or forming a tract into the subcutaneous soft tissues, creating a cutaneous fistula

# GASTROINTESTINAL (GI) BLEEDING: ARTERIOGRAPHY AND EMBOLIZATION

- **GI bleeding** from either an upper or lower GI source can cause symptomatic anemia or hemodynamic instability and could result in death if not treated.
- Presenting **symptoms** can vary from hematemesis, melena, or bright red blood per rectum *(hematochezia).*

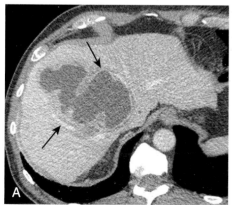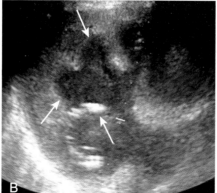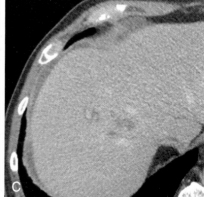

**Fig. 28.13 Hepatic Abscess with Drain.** (A) Contrast-enhanced CT of the abdomen demonstrates a large liver abscess *(arrows)* in a 74-year-old male patient with recurrent fevers. (B) Under ultrasound guidance, a percutaneous, pigtail-catheter drain was positioned in the collection *(arrows)* and was left in place to allow for resolution of the abscess while the patient simultaneously received antibiotic therapy. (C) A contrast-enhanced CT of the liver 2 months later shows resolution of the abscess.

- The initial **imaging study of choice** for a **lower GI bleed (LGIB)** is **CT-angiography** (Fig. 28.14A) or, possibly, a radionuclide tagged−red blood cell scan to assess for the location and presence of active bleeding.
- Frequently, **endoscopic evaluation** is the first diagnostic/therapeutic maneuver in patients with **upper GI bleeding (UGIB)** (proximal to the ligament of Treitz) to identify the source of bleeding that, if located, may be treated by the endoscopist.

## Indications for GI Arteriography and Embolization

- **Indications** for GI arteriography and embolization include:
  - **Positive bleeding scan** (abdominal CT-angiography or tagged-red blood cell study demonstrating active lower GI bleeding [see Fig. 28.14A]).
  - **Active upper GI bleeding** demonstrated on endoscopy with an inability to satisfactorily treat the bleeding from an endoscopic approach.
  - **Massive lower GI hemorrhage** with **hemodynamic instability** that generally warrants immediate interventional radiology and surgery consults and may bypass noninvasive diagnostic imaging.
  - Those who have ongoing symptomatic **anemia** with **melena**, requiring **frequent blood transfusions** despite negative or equivocal body imaging studies.

## Procedure for GI Arteriography and Embolization

- Review of preprocedural CT-angiography, tagged RBC scan, or endoscopy is done to aid in localization of the bleeding. Arterial access is then obtained and arteriography is performed in the branch arteries supplying the area of concern.
- If **initial arteriography is negative**, a stepwise approach can be performed to interrogate major branch vessels of the upper and lower bowel arterial anatomy (e.g., the

gastroduodenal artery in upper GI bleeding and the right colic artery in a LGIB).

- In the case of **upper GI bleeding, prophylactic embolization** of the blood vessel supplying the anatomic area of reported bleeding may be performed because of the **rich collateral supply** to the organs of the upper abdomen and the low incidence of visualizing active bleeding on angiography despite ongoing active bleeding.
- In the case of **lower GI bleeding, embolization** is usually **only performed if the source of active bleeding is identified.** This is because of the **increased risk of ischemia** compared with the upper GI tract (see Fig. 28.14).
- The type of embolic material used (e.g., metallic coil, cyanoacrylate glue, or Gelfoam™) depends on the location of the bleed, the patient's hemodynamic status, and comorbidities, as well as operator preference.
- Once embolization of the bleeding is complete, a **postembolization arteriogram** is performed to ensure the bleeding has stopped.

## Benefits and Potential Risks of GI Arteriography and Embolization

> **▶▶ IMPORTANT POINTS**
>
> - **GI arteriography and embolization** can provide diagnostic confirmation of the **location** of bleeding and then allow **intervention** that can lead to symptomatic relief and may be lifesaving in severe cases of GI bleeding.

- **Risks** of GI arteriography and embolization consist of the standard risks of arteriography, including vessel dissection from manipulation with guidewires, bleeding, and/or access site hematoma.

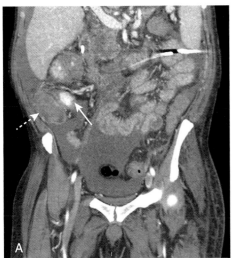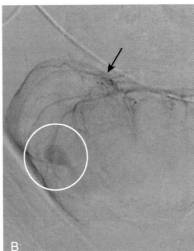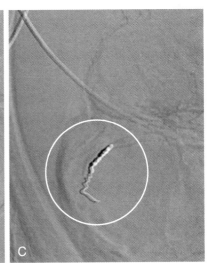

**Fig. 28.14 CT Angiogram Showing Lower GI Bleed.** A 36-year-old male presented to the emergency department with bright red blood per rectum. (A) CT-angiography (CTA) of the abdomen and pelvis displays a focal, active extravasation of contrast in the terminal ileum (*solid arrow*). The cecum is distended with densities representing stool and blood products (*dashed arrow*). (B) These **digital subtraction images** are produced by imaging an area before contrast is given and then using that image to electronically mask-out all but the contrast in subsequent images. Delayed digital subtraction imaging of the ileocolic artery (*arrow*) shows a focal blush of contrast (*circle*) in the region of the cecum and terminal ileum corresponding to the region of active extravasation on the CTA, originating from a branch of the ileocolic artery. (C) Status postinsertion of a coil for embolization of the bleeding vessel (*circle*), there is no further extravasation.

- *Nontarget embolization* can occur and refers to placement of embolic material in an unintended vessel because of catheter malpositioning or a technical issue in deploying the embolic agent.
- **Ischemia** can occur after embolization, which can result in bowel infarction that in turn can lead to perforation, possibly requiring surgical resection. This is more likely after embolization of lower GI bleeding, where the collateral blood supply is less robust compared with the upper GI tract.

## OBSTRUCTIVE UROPATHY: PERCUTANEOUS NEPHROSTOMY (PCN)/ NEPHROURETEROSTOMY (PCNU)

- **Obstructive uropathy,** or obstruction of the renal collecting system, can cause symptoms of renal colic and radiating flank pain and can lead to renal failure or urosepsis if not recognized and treated promptly.
- **Renal obstruction** can be secondary to **renal calculi** that become lodged within the ureter (see Fig. 16.7), **malignancy** within the abdomen or pelvis (including bladder or urothelial tumors of the ureter), or secondary to **ureteral inflammatory changes** (e.g., Crohn's disease, diverticulitis, or retroperitoneal fibrosis). Renal obstruction will demonstrate varying degrees of **hydronephrosis** on imaging.

### Indications for Percutaneous Nephrostomy/ Nephroureterostomy

- **Indications** for percutaneous nephrostomy/nephroureterostomy include:

- **Hydronephrosis,** either with or without signs of **renal failure,** infection, or secondary to renal/ureteral stones, malignancy, or inflammation
- **Urinary diversion** that is not amenable to urologic intervention in cases of ureteral rupture, leak, or fistula formation between the ureter and adjacent organs
- **Preoperative access** to the urinary collecting system prior to *ureteroplasty* (dilation of the ureter) or *nephrolithotomy* (stone removal)

### Procedure for Percutaneous Nephrostomy/ Nephroureterostomy

- Preprocedural imaging is reviewed to determine the best approach for percutaneous access to the desired renal calyx.
- **Ultrasound and/or fluoroscopic guidance** is used to help determine the approach to the target so as to deliver superficial and subcutaneous anesthetic along the approach route.
- An **access needle** is then used to course along the anesthetized tract under image guidance until the tip lies within a **renal calyx,** which is confirmed by aspiration of urine and often an injection of contrast.
- A guidewire is then inserted through the needle into the renal pelvis with subsequent **dilation** of the access tract prior to catheter placement.
- If *percutaneous nephrostomy (PCN)* placement is desired, the nephrostomy catheter is inserted over the wire with a **locking** *(retention)* **loop** formed within the renal pelvis (Fig. 28.15A).
- For *percutaneous nephroureterostomy (PCNU),* a series of catheters and guidewires are maneuvered from the kidney to **cross** the stricture/stenosis/obstruction to the urinary

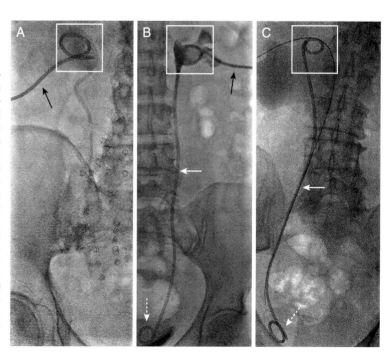

Fig. 28.15 Percutaneous Nephrostomy Tubes. (A) **A percutaneous nephrostomy tube (PCN)** includes a percutaneous component that enters through the skin, traverses the retroperitoneum *(arrow),* enters the kidney from a lower pole calyx, and contains a retention loop in the renal pelvis *(square).* This tube is connected externally to a bag to divert urine. (B) A **percutaneous nephroureteral stent (PCNU)** has a similar course to a PCN externally *(black arrow)* but has a longer internal component extending down the ureter *(solid white arrow)* to the urinary bladder. It has a retention loop in the renal pelvis *(square)* and another more caudal loop in the bladder *(dashed white arrow).* Side-holes along the internal part of the tube allow for this tube to drain into a bag or, after capping the tube, into the urinary bladder. (C) A **double-J stent** *(solid arrow)* can be placed by a urologist from a transurethral, retrograde approach or an interventional radiologist from an antegrade approach, as here. This tube has retention loops caudally in the bladder *(dashed arrow)* and cranially in the renal pelvis *(square)* and only allows for internal drainage. Once the percutaneous access is removed, a double-J stent can only be manipulated from below by a urologist or would require new percutaneous access to the kidney from above.

bladder, at which time the PCNU is advanced into the bladder and loops are formed in the bladder and renal pelvis (Fig. 28.15B).

- Alternatively, a *double-J stent* can be placed urologically (Fig. 28.15C).
- PCN and PCNU catheters are secured to the skin and **connected to a drainage bag** for urine collection. At some point a **cap** may be placed on the external portion in order to **promote internal drainage** through the bladder and urethra so long as there is antegrade drainage.

## Benefits and Potential Risks for Percutaneous Nephrostomy/ Nephroureterostomy

> ### ▶▶ IMPORTANT POINTS
>
> - PCN and PCNU placement can provide symptomatic relief of **obstructive uropathy;** allow for **urinary diversion;** decompress an obstructed, infected collecting system; or be used for preprocedural access in a minimally invasive manner.

- **Risks** of PCN and PCNU placement are bleeding, bacteremia through spread of infection during placement, peritonitis, and pneumothorax in cases where the approach is high enough to cross the pleura.
- Renal hemorrhage, pseudoaneurysm formation, or renal arteriovenous fistula formation can cause severe symptoms and in rare cases may require additional surgical or radiology intervention (e.g., embolization of a bleeding vessel).

## AORTIC ANEURYSM: ENDOVASCULAR ANEURYSM REPAIR (EVAR)

- An **aortic aneurysm** is a focal or segmental enlargement of the aorta resulting from weakening of all three layers of the arterial wall.
- **True aortic aneurysms** are defined by an enlargement that is greater than 1.5 to 2 times the aorta's normal size and can occur anywhere along the course of the aorta, although they are **more common** in the **abdominal aorta.**

> ### ▶▶ IMPORTANT POINTS
>
> - Small aortic aneurysms are usually periodically imaged because of the increasing risk of rupture if they enlarge. **Intervention** usually occurs if the patient is **symptomatic** or when the abdominal aortic aneurysm reaches **5.5 cm in diameter in men or 5.0 cm in women** or the aneurysm **grows** over a **short period** of time.

- **Aneurysm repair** can be achieved either with **open surgical repair** or through an **endovascular approach (EVAR)** with a covered stent placement *(endograft)*, which forms an **endoluminal channel** through which the blood flows with the purpose of **excluding flow through the aneurysm sac** itself.
  - *Covered stents* are generally metal stents wrapped with a fabric or graft material designed to **inhibit** the eventual growth of tissue that may **occlude the stent** and prevent flow of blood through the interstices of the stent.

## Indications for EVAR

- A thoracic or abdominal aneurysm that is **asymptomatic and ≥5.5 cm in men or ≥5.0 cm in women** or has a growth rate of >1 cm/year or >0.5 cm in 6 months
- A **symptomatic** thoracic or abdominal aneurysm, regardless of size
- Thoracic or abdominal aneurysm with **known or impending rupture**

## Procedure for EVAR

- In general, preprocedural imaging entails CT or MR angiography to fully characterize the aortic aneurysm and best determine the ideal location to place the endovascular stent graft.
- Either unilateral or bilateral common **femoral artery access** is achieved using the Seldinger technique **percutaneously** or by performing surgical *cut-downs* (surgical opening of subcutaneous tissues to expose the arteries).
- A *marking catheter* is advanced into the aorta and an **aortogram** is performed, which also allows for length measurement of the stent graft needed for adequate coverage of the aneurysm.

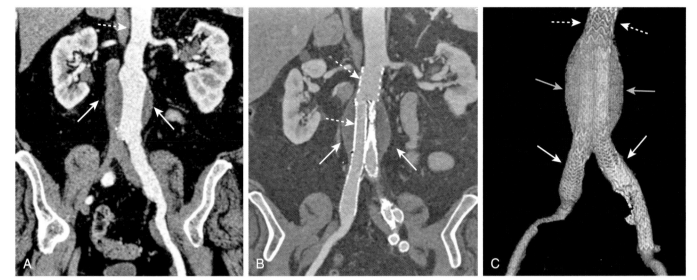

**Fig. 28.16 Endovascular Aneurysm Repair (EVAR).** A 65-year-old male presented with a history of an enlarging abdominal aortic aneurysm (AAA). (A) Coronal image from a CT angiogram demonstrates a fusiform infrarenal AAA *(solid arrows)* that measured 6.5 cm in maximum dimension (anterior to posterior). The aneurysm does not completely fill with contrast because it contains peripheral plaque/thrombus. The normal aortic caliber is noted above the level of the renal arteries *(dashed arrow).* (B) CT angiogram in the same patient after endovascular repair shows a covered stent (**stent graft**) *(dashed arrows)* that extends above and below the aneurysm sac *(solid arrows)* placed across the aneurysm to exclude it from the flow of blood. These covered stents are traditionally placed as several components that overlap and extend into the iliac arteries on both sides. Because of differing composition of materials for the components, their radiographic appearance can vary. (C) Color 3D reconstruction of the abdominal aorta after repair displays the aortic component of the covered stent *(dashed white arrows),* outline of the aneurysm that is being excluded *(blue arrows),* and inferior extension of the stents into both iliac arteries *(solid white arrows).*

- The stent graft is deployed over stiff guidewires to allow maximal control during placement (Fig. 28.16).
- The ideal placement ensures **no vital aortic branch vessels are occluded** during placement (e.g., superior mesenteric artery or renal arteries) or that a fenestrated stent graft is deployed to allow for patency of major arteries (e.g., renal arteries). The inferior mesenteric artery is often covered by the graft.
- A **completion aortogram** is performed to ensure that **no leak** exists around or through the new endograft.
- Surveillance imaging will look for any residual flow into the **excluded** part of the aneurysm, referred to as the *aneurysm sac.* Continued **flow** into the **excluded portion** of the aneurysm (i.e., the aneurysm sac) is referred to as an *endoleak.*
- Occasionally blood vessels that were excluded by the endograft can continue to bring blood **into** the **aneurysm sac.** This is most commonly seen with lumbar and inferior mesenteric arteries in abdominal endografts.

## Risks and Benefits of EVAR

- EVAR placement provides a minimally invasive option for repair of thoracic and abdominal aortic aneurysms, allowing patients to experience less intraprocedural blood loss and shorter hospital stays, all with comparable results to open repair in appropriately selected patients.
- **Risks** of EVAR placement are generally divided into two categories: **procedural-based** and **device-related.**

- **Procedural-based risks** include aneurysm perforation, organ ischemia, and groin and/or retroperitoneal hematoma.
- **Device-related risks** include stent-graft migration, stent fracture, stent thrombosis, and/or stenosis, and endoleak.

## UTERINE FIBROIDS: UTERINE FIBROID EMBOLIZATION (UFE)

- **Uterine fibroids (leiomyomas)** are benign uterine tumors. They may be markedly symptomatic and can be responsible for heavy menstrual bleeding (either **menorrhagia** or **meno-metrorrhagia**), abdominal and/or pelvic bloating, heaviness or discomfort, as well as urinary symptoms, and dyspareunia. They may also cause infertility.
- Uterine fibroids can be treated with **hormonal therapy,** excised individually through surgery (**myomectomy**), removed through a **hysterectomy,** or treated through **uterine fibroid embolization.**

### Indications for UFE

- UFE is indicated in women with documented uterine fibroids, causing symptoms of heavy menstrual bleeding, abdominal/pelvic pain/pressure/discomfort, urinary frequency or retention, dyspareunia, or any combination of these.

- UFE can be performed in patients with **adenomyosis**; however, current information shows that it is less effective than treating fibroids.

## Procedure for UFE

- Preprocedural evaluation includes review of imaging, which in most cases includes a gadolinium-enhanced pelvic MRI to best characterize the uterine fibroids and confirm their viability.
- Arterial access is achieved and uterine arteriography is performed bilaterally to establish the arterial distribution supplying the fibroids. The **uterine arteries** are usually a branch of the anterior division of the **internal iliac arteries** (Fig. 28.17).
- UFE is performed by injecting **embolic material** into the uterine arteries bilaterally to **slow** arterial flow. *Tris-acryl gelatin microspheres* (nonabsorbable) is a common product used for this purpose, but other materials, such as polyvinyl alcohol, have been described. The microspheres are injected until **stasis** within the artery is achieved, using angiography as a guide.

- Patients may undergo follow-up pelvic MRI as well as clinical evaluation to document fibroid size and character changes and interval change in symptoms (see Fig. 28.17C).

## Risks and Benefits of UFE

- UFE provides a minimally invasive approach toward treatment of uterine fibroids in patients who experience symptoms of heavy menstrual bleeding, abdominal pain, and/or discomfort, as well as urinary symptoms.
- **Risks** of UFE are much the same as other arterial interventions, including bleeding, infection, and vascular injury.
- Endometritis, uterine ischemia, and necrosis are also **rare** but reported complications that may require surgical intervention or hysterectomy and could be life-threatening, especially in the setting of infection.
- **Amenorrhea/early menopause** have been described as complications and tend to become more common as a woman gets closer to menopause. This may be caused by inadvertent ovarian embolization.
- **Fibroid passage** may occur in those individuals that have **intracavitary (endometrial cavity) or submucosal fibroids**

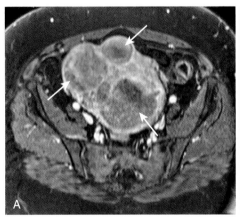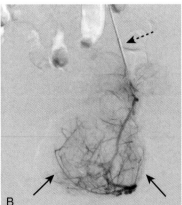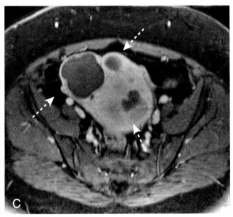

**Fig. 28.17 Uterine Fibroids and Uterine Fibroid Embolization (UFE).** (A) This 44-year-old woman, who presented with abdominal pain and menometrorrhagia, had multiple, hypoenhancing uterine masses consistent with uterine fibroids (*arrows*) seen on a T1-weighted, postcontrast MRI of the pelvis. (B) At the superior aspect of the angiogram image, the catheter (*dashed black arrow*) traverses the common iliac and internal iliac arteries, terminating in the uterine artery where a selective left uterine artery angiogram demonstrates significant arterial filling of the largest uterine fibroid (*solid black arrows*) when correlated with the preprocedural MRI. (C) A follow-up pelvic MRI done 4 months after uterine fibroid embolization shows the fibroids are smaller (*arrows*) and do not enhance now, a desired outcome that is consistent with the fibroids having undergone necrosis.

(see Fig. 18.18), as the ischemic changes cause sloughing of the fibroid. This may necessitate evaluation by a gynecologist to facilitate removal. Likewise **pedunculated subserosal fibroids** may detach from the uterus and migrate into the pelvis associated with infarction of their stalk.

## ACUTE ISCHEMIC STROKE: MECHANICAL THROMBECTOMY

- **Stroke** is the result of brain tissue death from a hemorrhagic or ischemic insult. It can result in permanent neurologic deficits or death.
- **Ischemic stroke**, if recognized early, can be treated with intravenous thrombolytics, most commonly **tissue plasminogen activator (tPA)** or **mechanical thrombectomy** to aid in revascularization of the affected brain before the infarct enlarges or undergoes hemorrhagic transformation, as neurons die quickly from ischemia.

### Indications for Thrombectomy in Stroke

- Therapy for acute ischemic stroke is a widely debated subject and is the topic of many research trials.
- Current data suggest that **mechanical thrombectomy,** with either a *stent retriever* (see below) or *thrombus aspiration,* may be performed in those with:

- A **good prestroke** functional status
- **Large-vessel occlusion** (internal carotid, middle cerebral, or first-branch of the middle cerebral arteries)
- An **onset of symptoms** that occurred <6 hours previously or did not respond to intravenous thrombolytic infusion (which is administered in ischemic stroke in patients with onset of symptoms within 4.5 hours of presentation). For posterior and possibly anterior circulation strokes, the intervention window may be considerably longer. **With new studies, these intervals may change.**
- **Significant neurologic deficit without** an extensive *infarct core* or **hemorrhage** on imaging of brain. The **infarct core** is that portion of the infarct that will not likely improve with reperfusion.

### Procedure for Mechanical Thrombectomy in Stroke

- Preprocedure imaging is **critical in directing therapy** in acute stroke and may entail noncontrast CT, CT-angiography, or CT or MRI perfusion imaging to identify the offending thrombus to be targeted for mechanical thrombectomy.
- Arterial access is obtained and a catheter is advanced into the internal carotid artery on the affected side. Angiography is performed. The thrombus is traversed using a microcatheter

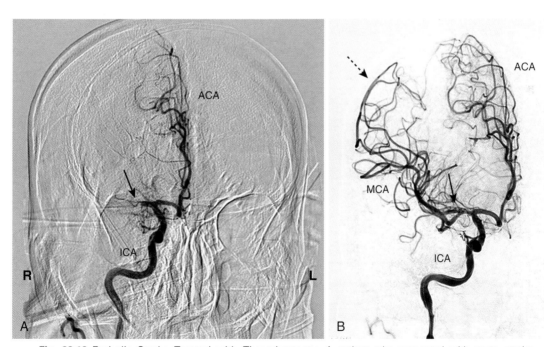

**Fig. 28.18 Embolic Stroke Treated with Thrombectomy.** A patient who presented with acute stroke symptoms was referred to angiography for evaluation. (A) This is a selective catheterization of the right internal carotid artery (ICA) that demonstrates abrupt cutoff (*arrow*) of the right middle cerebral artery (MCA) with no flow to most of the MCA's distribution. This correlates with an occlusive embolus in this segment, which was a potential target for intervention. Note that the anterior cerebral artery (ACA) and its branches are opacified. Because this is a selective catheterization of the right ICA, the left-sided vessels are not visualized. (B) In the same patient after mechanical thrombectomy, repeat right ICA arteriography shows perfusion of the entire right MCA distribution (*dashed arrow*) beyond the previously occluded point (*solid arrow*), signifying a technically successful intervention. *L,* Patient's left; *R,* patient's right.

and microwire, and a stent retriever device is passed through the microcatheter and unsheathed over the clot. The stent is allowed to dwell for a period of time and then pulled out through a larger guiding catheter. Aspiration systems also exist, which use suction to remove thrombus (Fig. 28.18).

- A ***stent retriever*** is a small stent that is permanently fused to a long wire. The stent can be deployed over a thrombus; it will incorporate the thrombus in its interstices and can then be removed while open to **pull the clot out** with it. Most devices can be used three times (three pulls) during a single procedure to remove clot.
- **Postprocedural arteriography** is performed to demonstrate **revascularization,** and follow-up CT imaging is done to assess the effects on the brain parenchyma after clot retrieval (e.g., hemorrhage).

## Risks and Benefits of Mechanical Thrombectomy in Stroke

- Mechanical thrombectomy is a critical treatment for eligible patients to prevent further neurologic deficits and salvage that part of the brain at risk of dying but is not already dead. Patient selection is key to having satisfactory clinical outcomes.
- **Risks** for mechanical thrombectomy are **significant** and include intracranial hemorrhage, arterial dissection or perforation during thrombectomy, embolization of clot fragments, reperfusion hemorrhage, and groin hematoma.

## CASE QUIZ 28 ANSWER

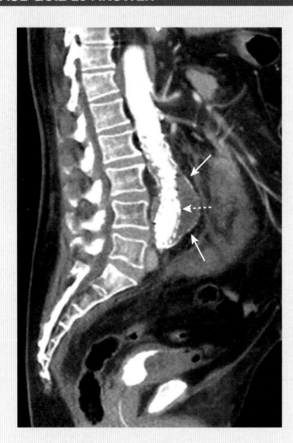

This is a CT angiogram in the same patient as the Case Quiz Question after an image-guided endovascular aneurysm repair (EVAR). A stent *(dashed arrow)* that extends above and below the aneurysm sac *(solid arrows)* was placed in the aorta to traverse the aneurysm in order to exclude it from the flow of blood and thus prevent subsequent rupture. EVAR is a technique that has transformed abdominal aortic aneurysm (AAA) repair, making intervention safer in high-surgical-risk patients.

## TAKE HOME POINTS

- The indications, procedures, and risks/benefits are described for a variety of procedures that form a part of **interventional radiology**, a medical specialty that uses image guidance to perform minimally invasive diagnostic and therapeutic procedures.
- Each procedure chosen highlights a different facet of the specialty: arterial access, central venous access, thrombolysis, image-guided biopsy, tumor ablation, shunt placement, percutaneous drainage, embolization, endovascular repairs, and thrombectomy.
- A **glossary** of terms applied to some of the more widely used tools in interventional radiology is included.
- **Arterial access** facilitates many other image-guided arterial interventions (e.g., embolization for active bleeding and angioplasty for arterial stenosis).
- **Central venous access** is used for venous intervention, pharmacotherapy, or hemodialysis. Tunneled catheters are used for long-term hemodialysis or pharmacotherapy (e.g., chemotherapy or parenteral nutrition).
- Patients who have a life-threatening, massive pulmonary embolism and are at high risk for developing a bleeding complication if they receive systemic intravenous thrombolytic medication may benefit from **catheter-directed thrombectomy/thrombolysis.**
- **Inferior vena caval filters** may be placed in patients with a pulmonary embolus when anticoagulation is contraindicated or when progression of the thromboembolic disease occurs despite use of anticoagulation as well as chronic, recurrent PE when anticoagulant therapy has failed.
- **Image-guided biopsy** is indicated for the minimally invasive sampling of a lesion previously identified on an imaging study or when the pathology of a lesion is in question.
- Common forms of **image-guided ablations** include radiofrequency and microwave ablation (through tissue heating), cryoablation (cooling), and chemical ablation. Pulmonary, hepatic, and renal tumors are those most frequently targeted.
- **Transjugular intrahepatic portosystemic shunt (TIPS)** placement is a minimally invasive procedure for lowering the portal pressure by creation of a portal-hepatic venous shunt. It is used most often to control recurrent variceal bleeding refractory to endoscopic and medical management and to control abdominal ascites secondary to cirrhosis.
- **Abscess aspiration and drain placement** can provide definitive diagnosis and offer curative relief for infected collections in locations accessible with image guidance.
- **GI bleeding,** either from upper or lower GI sources, can cause symptomatic anemia or possible hemodynamic instability and could result in death if not treated. In the case of lower GI bleeding, **embolization** can be performed if the source of active bleeding is identified.
- **Percutaneous nephrostomy (PCN)/nephroureterostomy (PCNU)** tubes can alleviate hydronephrosis secondary to renal/ureteral stones, malignancy, or inflammation. They can also be used for urinary diversion and preoperative access to the urinary collecting system.
- **Aneurysm repair** can be achieved with either open surgical repair or through an endovascular approach with a covered stent placement (endograft), which forms a new endoluminal channel through which the blood flows, the purpose being to exclude flow through the aneurysm itself and prevent rupture.
- **Uterine fibroid embolization** may be useful in women with documented uterine fibroids causing symptoms of heavy menstrual bleeding, abdominal or pelvic pain, pressure, discomfort, urinary frequency or retention, dyspareunia, or any combination of these symptoms.
- Image-guided intervention is used in patients with **strokes.** Mechanical thrombectomy may be performed in patients with a good prestroke functional status and large-vessel occlusion, and in those in whom certain temporal requirements from the onset of stroke symptoms are met.
- Each procedure described comes with its attendant **benefits** and certain **potential risks,** including—but not limited to—bleeding, infection, vessel or other organ injury, pneumothorax, and, rarely, radiation overexposure. In all cases, the potential benefits should outweigh the potential risks for a procedure to be performed.

Additional content is available online including chapters on Nuclear Medicine, Artificial Intelligence, Radiation Dose and Safety, an Early History of Radiology, and a compendium of 200 Diagnostic Radiology Signs.

# 29

# Recognizing the Findings in Breast Imaging

*Debra Copit, MD, FACR*

Breast imaging is the field of radiology dedicated to the detection and management of breast abnormalities, especially breast cancer. **Breast cancer** is second only to **skin cancer** as the **most common cancer** diagnosed in **women** and is the **second leading cause of cancer death in women,** behind lung cancer.

This is a view of both breasts from a mammogram of a 68-year-old female with a palpable breast mass. Based on the findings on this craniocaudal view of both breasts, what is the most likely diagnosis? The answer is at the end of the chapter.

- The **lifetime risk of breast cancer** is defined as the likelihood that a woman will develop cancer over an 80-year life span. For example, a woman with **no known risk factors** has a lifetime risk of developing breast cancer of **approximately 12%.**

- **Risk factors** for breast cancer include **early menarche, late menopause,** and other factors, some of which are shown in Table 29.1 and Box 29.1. Certain **histopathologic findings** also increase the risk of breast cancer.

**TABLE 29.1 Lifetime Risk Categories for Breast Cancer**

| Category | Percent Risk | Factors Affecting Risk |
|---|---|---|
| **Average** | <15% | No known risk factors |
| **Intermediate** | 15%—25% | Strong family history of breast cancer, but no *BRCA* mutation; those with a mutation in *CHEK2* (Box 29.1); those in the highest category of mammographic density; and those with a past history of lobular carcinoma *in situ* or atypical hyperplasia |
| **High** | >20% | *BRCA* mutation carriers and their untested first-degree relatives, such as a sister, mother, or daughter; women with histories of chest radiation between the ages of 10 and 30; a personal history of invasive breast cancer or ductal carcinoma *in situ* (DCIS) |

**BOX 29.1  *BRCA1* and *BRCA2* Genes**

- The most common cause of hereditary breast cancer is an inherited mutation damaging the *BRCA1* or *BRCA2* gene. **BRCA1** and **BRCA2** are human genes that are tumor suppressors. *BRCA* is an abbreviation for **BR**east **CA**ncer.
- Mutations in these genes correlate with an increased risk of breast cancer. If *BRCA1* or *BRCA2* are themselves damaged by a mutation, damaged DNA is not properly repaired.
- Females with a harmful variant of the *BRCA1* or *BRCA2* gene have up to an 80% risk of developing breast cancer by age 90. The increased risk of developing ovarian cancer is about 55% for females with *BRCA1* mutations and about 25% for females with *BRCA2* mutations.
- ***CHEK2*** (checkpoint kinase 2) is a tumor suppressor gene that encodes the protein CHK2. Inherited mutations in the *CHEK2* gene have been linked to certain cases of breast cancer.

# BREAST IMAGING MODALITIES: OVERVIEW

## Mammography

- The most widely studied and utilized of all breast imaging studies is *mammography*. A mammogram is a type of **low-dose x-ray imaging** developed to evaluate clinical breast abnormalities and to screen patients for breast cancer (Fig. 29.1).

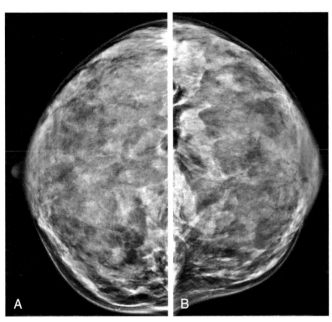

**Fig. 29.1 Mammogram.** Mammography, like all of radiography, uses the differential absorption of x-rays by fat, soft tissues, and calcifications to yield diagnostic images of the breast. It does this by using a very low dose of radiation. In this example of a right (A) and left (B) **craniocaudal view** of both breasts, the breast tissue is dense, which has diagnostic implications discussed in this chapter.

- Mammograms are performed on specialized radiographic units that produce **low-energy x-rays.** *Compression* is applied to the breast and used to improve image quality by reducing the **thickness** that the tissue x-rays must penetrate, decreasing radiation *scatter,* reducing the required radiation **dose**, and **preventing motion.** Mammographic images today are almost exclusively captured **digitally,** rather than on film.

- *Quality control* is an important part of any mammography program. Radiologists are evaluated with **regular audits** to determine how well they are performing. These include evaluation of **recall rate** (number of mammograms read that require additional views and/or ultrasound) and **positive predictive values** (how many patients that undergo biopsy return positive, i.e., cancerous, results).

- *Digital breast tomosynthesis (DBT)* (sometimes called *3D mammography*) is a type of mammography in which images are obtained at multiple different angles of the x-ray tube to create **thin slices** through the breast. It has been shown to reduce false-positive diagnoses while increasing invasive cancer detection (Fig. 29.2).

- Mammographic examinations are divided into *screening mammography* and *diagnostic mammography.* We discuss the differences between screening and diagnostic examinations later in this chapter.

## Contrast-Enhanced Mammography

- *Contrast-enhanced mammography (CEM)* is a developing technique that uses the same equipment as standard mammography and digital breast tomosynthesis but applies a principle of tumor enhancement similar to contrast-enhanced MRIs.

- After intravenous injection with iodinated contrast, a dual-energy mammogram is acquired. **Two images** of **each breast**

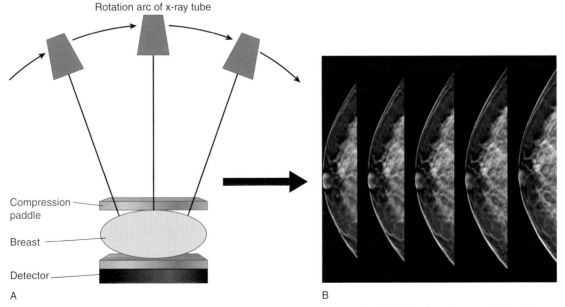

**Fig. 29.2 Digital Breast Tomosynthesis.** Digital breast tomosynthesis (DBT) involves the acquisition of multiple *slices* across an arc (A) that are then reconstructed into a series of stacked images (B). The stacked images provide localization information and improved lesion characterization, potentially decreasing or eliminating the need for additional diagnostic studies. (*Courtesy Hologic, Inc.,* https://www.hologic.com/)

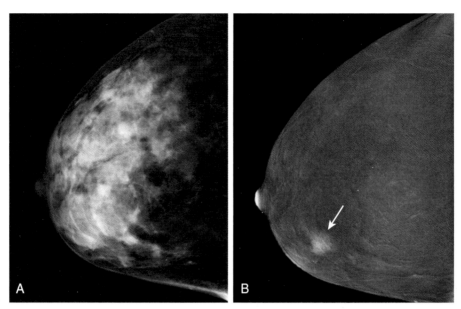

**Fig. 29.3 Contrast-enhanced Mammography (CEM).** The standard lower-energy mammographic image (A) shows dense tissue but no abnormality. (B) A second image obtained using higher energy x-rays better absorbed by the iodine in the contrast agent is digitally "subtracted" from the lower-energy image and the resultant mammographic image reveals a suspicious mass in the medial aspect of the same breast *(arrow)*.

are then available for display; one looks like a regular mammogram and the other highlights any areas that enhance with contrast after masking-out the tissues that do not enhance. Tumors are known to enhance because of tumor angiogenesis. (Fig. 29.3).

- CEM may be especially useful in women at increased risk for developing breast cancer or those with dense breasts.

## Ultrasound (US)

- **Breast ultrasound** is most commonly used in conjunction with **diagnostic mammography,** but may also be performed as an **additional screening method.**
- **Indications for US include:**
  - **Problem-solving** for asymptomatic patients **recalled** from a screening mammogram for additional breast imaging

- Evaluating **symptomatic patients** (Fig. 29.4)
- The initial study used in average-risk, symptomatic patients **under 30 years of age**
- Studies have shown that screening **high-risk patients** and patients with **dense breasts** with **ultrasound increases breast cancer detection** over mammography alone.

## Magnetic Resonance Imaging (MRI)

- Indications for MRI include:
  - Screening certain **high-risk patients** (Fig. 29.5)
  - Evaluating patients who have **breast implants** to determine the integrity of the implants

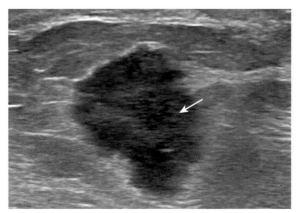

**Fig. 29.4 Ultrasound of the Breast.** In part because of the relatively superficial nature of breast lesions and sonography's absence of ionizing radiation, US is an ideal modality to study the breast. This patient displays a mass consistent with a breast cancer *(arrow)* discussed later in this chapter (see Fig. 29.14B).

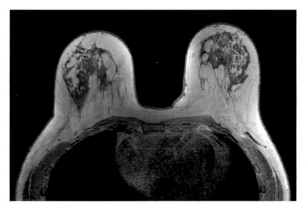

**Fig. 29.5 Breast MRI.** For a breast MRI, the patient lies prone with a gap in the table for the breasts, which are surrounded by a special magnetic coil dedicated to this type of imaging. Both breasts are imaged simultaneously. The MRI images can be reconstructed by computer to be visualized in any plane. Almost all studies use gadolinium enhancement as part of the protocol.

- Evaluating patients with positive lymph nodes and an **unknown primary** site
- Evaluating the response to *neoadjuvant chemotherapy*. **Neoadjuvant chemotherapy** refers to treatment that is given to reduce the size of a tumor in **advance** of more definitive therapy, such as surgery.
- In some cases, **newly diagnosed breast cancer** to look for extent of disease, contralateral disease, and multiple cancers
- Breast MRI is the **most sensitive** of all breast imaging modalities, but also the most expensive. Some patients cannot tolerate an MRI because of feelings of **claustrophobia** from the scanner or because they have certain **medical devices,** such as pacemakers, or ferromagnetic foreign bodies, such as some surgical clips.
- **MRI** is the **gold standard** for evaluating the **structural integrity** of *silicone breast implants* discussed later in this chapter.
- Other modalities included under the umbrella of breast imaging include **molecular breast imaging, positron emission tomography (PET),** and even **CT.**
- We will concentrate on the modalities of **mammography, US,** and **MRI,** the studies used most widely today.

## MAMMOGRAPHY: SCREENING VERSUS DIAGNOSTIC

### Screening Mammography

- The purpose of **screening mammography** is to try to detect breast cancer in **asymptomatic** patients.
- The **sensitivity of mammography** in detecting a breast abnormality depends on breast density: as **density increases** (tissue becomes whiter) **sensitivity decreases.** As with all conventional radiography, **fat appears gray** on mammography, whereas the imaging **signs of breast cancer are whiter.** This is why the denser ("whiter") a patient's underlying breast tissue is, the more difficult it is to detect a cancer among normal tissue. Finding cancer in a dense breast has been likened to looking for a polar bear in a snowstorm.
- **Breast density** is divided into four categories, ranging from almost **entirely fatty** to **very dense** (see Fig. 29.1).
- Every screening mammogram consists of two views of each breast, the *craniocaudal (CC) view* and the *mediolateral oblique (MLO) view* (Figs. 29.6 and 29.7).

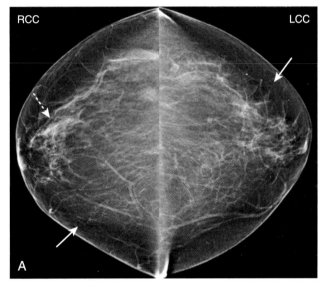

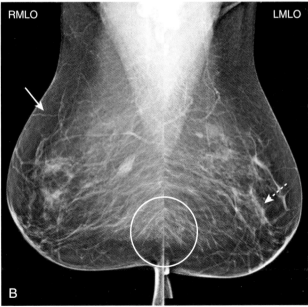

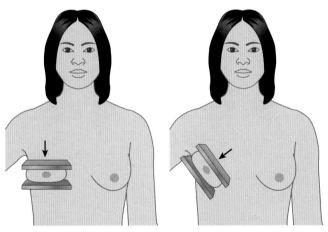

A. Craniocaudal (CC) view  B. Mediolateral oblique (MLO) view

**Fig. 29.6 Routine Views for Screening Mammography.** The screening examination includes two views of each breast, sometimes referred to as the *standard* or *routine* views (Fig. 29.7): a craniocaudal (CC) view and a mediolateral oblique (MLO) view. The CC view improves specificity and localization. The MLO view includes more breast tissue than any other single view. The two views are not orthogonal (i.e., 90 degrees) to each other.

**Fig. 29.7 Routine Mammographic Images.** (A) Craniocaudal (CC) views are displayed with the right side on your left (RCC) and the left on your right (LCC), just as most images in radiology. (B) Right and left mediolateral oblique (MLO) views. Normal structures include areas of fat (*solid arrows*), fibroglandular tissue (*dashed arrows*), and the suspensory Cooper's ligaments (*circle*).

## Screening Recommendations

- Multiple **randomized controlled trials** *(RCTs)* have shown at least a **22% reduction in breast cancer mortality** in women who undergo screening mammography versus those who do not. More **current and larger-scale observational studies** report a **38% mortality reduction** from breast cancer among those screened.
- The American College of Radiology (ACR) recommends **annual mammographic screening beginning at age 40** for women at **average risk** and **intermediate risk,** such as women with a personal history of breast cancer (Table 29.2). Other organizations also have guidelines.
- Some organizations point to the *risks* or *harms* of mammography. These include mammograms that are interpreted as abnormal, but turn out to be normal, or biopsy recommendations that reveal benign disease (false-positive) as well as the issue of *overdiagnosis,* meaning detecting cancers that may not be lethal.
- Although cancers may be low grade and grow slowly, they do not disappear without treatment. The ACR contends that overdiagnosis should not be a factor in deciding when to start screening or deciding the interval between examinations.
- Screening recommendations from the ACR have level-one evidence to support clear guidelines: **start** *yearly* **screening at age 40.** Other organizations vary in their recommendations, which may make it difficult for patients to decide when and how frequently they should be screened.
- At what age should screening mammograms stop? Randomized controlled trials proved the mortality reduction from screening stopped at age 74, but there have been numerous studies that show continued benefit for women over the age of 74. The ACR recommends that screening be stopped based on a **woman's health status** and **not on her age.**

## Diagnostic Mammography

- The indications for **diagnostic mammography** are listed in Box 29.2.

- A typical diagnostic imaging workup is shown in Fig. 29.8 for patients with **breast symptoms.**

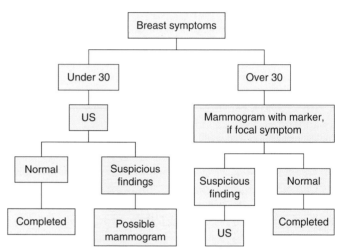

**Fig. 29.8** Flowchart for Diagnostic Mammography in Patients with Breast Symptoms. Any patient with **breast symptoms age 30 years or older** is first evaluated with **routine mammographic views.** Patients with a pertinent history (i.e., breast symptoms) who present for a diagnostic imaging examination and are **less than 30 years** of age undergo a US before a mammographic evaluation. Occasionally in this age group, a mammogram will be performed **after** the US if the sonographic findings are suspicious. If a patient has a **focal symptom** (e.g., pain in one spot), a small **radiopaque metal marker** is placed on the breast surface prior to imaging to assist the radiologist interpreting the images to identify the patient's area of concern. If the mammogram reveals anything other than a definitively benign finding, patients with a **focal** symptom will then undergo breast US. Patients with **generalized symptoms,** such as nonfocal pain, do not need further imaging after the mammogram.

| TABLE 29.2 **Mammography Screening Recommendations—American College of Radiology** | | |
|---|---|---|
| **Risk Factors** | **Start Screening** | **Frequency** |
| Average | Age 40 | Annual screening |
| Women with certain *BRCA1* or *BRCA2* mutations or who are untested but have first-degree relatives (mothers, sisters, or daughters) who are proved to have *BRCA* mutations | Age 30 | Annual screening |
| Women with histories of *mantle radiation* (usually for Hodgkin disease) received between the ages of 10 and 30 | Starting 8 years after the radiation therapy, but not before age 25 | Annual screening |
| Women with ≥20% lifetime risk for breast cancer on the basis of family history (both maternal and paternal) | Starting by age 30 (but not before age 25), or 10 years earlier than the age of diagnosis of the youngest affected relative, whichever is later | Annual screening |
| Women with mothers or sisters with premenopausal breast cancer | Starting by age 30 (but not before age 25), or 10 years earlier than the age of diagnosis of the youngest affected relative, whichever is later | Annual screening |
| Women with biopsy-proven lobular neoplasia (lobular carcinoma *in situ* and atypical lobular hyperplasia), atypical ductal hyperplasia (ADH), ductal carcinoma *in situ* (DCIS), invasive breast cancer, or ovarian cancer | From time of diagnosis, regardless of age | Annual screening |

- Patients **recalled** because of **prior screening mammography findings** or undergoing a diagnostic mammogram may be evaluated using a variety of **additional mammographic views.** Some of these additional views are spot compression images, spot compression magnification views, true lateral or 90-degree lateral views, rolled views, exaggerated views, and cleavage views, as well as US.
- Although the majority of **symptomatic** breast cancers **will** display an abnormality on mammography, US, or both, some cancers will have no imaging correlate to a clinically palpable finding or a reported symptom. For example, **invasive lobular carcinomas are classically difficult to detect** with imaging and can also be subtle clinically (Table 29.3).
- Therefore, anything that is **clinically palpable**, but has a **negative imaging** workup, should be evaluated **clinically,** often by a breast surgeon. The clinician can then decide whether to do follow-up studies or a biopsy.
- Patients who undergo diagnostic mammography typically receive their results at the conclusion of the examination(s) so that they understand what to do next and have the opportunity to ask questions.

# FUNDAMENTAL MAMMOGRAPHY FINDINGS

- There is no **typical** appearance of the breast in any age group. All breasts are composed of varying amounts of **fat, fibroglandular tissue,** and **connective tissue** *(Cooper's ligaments)* (see Fig. 29.7).
- Depending on the amount of fat and fibroglandular tissue, the breast will appear **less dense (more fat), more dense (less fat), or a combination of both.**

| TABLE 29.3 | **Types of Breast Cancer** | |
|---|---|---|
| **Noninvasive** | **Ductal Carcinoma In Situ (DCIS)** | |
| • Limited to basement membrane | • Spreads through ducts<br>• Typically presents as calcifications<br>• Usually does not produce palpable mass | |
| **Invasive** | **Invasive Ductal Carcinoma (IDC)** | **Invasive Lobular Carcinoma (ILC)** |
| • Breaks through basement membrane | • Can present with asymmetry, distortion, or mass<br>• Metastasizes through lymphatics | • Cancer composed of "single-file" cells, frequently not producing a mass<br>• May metastasize to GI tract, ovaries, uterus |

**Inflammatory Breast Cancer**
- Type of relatively uncommon invasive carcinoma (1%–3%), seen more in younger women and those of African ancestry
- Presents with swelling and redness of the breast
- Can resemble mastitis in early stages
- Poor prognosis

**Medullary Breast Cancer**
- Uncommon form of invasive carcinoma (3%) associated with *BRCA* gene abnormalities; more common in Japanese women
- Tends to affect women <50 years of age
- Produces palpable mass
- Good prognosis

**Tubular Carcinoma**
- Accounts for about 1%–4% of all invasive cancers
- Usually affects women older than 50 years
- Smallest spiculated mass on mammography
- Very favorable prognosis

**Other Types of Cancer**
Mucinous, papillary, and medullary carcinoma with not otherwise specified (NOS)

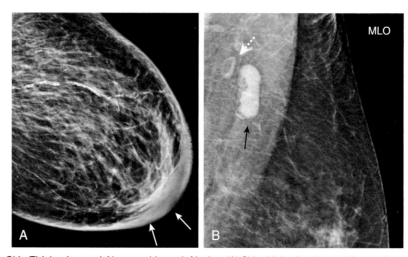

**Fig. 29.9 Skin Thickening and Abnormal Lymph Nodes.** (A) Skin thickening (*arrows*) in a patient with breast cancer. Compare the skin here with the normal skin thickness in Fig. 29.7. (B) Abnormal axillary lymph node (*black arrow*) adjacent to a normal lymph node (*white arrow*). The fatty interior (hilum) of the normal lymph node is visible.

- There is a tendency for breasts to become less dense with age, but there are many younger women with fatty breasts and a large number of elderly women with dense breasts.
- **Four basic signs of breast disease** can be seen on mammography. They are:
  - *Masses*
  - *Asymmetry*
  - *Architectural distortion*
  - *Calcifications*
  - Other important findings are **skin changes** and **abnormal lymph nodes** (Fig. 29.9).
- There is some overlap between the appearance of benign and malignant conditions. The ACR uses a standardized system called *BI-RADS,* which stands for **Breast Imaging Reporting and Data System,** to help describe findings, standardize reporting, and provide greater clarity to breast imaging interpretations. The final BI-RADS assessment categories help guide recommendations for biopsy or follow-up.

## Masses

- A **mass** is defined as a **space-occupying lesion** seen in at least **two different radiographic projections.** Masses are described by their **shape** (e.g., oval), **margins** (e.g., spiculated), and **density** (e.g., fat containing). These appearances help radiologists decide how suspicious a mass is for malignancy (Table 29.4).
- In general, a mass that is **irregular, spiculated,** and **high density** is more likely to be **malignant** (Fig. 29.10), whereas

| TABLE 29.4 | How Masses Are Described |
|---|---|
| **Shape** | Oval, round, irregular |
| **Margins** | Circumscribed, obscured, microlobulated, indistinct, spiculated |
| **Density** | High density, equal density, low density, fat containing |

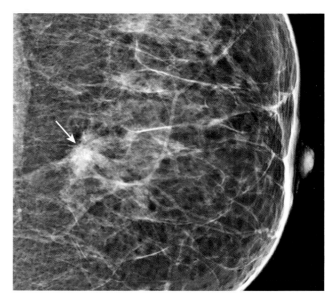

**Fig. 29.10 Spiculated Mass: Invasive Ductal Carcinoma.** There is a dense mass with spiculated margins (*arrow*). A spiculated mass is a principal finding in invasive ductal carcinoma, the most frequently encountered breast malignancy. They are most common in women ages 50 to 60 years.

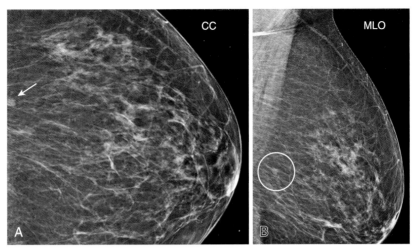

**Fig. 29.11 Cyst: Mammogram.** Craniocaudal (CC) and mediolateral oblique (MLO) views of the left breast show a small, oval, low-density mass (*arrow* in [A] and *circle* in [B]). Cysts are benign, may be single or multiple, and may change in size over time. They are most common in premenopausal women in their 30s or 40s.

a mass that is **oval, circumscribed,** and **low density** is more likely to be **benign** (Fig. 29.11). **Any fat-containing mass is typically benign** (Fig. 29.12).

## Asymmetry

- *Asymmetry* is a **unilateral** deposit of **fibroglandular tissue** that does not meet the definition of a mass. Asymmetries on mammography appear as an area of tissue that **does not** have a corresponding similar-appearing pattern in the

opposite breast. Asymmetries can be described as **global, focal, developing,** or simply **asymmetric.** Most asymmetry is **benign,** but it **may be a sign of breast cancer** (Fig. 29.13).

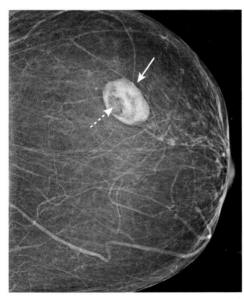

**Fig. 29.12 Hamartoma.** This mass (*solid arrow*) contains fat (*dashed arrow*), a finding that typically indicates benignity. Hamartomas are composed of benign dysplastic breast tissue that usually contains fat and may contain calcifications.

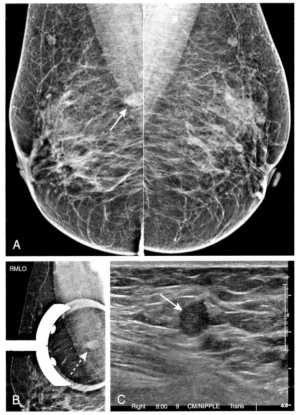

**Fig. 29.13 Asymmetry as a Sign of Cancer.** (A) A bilateral mammogram reveals a focal asymmetry in the right breast (*arrow*). (B) A special view called a **spot compression view** over the area of asymmetry (*white arrow*) again demonstrates and confirms the finding. (C) An ultrasound image shows a corresponding suspicious mass (*arrow*).

## Architectural Distortion

- *Architectural distortion* describes an alteration in the expected architecture of a breast with **no discrete mass** visible. It is one of the most subtle signs of breast cancer. It can be thought of as spiculation without a mass or a *tethering-in* of the tissue (Fig. 29.14).
- **Digital breast tomosynthesis** has been shown to be particularly helpful in identifying architectural distortion (Fig. 29.15; see also Fig. 29.2).

## Calcifications

- *Calcifications* in the breast fall into two major categories: those that appear **typically benign** (e.g., rod-like) and those that are **suspicious for malignancy** (e.g., pleomorphic). They are also described by their arrangement or **distribution** in the breast: **diffuse calcifications** throughout the

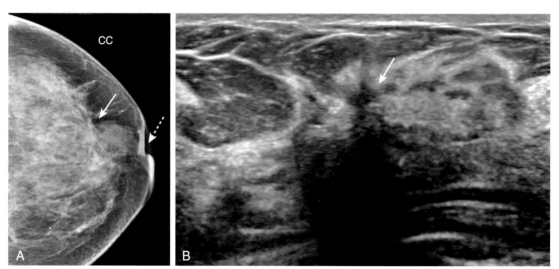

**Fig. 29.14 Architectural Distortion as a Sign of Cancer.** Architectural distortion can be a sign of breast cancer. It is caused by a ***desmoplastic reaction***—a growth of fibrous or connective tissue presumably in response to the neoplasm. (A) This craniocaudal view displays such distortion (*solid arrow*) described as "tethering-in" and associated retraction of the areola (*dashed arrow*). (B) Ultrasound shows corresponding distortion (*arrow*).

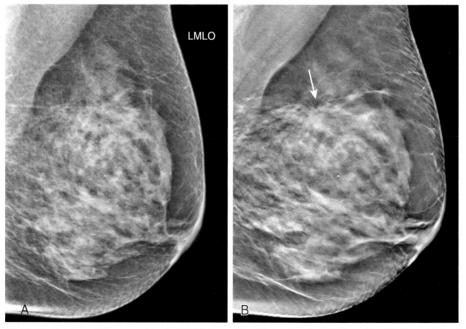

**Fig. 29.15 Digital Breast Tomosynthesis (DBT) Revealing Distortion.** In DBT (see Fig. 29.2), multiple views are acquired while the x-ray source traverses an arc. The views acquired are reconstructed to provide multiple *sections/slices* of the breast, which can be as thin as 1 mm. (A) The two-dimensional mediolateral oblique mammogram view shows dense fibroglandular tissue, but no abnormality. (B) A single tomosynthesis slice reveals an area of distortion (*arrow*) that proved to be an invasive carcinoma.

breast are less likely associated with malignancy than **grouped** calcifications (Table 29.5; Fig. 29.16).

| TABLE 29.5 | **Types of Breast Calcifications** | |
|---|---|---|
| **Classification** | **Morphology** | **Distribution** |
| **Typically benign** | Skin, vascular, coarse or *popcorn-like,* large rod-like, round, rim, dystrophic, milk of calcium, suture | Diffuse or regional |
| **Suspicious** | Amorphous, coarse heterogeneous, fine pleomorphic, fine linear, or fine-linear branching | Grouped, linear, segmental |

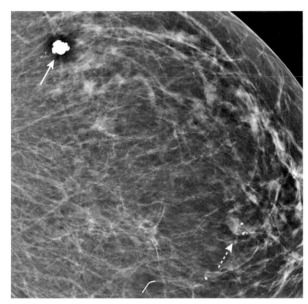

**Fig. 29.16 Breast Calcifications.** This image shows two examples of calcifications in degenerating fibroadenomas in the same breast. One has coarser calcifications (*solid arrow*) than the other (*dashed arrow*). Fibroadenomas are common benign tumors that form during adolescence, may enlarge during pregnancy and lactation, and regress—frequently with calcification—after menopause.

## ULTRASOUND

- Ultrasound is very important in the evaluation of breast lumps. It plays a key role in the differentiation between **cystic** and **solid** breast masses. A special high-frequency transducer is necessary for breast US because of the superficial nature of breast findings.
- For a **cyst** to meet the definition of **benign** by US, it must have the following criteria:
  - **Anechoic** (echo-free)
  - **Enhanced through transmission**
  - **Thin back wall** (Fig. 29.17)
- If the US does **not** demonstrate these criteria or shows a **solid mass**, then the lesion may still be benign but there is a chance of malignancy (Fig. 29.18).
- Ultrasound may also reveal a benign, prominent **ridge** of fibroglandular tissue that explains a patient's sensation of a

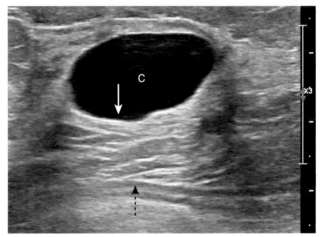

**Fig. 29.17 Benign Cyst: Ultrasound.** The cyst (C) itself is anechoic (contains no echoes), has a sharp back wall (*white arrow*), and has enhanced through transmission, as demonstrated by the strong echoes posterior to the cyst (*black arrow*). Cysts are the most common cause of a breast lump in women between ages 35 and 55 years.

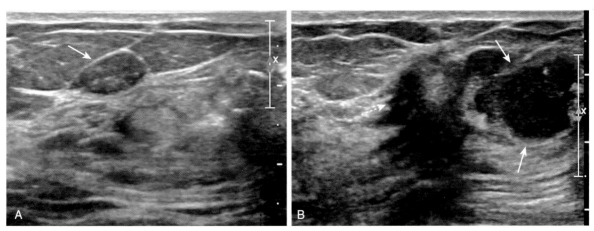

**Fig. 29.18 Sonograms of Solid Masses.** (A) The margins of the mass are well circumscribed (*solid arrow*). This represents a **fibroadenoma**. (B) In another patient, there are two adjacent **malignant** masses with both circumscribed (*solid arrows*) and spiculated margins (*dashed arrow*). Malignant lesions on ultrasound are commonly hypoechoic lesions with poorly defined borders. Typically a malignant lesion has spiculated margins and may have microcalcification. Compare these lesions to the appearance of the cyst in Fig. 29.17.

lump (Fig. 29.19). However, these patients should also be evaluated by a clinician, such as a breast surgeon, to ensure that the clinical findings correlate with the imaging results.

- A lesion that can be seen using US that requires a biopsy is best biopsied under image guidance using US (Fig. 29.20). A variety of biopsy devices and needle sizes are available for these procedures.

## MAGNETIC RESONANCE IMAGING

- When breast MRI is used to diagnose breast cancer, gadolinium-based intravenous contrast is administered and images are acquired over a period of several minutes (see Fig. 29.5).
- Breast cancer **typically enhances early** (within the first 2 minutes) after injection and the contrast will **wash-out rapidly**

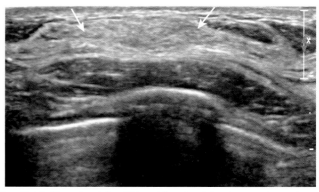

**Fig. 29.19 Fibroglandular Ridge.** Fibroglandular changes in the breast can produce lumps and ridges that may be worrisome to the patient. This ultrasound demonstrates a ridge of normal fibroglandular tissue (*arrows*) that accounts for a patient's lump.

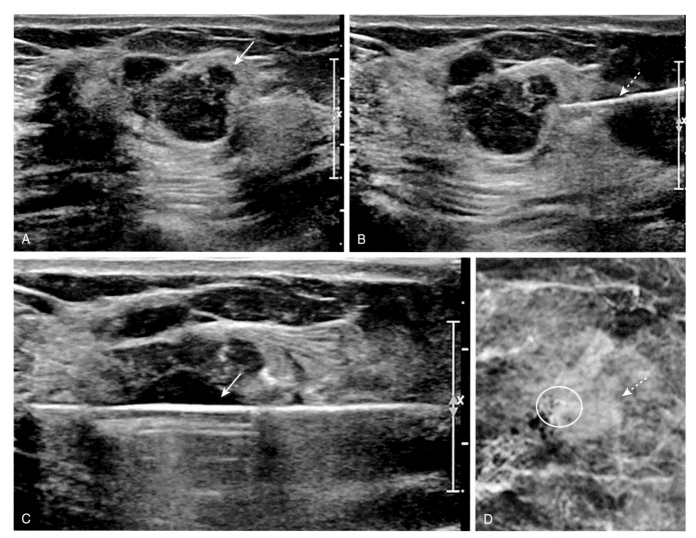

**Fig. 29.20 Ultrasound-Guided Biopsy.** (A) Ultrasound shows a suspicious mass with an irregular contour and internal echoes (*solid white arrow*). (B) The area is first anesthetized prior to biopsy. The biopsy is performed while watching the procedure in real time so that the **biopsy needle** (*dashed arrow*) can be seen in the appropriate position, that is, parallel to the chest wall. (C) The biopsy needle (*solid arrow*) passes through the mass. (D) A postbiopsy mammogram demonstrates a radiopaque clip in place (*circle*) within the mass (*dashed arrow*).

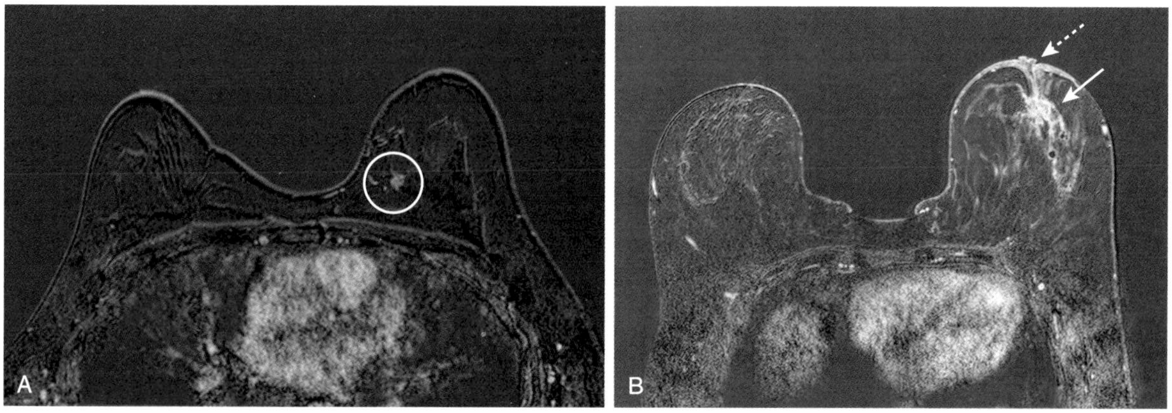

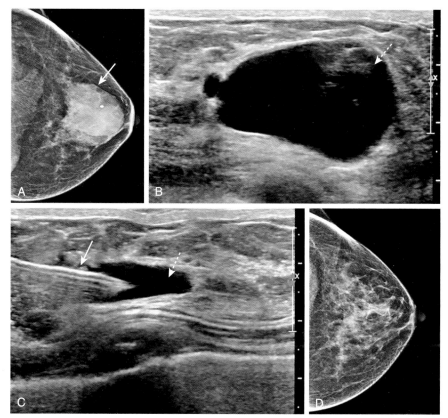

**Fig. 29.21** Breast Cancer: MRI. (A) This axial image shows a gadolinium-enhancing mass (*circle*). This patient had a history of *BRCA1* mutation. This was a breast cancer. (B) A different patient with a larger mass (*solid arrow*) that extends forward, involving the nipple (*dashed arrow*). Most breast cancers show a 90% increase in their signal intensity 90 seconds after gadolinium injection. A technique called fat suppression is used to reduce the signal from any fatty tissues in the breast and improve the ability to visualize masses (see Chapter 20).

(Fig. 29.21). Similar to mammography, an evaluation of the mass's morphology is important in diagnosis.

## MANAGEMENT OF BREAST ABNORMALITIES

- In general, breast abnormalities are managed with **percutaneous procedures** before any surgical intervention. These procedures include cyst aspiration, ultrasound-guided biopsy, stereotactic biopsy, and MRI-guided biopsy.

### Cyst Aspiration

- **Any cyst that does not fulfill strict criteria for a cyst** (see Fig. 29.18) **should undergo aspiration.** Cysts may also be aspirated to relieve symptoms such as pain.
- Aspiration is performed under US guidance after cleansing of the skin and use of a skin anesthetic (Fig. 29.22). The

**Fig. 29.22** Cyst Aspiration. This patient presented with a tender lump in the left breast. (A) Craniocaudal view of the left breast demonstrates a round mass (*arrow*). (B) Ultrasound revealed a cyst (*arrow*). (C) Another image during an ultrasound-guided aspiration of the cyst shows the aspiration needle (*solid arrow*) entering the cyst (*dashed arrow*). (D) A postaspiration mammogram displays resolution of the mass. After an **ultrasound-guided procedure, a postprocedure mammogram** is typically obtained to ensure that the aspirated cyst corresponded to the original mammographic finding.

color of cyst fluid varies; it may be blue, green, or yellow. Pure blood is sent for cytology, assuming the procedure was not traumatic (i.e., ruptured a blood vessel), but otherwise the fluid does not need to be sent for cytologic evaluation.

## Ultrasound-Guided Biopsy

- **The vast majority of findings**, particularly masses and other soft tissue abnormalities, for which biopsy is recommended **undergo ultrasound-guided breast biopsies.**
- A marker clip is typically placed at the site of the biopsy when the procedure is finished.
- **A postprocedure mammogram** is obtained to ensure correct placement of the clip and that the correct lesion was biopsied (see Fig. 29.20).

## Stereotactic Biopsies

- **Stereotactic biopsies** are performed **predominantly on calcifications** that are readily visible mammographically. A stereotactic biopsy uses x-ray to obtain images of the lesion at angles that are 30 degrees apart. A computer determines how much the lesion **shifts** on those images, allowing the **location** and **depth** of the lesion to be calculated (Fig. 29.23).
- After a percutaneous image-guided biopsy, the radiologist determines whether the pathology is **concordant** or **discordant** (Box 29.3).

## Surgical Excision

- Certain lesions (Box 29.4) require needle localization followed by **surgical excision** (Fig. 29.24). Other lesions

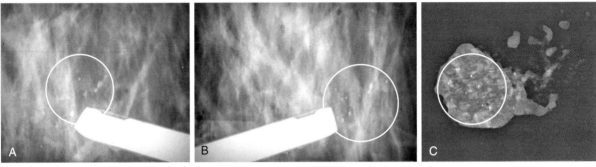

**Fig. 29.23 Stereotactic Biopsy of Calcifications.** (A, B) A close-up pair of prebiopsy images taken at an angle of 30 degrees from each other shows the needle tip adjacent to multiple calcifications (*circles*). (C) A radiograph of the excised specimen confirms that the tissue with numerous calcifications (*white circle*) has been obtained. Biopsy results returned ductal carcinoma *in situ*. Stereotactic breast biopsy is used especially for microcalcifications or nonpalpable lesions visible only on mammograms.

### BOX 29.3  Concordant Versus Discordant

- If the results are **concordant** (i.e., the radiologist thought the lesion looked like a fibroadenoma and the biopsy results revealed a fibroadenoma), then the patient may return to a routine screening protocol.
- If the results are **discordant** (i.e., the radiologist was expecting carcinoma but the biopsy results returned benign fibrocystic changes), rebiopsy or excisional biopsy is performed.

### BOX 29.4  Breast Lesions Requiring Surgical Excision

- Invasive carcinoma
- Ductal carcinoma *in situ* (DCIS)
- Atypical ductal hyperplasia
- Flat epithelial atypia
- Cellular fibroadenomas
- Fibroepithelial lesions

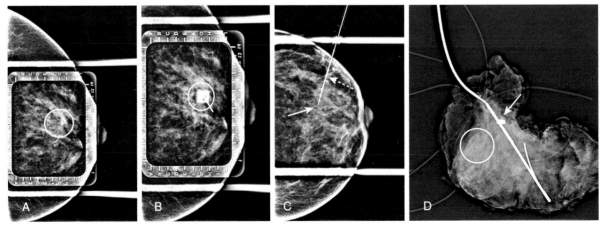

**Fig. 29.24 Needle Localization for Surgical Excision.** The patient had a prior stereotactic biopsy for calcifications that revealed ductal carcinoma *in situ*. (A) An image with a special alphanumeric paddle displays the marker clip from the previous biopsy (*circle*). (B) After needle placement, the hub of the needle is seen (*circle*). (C) The orthogonal (90-degree) view shows the needle (*dashed arrow*) passing adjacent to the clip and the tip of the hookwire engaged (*solid arrow*). The hook on the wire keeps the wire in place without moving and guides the surgeon in removing the correct tissue. (D) A specimen radiograph demonstrates the hookwire in the removed tissue with the surgical marker clip (*arrow*) and several calcifications (*circle*).

such as **papillary lesions** and **radial scars** may also need excision.

- The goal of needle localization is to guide the surgeon to the nonpalpable abnormality so that it may be successfully excised. General rules of needle localization include choosing the **shortest distance** from the skin to the lesion and obtaining a **specimen radiograph** after surgery to ensure that the lesion was removed.

- There are other ways to localize abnormalities using magnetic or radioactive *seeds,* often performed on a separate day from the surgery.

## SPECIAL CONSIDERATIONS

### Masses During Pregnancy

- Any **breast lump during pregnancy** needs to be evaluated, starting with a **mammogram** if the patient is **30 years of age or older** or with an US if **younger than 30.** The differential diagnosis includes benign etiologies such as normal breast tissue, cysts, fibroadenomas (which are hormone sensitive and therefore may grow with pregnancy), *galactoceles* (Fig. 29.25), and carcinoma.

### Nipple Discharge

- Most nipple discharges result from **benign** etiologies. Important clinical considerations are if the discharge is spontaneous, unilateral, or bilateral; emanates from a single or from multiple ducts; and if it is a certain color.

- In general, **pathologic** discharge is **spontaneous, unilateral,** and either **clear/serous or bloody.** The most common cause of bloody nipple discharge is a *solitary papilloma.* As with other breast symptoms, imaging starts with mammography if the patient is 30 years of age or older and often includes an US directed at the subareolar breast.

- A *ductogram* is a study that involves injecting a small amount of iodinated contrast into the duct from which discharge can be expressed and subsequently taking mammographic images looking for a filling defect(s), areas of narrowing, or irregularity of the duct. Ductograms are performed less frequently, having been replaced by **high-resolution ultrasound.**

### Mastitis and Breast Abscess

- *Mastitis* is inflammation of the breast and can be either **infectious** or **noninfectious.** The **most common cause of infectious mastitis** is *Staphylococcus aureus.* Mastitis and breast abscesses are defined as *puerperal* (related to childbirth) or *nonpuerperal.*

- **Puerperal infections are more common than nonpuerperal.** Risk factors for nonpuerperal infections include smoking, diabetes, and obesity.

- Mastitis is often **treated with antibiotics before any imaging.** It can look identical to **inflammatory carcinoma**

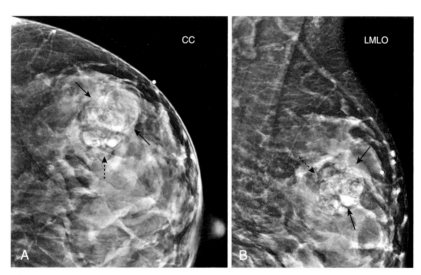

**Fig. 29.25 Galactocele.** This patient was breastfeeding and felt a lump in the left breast. Galactoceles typically occur during breastfeeding but may also be seen during pregnancy. (A) Craniocaudal and (B) mediolateral oblique views show a mass (*solid arrows*) that contains fat (*dashed arrows*). Galactoceles will contain fat on mammography because they represent the retention of fat in areas of cystic ductal dilatation.

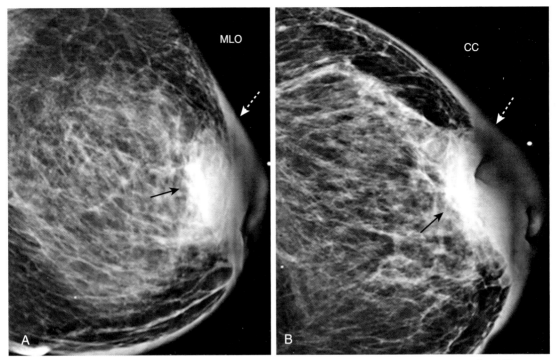

**Fig. 29.26 Breast Abscess.** Abscesses are almost always a complication of mastitis, usually nonlactational. They develop in those whose mastitis or cellulitis does not respond to antibiotic treatment. (A) Mediolateral oblique and (B) craniocaudal views display a mass (*solid arrows*) with associated skin thickening (*dashed arrows*).

of the breast, both clinically and mammographically, so if the patient does not completely respond to antibiotics, then a mammogram is performed. US can be helpful in trying to distinguish between the two by finding a suspicious mass.

- Mammography typically shows **edema, skin thickening, and prominence of Cooper's ligaments,** as lymphatics course along ligaments.
- Similarly, an **abscess** can be difficult to differentiate on imaging from **invasive carcinoma** as both present as masses. Typically, **breast cancer** is **not tender,** whereas an **abscess** is almost **always tender** (Fig. 29.26).

## Breast Trauma

- Trauma to the breast can result in a *hematoma* and/or *fat necrosis.* Initial imaging findings of fat necrosis may be subtle but often evolve on healing into classical *oil cysts* (fibrous-walled collections from focal fat necrosis) with or without calcifications.
- A *seatbelt injury* creates a specific pattern of trauma to the inner breast along the site of the seatbelt, with the driver injuring the upper-inner left breast and lower-inner right breast (Fig. 29.27). On a mammogram, a band-like

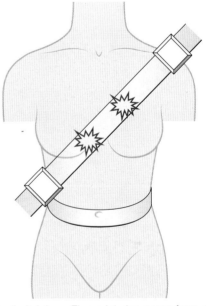

**Fig. 29.27 Seatbelt Injury.** These injuries occur from a three-point, lap-shoulder seatbelt during a motor vehicle collision. They can produce painful, chronic fat necrosis in the breast in a characteristic pattern across those areas the shoulder belt traverses, often the upper-inner quadrant of one breast and lower-inner quadrant of the opposite breast.

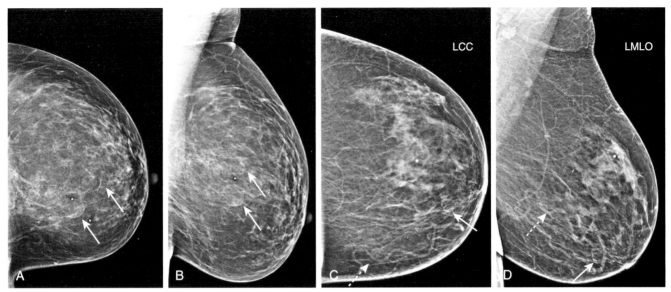

**Fig. 29.28 Seatbelt Injuries: Mammograms.** (A) Craniocaudal and (B) mediolateral oblique views show the typical pattern of multiple, thin-walled oil cysts (*arrows*) in a patient complaining of breast lumps after a motor vehicle accident. In another patient (C) craniocaudal and (D) mediolateral oblique views demonstrate a similar pattern of calcified (*solid arrows*) and noncalcified (*dashed arrows*) oil cysts along the inner breast.

asymmetry and/or hematoma may be seen, and later there are often multiple **oil cysts** along the path of the seatbelt's impact (Fig. 29.28).

## Dense Breasts

- **Dense breasts** (heterogeneously dense or extremely dense), which occur in approximately 50% of the population, create challenges for breast cancer diagnosis. Although concern for the difficulties of imaging dense breast tissue has been cited as a reason not to screen young women, many young women **do not have** dense breasts.
- The use of **digital breast tomosynthesis** has been shown to be **helpful** for women with dense breasts and **can be**

performed as part of a routine screening or diagnostic mammogram. Other studies, such as breast MRI and breast US, can be useful but are not routinely recommended for average-risk patients.

## Postoperative Breast

- The postoperative breast includes the breast in patients with a history of reduction mammoplasty, breast augmentation, lumpectomy or breast-conserving therapy, and benign breast biopsies.
- **Reductions** often have typical findings on mammography related to surgery as well as signs of fat necrosis (Fig. 29.29).

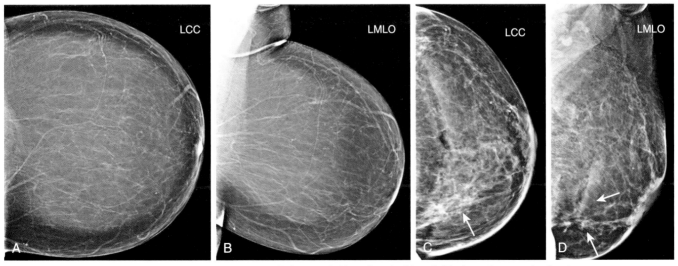

**Fig. 29.29 Reduction Mammoplasty, Before and After.** Panels (A) and (B) show the prereduction fatty breast. (C, D) After reduction the breast has decreased in size and there are postsurgical changes (*arrows*). Postsurgical distortion and fat necrosis may be seen in postoperative mammoplasties, especially in the inferior part of the breast.

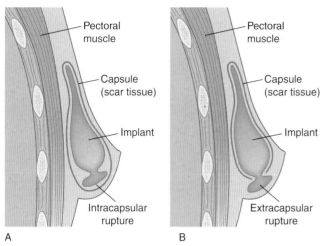

**Fig. 29.30 Intracapsular and Extracapsular Ruptures of Breast Implants.** A fibrous capsule normally forms around the shell of silicone implants. (A) Intracapsular ruptures leak from the implant shell but are contained by the capsule. Mammographic findings of an **intracapsular rupture** can be subtle. The shell of the implant itself can collapse inward (see Fig. 29.31). (B) An **extracapsular rupture** will display silicone outside of the capsule, within the breast tissue, and/or within axillary lymph nodes that will look denser than normal (see Fig. 29.32).

- *Breast implants* most commonly contain either **saline** or **silicone** and may be placed behind the pectoralis muscle *(subpectoral)* or in front of the pectoralis muscle *(subglandular)* (Fig. 29.30).
- **Saline implants** are either intact (normal) or deflated; **silicone implants** rupture by leaking silicone within the *fibrous capsule* that normally forms around the implant *(intracapsular rupture)* (Fig. 29.31) or by leaking silicone outside the capsule *(extracapsular rupture)* (Fig. 29.32).

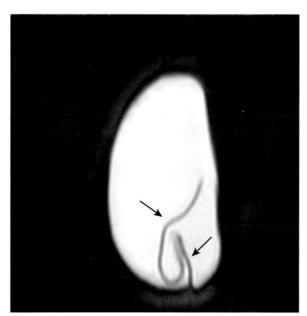

**Fig. 29.31 Intracapsular Breast Implant Rupture: MRI.** A sagittal image of an implant (the breast tissue surrounding the implant is dark on this MRI image) shows a hypointense, wavy line within the implant (*arrows*), which is a piece of the free-floating, collapsed implant shell (envelope). This has been called the ***linguine sign.***

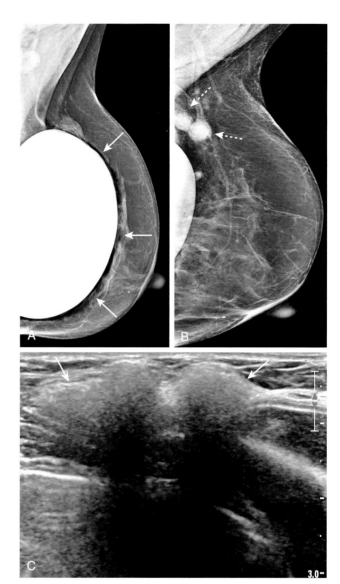

**Fig. 29.32 Extracapsular Silicone Implant Rupture.** (A) Mediolateral oblique view with implant shows a silicone subglandular implant (*arrows*). (B) A special implant-displaced view helps to reveal more breast tissue and, in this case, displays dense white material (*arrows*), indicating free silicone. (C) Ultrasound image demonstrates what is called the ***snowstorm*** appearance, markedly echogenic areas with sharp anterior margins and indistinct posterior margins from the free silicone (*arrows*).

- **MRI is the gold standard for evaluating the integrity of silicone breast implants.** Contrast is not used in these studies. The older an implant is, the more likely it is to rupture or leak.
- Patients with a history of a **surgical biopsy** or **lumpectomy** may have distortion, asymmetry, and calcifications. These findings tend to be more pronounced in breast cancer patients because of the addition of **radiation** to the treated breast. At times, patients may also have a seroma or hematoma at their surgical site.
- Careful follow-up of these patients is required to ensure that the postoperative findings stabilize by 2 years. **Recurrences are not common within the first 2 years, with the exception of triple negative breast cancer** (i.e., cancer that tests negative for estrogen receptors, progesterone receptors, and excess HER2 protein do not respond to hormonal therapy medicines or medicines that target HER2 protein).

## CASE QUIZ 29 ANSWER

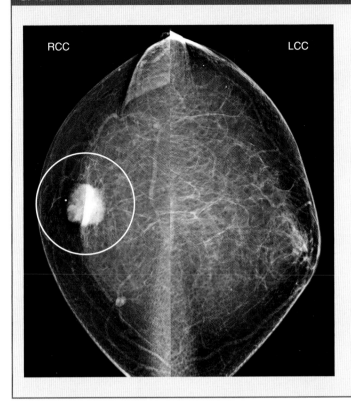

Craniocaudal views of both breasts demonstrate a predominantly spiculated, partially circumscribed, dense mass in the right breast *(circle)*. The findings are consistent with a carcinoma, and biopsy confirmed an invasive ductal cell carcinoma. Invasive ductal carcinoma accounts for about 70% to 80% of all breast cancers.

## 🏠 TAKE HOME POINTS

- Breast imaging primarily employs mammography, ultrasound, and MRI for the evaluation of various breast symptoms and for the detection of breast cancer.
- Mammographic examinations are divided into two different categories: **screening,** done primarily on asymptomatic women, and **diagnostic mammography,** done in women with breast symptoms, patients recalled for a more extensive examination, and often those with a history of breast cancer or with breast implants.
- **Screening mammograms** consist of two views of each breast: the craniocaudal (CC) view and the mediolateral oblique (MLO) view.
- The American College of Radiology's (ACR) recommendations for screening mammography are described.
- **Diagnostic mammograms** may involve a variety of additional mammographic views to those used in a standard screening protocol, such as compression or spot views, as well as the use of ultrasound.
- Dense breasts produce challenges for imaging because they might mask a carcinoma. Digital breast tomosynthesis and breast MRI may be helpful.
- **Breast ultrasound** is the initial study used in average-risk, symptomatic patients under 30 years of age. It is most commonly used in conjunction with diagnostic mammography and is helpful in distinguishing cystic from solid breast masses and as a problem-solving tool.
- **Breast MRI**, the most sensitive of all breast imaging modalities, is used with gadolinium enhancement for screening certain high-risk patients, evaluating patients who have received breast implants, or adjuvant chemotherapy.

- **Four basic signs** of breast disease on mammography are described and illustrated. They are masses, asymmetry, architectural distortion, and calcifications.
- Several characteristics of preinvasive and invasive breast cancers are described.
- **Ultrasound** plays a key role in the differentiation between cystic and solid breast masses.
- **Cyst aspiration** is used to relieve symptoms, such as pain, and to further study any presumed cyst that does not fulfill the strict criteria for a benign cyst.
- Lesions such as ductal carcinoma *in situ* (DCIS) and invasive carcinoma require **surgical excision** with needle localization of the lesion helping guide the surgeon to the abnormality.
- **Galactoceles** are one of the abnormalities that can occur during lactation (or pregnancy). They characteristically contain fat seen on mammography.
- Most **nipple discharges** are a consequence of a benign etiology. Solitary papillomas can cause a bloody nipple discharge.
- **Mastitis** is an inflammation of the breast most often caused by *Staphylococcus aureus*. **Breast abscesses** tend to form from mastitis. Both can appear clinically similar to inflammatory carcinoma of the breast.
- **Breast trauma** can lead to hematomas and fat necrosis. Seatbelt shoulder restraints can produce a characteristic pattern of injury from a motor vehicle collision.
- MRI is the gold standard for evaluating **silicone breast implants.** Implant ruptures are divided into intracapsular or extracapsular.

 Additional content is available online including chapters on Nuclear Medicine, Artificial Intelligence, Radiation Dose and Safety, an Early History of Radiology, and a compendium of 200 Diagnostic Radiology Signs.

# BIBLIOGRAPHY

## TEXTS

Fraser RS, Pare P, Fraser R, Pare PD. *Synopsis of Diseases of the Chest.* 2nd ed. Philadelphia: Saunders; 1994.

Goodman LR. *Principles of Chest Roentgenology.* 3rd ed. Philadelphia: Elsevier; 2007.

Greenspan A. *Orthopedic Radiology: A Practical Approach.* 3rd ed. Philadelphia: Lippincott Williams and Wilkins; 2000.

Grossman RL, Yousem DM. *Neuroradiology: The Requisites.* St. Louis: Mosby; 1994.

Guyton AC, Hall J. *Textbook of Medical Physiology.* 11th ed. Philadelphia: Saunders; 2005.

Harris JH, Harris WH. *The Radiology of Emergency Medicine.* 4th ed. Philadelphia: Lippincott Williams and Wilkins; 2000.

Juhl JH, Crummy AB. *Essentials of Radiologic Imaging.* 6th ed. Philadelphia: Lippincott; 1993.

Love M. *An Introduction to Diagnostic Ultrasound.* 1st ed. Springfield: Charles C. Thomas; 1980.

Manaster BJ, Disler DG, May DA. *Musculoskeletal Imaging: The Requisites.* 2nd ed. St. Louis: Mosby; 2002.

McCloud T. *Thoracic Radiology: The Requisites.* 1st ed. St. Louis: Mosby; 1998.

Mettler F, Guiberteau M. *Essentials of Nuclear Medicine Imaging E-Book.* 6th ed. Philadelphia: Saunders; 2012.

Nutritional Considerations in the Intensive Care Unit: Science, Rationale, and Practice. American Society for Parental and Enteral Nutrition. April 2002.

Ranschaert E, Morozov S, Algra PR. *Artificial Intelligence in Medical Imaging: Opportunities, Applications and Risks.* Springer Nature; 2019.

Resnick D. *Diagnosis of Bone and Joint Disorders.* 4th ed. Philadelphia: Saunders; 2002.

Rumack C, Wilson S, Charboneau WJ. *Diagnostic Ultrasound.* 2nd ed. St. Louis: Mosby; 1998.

Schultz RJ. *The Language of Fractures.* Huntington, NY: Robert E. Krieger; 1972.

Swischuk L. *Imaging of the Newborn, Infant, and Young Child.* 5th ed. Lippincott Williams & Wilkins; 2003.

Webb WR, Brant WE, Helms CA. *Fundamentals of Body CT.* Philadelphia: Saunders; 1991.

Weissleder R, Wittenberg J, Harisinghani MG. *Primer of Diagnostic Imaging.* 3rd ed. St. Louis: Mosby; 2003.

## JOURNAL ARTICLES

Aberle DR, Wiener-Kronish JP, Webb WR, Matthay MA. Hydrostatic versus increased permeability pulmonary edema: diagnosis based on radiographic data in critically ill patients. *Radiology.* 1988;168:73−79.

ACR Manual on Contrast Media, 2021 Version, American College of Radiology Committee on Drugs and Contrast Media.

Almeida A, Roberts I. Bone involvement in sickle cell disease. *Br J Haematol.* 2005;129:482−490.

American Society for Gastrointestinal Endoscopy. Management of ingested foreign bodies and food impactions, position paper. *Gastrointest Endosc.* 2011;73(6):1085−1091.

Amjadi K, Alvarez GG, Vanderhelst E, Velkeniers B, Lam M, Noppen M. The prevalence of blebs or bullae among young healthy adults: a thoracoscopic investigation. *Chest.* 2007;132(4): 1140−1145.

Baskin KM, Jimenez RM, Cahill AM, et al. Cavoatrial junction and central venous anatomy: implications for central venous access tip position. *J Vasc Interv Radiol.* 2008;19(3):359−365.

Bates D, Ruggieri P. Imaging modalities for evaluation of the spine. *Radiol Clin North Am.* 1991;29(4):675−690.

Bonner A. The Complete Beginner's Guide to Deep Learning: Convolutional Neural Networks and Image Classification; Towards Data Science. Feb. 2, 2019.

Boudiaf M, Soyer P, Terem C, Pelage J, Maissiat E, Rymer R. CT Evaluation of small bowel obstruction. *Radiographics.* 2001;21: 613−624.

Boyse TD, et al. US of soft-tissue foreign bodies and associated complications with surgical correlation. *Radiographics.* 2001;21: 1251−1256.

Burney K, Burchard F, Papouchado M, Wilde P. Cardiac pacing systems and implantable cardiac defibrillators (ICDs): a radiological perspective of equipment, anatomy, and complications. *Clin Radiol.* 2004;59(8):699−708.

Connolly B, Mawson JB, MacDonald CE, Chait P, Mikailian H. Fluoroscopic landmark for SVC-RA junction for central venous catheter placement in children. *Pediatr Radiol.* 2000;10:692−695.

Cury RC. Coronary CT angiography versus standard of care for assessment of chest pain in the emergency department. *J Cardiovasc Comput Tomogr.* 2013;7(2):79−82.

Dalinka MK, Reginato AJ, Golden DA. Calcium deposition disease. *Semin Roentgenol.* 1982;17(1):39−47.

de Jong EM, Felix JF, de Klein A, Tibboel D. Etiology of esophageal atresia and tracheoesophageal fistula: "Mind the gap. *Curr Gastroenterol Rep.* 2010;12(3):215−222.

Doubilet PM, Benson CB, Bourne T, Blaivas M. Society of Radiologists in Ultrasound Multispecialty Panel on Early First Trimester Diagnosis of Miscarriage and Exclusion of a Viable Intrauterine Pregnancy, et al. Diagnostic criteria for nonviable pregnancy early in the first trimester. *N Engl J Med.* 2013;369:15.

Dyer DS, Moore EE, Mestek MF, et al. Can chest CT be used to exclude aortic injury? *Radiology.* 1999;213:195−202.

Edeiken J. Radiologic approach to arthritis. *Semin Roentgenol.* 1982;17(1):8−15.

Edwards MO, Kotecha SJ, Kotecha S. Respiratory distress of the term newborn infant. *Paediatr Respir Rev.* 2013;14(1):29−37.

Ellis K, Austin J, Jaretzki A. Radiologic detection of thymoma in patients with myasthenia gravis. *AJR Am J Roentgenol.* 1988;151: 873−881.

Epelman M, et al. Necrotizing enterocolitis: review of state-of-the-art imaging findings with pathologic correlation. *Radiographics.* 2007;27:285−305.

European Society of Radiology (ESR). What the radiologist should know about artificial intelligence − an ESR white paper. *Insights Imaging.* 2019;10(1):44.

Garcia MJ. Could cardiac CT revolutionize the practice of cardiology? *Cleve Clin J Med.* 2005;72(2):88−89.

Gaube S, Suresh H, Raue M, et al. Do as I say: susceptibility in deployment of clinical decision-aids. *npj Digit. Med.* 2021;4:31.

Gilardi BR, López JIM, Villegas ACH, Mora JAG, Rodríguez OCR, Appendini RC, Malváez MDM, Calleja JAH. Types of cerebral herniation and their imaging features. *RadioGraphics*. 2019;39(6):1598−1610.

Gluecker T, Patrizio C, Schnyder P, et al. Clinical and radiologic features of pulmonary edema. *Radiographics*. 1999;19:1507−1531.

Goodman A, Perera P, Mailhot T, Mandavia D. The role of bedside ultrasound in the diagnosis of pericardial effusion and cardiac tamponade. *J Emerg Trauma Shock*. 2012;5(1):72−75.

Gould MK, Tang T, Liu IL, et al. Recent trends in the identification of incidental pulmonary nodules. *Am J Respir Crit Care Med*. 2015;192(10):1208−1214.

Gundepalli SG, Tadi P. *Lung Pancoast Tumor*. StatPearls. StatPearls Publishing; Jan. 2021.

Haus BM, Stark P, Shofer SL, Kuschner WG. Massive pulmonary pseudotumor. *Chest*. 2003;124(2):758−760.

Hendrix RW, Rogers LF. Diagnostic imaging of fracture complications. *Radiol Clin North Am*. 1989;27(5):1023−1033.

Henry M, Arnold T, Harvey J. British Thoracic Society's guidelines for the management of spontaneous pneumothorax. *Thorax*. 2003;58(suppl 2):39−52.

Henry-Tillman RS, Klimberg VS. In situ breast cancer. *Curr Treat Options Oncol*. 2000;1:199−209.

Henschke CI, Yankelevitz DF, Wand A, Davis SD, Shiau M. Accuracy and efficacy of chest radiography in the intensive care unit. *Radiol Clin North Am*. 1996;34(1):21−31.

Hergueta-Redondo HR, Palacios J, Cano A, Moreno-Bueno G. "New" molecular taxonomy in breast cancer. *Clin Trans Oncol*. 2008;10(12):777−785.

Herold CJ. Management of solid and sub-solid lung nodules. *Cancer Imaging*. 2014;14(suppl 1).

Horrow MM. Ultrasound of the extrahepatic bile duct: issues of size. *Ultrasound Q*. 2010;26(2):67−74.

Hosny A, Parmar C, Quackenbush J, Schwartz LH, Aerts HJWL. Artificial intelligence in radiology. *Nat Rev Cancer*. 2018;18(8):500−510.

Husain LF, Hagopian L, Wayman D, Baker WE, Carmody KA. Sonographic diagnosis of pneumothorax. *J Emerg Trauma Shock*. 2012;5(1):76−81.

Indrajit IK, Shreeram MN, d'Souza JD, Multislice CT. A quantum leap in whole body imaging. *Indian J Radiol Imaging*. 2004;14(2):209−216.

Ingram MD, Watson SG, Skippage PL, Patel U. Urethral injuries after pelvic trauma: evaluation with urethrography. *Radiographics*. 2008;28:1631−1643.

Iqbal J, Narod SA. Choices for young women at intermediate risk of breast cancer. *Curr Oncol*. 2012;19(3):e112−e114.

Johnson JL. Pleural effusions in cardiovascular disease. *Postgrad Med*. 2000;107(4):95−101.

Karlo CA, Leschka S, Stolzmann P, Glaser-Gallion N, Wildermuth S, Alkadhi H. A systematic approach for analysis, interpretation, and reporting of coronary CTA studies. *Insights Imaging*. 2012;3(3):215−228.

Kim H, Min Park C, Koh JM, Lee SM, Goo JM. Pulmonary subsolid nodules: what radiologists need to know about the imaging features and management strategy. *Diagn Interv Radiol*. 2014;20(1):47−57.

Kim HE, Kim HH, Han BK, Kim KH, Han K, Nam H, et al. Changes in cancer detection and false-positive recall in mammography using artificial intelligence: a retrospective, multireader study. *The Lancet Online*. 2020;2(3):e138−e148.

King JB. Calcification of the costal cartilages. *Br J Radiol*. 1939;12(133):2−12.

Kundel HL, Wright DJ. The influence of prior knowledge on visual search strategies during the viewing of chest radiographs. *Radiology*. 1969;93:315−320.

Leonard-Lorant I, Severac F, Bilbault P, Muller J, Leyendecker P, Roy C, Ohana M. Normal chest CT in 1091 symptomatic patients with confirmed Covid-19: frequency, characteristics and outcome. *Eur Radiol*. 2021;31(7):5172−5177.

Li X, Wang X, Yang X, Lin Y, Huang Z. Preliminary study on artificial intelligence diagnosis of pulmonary embolism based on computer in-depth study. *Ann Transl Med*. 2021;9(10):838.

Lingawi SS. The naked facet sign. *Radiology*. 2001;219:366−367.

Lu MT, Ivanov A, Mayrhofer T, Hosny A, Aerts HJWL, Hoffmann U. Deep learning to assess long-term mortality from chest radiographs. *JAMA Netw Open*. 2019;2(7), e197416.

National Comprehensive Cancer Network. *National Clinical Practice Guidelines in Oncology*. 2007;4(9):516−525.

Neu J, Walker WA. Necrotizing enterocolitis. *N Engl J Med*. 2011;364:255−264.

Old JL, Calvert M. Vertebral compression fractures in the elderly. *Am Fam Physician*. 2004;69(1):111−116.

Pathria MN, Petersilge CA. Spinal trauma. *Radiol Clin North Am*. 1991;29(4):847−865.

Pooley RA. Fundamental physics of MR imaging. *Radiographics*. 2005;25(4):1087−1099.

Riddervold HO. Easily missed fractures. *Radiol Clin North Am*. 1992;30(2):475−494.

Rubin DL. Artificial intelligence in imaging: The radiologist's role. *JACR*. 2019;16(9):P1309−1317.

Sechopoulos I, Teuwen J, Mann R. Artificial intelligence for breast cancer detection in mammography and digital breast tomosynthesis: State of the art. *Seminars in Cancer Biology*. 2021;72:214−225.

Shifrin RY, Choplin RH. Aspiration in patients in critical care units. *Radiol Clin North Am*. 1996;34(1):83−95.

Sik B, Kim M, Li BT, et al. Diagnosis of gastrointestinal bleeding: a practical guide for clinicians. *World J Gastrointest Pathophysiol*. 2014;5(4):467−478.

Smith-Bindman R, Miglioretti DL, Larson EB. Rising use of diagnostic medical imaging in a large integrated health system. *Health Aff (Millwood)*. 2008;27(6):1491−1502.

Soffer S, Klang E, Shimon O, et al. Deep learning for pulmonary embolism detection on computed tomography pulmonary angiogram: a systematic review and meta-analysis. *Sci Rep*. 2021;11, 15814.

Steenburg SD, Ravenel JG. Acute traumatic thoracic aortic injuries: experience with 64-MDCT. *AJR Am J Roentgenol*. 2008;191:1564−1569.

Sutton RT, Pincock D, Baumgart DC, et al. An overview of clinical decision support systems: benefits, risks, and strategies for success. *npj Digit. Med*. 2020;3:17.

Thomas EL, Lansdown EL. Visual search patterns of radiologists in training. *Radiology*. 1963;81:288−292.

Tie MLH. Basic head CT for intensivists. *Crit Care Res*. 2001;3:35−44.

Tocino I, Westcott JL. Barotrauma. *Radiol Clin North Am*. 1996;34(1):59−81.

Veltman CE, de Graaf FR, Schuijf JD, et al. Prognostic value of coronary vessel dominance in relation to significant coronary artery disease determined with non-invasive computed tomography coronary angiography. *Eur Heart J.* 2012;33:1367–1377.

Wu A, March L, Zheng X, Huang J, Wang X, Zhao J, Blyth FM, Smith E, Buchbinder R, Hoy D. Global low back pain prevalence and years lived with disability from 1990 to 2017: estimates from the Global Burden of Disease Study 2017. *Annals Translational Medicine.* 2020;8(6):299.

Yamashita R, Nishio M, Kinh R, Do G, Togashi K. Convolutional Neural Networks: an Overview and Application in Radiology. *Insights into Imaging.* 2019;9:611–629.

Yu S, Haughton VM, Rosenbaum AE. Magnetic resonance imaging and anatomy of the spine. *Radiol Clin North Am.* 1991;29(4): 675–690.

Yuh W, Quets J, Lee H, et al. Anatomic distribution of metastases in the vertebral body and modes of hematogenous spread. *Spine.* 1996;21(19):2243–2250.